THE MEASUREMENT OF INTELLIGENCE

THE MEASUREMENT OF INTELLIGENCE

Readings selected and comments written by
H. J. Eysenck, Ph.D., D.Sc.
Professor of Psychology, University of London

The Williams & Wilkins Company

Baltimore

SANS TACHE

To the Memory of Cyril Burt, who taught me

Published by
MTP
Medical and Technical Publishing Co. Ltd.,
St. Leonard's House, St. Leonard's Gate,
Lancaster, England

Copyright 1973 © H. J. Eysenck

SBN 852 00059 6

Printed in Great Britain by
C. Tinling & Co., Ltd., London and Prescot.

CONTENTS

"As the ear is made to perceive sound and the eye to perceive colour, so the mind of man has been found to understand not all sorts of things, but quantities. It perceives any given thing more clearly in proportion as that thing is close to bare quantities as to its origin, but the further a thing recedes from quantities, the more darkness and error inheres in it."

Johannes Kepler, Opera, 1, 14. (1595).

"We owe all the great advances in knowledge to those who endeavour to find out how much there is of anything."

Clerk Maxwell

"One's knowledge of science begins when he can measure what he is speaking about, and express it in numbers."

Lord Kelvin

FOREWORD

This book deals with one aspect of the modern, scientific study of intelligence, namely its measurement. The term, *measurement*, has difficulties attached to it which rival those attached to the term, *intelligence*; many psychologists have little idea of what the word means, and what are the requirements which must be fulfilled in order to enable "measurement" to take place. Krantz, Luce, Suppes and Tversky (1971) have tried to provide us with an introduction to the "Foundations of Measurement"; these two volumes outline the background against which attempts to measure intelligence must be evaluated.* No short excerpt or set of readings could suffice to bring home to the "innumerate" reader the implications of scientific measurement, and no attempt has been made accordingly to treat this concept systematically, although occasional discussions will alert the reader to problems and possible solutions. Instead we have concentrated on selecting papers for reprinting which are historically valuable, and which mark milestones in the development of the concept of intelligence as a scientific variable, or alternatively which summarize in an acceptable fashion research in an important field.

We have not dealt at all with another aspect of modern intelligence testing which has attracted more and more attention in recent years, namely the social, ethical and political side. As with all other scientific discoveries and inventions, there is a clear difference between the scientific aspect, which is concerned with the validity of the theories involved, their proof and dis-

* In view of the importance of the concept of "measurement", and the many problems and questions it gives rise to, it may be useful to mention a few of the numerous sources which the interested reader may consult, both with respect to measurement in general, and the measurement of intelligence, in particular. Among the better known sources are Bridgman (1927), Churchman and Ratoosh (1959), Campbell (1957); Carnap (1955), Dingle (1950), Ellis (1966), Ipsen (1960, Suppes and Zinnes (1963), Thorndike (1927), Torgerson (1958), and Woolf (1961).

proof, and the deductions to which they give rise, and the social aspect, which is concerned with the "good" or "evil" consequences which follow from the scientific discovery or invention. Thus IQ testing would appear to many people to give rise to desirable and "good" consequences when it enables us to pick out bright "disadvantaged" children for higher educational and university training who would otherwise not have been educated up to the level of their ability. On the other hand, IQ testing would appear to many people to give rise to undesirable and "bad" consequences when it enables trade unions to exclude coloured workers by the imposition of unrealistic and irrelevant intellectual requirements for membership. It is not suggested that such concerns with social consequences and ethical considerations are undesirable or irrelevant; on the contrary, to most psychologists they will undoubtedly appear extremely important. The social consequences of IQ testing are of vital importance to us all, but they must form the substance of another, different book; one volume is hardly sufficient to include all that is relevant to the simple scientific problem.

The measurement of intelligence has provided psychology with one of its most successful paradigms, to use Kuhn's (1962) phrase; yet one might not think so in looking at typical modern text-books of psychology. None of these present the paradigm in its proper form, and none discuss the evidence for the paradigm in any systematic fashion. Selection of evidence is usually arbitrary, and far from up-to-date; proper critical discussion is almost entirely missing; and the essentially quantitative nature of the paradigm is not even hinted at. This last fault extends particularly to the criticisms often made of the paradigm; these are usually verbal and semantic, based on philosophical or political ideas, rather than scientific or quantitative. We shall return to this point in the section dealing with criticisms of the paradigm. It is in fact one of the reasons for the appearance of this book that it seemed desirable to put together in one volume a cogent yet detailed statement of the various parts which go to make up this paradigm, and to do so in as quantitative a fashion as possible. The reader may weary of the repeated insistence on the *quantitative* nature of the theory underlying modern work on intelligence, yet it is precisely this which singles it out from the many purely semantic solutions to the problems posed which have been suggested in the past, and which have failed conspicuously to provide us with testable hypotheses. "Everything that exists, exists in some quantity, and can therefore be measured," asserted E. L. Thorndike,* and while philosophers will no doubt raise their eyebrows at the implied notion of existence, this dictum has proved extremely useful in psychology.

I have been fortunate in knowing personally, and often being friendly with, many of the giants whose work has created this paradigm. Spearman, and after him Burt, were my teachers at University College, London; I later met Thurstone and Guilford on many occasions, as well as Godfrey Thompson and R. B. Cattell. Of more recent writers I have worked with such men as A. Jensen and J. L. Horn, and during my stay at Berkley I met R. C. Tryon, D. Krech and M. R. Rosenzweig. These and many others, like J. Piaget whose views are more "environmentalistic" than mine, have been instrumental through their work and their discussion, in forming my present views; they are not, of course, responsible for any errors that may have crept into this book. On the whole I have avoided controversial topics; I believe that the evidence presented is sufficient in each case to make sure that the conclusions presented are at least in the right direction, even though adjustment will certainly be needed in many of the precise numerical values. Some topics, such as those associated with the so-called nature-nurture problem, will no doubt be considered controversial by those not intimately acquainted with the facts; I know of no-one actually working in the field who would not acknowledge the importance of the facts quoted, or the

---

* While this statement certainly represents Thorndike's view, and is often quoted, I have been unable to find it in his writings. In an article published in 1918, Thorndike wrote: "Whatever exists at all exists in some amount. To know it thoroughly involves knowing its quantity as well as its quality." McCall (1923) quoted the first part of Thorndike's 1918 statement to head one of the sections of his own book; he began another with "Anything that exists in amount can be measured;" this time without credit, presumably as his own. Thus the alleged Thorndike statement puts together two rather different ideas advanced by different writers (Jonçich, 1968). Another form of the statement was advanced by Thorndike in 1936 when he said: "I am not prepared to say that there is any quality so spiritual or so refined or subtle that it may not yield itself to objective measurement." These views are now widely accepted among psychometrists, although behaviourists, following another line of Thorndike's theoretical teaching, often reject the very notion of "qualities" and instead prefer to think in terms of simple S-R bonds (Eysenck, 1970).

truth of the conclusions drawn. Again, I am fortunate in knowing personally the leading workers in this field, such as K. Holzinger, L. Penrose, and J. Jinks and D. W. Fulker, whose application to this problem of the theories and formulae of Fisher and Mather have revolutionized the field and rendered many traditional criticisms out of date.

The only section in which I have included material which has not received the general approval of the "establishment" is that entitled "Analysis of IQ performance," which deals with certain theories of my own, and the empirical and theoretical work of two of my collaborators, D. W. Furneaux and Owen White. My own belief that the future development of intelligence testing will follow the path outlined in this section is probably not shared by many of the experts working in the field at the moment; this is not surprising when it is realised that these new theories carry in them the germ, not only of crucial criticisms of the old paradigm, but also of an entirely new one. As Kuhn pointed out, such criticisms and such changes are not readily accepted; quite rightly, evidence to support such revolutionary developments has to be much more convincing than is usual in order to win assent. It seemed only fair to point out to the reader that this section differs from the rest in this important fashion, and that its contents are not covered by the mantle of the establishment; this fact does not alter my view of the essential correctness of the analysis there given, but it may affect profoundly the reception given to it by the reader.

One important point may with advantage be dealt with here, as it is relevant to the general question of the *validity* of applying the term "intelligence" to the theoretical concept underlying observed scores on IQ tests; it is also relevant to the problem of whether in fact "intelligence" so measured has any great social importance. The value of the work done does not of course depend on a positive answer to both these questions; substitute a different term, or even a letter, such as Spearman's g, for intelligence, and the remainder of the book would remain unaffected. Yet such a course would not be reasonable if we could agree that what is measured by IQ tests resembles in important ways what is commonly regarded as "intelligence," and that whatever this may be, it is important in our society. It is suggested here that our society (like the Chinese culture and the Greek culture before it) is oriented towards, and dominated by, intelligence and intellectual achievement; that its success is dependent upon this orientation and this dominance; and that it values and rewards people generally in direct proportion to the extent of their intellectual performance. It is not necessary to point out that this correspondence is not perfect; luck, personality qualities, social background, and many other factors obviously play an important part in a person's final status in our social hierarchy. Nor is it necessary to point out that other cultures have been oriented towards, and dominated by, other values.

Many societies have been glorifying the warrior, and have rewarded and valued strength, courage and agility in battle. Others, like many Negro groups in Africa, have placed great value on rote memory, no doubt influenced by the great importance of ritual in these societies, and the absence of a written record. However that may be, there is little doubt about the stress on intelligence in our own society; Table 1 shows just how close IQ and social status are in fact related. This Table is a summary of information contained in papers published by Burt (1961), Cattell (1934, 1971), Fryer (1922), Harrell and Harrell (1945), Himmelweit and Whitfield (1949), with IQ values reduced to a common SD of 16 points.

TABLE 1

140	Higher Professional; Top Civil Servants; Professors and Research Scientists.
130	Lower Professional; Physicians and Surgeons; Lawyers; Engineers (Civil and Mechanical).
120	School Teachers; Pharmacists; Accountants; Nurses; Stenographers; Managers.
110	Foremen; Clerks; Telephone Operators; Salesmen; Policemen; Electricians; Precision Fitters.
100+	Machine Operators; Shopkeepers; Butchers; Welders; Sheet Metal workers.
100−	Warehousemen; Carpenters; Cooks and Bakers; Small Farmers; Truck and Van Drivers.
90	Labourers; Gardeners; Upholsterers; Farmhands; Miners; Factory Packers and Sorters.

*Mean IQ of different professional
and occupational groups.*

It will be clear, and has been established in a number of empirical studies, that the order of professions and occupations in terms of IQ coincides well with the popular view of intellectual requirements of these professions and occupations, and also with the social value placed upon them by the majority. There are of course slight misplacements; physicians and surgeons are slightly below research scientists in IQ, but slightly above them in popular esteem. But on the whole the coincidence is reasonably close. It is of course true, and should be emphasized, that these are mean values; when the IQ's of different occupations are compared in terms of distributions, there is nearly always some overlap. Some of the gardeners, miners, cooks or truck drivers studied have IQ's as high as some of the physicians and lawyers, top civil servants or research scientists. Generally there is a reduction in the S.D. of these professional and occupational distributions of 35%; for the top professions the reduction is considerably greater. This means that there are many persons with IQ's considerably in excess of the mean of their group in the lower social classes, but relatively few persons with IQ's considerably below the mean of their group in the upper social classes. This is understandable; a person with a high IQ may fail to rise in the social scale because of laziness, personality defects, mental disorder, bad luck, ill health, poor schooling and generally social deprivation of one kind or another. A person with a low IQ is much less likely to succeed in overcoming all the hurdles which society puts between aspiration and achievement in the higher professions. Hence a high position is almost a guarantee of high IQ; a low position is by no means a guarantee of low IQ.

Nor, of course, does the Table include all the occupations; there are groups (of which the entertainment industry is the most obvious) which do not fit in too well with our generalization. Top singers, performers in certain sports, actors, TV personalities, strippers, and kings and queens (who for our purpose may be regarded as part of the entertainment industry in its wider aspects) are not on the whole renowned for high IQ's, but are extremely well paid. However, what is true of top performers is not true in general; the average earnings of actors, singers, football players, etc. are not high, and even for top performers in sport the duration of their top earning capacity is short. Furthermore, the social estimation of entertainers is not as high as their top earnings would suggest (nor is it as low, perhaps, as their average earnings would suggest). Although only a very small group, the existence of entertainers may remind us that the generalization linking IQ with social class, esteem and earning capacity is true on the average, but has important exceptions.*

We have dealt with a factual account of the position as it actually exists at present, both in the countries of the West, and also in the U.S.S.R.; while it is true that Stalin, like Hitler, banned IQ testing for political reasons, this ban has recently been rescinded, and the obvious usefulness of IQ testing in an educational and industrial context has been recognized in the communist countries also. It is of course open to social critics to say that this position is undesirable, and that society should not be based so explicitly on intellectual ability. The rulers of modern China seem to have adopted such a position, deemphasizing intelligence and stressing

* The correlation between IQ and earning capacity is clearly lower than that between IQ and social esteem. The teacher earns less than a docker, yet his social esteem is higher; the research scientist earns less than the shopkeeper, yet his social esteem, too, is higher. Society honours high intelligence, even though it is not always prepared to translate this feeling into hard cash. Stenographers and telephone operators are greatly underpaid, taking their IQ into account; possibly this, as well as the failure of social esteem to keep pace with their IQ, is due in part to the general devaluation of the female sex which is unfortunately characteristic of our society. This factor may also play a part in the low remuneration received by teachers, most of whom are female.

Some references to the work done on the relation between IQ and social esteem of jobs and professions are: Haller et al. (1972), Hodge et al. (1966), Reiss (1961), Scase (1972), Sigal et al. (1966), Simpson et al. (1960), Smith (1943), Soalstoga (1959), and Yichtman & Fistelson (1972).

physical work and political attitude. Unfortunately we do not know anything about the IQ's of their leading politicians, military leaders, factory directors, scientists, etc., but it would be very surprising if these were not on a par with those of Western leaders in these fields. It would be very interesting indeed if information could be provided about conditions in China in this respect; in the complete absence of such factual information, speculation would be useless. One point should, perhaps, be borne in mind by those who condemn the stress on intellectual excellence in modern society: such societies could not exist in the absence of a science and technology, a political system and a civil service, a manufacturing and distributing industry created and run by exceptionally able people. It is quite open to critics to say that our society is far from perfect, and indeed such criticism is clearly justified and needed; it is quite another thing to say that our society could be improved by deemphasizing intelligence.

Our Table presents certain facts, but it is purely descriptive; no conclusions can be derived from these facts regarding the causation of the observed differentials. To enable us to say that the IQ differences between different occupations play a causal part in selecting people for these occupations, or else that coming from a certain social class which is associated with a given occupation plays a causal part in determining a person's IQ, requires a much more complex type of experimental design and analysis; studies relevant to this problem will be reprinted in later sections of this volume. There is no point in anticipating the conclusion here; the reader may suspect that both causal factors are in fact active in our society, but he may well suspend judgment until after studying the relevant documents. Altogether, most of the problems mentioned in the last few pages require the sort of factual information contained in the readings which go to make up the body of this book; these facts do not by themselves enable us to give an answer, which must include ethical, social and political considerations as well as factual psychological statements. But it must be stated once and for all that attempts to give answers to these problems which do not take into account the facts as we know them do a disservice to society, and make the achievement of a better society that much harder. This belief that facts are essential in coming to reasonable judgments is the main justification for putting together this book.

REFERENCES

BRIDGMAN, P. V. *The logic of modern physics*. London: Macmillan, 1927.

BURT, C. Intelligence and social mobility. *Brit. J. Statist. Psychol.*, 1961, *14*, 3–24.

CATTELL, R. B. Occupational norms of intelligence, and the standardization of an adult intelligence test. *Brit. J. Psychol.*, 1934, *25*, 1–28.

CATTELL, R. B. *Abilities: their structure, growth and action*. New York: Houghton Mifflin, 1971.

CAMPBELL, N. R. *Foundation of sciences*. New York: Dover, 1957.

CARNAP, R. Foundations of logic and measurement. *Internat. Encyclop. of Unified Science*, Vol. 1. Chicago: Univ. Press, 1955.

CHURCHMAN, C. W. & RATOOSH, P. (Eds.) *Measurement: Definition and theories*. New York: Wiley, 1959.

DINGLE, H. A theory of measurement. *Brit. J. Phil. Soc.*, 1950, *1*, 5–26.

ELLIS, B. *Basic concepts of measurement*. Cambridge: Univ. Press, 1966.

EYSENCK, H. J. *The Structure of Human Personality*. (3rd edition). London: Methuen, 1970.

FRYER, D. Occupational intelligence levels. *School & Soc.*, 1922, *16*, 273–277.

HALLER, S. O., HOLSINGER, D. B. & SARAIVA, H. U. Variations in occupational prestige hierarchies: Brazilian data. *Amer. J. Social.*, 1972, *77*, 941–956.

HARRELL, T. W., & HARRELL, M. G. Army General Classification Test scores for civilian occupations. *Educ. & Psychol. Measment.*, 1945, *5*, 229–240.

HIMMELWEIT, H., & WHITFIELD, J. Mean intelligence scores on a random sample of occupations. *Brit. J. Indust. Psychol.*, 1949, *1*, 224–276.

HODGE, R. W., TRIEMAN, D. S., & ROSSI, P. A comparative study of occupation prestige. In: R. Bendix & S. Lipset (Eds.) *Class, Status and Power*. New York: Free Press, 1966.

IPSLEY, D. C. *Units, dimensions and dimensionless numbers*. New York: McGraw-Hill, 1960.

JONCICH, G. *The Sane Positivist*. Middletown: Wesleyan Univ. Press, 1968.

KRANTZ, D. H., LUCE, R. D., SUPPER, P., & TVERSKY, S. *Foundations of measurement*. 2 Vols. New York: Academic Press, 1971.

KUHN, T. S. *The structure of scientific revolutions*. Chicago: University Press, 1962.

McCALL, W. *How to measure in education*. New York: Macmillan, 1923.

REISS, S. F. *Occupations and social status*. Glencoe: Free Press, 1961.

SCASE, R. "Industrial man": a reassessment with English. *Brit. J. Sociology*, 1972, *23*, 204–220.

SIEGAL, P. M., & ROSSI, P. H. Occupational prestige in the United States: 1925–1963. In: R. Bendix & S. Lipset (Eds.) *Class, Status and Power*. New York: Free Press, 1966.

SIMPSON, R. L., & SIMPSON, J. H. Correlates and estimates of occupational prestige. *Amer. J. Sociol.*, 1960, *66*, 135–140.

SMITH, M. An empirical scale of prestige status of occupation. *Amer. Sociol. Ther.*, 1943, *8*, 185–193.

SOALSTOGA, K. *Prestige, class and mobility*. Copenhagen: Gyldental, 1959.

SUPPES, P., & ZINNES, J. L. Basic measurement theory. In: R. D. Luce, R. R. Bush & E. Galcurter (Eds.) *Handbook of Mathematical psychology*, Vol. I. New York: Wiley, 1963.

THORNDIKE, E. L. et al. *The measurement of intelligence*. New York: Columbia Univ. 1927.

TORGERSON, W. S. *Theory and methods of scaling*. New York: Wiley, 1958.

WOOLF, H. (Ed.) *Quantification*. New York: Bobbs-Merrill, 1961.

YICHTMAN, E., & FISTELSON, G. Some problems in the study of occupational prestige with an illustration from Israel. *Brit. J. Sociol.*, 1972, *23*, 159–171.

PART I

HISTORY AND DEFINITION OF THE CONCEPT

The two papers in this section may serve as an introduction to the more experimental papers which follow. They set the scene, and give a general overview of the paradigm mentioned in the Foreword; they also deal with certain questions and problems relating to the definition of the term "intelligence". Questions of definition usually worry the scientist much less than the interested layman; the former realizes, as the latter does not, that a proper definition comes at the end, not at the beginning, of a scientific quest. The notion that a scientist must be able to give a definition of the terms he uses which would be understandable to the layman, and which would encompass all the important and relevant properties of the concept in question is not one which can be seriously maintained. Ever since Newton framed the law of universal attraction to account for the facts of "gravitation" have there been discussions and acrimonious disputes about the meaning and definition of the term (Janner, 1954, 1957); for hundreds of years the most prominent physicists and astronomers have argued about "action at a distance", without coming to any agreed conclusion. Yet nobody would deny the importance of Newton's law, or the very real progress made in physics and astronomy following its publication. So much nonsense is being talked in this connection that a thorough, painstaking and philosophically sound discussion, like that by T. R. Miles, seems overdue. Essentially, the definition of a scientific term is to be found in the whole "nomological network" within which it is enfolded, i.e. the whole set of theories and facts which constitute the paramount paradigm at a given time. Thus in a very real sense, the definition of "intelligence" is to be found in the body of knowledge enclosed within the covers of a book such as this; si vis definitionem, circumspice!

This modern paradigm did not, of course, emerge suddenly and without warning; there is a long history going back to Plato, Aristotle and Cicero, and leading through Spencer and Galton to the more modern figures of Binet, Spearman and Burt. There are many reasons why the latter has been chosen here to set out this history in brief, and to introduce the paradigm in some detail. Sir Cyril Burt was the first to introduce the modern paradigm in the 1911 paper referred to in his article here reprinted; he has steadfastly kept before him the vision of a general theory encompassing all the relevant facts which go to make up our paradigm, and worked to add crucial facts to the picture. He combines in a fashion all too rare the numerate and literate abilities of Snow's "two cultures"; in addition to being one of the recognised leaders of the psychometric school, he also writes prose which is a pleasure to read. Most of all, he is a link with the past he describes, having known such men as Sir Francis Galton in his youth; it is this historical knowledge which gives "bottom" to his writings. Burt's definition of intelligence as "innate, general, cognitive ability" encapsulates the various strands which are woven together to create the modern paradigm; he describes the way in which they originated and coalesced, and he mentions some of the experimental proofs which we shall have occasion to look at in more detail in the remainder of this book.

One point is agreed by both our authors, and it is so important that it may usefully be spelled out again in this brief introduction to the first section. The man in the street, and often the unwary psychologist too, thinks of intelligence as something really existing "out there"; something which the psychologist may or may not recognize successfully, and measure with more or less success. In these terms it would make sense to argue about whether a particular test "really" measures intelligence. Such reification is utterly mistaken; there is nothing "out there" which could be called intelligence, just as there is nothing "out there" which could be called gravitation. Intelligence and gravitation are *concepts*, and concepts only exist in the minds of scientists; they are useful or useless, appropriate or inappropriate, in terms of their success in enabling us to form generalizations, discover invariances, and predict future events.

In this sense Thorndike was wrong in the dictum quoted in the Foreword; intelligence does not exist, but that does not mean that it cannot be measured. Gravitation, after all does not exist either; yet it can be measured very accurately. Individuals exist and their behaviour can be observed and measured; these observations and measurements give rise to concepts which we reify at our peril. It makes sense to argue about the usefulness of the resulting concepts; it makes no sense to argue about the "existence" of these conceptualizations. As we shall see, intelligence passes this hurdle triumphantly, and this is the only question we may pose, and the only answer we require.

We have already raised the question of whether intelligence, as conceived by the psychologist, is sufficiently like the intelligence talked about by the man in the street, and we have suggested that there is sufficient similarity to make it unnecessary to change the word, or to have recourse to a single letter to designate the concept. Yet there is one aspect on which there is likelihood of confusion arising, and it may be useful to discuss the issues involved. Intelligence, as the psychologist perceives it, is a hypothetical entity, a force, which is posited in order to explain certain types of behaviour. These behaviours are quite variable, and include such items as problem solving, learning of complex material, and the speedy discovery of relations between elements. Intelligence, as the man in the street sees it, is concerned more with the products of the force involved, i.e. with knowledge. Now obviously there is a close connection between the ability to acquire knowledge, which is the psychologist's kind of concept, and the amount of knowledge acquired, which is the layman's concern. But in particular cases this consensus may break down; an extreme case is the ancient and not very good joke about the Englishman who goes abroad for the first time in his life and tells his cronies in the pub: "Very smart these dagoes—even the kids speak French!" These are commonsense observations; they have given rise to the important concepts of fluid and crystallized ability which are treated in another section; here, mention is made of this point because it has proved bothersome to many people.

Another point, also frequently an obstacle to clear understanding, relates to the often heard remark that intelligence is what intelligence tests measure. Miles, in his paper, discusses the implications of this definition; it is not always realized that in this respect, as in so many others, intelligence does not in fact differ at all from such physical concepts as gravitation. A textbook of physics does not define gravitation; it (1) refers to examples of the action of this hypostatized force, such as the apple falling, and then (2) goes on to describe the means of measuring the effects of gravitation. It would not be a caricature of the usual method of treating the subject to say that apparently gravitation is what tests of gravitation measure. Up to that point, of course, physicists are in agreement; when we come to a fundamental discussion of the nature of gravitation, of field theory, curved space, and space-time coordinates, then we find at least as much disagreement as critics are delighted to find in the field of intelligence testing. There is in science an inevitable circularity; concepts are always based on factual observations, and these factual observations are then "explained" in terms of these self-same concepts. We postulate "gravitation" to explain the falling of the apple, and the movement of the planets; we explain the falling of the apple, and the movements of the planets, in terms of gravitation. It is only in the case of intelligence testing that this customary process of scientific theory-building is held up to ridicule.

The term "circular" in this connection is perhaps a misnomer; progress in science is more nearly reminiscent of a spiral, approaching some ideal "truth" ever more closely. We start with haphazard and scarcely quantified observations, like Plato and Aristotle; we invent terms to generalize our findings. These terms suggest better observations, and these in turn lead us to improve our concepts, and state our theories in slightly more precise fashion, like Spencer and Galton. The next turn of the spiral leads to a testing of these theories in a more precise fashion, and the construction of a proper paradigm, quantified and reasonably precise, like the work of Spearman, Binet and Burt. This paradigm is then taken up and subjected to close empirical scrutiny, leading to modifications and quantitative improvements, as in the case of Thurstone, Cattell and Guilford. Each turn of the spiral leads to a model which approaches reality more closely, which takes into account more and more facts, and which enables us to perfect our theories and improve our predictions. This is the usual fashion of science, and psychology does not seem to have anything to reproach itself with in following this fashion. To say that intelligence is what intelligence tests measure is only a half-truth, but it does not invalidate either the use of such tests, or the value of the concept so defined. "Intelligence tests" are not constructed arbitrarily or at random; they are specially made up in conformity with some implicit or explicit theory, and the quantitative results to which their use gives rise serve to verify or disprove that theory. Critics must go beyond verbal methods of ridiculing the results if they wish to be taken seriously; they must deal with the whole set of theories and quantitative observations based upon, and buttressing these theories.

REFERENCES

JANNER, M. *Concepts of space*. Cambridge: Harvard Univ. Press, 1954.

JANNER, M. *Concepts of force*. Cambridge: Harvard Univ. Press, 1957.

From C. Burt (1955). Brit. J. Educ. Psychol., **25,** 158–177, *by kind permission of the authors and Scottish Academic Press*

THE EVIDENCE FOR THE CONCEPT OF INTELLIGENCE

By CYRIL BURT

I.—*The non-statistical evidence* : (1) *observational* ; (2) *biological* ; (3) *physiological* ; (4) *individual psychology.* II.—*The statistical evidence* : (1) *the general factor* ; (2) *the factor as cognitive* ; (3) *the factor as innate—the hypothesis of multi-factorial inheritance.* III.—*Summary.* IV.—*References.*

I.—THE NON-STATISTICAL EVIDENCE.

Current Criticisms.—The concept of intelligence, and the attempt to measure intelligence by standardized tests, have of late furnished a target for vigorous attack. The objections urged are partly practical and partly theoretical. Yet few of the critics show a clear or correct understanding of what the term really designates or of the reasons that have led to its introduction. Two misconceptions have become widely current.

(i) Those writers who are chiefly interested in the more practical issues, like Dr. Heim and Dr. Blackburn, explain that intelligence " is a popular and relatively unambiguous word," and denotes a quality that " all can recognize, though few can define.[1] " It follows that, instead of pinning I.Qs. on to the coat of each child, we should leave any decisions that may be necessary to the intuitive insight of the teacher. Unfortunately, in a vain effort to measure the immeasurable, the modern psychologist " has been induced to restrict the meaning of the term to a vague quantitative abstraction." No two of them, however, agree as to how that abstraction is to be defined. Hence " those who go chasing this *ignis fatuus* get quickly bogged down in mathematical abstruseness." Meanwhile, the layman, so Mr. Richmond assures us, has begun to " sense a certain absurdity in measuring something called ' intelligence ' without knowing what that something is or how it is defined."[2]

(ii) Those who are concerned with the more technical aspects of the subject apparently suppose that the concept was invented by a small band of statistical enthusiasts—Dr. Kirman (13) mentions Spearman, Pearson, and myself—who deduced their theories by primitive factorial procedures that have since been " publicly discredited." The more accurate methods of Thurstone and his American followers, it is said, have since clearly shown that the intellectual achievements of different individuals are the product, not of a single general factor, but of a number of more specialized ' primary abilities.'[3] And this at once accounts for the difficulties that beset all attempts to define intelligence. As Captain Kettle observed, when asked why the pictures of the Saghalien sea-serpent showed such incredible differences : " ' Spects it's because there's no such crittur ' ; so each just draws his own fancy."

The Definition of Intelligence.—Now the critics who protest about " the spate of incongruous definitions " usually rest their complaint on the results of the famous Symposium organized some twenty years ago.[4] The Editor of an

---

[1] (11), pp. 30f. Cf. also J. BLACKBURN : *Psychology and the Social Pattern* (1945), p. 61.

[2] (18), p. 227. Similar criticisms have also been put forward by Dr. E. G. Chambers, Dr. D. H. Stott, and Dr. C. M. Fleming.

[3] For a recent statement of the American view, see A. ANASTASI : *Psychological Testing* (1955), pp. 15, 353f.

[4] " Symposium on Intelligence and its Measurement," *J. Educ. Psych.,* XII, 1921, pp. 123-147 and 195-216. In framing his question, the Editor specifically asked, not how is intelligence to be defined, but " what do you conceive intelligence to be, and how can it best be measured : should the test material call into play analytical and higher thought processes, or should it deal rather with simple, with associative, or with perceptual processes, etc. ? "

American journal submitted two searching questions about the nature of intelligence to a dozen different psychologists, and received a dozen different replies. But the varying descriptions suggested were not, as Dr. Heim and others have supposed, intended to be ' definitions ' in the strict logical sense : they were, in the language of J. S. Mill, merely " attempts to explain the thing," not " attempts to interpret the word." As the editorial letter shows, the purpose of the discussion was primarily a practical one—to determine how intelligence appears to operate, with a view to ascertaining " what material may most profitably be used in constructing tests." But that is quite a separate question, and except incidentally will not concern us here. Nor shall I discuss the validity of mental measurement or the practical value of the I.Q.[1]—problems that are continually confused with the fundamental issue. The questions I now want to settle are prior to all these, namely, (i) how precisely should the term , be defined, and (ii) what evidence is there for believing that something really exists corresponding to the definition proposed ? However, instead of taking the term for granted and hunting round for a plausible formula, as is most frequently done, a sound scientific procedure requires us to start with the relevant facts. Let us, therefore, take the second of our two questions first.

History of the Concept.—Many of the criticisms to which I have alluded spring largely from a manifest ignorance as to how the concept originated. A rapid glance at the literature is, therefore, needed first of all.[2] As a brief historical review will show, long before the advent of statistical analysis, several converging lines of evidence had already drawn attention to an important property of the mind, for which some special name seemed desirable. How its nature was envisaged can best be gathered by recalling the actual statements of leading authorities in each field.

(1) *Observational*.

The earliest attempts to analyse and classify the activities of the mind were based partly on the observation of various types of person in everyday life and partly on introspection. Plato, to whom we owe the basic distinctions, draws a clear contrast between ' nature ' and ' nurture ' ($\phi\acute{v}\sigma\iota\varsigma$ and $\tau\rho\upsilon\phi\acute{\eta}$) ; and then distinguishes three parts or aspects of the soul—$\tau\grave{o}$ $\lambda o\gamma\iota\sigma\tau\iota\kappa\acute{o}\nu$, $\grave{\epsilon}\pi\iota\theta\upsilon\mu\acute{\iota}\alpha$, $\theta\upsilon\mu\acute{o}\varsigma$ (*Republic*, 435Af.). The modern terms—intellectual, emotional, and moral, cognition, affection, and conation—suggest rough but somewhat inexact equivalents for these untranslatable expressions. In a celebrated passage (*Phaedrus*, 253D) he sketches a picturesque analogy which conveys a better notion of the fundamental difference : the first component he compares to a charioteer who holds the reins, and the other two to a pair of horses who draw the vehicle ; the former guides, the latter supply the power ; the former is the *cybernetic* element, the latter the *dynamic*.

Aristotle makes a further contribution of lasting importance. He

---

[1] For a discussion of these questions I may refer to Professor Vernon's address on ' The Psychology of Intelligence and G ' in the current *Bulletin* of the Brit. Psychol. Society (No. 20, pp. 1-14), which I had not seen before this article was written.
[2] A more detailed account will be found in my " Historical Sketch," which forms the first chapter of the Board of Education Report on *Psychological Tests of Educable Capacity* (2, pp. 1-61) and in a recent Galton Lecture on " The Meaning and Assessment of Intelligence " (5). The antecedent evidence, drawn from the four main fields reviewed below, was briefly summarized in my earliest papers on general intelligence (e.g., *J. Exp. Pedag.*, I, 1911, pp. 96). If the reader refers to that article, he will see that the criticism made by Dr. Maberley, and repeated in varying terms by several later writers—namely, that I " claimed to deduce the general factor from a statistical analysis of test-data "—quite misrepresents my argument : the statistical analysis was intended merely to confirm a hypothesis reached on far more concrete grounds.

contrasts the actual or concrete activity with the hypothetical capacity[1] on which it depends (δύναμις), and thus introduces the idea of an ' ability.' Plato's threefold classification he reduces to a twofold. For him the main distinction is between what he calls the ' dianoetic ' (cognitive or intellectual) capacities of the mind and the ' orectic ' (emotional and moral).[1] Finally, Cicero, in an endeavour to supply a Latin terminology for Greek philosophy, translates δύναμις by *facultas*, and ὄρεξις by *appetitio* or sometimes *conatus* ; while to designate διάνοια he coins a new word, rendering the Greek term almost literally by the compound ' *intellegentia*.'

Here then we have the origin of both the concept and the term. So far from being a ' word of popular speech,' whose meaning has been restricted and distorted by the modern psychologist, intelligence is a highly technical expression invented to denote a highly technical abstraction. From Aristotle and Cicero it descended to the mediaeval schoolmen ; and the scholastic theories in turn became elaborated into the cut-and-dried schemes of the faculty psychologists and their phrenological followers.

(2) *Biological*.

As Guilford has reminded us, the modern notion of " intelligence as a unitary entity " was " a gift to psychology from biology through the instrumentality of Herbert Spencer." Following Aristotle and the later Scottish school, Spencer recognizes two main aspects of mental life—the cognitive and the affective. All cognition (he explains) involves both an analytic or discriminative and a synthetic or integrative process ; and its essential function is to enable the organism to adjust itself more effectively to a complex and ever-changing environment. During the evolution of the animal kingdom, and during the growth of the individual child, the fundamental capacity of cognition " progressively differentiates into a hierarchy of more specialized abilities "— sensory, perceptual, associative, and relational, much as the trunk of a tree sprouts into boughs, branches, and twigs. To designate the basic characteristic he revives the term ' intelligence.'[2]

Evidence favouring Spencer's somewhat speculative theories was adduced by Romanes, Lloyd Morgan, and other pioneers of comparative psychology ; and his views on intelligence were accepted, not only by British biologists like Darwin, but also by continental writers, like Binet and Claparède.[3] Certainly, Mendel's earliest disciples maintained that the doctrine of unit-characters was utterly irreconcilable with the inheritability of a graded trait, such as intelligence (cf. 6, pp. 333f.) ; but, as we shall see in a moment, the later developments of the Mendelian hypothesis not only permit it, but actually suggest it.

(3) *Physiological*.

The clinical work of Hughlings Jackson, the experimental investigations of Sherrington, and the microscopical studies of the brain carried out by Campbell, Brodmann, and others, have done much to confirm Spencer's theory of a

---

[1] DE ANIMA, II, 3, 414a, 31. *Eth. Nic.*, 1, 13, 18, 1102b, 30. The usual rendering ' power ' must not be taken to imply causal agency : Aristotle is simply describing what Professor Broad has called a ' dispositional property.'

[2] H. SPENCER : *Principles of Psychology* (1870). I have summarized Spencer's views more fully in a recent article (" The Differentiation of Intellectual Ability," this *Journal*, XXIV, 1954, pp. 76f).

[3] Cf. C. DARWIN : *The Descent of Man* (1888), I, pp. 101f. ; G. J. ROMANES : *Animal Intelligence* (1890) ; and LLOYD MORGAN : *Animal Life and Intelligence* (1796).

Sir Cyril Burt

' hierarchy of neural functions,'[1] with a basic type of activity developing by fairly definite stages into higher and more specialized forms. In particular, the examination of the cortex, both in mental defectives and in normal persons, suggests that the quality of the nervous tissue in any given individual tends to be predominantly the same throughout. Defectives, for example, exhibit a " general cerebral immaturity " ; their nerve-cells tend to be " visibly deficient in number, branching, and regularity of arrangement in every part of the cortex."[2] After all, as Sherrington himself points out, much the same is true of almost every tissue of which the human frame is composed—of a man's skin, bones, hair, or muscles : each is of the same general character all over the body, although minor local variations are usually discernible. In the adult human brain marked differences in the architecture of different areas and of different cell-layers are perceptible under the microscope ; but these specializations appear and develop progressively during the early months of infant life. And, of course, such differentiation is precisely what the Spencerian theory would entail.

The experimental study of the brain leads to the same conclusion. The intact brain acts always as a whole. No part of the brain functions in total isolation from the rest, as the older champions of cortical localization originally assumed. The activity, in Sherrington's phrase, is " patterned not indifferently diffuse " ; but the patterning itself " involves and implies integration." Lashley's[3] conclusions about the ' mass action ' of the brain seem to lend further corroboration to that view ; and, as several writers have suggested, this ' mass-action ' might well be identified with g.[4]

The evidence of neurology, therefore, itself suggests something very like a theory of general ability, which gradually differentiates into more specific functions, though we must beware of picturing such functions as separate ' faculties ' located in certain centres or compartments of the brain, after the fashion of the older phrenologists and of several recent writers on so-called ' physiological ' or ' medical ' psychology.

(4) Individual Psychology.

All these earlier writers were interested primarily in the working of the mind as such, that is to say, in problems of *general* psychology. The first to apply scientific methods to the problems of *individual* psychology was Galton. Darwin and Spencer had maintained that the basic capacities of the human mind were hereditary, transmitted as part of our common racial endowment. Galton went farther and maintained that individual differences in these capacities were also innate. As a result of his investigations into ' hereditary genius,' he was led to discard the traditional explanation in terms of faculties and types, and to substitute a classification in terms of ' general ability ' and 'special aptitudes' :

[1] The phrase is Sherrington's. Cf. C. S. SHERRINGTON : *Integrative Action of the Nervous System* (1906), pp. 314f ; HUGHLINGS JACKSON : *Brain* (1899), XXII, pp. 621f. ; M. DE CRINIS, " Die Entwickelung der Grosshirnrinde in ihren Beziehungen zur intellektuellen Ausreifung des Kindes," *Wiener Klinische Wochenschrift*, 1932, XLV, pp. 1163f. ; J. L. CONEL : *The Post-Natal Development of the Human Cerebral Cortex* (1941).

[2] J. S. BOLTON : *The Brain in Health and Disease* (1914).

[3] K. S. LASHLEY : *Brain Mechanisms and Intelligence* (1929). The experiments of Lashley and his colleagues consisted in training animals to perform definite tasks, and then removing parts of their brains : the animals were then re-tested, and in some instances re-trained. The main conclusion was that ability to learn depends, not so much on the nature or location of the tissue remaining, but upon its amount.

[4] This identification is suggested by SHERRINGTON (*Man on His Nature*, 1940, p. 288). It should be added that the details of Lashley's conclusions are not entirely free from criticism ; but here we are concerned only with the major principle.

of the two he considered that general ability was " by far the most powerful ".[1] The differences between individuals formed, so he believed, not a set of distinct and discontinuous classes, as the type-theory assumed, but a series of continuously varying gradations, distributed more or less in accordance with the normal curve, i.e., much like differences in head-length, arm-length, or stature (10, pp. 23f., 35f.).

The Definition Implied.—These converging lines of inquiry, therefore, furnished strong presumptive evidence for a mental trait of fundamental importance defined by three verifiable attributes : first, it is a general quality ; it enters into every form of mental activity ; secondly, it is (in a broad sense of the word) an intellectual quality—that is, it characterizes the cognitive rather than the affective or conative aspects of conscious behaviour ; thirdly, it is inherited or at least innate ; differences in its strength or amount are due to differences in the individual's genetic constitution. We thus arrive at the concept of an *innate, general, cognitive ability.* We cannot, however, keep repeating a cumbersome phrase of twelve syllables every time we wish to mention it. And, since a name that suggests its own meaning seems preferable to a brand-new esoteric symbol, what better label can be found than the traditional term ' intelligence ' ?[2]

Here then is a clearly formulated hypothesis, the outcome of centuries of shrewd observation and plausible conjecture—a psychological hypothesis fully in accord with the findings of the biologist and neurologist. Nevertheless, each of the three propositions that I have just laid down has been vigorously challenged ; and each has started off a protracted controversy that still remains unresolved.

At this point, therefore, the need for *ad hoc* inquiries based on rigorous statistical analysis becomes obvious. It is the function of statistical procedures to decide between alternative hypotheses by testing their verifiable corollaries. The claim of the factorist is not, as his critics so often imagine, to ' discover ' mental abilities, running round with a cry of ' Eureka' whenever he has extracted a fresh factor : his object is merely to confirm or refute certain hypothetical concepts or components that have been tentatively reached on more concrete grounds. Let us then take each of the three foregoing propositions in turn, and consider what evidence, if any, is provided by these more cogent techniques.

[1] Many contemporary writers, particularly in the field of education, attribute the antithesis between ' general ' and ' special ' abilities to Spearman, and identify it with the contrast between what he called *g* and *s*. Spearman himself, however, frankly admits that his own theories were prompted by those of Galton and Spencer. However, in his earlier papers he eventually rejected the notion of ' special aptitudes,' as merely a relic of ' the discredited faculties of the older school ' : the only ' specific ' capacities that he recognized were those ' specific ' to each particular test (cf. *Amer. J. Psych.*, XV, 1904, pp. 74f, and 206f, and 20, pp. 6f.).

[2] In educational psychology the popularity of the term is due to the work of Alfred Binet, himself an avowed follower of Spencer and Galton. Like Galton, Binet firmly believed in the existence of a ' general ability,' and repeatedly distinguished it from what he called ' partial aptitudes.' This ability, he says, enters into " nearly all the phenomena with which the experimental psychologist has previously concerned himself—sensation, perception, memory, as well as reasoning," i.e., it is essentially a cognitive capacity. Finally, he explains that his intelligence tests were deliberately constructed to measure innate differences, in contrast to his pedagogical tests which measure acquired attainments (cf. esp., *L'Année Psychologique*, XI, 1905, pp. 191f., 245f.).

Galton himself more frequently spoke of ' general ability.' But at times he used ' intelligence ' as a synonym, especially when the context called for the adjective (e.g., 9, p. 336). Those who fear the ambiguities of the more familiar term can use a literal symbol : I have suggested using γ for the hypothetical quality defined as above, and keeping *g* for the empirical measurement, with a subscript to indicate the method of measurement.

Sir Cyril Burt

The logic of the argument should be carefully noted. In the natural sciences a direct deductive proof is out of the question: the mode of proof must be indirect and inductive. Hence, the conclusions reached can never be certain, but only probable. The critic commonly misses this point. He revels in demonstrating that some alternative interpretation can readily be conceived. But one can always think up alternatives. The verdict must depend on determining and balancing the crucial facts. A probable hypothesis can only be overthrown by showing that its rival is still *more probable*. And equally, of course, the defender of a hypothesis must prove that every alternative that is worth considering is *less probable* than his own.

II.—The statistical evidence.
(1) *The General Factor*.

At the beginning of the century, the problem which chiefly exercised students of individual psychology was, in Bain's phrase, 'the classification of intellectual abilities or powers.' (i) Were there, as the faculty psychologists maintained, a number of specialized abilities, each independent of the rest—observation, practical ability, memory, language, reasoning, and the like? (ii) Or was there, as Ward maintained, "not a congeries of faculties, but only a single subjective activity"—a general capacity for cognition as such? (iii) Were there, as Galton believed, both a general ability and a number of more or less specialized capacities? (iv) Or, finally, might there be, as the earlier associationists and most of the later behaviourists alleged, no discernible structure in the mind at all?

Each hypothesis entailed its own distinctive corollaries; and Galton's technique of correlation offered a ready-made method of checking them. Thus, the obvious plan for attacking such a many-sided issue was to devise and apply suitable tests for the main forms of mental activity, and then calculate the correlations between each test and the rest. If, for example, the orthodox behaviourist is right, and there is "no organized structure in the mind—no ground for classifying mental performances under one or more broad headings, no basis for inferring efficiency in one type of activity from efficiency in another," then we should expect *all the intercorrelations to be zero* or at least non-significant.[1]

---

[1] Spearman, writing of the "momentous investigation by Cattell and Wissler"—the first to apply 'the Galton-Pearson coefficient of correlation' to the results obtained with psychological tests—evidently understands them to have accepted this inference (20, p. 56). Wissler, it is true, says that at first sight the low coefficients suggest that "every act measured by the tests is special and unrelated to every other act" (22, p. 55): but he plainly does not intend this conclusion to be final: he speaks of a "deep conviction that we are otherwise constituted," and points out that certain correlations (e.g., for memory and College grades) are positive and significant. Thorndike also said it was tempting to infer from the data that "there is *nothing whatever* (his italics) common to all mental functions or to any part of them" (*Amer. J. Psych.*, XX, 1909, p. 368): but he, too, quickly abandoned this view. The reasons for the low correlations obtained in these earlier researches are now quite clear: (*a*) the earlier tests had a low reliability; (*b*) the functions tested were extremely simple, and the size of the correlation tends to increase with the complexity of the function; (*c*) the groups tested (students or school classes rather than complete age groups) were already highly selected for general intelligence.

Thomson's sampling theory, though expressed in language similar to that of the 'anti-structural psychologists,' leads to very different corollaries. "The Mind," he says, "has little structure: unlike the body, it is not sub-divided into distinct organs, but forms a comparatively undifferentiated complex of innumerable elements." These he pictures as 'bonds,' i.e., interconnecting neural paths: they have the same character or quality throughout the brain. But, so far from the effects of specific stimuli being limited to specific neural paths (as the earlier opponents of structure assumed), "*any* sample whatever of these elements can be assembled in the activity called for by a 'test'" (21, pp. 303, 306). Now

Evidence for the Concept of Intelligence

If, on the other hand, the mind consists of a number of specialized faculties or abilities, such as ' observation ' (assessed by tests of sensory capacity) or ' practical ability ' (assessed by tests of motor capacity), then we should expect that all the inter-correlations between the sensory tests would be positive and similarly that all the inter-correlations between the motor tests would be positive ; on the other hand, we should expect that *all the cross-correlations between the one group and the other would be approximately zero*. If what Thorndike called ' the theory of natural compensation ' held good, then the cross-correlations would actually become negative, since the ' sensory type ' would be deficient in the characteristic capacities of the ' motor type ' and *vice versa*. Lastly, if there were no specific faculties at all, but only ' a single cognitive activity '—' attention,' as Ward believed, ' sensory discrimination ' as Sully maintained—then we should expect the entire table of correlations to exhibit what Spearman called a ' perfect hierarchical order,' or (in the more precise language of the mathematical textbook) to have ' a rank of one '—apart, of course, from minor aberrations due to sampling errors.

The results of the earlier inquiries revealed, almost without exception, *positive and significant correlations between every form of cognitive activity*. This disproves hypotheses (i) and (iv). Further, except when the sample was small and the sampling errors large, there were nearly always *well-marked clusters of augmented correlations confined to similar forms of cognitive activity*, and leaving significant residuals after the general factor was removed. This rules out hypothesis (ii). We are thus left with hypothesis (iii) as the only alternative consistent with the facts. And, accordingly, the unavoidable inference is that *both* a ' general factor ' *and* a number of ' group factors ' must be at work.[1]

But we are not yet justified in identifying this abstract ' general factor ' with anything so concrete as ' general intelligence.' In Spearman's investigations ' general intelligence ' is always represented by an *external* criterion, i.e., either by direct assessments for intelligence as popularly understood or (in later researches) by standard tests, selected as furnishing accredited ' reference values.' In my own investigations, the ' general cognitive factor ' forms an *internal* criterion, namely, what I called the ' highest common factor ' in the battery of tests. And to determine the concrete nature of such a factor, or

this (as Thomson recognizes) is merely another version of the general factor theory : the chief difference is that with Spearman the general factor is identified with something concrete (mental energy) ; with Thomson it represents something abstract (the fact that the neural elements have the same general character throughout). The corollaries are plain. First, since " the physical body has an obvious structure," the contribution of the general physical factor should be much smaller for correlations between bodily measurements than for correlations between mental ; indeed, it was this supposed ' contrast with physical measurements ' that led Thomson to promulgate his theory. Secondly, with mental measurements, the correlation table, even if not as completely hierarchical as Spearman believed, ought always to exhibit a ' low rank.' Recent work has falsified both these corollaries. To begin with, in the very table for physical measurements which Thomson cites, the contribution of the general factor is practically the same as for mental measurements (50 per cent. or rather more, *Brit. J. Psych., Stat. Sec.*, II, p. 116) ; secondly, the application of mental tests to much larger samples shows that the low rank of the tables Thomson has in mind resulted from the small numbers tested, whereas the physical measurements were obtained from 3,000 persons. It may be added that no neurologist would subscribe to the view that a stimulus, whether simple or complex, merely ' sampled ' the neural elements : the responses to the simpler stimuli are relatively specific and selective; the response to more complex stimulation essentially involves the integration or organization of the neural elements.

[1] C. Burt : '' Experimental Tests of General Intelligence,'' *Brit. J. Psych.*, III, 1909, pp. 94-177.

Sir Cyril Burt

rather of the processes that give rise to it, a supplementary investigation is requisite, based on observations or introspections, or on the correlation of the factor measurements with independent gradings.[1]

Later investigators, notably Brown, Thomson, and more recently Thurstone, have argued that, if we accept the existence of group factors or ' primary abilities,' we can dispense with the hypothesis of a general factor by assuming that the group factors overlap.   But this solution has proved unworkable both in theory and in practice.   When the general factor accounts for much more of the variance than any single group factor, or indeed than all the group factors put together, there is no theoretical gain in closing one's eyes to its presence. And in educational practice the rash assumption that the general factor has at length been demolished has done much to sanction the impracticable idea that, in classifying children according to their varying capacities, we need no longer consider their degree of general ability, and have only to allot them to schools of different types according to their special aptitudes ; in short, that the examination at eleven plus can best be run on the principle of the caucus-race in Wonderland, where everybody wins and each gets some kind of prize.[2]

In their more recent writings, most of the opponents of the ' general factor hypothesis ' have, more or less openly, withdrawn their opposition.   Brown, for example, ultimately acknowledged that " the evidence for a general factor now seems conclusive."   Thomson himself has constructed numerous booklets for testing intelligence.   And Thurstone has proposed a scheme of ' second order factors ' which shall expressly include a ' general factor ' and so account for the correlations between the ' first order factors ' or ' primary abilities.'[3]

(2) *The Factor as ' Cognitive.'*

Merely to demonstrate the presence of a general factor common to all cognitive activities does not (as is usually assumed) prove that this factor is specifically cognitive.   One might as well argue that, because a general factor can be demonstrated common to all sensory activities, therefore this factor is simply and solely a capacity for sensory discrimination.   Impressed by this obvious fallacy, a number of writers went on to argue that in all probability the factor common to mental and scholastic activities was not cognitive but conative.   Such an interpretation had a warm appeal for those who cherished the doctrine of intellectual equality.   When a pupil lagged behindhand in nearly

[1] Actually teachers' gradings for ' intelligence ' (as I showed in my 1909 research) are markedly biased in favour of memory or capacity to learn ; and many psychologists (e.g., Colvin) adopted this as a definition of intelligence.   Spearman, following Sully and the sensationalist school, originally equated intelligence with ' sensory discrimination,' as the basic form of mental *analysis*.   Ward, Stout, and others inclined to identify it with ' attention ' or ' apperception,' i.e., mental or ' neotic ' *synthesis*.   This early disagreement about the ' nature of intelligence ' is no reason for repudiating the concept : after all, there is little agreement about the ' nature ' of gravity : but that is no reason for discarding the principle. And, in point of fact, the conflict can easily be reconciled if we borrow the suggestion of the neurologists and suppose its function to be that of ' integration,' i.e., organization (which involves both analysis and synthesis).

[2] For a fuller discussion of these practical consequences, see this *Journal*, XIII, p. 136, and XXIV, p. 87.

[3] Cf. W. Brown and W. Stephenson : " A Test of the Theory of Two Factors," *Brit. J. Pysch.*, XXIII, 1933, pp. 352-370 ; G. Thomson, *loc. cit. sup* ; L. L. Thurstone : *Multiple Factor Analysis*, 1947, pp. 421f. As both Brown and Thomson indicated, their change of front was partly the effect of the change in physiological views regarding cerebral localization (notably the conclusions of Lashley in regard to ' mass action ' to which they both refer, and Head's drastic criticisms of the ' cerebral map-makers '). Thurstone and his followers, on the other hand, seem indifferent to biological, physiological, or experimental evidence, and prefer to rely exclusively on statistical analysis.

Evidence for the Concept of Intelligence

every subject, the teacher was apt to lay the blame on what Dr. Ballard dubbed the ' general factor of laziness.' Conversely, when a bright child forged ahead in all he undertook, he found himself applauded as a paragon of industry and held up to his fellows as a model of zeal : " genius," said the apostles of the gospel of work, " is just an infinite capacity for taking pains."

This interpretation was elaborated in some detail by Maxwell Garnett, Pearson's brilliant assistant, and one of the ablest champions of the doctrine of a general factor. After re-analysing a good deal of the available data, he came to the conclusion that the factor was after all a factor of Will rather than of Intelligence, and affected moral behaviour quite as much as intellectual success.[1] It was largely as a result of his discussions with Garnett that Spearman eventually dropped his earlier interpretations (' sensory discrimination ' in his first paper, ' neural plasticity ' in the second) and proposed instead a hypothesis of ' mental energy.'

But a re-analysis of existing data, coupled with a priori arguments, could scarcely suffice to settle the question, either one way or the other. Accordingly, in our later experiments, Mr. Moore and I correlated assessments for intellectual performances with assessments for physical, temperamental, and moral qualities. This time most of the cross-correlations were certainly positive, though never very large : it seemed, in fact, as if there was a small but far more comprehensive general factor—a super-factor, as it were—making for excellence in every direction, while the older and more conspicuous factor for cognitive efficiency now appeared simply as a broad group factor, confined to cognitive activities alone : in short, the so-called ' general cognitive factor ' turned out to be merely one of the largest of a number of ' group factors ' varying in extent and size (2, p. 19). At the same time, another broad group factor emerged underlying the temperamental and moral assessments : this was obviously identifiable with what we had previously called ' the general factor for emotionality.' No sharp division appeared, separating affective characteristics from conative. And the so-called cognitive factor was found to be quite as prominent in tests of practical efficiency as in tests of intellectual activity in the narrower sense.

In the light of this further evidence, Garnett's arguments no longer required us to surrender the idea of a cognitive factor. But it certainly seemed necessary to revise the implications conveyed by the word cognition. The basic contrast seems to lie, not so much between cognitive processes and non-cognitive (i.e., affective or conative) in the old introspective sense of those terms, but rather between the capacity for adapting, guiding, or directing mental activities, by means of discriminative and integrative processes, and the capacity for responding promptly, actively, and energetically. Some such distinction was implicit in Spencer's antithesis between mental mechanism and mental force (or, as the Americans preferred to call it, ' drive '). It was, indeed, the distinction originally laid down by Plato. And, in the absence of more appropriate English names, it is tempting to borrow from the Greek, and speak of a general ' cybernetic '[2] factor and a general ' dynamic ' factor.

[1] J. C. M. Garnett : *Proc. Roy. Soc.*, A, XCVI (1919), pp. 102f. Cf. also *id.*, *Education and Citizenship*, 1921, pp. 476f. It should be noted that in all his writings Garnett, one of the noblest quakers of his day, invariably placed ethical considerations first.

[2] I.e., a factor for guiding or controlling : see above, Sect. I (1). On the basis of purely observational and experimental work with children, Professor Piaget seems to have reached a very similar interpretation of the traditional antithesis between cognitive and affective processes : cf. *The Psychology of Intelligence*, 1950, pp. 4f.

(3) *The Factor as 'Innate.'*

The evidence we have so far considered seems fully to vindicate the notion of a 'general cognitive factor.' However, during the last fifteen years or so, the most frequent object of attack has been the assertion that this general factor is largely, if not wholly, innate. This line of criticism is partly an after-effect of the doctrines popularized by the behaviourist school, which dominated psychology for so long in the United States. Educational writers in this country still quote Watson's well-known pronouncements: "We no longer believe in inherited capacities . . . All have equal chances at birth."[1] Watson, however, overstated his case. A doctrine of perfect equality in regard to innate mental traits would fly in the face of all biological experience: throughout the animal kingdom, except where the characteristic is absolutely essential to life, innate differences between individuals are the invariable rule.

Twins and Siblings Reared Together and Apart.—In an earlier issue of this *Journal*[2] I summarized the six or seven converging arguments which can be adduced in support of the inheritance of general ability. The most logical method of investigating such a problem is to keep each of the two variables constant in turn, and compare the results. Let us, therefore, take measurements first for children of identical heredity brought up in different environments and secondly for children of different heredity brought up in the same environment.

In the paper just cited, I gave correlations obtained originally from surveys in the London schools, and supplemented them by further data collected by Miss Conway, who had been responsible for the final computations. Thanks to numerous correspondents, she has since been able to increase the number of cases, particularly for the small but crucial groups of monozygotic twins reared together or apart. The total numbers now amount to 984 siblings, of whom 131 were reared apart; 172 dizygotic or two-egg twins, all reared together; 83 monozygotic or one-egg twins reared together, and 21 reared apart.[3] By way of contrast, she has also secured data for 287 foster children.

[1] *Behaviourism* (1931), pp. 99f. Watson goes on to guarantee that "given my own world to bring them up in," he could train any healthy infant to follow any type of profession—"doctor, lawyer, artist, regardless of abilities or ancestors." Without going so far as this, Dr. Blackburn, Dr. Fleming, Dr. Heim, and a large number of sociological writers, appear to accept the general behaviourist view; but it should be noted that even Watson slipped in a few reservations which his more ardent disciples commonly omit. So far as individual psychology is concerned—apart from the discredited claims of the Iowa school—no new facts have been responsible for this remarkable change of view: it seems rather to be an incidental symptom or consequence of an equally remarkable change in the general climate of opinion. In psychology as in politics, the pendulum of fashion swings to and fro; and the vacillations roughly synchronize. During the nineteenth century, the associationists preached an egalitarian doctrine, and three reform bills were passed. Then the close of the century witnessed a reaction; and we ourselves are witnessing the counter-reaction. An excessive emphasis on heredity has now been succeeded by an equally excessive emphasis on environment. Apparently it is difficult to give due weight simultaneously to each.

[2] "Ability and Income," *Brit. J. Educ. Psych.*, XIII, 1943, pp. 89-91.

[3] Of the monozygotic twins, only nineteen were found in London; and, owing to the distances involved, we have been obliged to depend for measurements of the rest either on research-students or on local teachers and doctors (to whom we must extend our sincerest thanks). As a result, the correlations for this group may have been somewhat reduced. There is a natural prejudice against separating twins, especially if their sex is the same; and we should like to repeat our appeal for further cases. Although the handful of monozygotic twins reared apart is decidedly small (and it is the outcome of a quest that has lasted for over forty years), the differences between the correlations for this group and the rest are for the most part statistically significant. The figures for head-length, head-breadth, and eye-colour are based on much smaller numbers in every batch. Eye-colour (assessed by the methods described in my paper in the *Eugenics Review*, XXXVII, 1946, pp. 149f.) was added because, of all readily observable traits, it is immune from environmental influence.

Evidence for the Concept of Intelligence

The correlations are set out in Table I. Since one or two writers apparently think that the figures obtained by American investigators imply different conclusions from those that I have drawn, I have also included the correlations obtained by Newman, Freeman, and Holzinger (15).[1]

TABLE I

CORRELATIONS BETWEEN TESTS OF MENTAL, SCHOLASTIC AND PHYSICAL MEASUREMENTS.

Measurement	A—BURT AND CONWAY						B—NEWMAN, FREEMAN & HOLZINGER.		
	Identical Twins reared together	Identical Twins reared apart	Non-identical Twins reared together	Siblings reared together	Siblings reared apart	Un-related children reared together	Identical Twins reared together	Identical Twins reared apart	Non-identical Twins reared together
MENTAL (INTELLIGENCE) Intelligence :									
Group Test	·944	·771	·542	·515	·441	·281	·922	·727	·621
Individual Test ..	·921	·843	·526	·491	·463	·252	·910	·670	·640
Final Assessment ..	**925**	**876**	**551**	**538**	**517**	**269**	—·	—	—·
SCHOLASTIC									
General Attainments	**898**	**681**	**831**	**814**	**526**	**535**	·955	·507	·883
Reading and Spelling	·944	·647	·915	·853	·490	·548	—·	—	—·
Arithmetic	·862	·723	·748	·769	·563	·476	—·	—	—
PHYSICAL									
Height	·957	·951	·472	·503	·536	·069	·981	·969	·930
Weight	·932	·897	·586	·568	·427	·243	·973	·886	·900
Head Length	·963	·959	·495	·481	·536	·116	·910	·917	·691
Head Breadth	·978	·962	·541	·507	·472	·082	·908	·880	·654
Eye Colour	1·000	1·000	·516	·553	·504	·104	—	—·	—

As regards intelligence, the outstanding feature of the table is the high correlation between the assessments for identical twins even when they have been reared apart : it is almost as high as the correlation between two successive testings for the same individuals. Between non-identical twins the resemblances (at any rate with our own data) are not much closer than those between ordinary brothers and sisters. Nevertheless, environment is not entirely without effect, particularly when the assessments have been obtained by written tests applied

[1] Dr. Heim, referring to the American inquiry, states that " when young monozygotic twins are separated . . . the differences between their scores are as great as those between unseparated dizygotic twins." But it will be seen that, in point of fact, both with the group test (Otis) and with the individual test (Stanford-Binet) the figures there given for the separated monozygotic twins are appreciably higher than those for the unseparated dizygotic twins, even though their figures for the latter are larger than those of most other investigators.

The figures obtained for twins in the most recent and extensive studies of twins carried out in Great Britain seem in the main to agree with our own. Herman and Hogben report with the Otis group test a correlation of 0·66 for twins of like sex and only 0·53 for twins of unlike sex : if we suppose that about half those of like sex were non-identical, this suggests a figure of about ·80 for the identical twins (12). Maxwell analysed data obtained with group tests for 468 twins during the Scottish Survey, and found correlations of 0·73 for twins of like sex and 0·63 for twins of unlike sex : as he observes, the latter value is " a little higher than that found in most other studies " (19).

to whole groups. The effect is obvious when we compare the correlations for children reared together and children reared apart. And it might be thought that in the correlations obtained from unrelated children reared in the same homes we have a direct indication of its actual amount. In all probability, however, such correlations mainly reflect the method of placement : a dull or defective orphan would not be boarded out with a highly intellectual family.

The figures for physical measurements, at least in our own data, show very similar trends : with the American data the correlations are somewhat higher, but the disparity is seldom large.[1]

The results obtained for the scholastic tests, both in the American inquiry and in our own, present a striking contrast. In our own inquiry the correlations for siblings and non-identical twins reared together are actually higher than those for the identical twins who have been reared apart. And it may be instructive to note that the correlations which are most conspicuously increased by similarity of home environment are those for verbal or literary attainments ; those for arithmetical attainments are, if anything, increased more by similarity of genetic constitution.

Figures like the foregoing provide ample evidence that individual differences in general intelligence are in part at least inherited, and that they are affected by environmental differences much less than are school attainments. However, the mere fact of hereditary influence the more sober critics do not deny. What they question is whether its amount is really large enough to be of any practical consequence either in the sphere of education or in later civic life.

Now I believe that a good deal of the difficulty arises because both the opponents of mental inheritance and its advocates still cling to wholly out-of-date notions of what is to be understood by such a phrase. Terms like heredity and variation, which played such crucial roles in the theories of Darwin, Spencer and the earlier biometricians, continue to be used by modern biologists, but their implications have radically changed. Moreover, the few educationists who appreciate the relevance of this change seem to be quite uncertain how far the newer theories have undermined the older inferences of the Galton-Pearson school.

The Hypothesis of Multifactor Inheritance.—Galton at the very outset of his work noted that in nearly all mental characteristics the observable differences between individuals are differences of degree rather than of kind, and proposed a scale of continuous variation in place of the traditional schemes of discontinuous types. Now, during the first two decades of the century, both the advocates of the new Mendelian hypothesis, and its opponents, originally supposed that the particulate theory of heredity, and the basic principle of segregation, were incompatible with continuous variation in an inheritable trait. Thus, Pearson and the biometric school contended that, even if true, the Mendelian hypothesis must be exceedingly limited in its application, and could have little or no bearing on normal psychology. On the other hand, the earlier Mendelians, De Vries, for example, believed that, since the Mendelian mechanism must underlie all forms of inheritance, no continuous variations could ever be inheritable ; and this argument is still adduced by those who reject the inheritability of intelligence, because (so they assume) the very fact that variations in intelligence are continuous shows that they are produced by purely environmental agency.

---

[1] The high correlation for physical measurements obtained by Newman and his colleagues with non-identical twins is a little surprising. Lauterbach's figures agree more closely with my own. His correlations for twins of like and unlike sex are, for height, 0·80 and 0·53 ; for weight, 0·89 and 0·50 (*Genetics*, X, 1925, pp. 525-568).

Evidence for the Concept of Intelligence

Now, in spite of their undoubted importance for genetic and agricultural research, analogies drawn from the study of domesticated animals and plants may be highly misleading when we turn to human genetics. Very naturally, the characters that first caught the eye of the Mendelian experimentalist were qualitative traits, attributable each to some single factor or 'gene' which produces its own visible and distinctive effect. But there is no reason why genes should not exist whose separate manifestations evade our present methods of discrimination-systems of polygenes, and whose effects are *small, similar,* and *cumulative*.[1] If the number affecting the same trait were large, the result would be that observable variations in that trait would appear continuous, and the frequency-distribution of the measurements would approximate to the normal curve.[2] This is fully in keeping with the conclusions reached by Galton and his followers. It may be shown, says Galton, "that the distribution of human qualities and faculties (qualities like height and head-length, faculties like strength, visual acuity, or general ability) is approximately normal "(9, p. 32 ; (10, pp. 59, 201).

Manifestly it is impossible to check the existence of such genes by direct Mendelian *methods* ; but, with the aid of statistics, we can discover whether the apparent effects are in accordance with Mendelian *principles*. Suppose, then, that a child's endowment of intelligence is dependent, not on a single pair of genes, but on many such pairs, each segregating in the usual fashion, and all affecting the same observable trait ; and suppose too that one member of each pair (designated by a capital letter) would, if present, *add* a small quantity to the net result, while the other (designated by a small letter) would *deduct* an equal quantity. Then, for any given individual (or 'phenotype'), the total mount of intelligence would be proportional to the number of capital letters specifying the 'genotype.' Hence, if there were only three pairs of genes, the brightest individual would have a genetic constitution represented by $AABBCC$, the dullest a constitution represented by $aabbcc$, and the average person a constitution represented by $AaBbCc$. Assuming that mating is random and that there is no 'dominance,' the frequency of each genotype could be deduced by expanding the product $(A+a)^2 (B+b)^2 (C+c)^2$: it would, in fact, be proportional to the binomial coefficients, 1, 6, 15, 20, 15, 6, 1. With n such pairs of genes there would be $2n \pm 1$ classes. And, as n increases, the binomial distribution will approach

[1] The possibility of multi-factor inheritance was mentioned by Mendel in his discussion of the colouring of white, red, and purple flowering beans. It was first demonstrated by H. Nilsson-Ehle in hybridization experiments on oats and wheat (*Kreuzungsuntersuchungen an Hafer und Weizen*, 1909) ; and the cardinal principles were elucidated more fully by E. M. East in studies of the corolla-length in the tobacco-plant ('Size-inheritance in Nicotiana' *Genetics*, I, 1915, pp. 164-176). The first to point out the importance of such a theory for human genetics appears to have been C. B. Davenport ("Inheritance of Stature," *Genetics*, II, 1917, pp. 313f.). The number of genes which the theorist may legitimately postulate is now known to be far larger than was formerly thought : the banana-fly, *Drosophila*, is estimated to possess between 5,000 and 10,000 ; and man may have six times as many.

[2] For those who are not familiar with recent work in genetics, a brief explanation may be helpful. H. G. Wells, in one of his short stories, tells how an engaged couple hailing from North Wales—a Mr. Price-Jones and a Miss Evan-Roberts—plume themselves on bearing the family names of both their fathers and their mothers. But, they ask, how are they to christen their prospective children ? The minister who is to marry them suggests that each child should take *one* surname from the male parent and *one* from the female, and that a coin should be tossed to decide the choice. Now let us apply the same principle to the case where a Mr. Price-Jones had married a Miss Price-Jones : the possible names for the children would be Price-Price, Price-Jones, Jones-Price, and Jones-Jones. This is exactly parallel to the way single genes are transmitted. Put A for Price and a for Jones. Then, when Mr. Aa marries Miss Aa, the possible recombinations are AA, Aa, aA, and aa : since Aa and aA are equivalent, the resulting proportions given by the toss will be 1 : 2 : 1.

Sir Cyril Burt

more and more closely to the normal curve. But this, as we shall see, is only part of the story.

The Frequency-distribution for the General Population.—Modern critics of the Galtonian view usually start by attacking the theory of normal distribution. Dr. Heim, for example, assures us that it is a sheer assumption, " though not explicitly recognized as an assumption " ; quite unwarrantably (she says) it has got " hailed as a scientific discovery, despite the fact that frequency distributions depend mainly on the system of scoring adopted." Mr. Richmond makes much the same point. To ensure this " a priori principle " (he says) the psychometrist " tinkers with the test material " ; as a result " measurements are normally distributed, simply because the test has been so constructed that they must be so distributed " (11, 18).

Such arguments betray a singular indifference to the facts. In this country the first attempts to secure objective evidence about the distribution of test measurements were those made during my surveys of London schools. The chi-squared test was applied ; and (as I pointed out at the time) the results disclosed quite plainly that such measurements are *not* distributed in exact conformity with the normal curve. The most conspicuous departure appeared in the lower tail of the curve, where, owing to an excess of dull and defective pupils (by no means invariably of a pathological type), the frequencies were much larger than the expected values.[1] When the defectives are omitted, then the resulting curve approximates more nearly to the normal, though the fit is still far from perfect. This *approximate* normality (which was all that Galton claimed) is thus not ' an a priori assumption ' but an empirically demonstrated fact.

On examining the frequency curves for intelligence, therefore, we seem compelled to envisage two kinds of inheritance—unifactor inheritance and multifactor inheritance. If I may repeat what I have said elsewhere, " both the form of the distribution and the correlations obtained are very much what we should theoretically expect were these graded measurements, mainly though not wholly, determined by a very large number of similar genes ; while in certain instances and in certain forms (as independent evidence from pedigrees suggests) mental dificiency may occasionally act like a dominant, or, still more frequently, like a recessive, and in some even be sex-linked " : in this double mode of transmission, so I suggested, the inheritance of intelligence seems to resemble the inheritance of stature (3, p. 81). Moreover, as with stature so with intelligence, the observable measurements are in some degree modified by non-heritable influences. In the case of stature, the excessive frequency of very short persons is due partly to single genes (as with the achondroplastic dwarf, where the condition is dominant, and the ateleiotic dwarf, where it is apparently recessive), partly to environmental and pathological causes (as with rachitic or under-nourished children), and sometimes to both (as with the cretin) ; and precisely the same types of causation are traceable in the dull and mentally deficient.

---

[1] A typical curve is that printed by Mayer Gross, Eliot Slater, and Martin Roth in their recent textbook on *Clinical Psychiatry* (1954, p. 56) : the diagram is reproduced from one of my earlier surveys and based on over 3,000 cases ; the irregularities are clearly visible.

Mr. Richmond cites as an example of ' tinkering ' the revised version of the Binet-Simon Scale. But the tests were standardized with no reference whatever to normality : the assumption made was that, between the ages of 5 and 12, the annual increments are approximately equal. With properly constructed group tests, the items are selected (often by elaborate scaling techniques, such as paired comparison or its equivalents) so as to increase more or less uniformly in difficulty. Even in mechanical tests like erasing *o*'s and *e*'s in a page of pied print, where there can be no suspicion of ' tinkering with the scale,' the distributions are still approximately normal.

Evidence for the Concept of Intelligence

The Frequency-distributions for Parents and Siblings.—The possibility of polygenic determination was not overlooked by the biometric school. Galton himself was convinced that " inheritance may be described as largely, if not wholly ' particulate ' " (10, p. 7). And Karl Pearson carried out a theoretical study of the statistical consequences of multifactorial inheritance (16). He concluded, however, that the correlations actually observed both between parents and their offspring and between children and their own brothers or sisters were far too high to be explicable by any such hypothesis. But, as now seems plain, his deductions were partly invalidated by certain untenable assumptions and several undue simplifications. To begin with, he tacitly assumed that dominance would be complete ; furthermore, though keenly aware of the facts of assortative mating, he failed to make correct allowance for its influence ; and above all, like most of the earlier biometricians, he failed to recognize the clear distinction between the causes of inheritable variation and their observable effects, between the carriers of heredity and the manifestations of heredity, in short, between what is conveniently called the ' genotype ' (the hereditary determinants considered as a system typical of certain individuals) and the ' phenotype ' (the kind of individual organism eventually produced by the interaction of the genotype with its particular environment) ; and it is a failure to recognize the same distinction that is largely responsible for the misconceptions and criticisms which the genetical psychologist encounters to-day.

The examination of the bivariate distributions is greatly simplified if we work with grouped frequencies. It is not difficult to show that, if a large number of genes combine, in the manner described above, to determine the measurements for two related members in a random sample of families (e.g., for parents and their children or for children and their sibs), and the measurements are suitably grouped to yield classes instead of continuous variates, then the frequencies to be expected will be similar to those deducible from a single pair of genes, for which the hybrid state (Aa or aA) is intermediate. Such frequencies, of course, can be readily computed by applying the ordinary principles of probability. The detailed values for multifactor inheritance have, in fact, been deduced by Fisher in his classical paper on ' The Correlation between Relatives on the Supposition of Mendelian Inheritance ' (7) : a non-technical account will be found in (8).

To ascertain how far the actual results for general intelligence conform with those which are required by the multifactor hypothesis, I have collected assessments for a 1,000 pairs of sibs, representing, so far as possible, a random selection of the London school population.[1] At the same time I have endeavoured, though with poorer success, to secure assessments for at least one parent. Since these proved obtainable for only 954 cases, the analysis has to be limited to this smaller number. On the basis of the measurements, the children were divided

[1] The inquiry was limited to children between the ages of 8 and 13, and was based primarily on verbal and non-verbal tests of intelligence. The actual measurements were transformed into standard scores (i.e., deviations divided by the standard deviation for each age) ; and these scores in turn were converted to terms of an I.Q. scale with a standard deviation of 15. Thus, the dividing lines for the three groups are approximately I.Q's of 90 and 110. Borderline cases were specially investigated in the light of the teachers' reports, and doubts resolved by individual testing. For the assessments of the parents we relied chiefly on personal interviews ; but in doubtful and borderline cases an open or a camouflaged test was employed. The entire set of data on which the following tables are based were derived from four successive surveys carried out with the assistance of Miss Pelling, Mr. Seymour, Miss Richardson, and Miss Howard respectively. The methods adopted were slightly different in each ; and the last was the most accurate. But, so far as the grouped frequencies are concerned, the results disclose no significant changes ; hence, it seems legitimate to lump the whole series together for purposes of the present analysis.

Sir Cyril Burt

into three groups—bright, average, and dull—in the proportions 1 : 2 : 1 ; and a similar classification was adopted for the parents. The percentages we should expect for the bivariate distribution, based on the triple assumption of random mating, Mendelian segregation, and no tendency to dominance, are shown below in Tables IIA and IIIA. They are, it will be noted, in the proportions 1, 1, 0 ; 1, 2, 1 ; 0, 1, 1 for parent and child, and 9, 6, 1 ; 6, 20, 6 ; 1, 6, 9 for pairs of sibs. On calculating the product-moment correlation for each hypothetical table, the value will be found to be exactly 0·500.

The observed frequencies, also reduced to percentages, are shown in Tables IIB and IIIB : (the perfect symmetry of the latter results from the procedure regularly followed in constructing a table for an intra-class correlation). It will be seen that the observed proportions agree tolerably well with the hypothetical; and, as we shall learn in a moment, the divergences themselves are very much what we should anticipate. The actual correlations, computed from the original data, were, for parent and child, 0·481, and for sibs 0·507 (computed from the pooled frequencies tabulated below, the values would be slightly different owing to the ‘ coarse grouping ’).

TABLE II
BIVARIATE DISTRIBUTIONS FOR PARENTS AND THEIR CHILDREN.

| Parents | A.—Theoretical Frequencies | | | | B.—Observed Frequencies | | | |
| | Children | | | | Children | | | |
	Bright	Average	Dull	Total	Bright	Average	Dull	Total
Bright	12·5	12·5	0·0	25·0	10·8	12·3	1·9	25·0
Average	12·5	25·0	12·5	50·0	13·4	26·5	10·1	50·0
Dull	0·0	12·5	12·5	25·0	0·8	11·2	13·0	25·0
Total	25·0	50·0	25·0	100·0	25·0	50·0	25·0	100·0

TABLE III
BIVARIATE DISTRIBUTIONS FOR SIBLINGS.

| Children | A.—Theoretical Frequencies | | | | B.—Observed Frequencies | | | |
| | Children | | | | Children | | | |
	Bright	Average	Dull	Total	Bright	Average	Dull	Total
Bright	14·1	9·4	1·5	25·0	14·7	8·2	2·1	25·0
Average ..	9·4	31·2	9·4	50·0	8·2	34·7	7·1	50·0
Dull	1·5	9·4	14·1	25·0	2·1	7·1	15·8	25·0
Total	25·0	50·0	25·0	100·0	25·0	50·0	25·0	100·0

A perfect agreement between the observed frequencies and the theoretical cannot possibly be expected, since there must be numerous unavoidable influences, tending partly to increase and partly to diminish the apparent correlation. (i) To begin with, like all mental measurements, assessments for intelligence, however scrupulously checked and adjusted, are in some degree distorted by the *unreliability* of the methods available. The best estimate for the reliability coefficient is 0·916. If we apply the usual correction for unreliability, the observed values would be raised to 0·525 and 0·554 respectively. (ii) But, as we have seen, the most punctilious attempts to assess ‘ innate ability ’

Evidence for the Concept of Intelligence

(itself a purely hypothetical quantity) cannot entirely escape the effects of different *environmental conditions* ; and, of course, for members of the same family the effects must generally tend in the same direction. How far this may have augmented the apparent correlation it would be hard to say : but the increase must almost certainly have been smaller than the decrease due to unreliability.[1]

(iii) The most elusive tendencies to allow for are those of dominance and assortative mating. Were *dominance* complete, the expected correlations would be altered to $\dfrac{q}{1+q}$ and $\dfrac{1+3q}{4(1+q)}$ respectively, where p^2, $2pq$, and q^2 denote the proportions of pure dominants, mixed dominants, and pure recessives respectively, and $q+p=1$. Thus, the effect of dominance is once again to lower the apparent correlations ; but, unlike that of unreliability, it lowers them by widely differing amounts. Now the initial classification we have adopted makes $p=q=\frac{1}{2}$. Substituting this value in the fractions given above, we obtain, for the expected correlation between parents and their children, a coefficient of 1/3, that is 0·333, and for the expected correlation between children and their brothers or sisters a coefficient of 5/12, that is 0·416.[2] The observed values are significantly higher.

(iv) What then can have raised the absolute values to this high level ? The most likely answer is *assortative mating*. How then can its presence be verified and its influence assessed ? One of its calculable results would be to increase the variance of the younger generation. Now, if we may trust our rather crude measurements, the variance of the parents is only 12·3 I.Q., whereas (in virtue of the mode of standardization) the variance of the children is 15 I.Q. This is tantamount to an increase in the filial generation of about 22 per cent. Spouses, it appears, prefer partners whose intelligence in some degree resembles their own. The actual amount of the resemblance can be estimated by calculating the correlation between husband and wife. In the earlier surveys it was well over 0·40 ; in the later somewhat below.

Now, as we have seen, dominance, like unreliability, tends to reduce the correlations between parent and child and between one sib and another ; but, unlike unreliability, it reduces them to different extents. On the other hand, the effect of assortative mating, like that of similar environment, is to increase the correlations, and to increase them by amounts that make them more nearly equal. The net result can be estimated, if we treat the contributory variances as additive components, and then apply the ordinary principles of factor analysis. A little calculation indicates that the ultimate effect of assortative mating would be to *add a small amount to both correlations*, viz., in the present

---

[1] The critic usually supposes that intelligence-tests are considerably affected by cultural differences in the testees' environment. But, if the tests have been properly constructed and their pronouncements properly checked and adjusted, such effects are almost negligible. The influence of unhygienic conditions in early infancy is a more likely source of error, for which it is difficult to allow. The statement in the text was based on indirect attempts to estimate the upper limit for environmental influences by methods which need not be detailed here.

[2] These are the theoretical values deduced by Pearson in the paper already cited (16). He rejected them, and with them the assumptions on which they were based, because they fall far below the correlations he had empirically obtained for numerous traits showing continuous variation. Yule, however, pointed out that if, instead of postulating complete dominance (as Pearson had tacitly done), we postulate complete absence of dominance, both the theoretical values would be raised to 0·500 ; and this would accord far better with Pearson's own figures (*Report of Conference on Genetics*, 1906). Yule's assumptions make the relevant conditions even simpler than Pearson's ; but in view of recent results, it seems pretty certain that they are far more complex.

Sir Cyril Burt

instance about 0·15 and 0·09. With complete dominance, this would raise the theoretical values from 0·333 and 0·416 to about 0·48 and 0·52 respectively. And these figures tally reasonably well with those observed.[1]

The Relative Importance of Heredity and Environment.—We now reach our final problem : what proportion of the total variance shown by the children is attributable to genetic conditions as contrasted with environmental ? In recent discussions on this point, two important considerations are frequently ignored.

(i) If the observed correlation between parent and child is 0·481, we might infer that each parent contributes $0·481^2 = 23$ per cent. to the total variance. And if the mating were random, the two parents together would contribute $2 \times 23 = 46$ per cent. But since, as we have seen, there is a correlation of at least 0·40 between fathers and mothers, part of the influence of one parent must overlap with that of the other, and consequently should not be included twice. Making due allowance for the overlap, we may estimate the contribution deducible from the assessments for the two parents as about 45 per cent. at most. Now it is often inferred that the remainder of the variance must, therefore, be ascribed to non-inheritable factors, that is, to the influence of the environment. But with the mode of transmission we have assumed, not only the parents but also the grandparents and remoter ancestry must contribute something to the variance. A simple algebraic deduction from the postulates of multifactorial inheritance will show that the total effect of parentage and ancestry may be directly measured by the correlation between sibs. The observed correlation, it will be remembered, was 0·507. According to our findings, therefore, about 51 per cent. of the variance must be contributed by such factors.

(ii) But, even so, it would be quite mistaken to assign the whole of the residue (49 per cent.) to environmental influences. By an odd paradox, not only the similarity between siblings, but also their differences are largely the outcome of their genetic constitution. Thus, arguing from Mendelian principles, we should definitely anticipate a frequent lack of resemblance between one sib and another owing to the segregation of those factors in respect of which the parents are heterozygous. After computing a rough estimate for this additional contribution, I calculate that *in all at least 75 per cent. of the entire variance must be due to genetic influences, probably far more.*[2]

It must be frankly owned that, with a sample covering under a thousand cases, the somewhat speculative balancing of the accessory factors that affect the correlations here obtained can make no pretence to be either accurate or

---

[1] It might be suggested that the resemblance between brothers and sisters appears greater than that between parents and their children, because children of the same family are brought up together and may even go to the same school. Similarity of schooling might no doubt affect the correlations for cultural and educational tests, as indeed the figures in Table I suggest ; but (for the reasons given above) it cannot appreciably affect the results obtained for intelligence. Certainly the assessments for siblings who have gone to the same schools reveal no higher correlation than the assessments for those who have gone to different schools.

[2] The theoretical considerations on which such calculations should be based are clearly set out by Fisher in the paper already cited (7). It may be observed that the figure for the residual contribution which we have thus reached, namely 25 per cent., would imply a correlation with the conditions causing it amounting to $\sqrt{0·25} = 0·50$. But a direct calculation of the partial correlation between favourable environmental conditions and the assessments for intelligence proves to be well under this figure. Hence, the final figure reached above for genetic influence leans definitely to the conservative side. Fisher's formulae would subdivide the contributions to the total variance into (i) genotypes 49 per cent., (ii) dominance 28 per cent., (iii) assortative mating 19 per cent., leaving for (iv) environment only 4 per cent.

Evidence for the Concept of Intelligence

conclusive. My aim has rather been to adumbrate a line of reasoning that merits closer consideration and further research. But, even as it stands, the analysis I have made, supplemented by the other evidence that I have mentioned, seems to me to afford a strong corroboration for the view I have indicated, namely, that *human intelligence, like human stature, is determined largely though not wholly by multifactorial inheritance.*[1]

Conclusion.—I have now reviewed the wide variety of evidence—observational, introspective, and experimental, biological, physiological, and statistical, bearing on our initial question. The results are mutually supporting ; and, apart from certain minor modifications or extensions, seem abundantly to confirm the threefold hypothesis that I tentatively put forward over forty years ago in the forerunner of this *Journal*[2] : namely, that there is a general factor making for efficiency in all mental activities, that this factor is essentially cognitive or directive, and that the greater part of the individual variance found in this factor is attributable to differences in genetic constitution. This triple conclusion suggested a modernized formula for the abstract conception to which so many different writers had been led, viz., ' innate, general, cognitive ability.' If, therefore, we are to retain the word ' intelligence ' as a technical term in psychology, this still seems the best definition.

III.—SUMMARY.

The main steps in the argument may be epitomized as follows :

1.—Evidence from different branches of psychology leads to the notion of a mental capacity that is (i) cognitive, (ii) general, (iii) innate.

2.—Each of these three characteristics has been amply verified by statistical research.

3.—As the history of the word shows, intelligence was a technical term put forward to designate a technical concept : and the meaning given it, implicitly or explicitly, by leading authorities from Cicero and the scholastics to Spencer, Galton, and Binet, suggests that it furnishes the most convenient name for the concept thus reached.

---

[1] As I suggested in my earlier paper, it is urgently desirable that similar methods should be employed to investigate the presence of a general cognitive factor in lowlier animals, and, if possible, to determine its mode of inheritance. The few researches so far carried out point to conclusions similar to those reached above. R. L. Thorndike has calculated correlations between tests of learning, strength of drive, etc., in albino rats, and finds a general factor of learning ability and two supplementary factors (*Genet. Psych. Monogr.*, XVII, 1935, pp. 1-70). Vaughn (*Comp. Psych. Monogr.*, XIV, 1937, pp. 1-41) and Tolman and others (*ibid.*, XVII, 1941, pp. 1-20) have also published tables of correlations for the performances of rats ; their figures are fully consistent with the theory of a general factor, though the investigators themselves prefer an analysis in terms of overlapping group factors.

To test the hypothesis of multifactorial inheritance, Tryon has carried out experiments on maze-learning, which he regards as a test of general ability, and has repeated them with successive generations. He attempted first to secure two strains, of bright and dull rats respectively, by selective inbreeding. After seven selections and seven generations, he found practically no overlapping between the distribution-curves for bright and for dull. He then, as it were, reversed the procedure, crossing the two strains, and testing two further generations. It is true that the variance exhibited by the F_1-generation seemed too great to be explained wholly by non-genetic influences, and much greater than would be expected had the method of inbreeding been successful. Yet, on the whole, as he contends, the results seem to support the multifactorial hypothesis (R. C. Tryon, " Genetic Differences in Maze-Learning in Rats," *Thirty-ninth Yearbook of Nat. Soc. Study of Education*, 1940, pp. 113f. ; cf. also E. G. Brody, " Genetic Basis of Spontaneous Activity in the Albino Rat," *Com. Psych. Monogr.*, XVII, 1942, No. 5.).

[2] See *J. Exp. Pedag.*, I, 1911, pp. 93f ; Cf. also [1].

Sir Cyril Burt

4.—Apart from comparatively rare and abnormal variations, differences in intelligence as thus defined seem to depend on the combined action of numerous genes whose influence is similar, small, and cumulative—a hypothesis that is fully borne out by the frequency-distributions obtained for parents, siblings, and the population as a whole. And on this hypothesis not only the similarities between relatives but also their dissimilarities will be largely due to genetic factors.

5.—It is essential to distinguish between intelligence as an abstract component of the individual's genetic constitution (γ) and intelligence as an observable and empirically measurable trait (g). The evidence indicates that at least 75 per cent. of the measurable variance (based on carefully checked assessments) is attributable to differences in genetic constitution, and less than 25 per cent. to environmental conditions.

IV.—References.

(1) Burt, C. (1912): " The Inheritance of Mental Characteristics," *Eugenics Review*, IV, pp. 1-33.

(2) Burt, C. (1924): " History of the Development of Psychological Tests," Ap. Board of Education, *Report on Psychological Tests of Educable Capacity*. (London : H.M. Stationery Office.)

(3) Burt, C. (1935): *The Subnormal Mind*. (Oxford : The Oxford University Press.)

(4) Burt, C. (1946): *Intelligence and Fertility*. (London : Hamish Hamilton.)

(5) Burt, C. (1955): " The Meaning and Assessment of Intelligence " (Galton Lecture for 1955), *Eugenics Review*, XLVII, pp. 81-91.

(6) Carmichael, L. (ed). (1946): *Manual of Child Psychology*. (New York : Wiley.)

(7) Fisher, R. A. (1918): " The Correlation between Relations on the Supposition of Mendelian Inheritance," *Trans. Roy. Soc. Edin.*, LII, pp. 399-434.

(8) Fisher, R. A. (1919): " The Causes of Human Variability," *Eugenics Review*, X, pp. 213-220.

(9) Galton, F. (1869): *Hereditary Genius*. (London : Macmillan.)

(10) Galton, F. (1889): *Natural Inheritance*. (London : Macmillan.)

(11) Heim, A. W. (1954): *The Appraisal of Intelligence*. (London : Methuen.)

(12) Hogben, L. and Herman, L. (1933): " The Intellectual Resemblance of Twins," *Proc. Roy. Soc. Edin.*, LIII, pp. 105-129.

(13) Kirman, B. H. (1952): *This Matter of Mind*. (London : Watts.)

(14) Newman, H. H., Freeman, F. N., and Holzinger, K. J. (1937): *Twins : A Study of Heredity and Environment*. (Chicago : University of Chicago Press.)

(15) Newman, H. H. (1942): *Twins and Super-Twins*. (London : Hutchinson).

(16) Pearson, K. (1903): " On a Generalized Theory of Alternative Inheritance with Special Reference to Mendel's Laws," *Phil. Trans.*, CCIII, 53-87.

(17) Piaget, J. (1950): *The Psychology of Intelligence*. (London : Routledge and Kegan Paul.)

(18) Richmond, W. K. (1953): " Educational Measurement : Its Scope and Limitations : A Critique," *Brit. J. Psych.*, XLIV, pp. 221-231.

(19) Scottish Council for Research in Education (1953): *Social Implications of the 1947 Scottish Mental Survey*. (London : University of London Press.)

(20) Spearman, C. (1927): *The Abilities of Man*. (London : Macmillan.)

(21) Thomson, G. H. (1948). *The Factorial Analysis of Human Ability*. (London : University of London Press.)

(22) Wissler, C. (1901): " The Correlation of Mental and Physical Tests," *Psych. Rev. Monogr. Supp.*, III, vi.

From T. R. Miles (1957). Brit. J. Educ. Psychol., *27*, 153-165, *by kind permission of the authors and Scottish Academic Press*

CONTRIBUTIONS TO INTELLIGENCE TESTING AND THE THEORY OF INTELLIGENCE

I.—ON DEFINING INTELLIGENCE.

BY T. R. MILES
(University College of North Wales).

I.—*Introduction.* II.—*Different senses of the word ' definition.'* III.—*Application to the study of intelligence.* IV.—*Wechsler's definition.* V.—*Burt's definition.* VI.—*References.*

" We have first raised a dust and then complain that we cannot see."
—BISHOP BERKELEY.

SUMMARY.—In offering what purport to be definitions of intelligence, psychologists do not always seem to have worked out what sense of the word ' definition ' they have in 'mind. Six possible senses of the word ' definition ' are here distinguished. Each sense is then discussed with special reference to the problem of defining intelligence. In the light of the distinctions made, the definitions of intelligence offered by Wechsler and Burt are critically examined from the point of view of methodology.

I.—INTRODUCTION.

IT is commonly thought to be a great scandal that psychologists cannot agree on a definition of intelligence. People then draw the conclusion that intelligence must be something very obscure and elusive to provoke such controversy. I do not dispute that there are many disagreements on matters of fundamental principle, but it seems to me that the issue has often been confused by *unnecessary* disputation and by argument at cross purposes.

I shall not, in this paper, offer any definition of intelligence of my own, nor shall I take sides on the question of whether a particular definition is a good or bad one. My task is the preliminary one of clearing the ground. The question towards which I wish to focus attention is : *By what arguments do we establish that one definition of intelligence is better than another ?*

I shall suggest in answer to this question that the word ' definition ' is ambiguous, and that different arguments are appropriate according to the sense in which the word ' definition ' is being used.*

II.—DIFFERENT SENSES OF THE WORD ' DEFINITION.'

In distinguishing different senses of the word ' definition ' I have relied largely on the work of Robinson (1950).† A distinction needs to be drawn in the

---

* I have used throughout the phrase " different *senses of the word* ' definition ' " in preference to the more familiar " different *kinds* of definition." Neither phrase is wholly satisfactory. The important point is that ' defining ' is not the name of a single procedure, but refers to a group of procedures having a certain " family-resemblance " (to use Wittgenstein's phrase) between them.

† This must not be taken as a suggestion that the work of earlier writers on the subject of definition can simply be dismissed. Many of the traditional ' rules ', e.g., that a definition should be *per proximum genus et differentiam specificam* seem to me not so much wrong as in need of reformulation.

On Defining Intelligence

first place between *nominal* and *real* definition.* Nominal definition is concerned in the main with the meaning of words rather than with the things for which the words appear to stand.† Robinson sub-divides nominal definition into two classes, (1) lexical definition and (2) stipulative definition. A lexical definition gives an account of how a word has in fact been used by a particular group of people ; a stipulative definition states how the speaker proposes to use the word, irrespective of how that word has been used in the past.

In contrast, ' real definition ' is commonly taken to be definition of *things*. A real definition is supposed to tell us the ' nature of the thing defined.' It is here that some of the biggest pitfalls in argument occur. Robinson distinguishes no less than twelve different activities, all of which have been bunched, very confusedly, under the general title ' real definition.' Of these twelve I shall mention three : (1) *The search for the essence or essential nature of a thing*. This notion Robinson regards as misleading, on the grounds that there are no such things as essences in the sense given to the word ' essence ' by Aristotle. In Robinson's view, " Is it part of the essence of a swan to be white ? " is a disguised request for a nominal, not a real definition, and means no more than " If I were to see a creature otherwise like a swan but black, should I continue to give it the label ' swan ' ? " (2) " *Description plus naming*." Robinson writes " Many so-called ' real definitions ' of the form x is yz are equivalent to the statement that : ' The character yz occurs and I call this character (or it is commmonly called) by the name ' x '." Robinson regards this as a legitimate and useful activity, but suggests that ' real definition ' is a misleading name for this activity. It suggests the hopeless search for real essences, and invites confusion with other activities also grouped under the heading of ' real definition.' (3) *The search for a key*. A definition of x, on this showing, involves a single short sentence from which follow all the things which we need to know about x. The stock example is geometry, where all the important things we know about triangles—so it was supposed—follow from the definition of a triangle as a plane figure bounded by three straight lines. This account of a triangle thus provides the key to understanding a wide range of other true sentences about triangles. Again Robinson is hesitant to call such procedure ' real definition,' partly, once more, because it might be confused with his other eleven possible senses of ' real definition,' and also because it tends to conceal from us the fact that in some cases no such key may be discoverable.

There is a further procedure, not discussed in any detail by Robinson, but playing quite a large part in modern psychology—the so-called ' operational ' definition. This is an attempt to define the meaning of a word in terms of the observations, or scientific ' operations,' necessary if that word is to form part of a true sentence. Thus it might be said that the word ' length ' requires to be defined in terms of the operations involved in measuring length, and that " This rod is 6-in. long " is meaningful in virtue of the possibility of specifying in detail the appropriate operations.‡

This classification of definitions must not be regarded as exhaustive, nor need the different activities which I have distinguished be regarded as mutually exclusive. The important point which I wish to stress is that, until we know the sense in which the word ' definition ' is being used, attempts to assess the merits or de-merits of a defintion of intelligence are liable to lead to argument at cross-purposes.

* Compare Burt (1947, p. 129).
† This statement requires qualification, but is accurate enough for present purposes.
‡ For further discussion, see Bridgman (1927), esp. Chapter 1.

T. R. Miles

III.—Application to the Study of Intelligence.

(i) *The 'real essence' of intelligence.* If we agree with Robinson that the notion of 'real essences' is a mistaken one,* then sentences which refer to "the real essence of intelligence" are either illegitimate or in need of reformulation. Few, if any, writers at the present time speak in as many words of the 'essence' of intelligence.† But there are plenty of people who ask about its 'real nature' or 'real meaning,' which comes to much the same thing. The presupposition underlying such questions is that there is one thing and one only which intelligence *is*, and that the task of psychologists is to discover it. Any sentence starting " intelligence is . . . " justifiably arouses one's suspicions.

The assumption behind the mistake seems to be that every word has one settled and precise meaning, or, more strictly, that classifications of things in nature are somehow done *for* us. The truth is surely that *we* must classify as suits our purposes. For many purposes it is helpful to classify behaviour into 'intelligent' and 'unintelligent,' but it does not follow that there is to be found in the universe one permanently existing 'thing' which intelligence *is*.

It is important in this connection to pay attention to inverted commas. One function of inverted commas—there are others—is to indicate that a word is being mentioned as opposed to used. Thus, when I say "This table is brown," I am *using* the word 'table' not mentioning it, and no inverted commas are needed. On the other hand, if I say "'Table' is the English equivalent of the Latin 'mensa ','" I am *mentioning* the words 'table' and 'mensa' and both require inverted commas. In exactly the same way, if we are *using* the word 'intelligence,' as in "Intelligence increases up to age 15," there are no inverted commas ; but if we say, "I recommend that the word 'intelligence' be defined in a particular way," we are mentioning the word 'intelligence,' not using it, and the inverted commas are indispensable.

When Piaget (1950, p. 7), says, "Intelligence is thus only a generic term to indicate the superior forms of organisation or equilibrium of cognitive structurings," it seems fair to point out that the word 'intelligence' is being *mentioned* here, not *used*, and that inverted commas round the word 'intelligence' would make his formidable statement, if not crystal-clear, at least easier. In general, it may be said that the surest way of avoiding muddle about 'real essences' is to pay strict attention to inverted commas.

(ii) *Lexical definitions and the appeal to ordinary usage.* I propose to argue in this section that, as far as lexical definitions of intelligence are concerned, there need be no serious disputes among psychologists. It is implicit in the notion of a lexical definition that its merits should be decidable by an appeal to ordinary usage. This appeal presents certain problems which require discussion ; but even if two psychologists did in fact disagree on what constituted ordinary usage, no important theoretical consequences would follow.

I shall begin by considering certain points about the way in which the word 'intelligence' normally functions, and I shall then attempt to remove some of the confusions and difficulties that are liable to arise in connection with discussions about the lexical definition of intelligence.

(*a*) The word 'intelligence' is the noun of the adjective 'intelligent.'

---

* For the arguments which he gives in support of this view, see pp. 153-6. The relevant passage in Aristotle is *Metaphysics*, Z, 4-6.

† The word 'essence' does occur, however, in the earlier literature on the subject of intelligence. Thus, Spearman (1927, p. 15) quotes an earlier writer, Bobertag, as saying, "The knowledge of the essence of intelligence is *naturally* a thing that merits profound research " (my italics).

On Defining Intelligence

This point seems obvious, but is none-the-less informative. If we are not careful, we are liable to suppose that all nouns refer to 'things,' whereas it is by no means obvious that the word 'intelligence' can correctly be said to refer to a 'thing.' By using the adjective 'intelligent' any temptation towards misleading hypostatisation (i.e., treating words as 'thing'-words when they are not) can be avoided. Instead of the unsatisfactory "What is intelligence?" we can now ask "What is the meaning of the word 'intelligent'?" or, perhaps better, "How does one test if a person is intelligent? i.e., what constitute samples of intelligent behaviour?"

(*b*) The word 'intelligent' may be labelled a *disposition-word*.* Here are further examples of disposition-words—'Lazy,' 'bad-tempered,' 'cheerful,' 'kind-hearted,' 'punctual.' In all these cases there is no necessary suggestion of a person's actually doing something here and now. "X is very kind-hearted" may be true even though at this moment X happens to be asleep. The suggestion is rather that a person to whom any of these adjectives applies is *disposed* to act in certain ways, i.e., that if certain conditions are fulfilled, certain behaviour will follow. Thus "X is lazy" is approximately equivalent to "If X is given any hard tasks he usually tries to shirk them." In general, sentences containing disposition-words can be replaced by sentences containing the words "if . . . then." Similarly, "X is intelligent" can be taken as equivalent to "If X is placed in particular circumstances he produces responses of a particular kind"—e.g., if he is present at a group discussion he makes appropriate remarks, if presented with a difficult crossword puzzle he can usually solve it, and so on.

I want now to introduce three further technical terms in addition to 'disposition-word.' The word ascribing the disposition, such as 'lazy' or 'punctual,' I shall refer to as the *substrate*; the actual or possible manifestations of the disposition I shall refer to as the *exemplaries*. Thus the exemplaries of "X is kind-hearted" are the particular occasions when he is kind to people, the exemplaries of "X is lazy" are the particular occasions when he shirks tasks, and so on. Thirdly, I shall make use of the term *polymorphous*.† The concepts 'grocer' and 'solicitor' are, we might say, polymorphous as compared with the concept 'baker.' A baker, *qua* baker, does one thing only—he bakes. A grocer does all sorts of different things—he weighs out sugar, he sells butter, he cuts bacon, and so on. A solicitor draws up wills, advises clients, etc., etc. There is no one way to manifest being a grocer or a solicitor. Similarly, 'lazy' and 'bad-tempered' are polymorphous concepts as compared with 'punctual.' The exemplaries of being punctual are an unvaried series of arrivals on time, the exemplaries of being lazy or bad-tempered cover a wide range of different sorts of behaviour.

(*c*) Using this terminology we may say that 'intelligent' is a polymorphous concept. In other words there are many different exemplaries which the substrate 'intelligent' carries; intelligence may manifest itself altogether differently on different occasions.

(*d*) Finally, it should be stressed that the list of exemplaries carried by the word 'intelligent' is *open*. In other words, no one has ever made any precise legislation as to what shall or shall not count as exemplaries of the word 'intelligent'; nor is there any precise list laid up in heaven for the discerning to discover. Just now I mentioned two examples—making appropriate remarks in a discussion and being able to solve difficult crossword puzzles. But clearly these are only two exemplaries among many. By making stipulative definitions

* Compare Ryle (1949), Chapter 5.
  † This term, and the following examples, are due to Ryle. There is no reference to Freud's use of the word.

T. R. MILES

we can formulate a precise list of exemplaries if we wish, but 'intelligence,' as it functions in ordinary speech, carries no such list.

Now the fact that the list of exemplaries carried by the word ' intelligent ' is ' open ' may give rise to disputes in the less straightforward type of case. Sometimes, of course, disputes may be genuinely factual. Thus, if it is known that X has an extraordinary facility for rapid calculation in his head, someone may still say, " But he may not be intelligent," the suggestion being that other exemplaries carried by the word ' intelligent,' will not be satisfied. In other cases the dispute is in a sense a verbal one—a matter for linguistic decision. Spearman (1927, p. 10) quotes an amusing example in this connection : " Trabue . . . told of a woman who, although making a bad record with the tests, nevertheless became ' the housekeeper at one of the finest Fifth Avenue hotels, where she successfully directed the work of a corps of approximately fifty maids, three carpenters, two decorators, and a plumber.' He was moved to conclude as follows : ' In spite of the evidence of the tests I insist that she is intelligent '." Perhaps there is *some* factual dispute here as to how the woman would behave in different circumstances, but Trabue's words suggest that the point at issue is not how the woman is likely to behave in different circumstances, but whether ability to supervise fifty maids, etc., constitute exemplaries of the word ' intelligent.' To this question there is no uncontroversial answer, not because we are incompetent psychologists, but because the inexactness of ordinary language makes a conclusive answer impossible.*

Even, however, if a psychologist is accused in his definition of intelligence of doing extreme violence to ordinary usage, no important principle is at stake. All that he need do is to leave the word ' intelligence ' imprecise and invent a special technical term of his own. Thus, if we are sure in advance that it is informative to test a person's memory span for digits, and if, as a result, we include such an item in what we call an ' intelligence-test,' we will not be seriously worried if someone says, " But this is a test of memory, not intelligence." All that is required is to invent a new technical term and to say that *that* is what we are measuring. The important point is not whether what we measure can appropriately be labelled ' intelligence,' but whether we have discovered something worth measuring. And this is not a matter that can be settled by an appeal to what is or is not the correct use of the word ' intelligent.'

One final point should be made in connection with lexical definitions. When it is said that psychologists do not agree on the definitions of intelligence, the position may seem all the more absurd if we unwittingly assume that they disagree about its lexical definition. Psychologists in that case are guilty of using a word without explaining its meaning and perhaps without being able to do so. It is as though someone attempted to give a talk on armadillos when neither he not his audience knew what the word ' armadillo ' meant. Clearly, explanation of any new or unfamiliar word is obligatory as soon as that word is introduced.† In the case of the word ' intelligence,' however, no one, surely, wants a definition in *this* sense. In the standard sense of ' know the meaning of,' the great majority of English-speaking adults, including psychologists, know the meaning of the word ' intelligence ' already. To put the matter somewhat more precisely, they can recognise particular pieces of behaviour as constituting

* Spearman seems to me to have shown himself extremely sensitive to this sort of problem. Compare his well-known dictum that ' intelligence ' is " a word with so many meanings that finally it has none " (1927, p. 14).

† Compare Robinson (1950, p. 41). As Robinson in effect points out, the question whether definitions should come at the beginning or at the end of an enquiry cannot be answered unless we are told the sense in which the word ' definition ' is being used.

On Defining Intelligence

exemplaries of the word 'intelligent.' No one thinks that, if the word 'intelligence' figured in the Terman-Merrill vocabulary test, most professional psychologists would fail to secure a pass. Psychologists may disagree as to what general formula, if any, will lead to significant advances in our understanding of intelligent behaviour ; but, as far as lexical definitions are concerned, there is very little that they *could* disagree about, and certainly nothing of major importance.

(iii) *Stipulative definition* ; (iv) *Description plus naming* ; and (v) *The search for a key*. These three processes will be considered under the same heading since there is considerable overlap between them.

To frame a stipulative definition involves either coining a new word or announcing that one intends to use an existing word in a special way. Stipulative definitions of intelligence clearly involve the latter. In all uses the *purpose* of the stipulation needs to be considered. The need, in this case, is for concepts which help our understanding of intelligent behaviour.

'Description plus naming' is a helpful activity in psychology, provided what is named is something worth investigating. Similarly, to 'search for a key' is helpful, provided that the key, when we find it, really does unlock the requisite doors. Both these activities (which can legitimately be regarded as varieties of stipulative definition) involve, in effect, the commendation of a policy. Using our earlier terminology, we may say that to make a stipulative definition is to formulate a substrate—a substrate whose exemplaries are thereby assumed to be worh investigating. Differences of opinion on policy are *serious* differences, and give rise to heated controversy. In the study of intelligence, as in any other study of personality, the crucial question is the choice of substrates. Thus, the substrates 'extraversion-introversion' are helpful if there is a suggestive association between people's scores on extraversion-introversion tests and their other independently observed behaviour. In the same way those who study intellectual differences need to produce substrates that are *worth-while*. Disagreements over *stipulative* definitions of intelligence are far more fundamental and serious than disagreements over lexical definition.

It does not, of course, follow, because the substrate 'intelligent' is helpful for workaday purposes, that it necessarily holds the key to any great scientific advance. It may do so ; but we have no right to assume it.*

(vi) *Operational definitions.* Those who insist on the importance of operational definitions for scientific method are in effect pointing out that a substrate has meaning only in relation to its exemplaries. The relation between exemplaries and substrate is not that of effects to an unknown cause, but of a series of occurrences to a general law under which they can be subsumed. It is pointless to assume the existence of an unknown entity lying behind or beyond the exemplaries.†

Applied to the notion of 'intelligence,' this is, in effect, to say that the word 'intelligence' does not refer to a 'real thing' lying behind or beyond the manifestations of intelligence. Instead of " *What is* intelligence ? " or even " What does the word 'intelligence' *really mean* ? " we need to ask instead, " How do you test—or what operations are involved in testing—whether a person is intelligent ? "

---

* Compare Heim (1954, p. 46) : " A majority of the factorists appear agreed that a clear-cut key to these problems exists and is in their hands."

† Compare Berkeley's attack on the notion of *material substance*, passim.

T. R. Miles

This question can readily be answered. Psychologists have devised *standardised* tests. It is the items in these tests (or, more strictly, the person's behaviour in producing correct responses to these items) that are regarded as constituting the exemplaries of the word ' intelligent.' Intelligence, in other words, *is what intelligence tests measure.* This definition is a stipulative one. What is being said is, in effect, that correct responses to the test items *shall be deemed to constitute* exemplaries of the word ' intelligent.' To give a tidy list of exemplaries all that is needed is to specify what particular test we have in mind.

" Intelligence is what intelligence tests measure " does not, of course, tell us what test items are *good* ones, but this is not a ground for criticism since it does not set out to do this. Whether a list of exemplaries should be as tidy as this stipulation makes them is perhaps questionable. Some would say that a substrate should only *suggest* exemplaries, not specify them to the last detail, and that details of exemplaries can be worked out and modified in the course of future research. Despite this, however, the ' operational ' approach to the study of intelligence seems to me fundamentally sound, and a great improvement on the traditional search for " what intelligence really is."

IV.—Wechsler's definition.

In this section I shall examine Wechsler's introductory remarks on the subject of intelligence.* I shall argue that, whatever the merits of his policy, his formulation of that policy is unnecessarily puzzling and difficult simply through failure to distinguish the ambiguities of the word ' definition.'

Wechsler begins by discussing the dictum that intelligence is " what intelligence tests measure." He refers disparagingly to it as " this circular position " (p. 3), without, apparently, having noticed, that, if in the definiens we substitute the names of *particular* intelligence tests—the Terman-Merrill or his own, for instance, any trace of circularity disappears.†

He reinforces his argument by saying that the lay person " is entirely justified in asking, ' Do your tests really test intelligence ? ' " (p. 3). This seems to me to be putting the cart before the horse. If we agree to define the word ' intelligence' as " what intelligence tests measure," then admittedly " Do your tests really test intelligence ? " becomes pointless. But it is very perverse, surely, to argue, on the grounds that " Do your tests really test ingelligence ? " is *not* pointless, that " intelligence is what intelligence tests measure " *must therefore* be unhelpful. Why anyone should even have *wanted* to say that intelligence is what intelligence tests measure is a question that Wechsler does not seem to have seriously considered.

The purpose of this dictum, as we have seen, is to warn us against asking meaningless questions about the ' real nature ' of intelligence. Having ignored the warning notice, Wechsler not surprisingly falls head-foremost into the abyss of muddle against which he was warned. " General intelligence," he says (p. 4), " like electricity, may be regarded as a kind of energy. We do not know what the *ultimate nature* of this energy is, but as in the case of electricity, *we know*

---

* Wechsler (1944, pp. 3-4).

† A further difficulty is that Wechsler does not seem to have considered for what reasons and in what circumstances a definition should not be circular. If a child asks the meaning of the word ' armadillo ' and is told " It's a—well, it's an armadillo," we would rightly condemn such procedure as uninformative. But if we are told that the symbols bc can be substituted for the symbol a, that xyz can be substituted for bc, and that a can be substituted for xyz, this is not necessarily a futile procedure. Not only may it teach us the rules for the interchange of certain words, but, in addition, provided we can relate one of the three groups to the actual word, we will then be able to relate the other two groups to the actual world also. Circularity of this sort is not necessarily a vice.

On Defining Intelligence

it by the things it does " (my italics). Just what use it is to postulate such energy is unexplained, and its existence or non-existence would make no difference whatever to the value of Wechsler's tests. The concepts ' intelligence' and ' electricity ' are similar (in so far as they are similar at all) not because both refer to some unknown ' energy ' but because both require to be understood in terms of their exemplaries.

Finally, what are we to make of Wechsler's own definition ? Intelligence, he tells us, is " the aggregate or global capacity of the individual to act purposefully, to think rationally, and to deal effectively with his environment," (p. 3). In what sense is this a definition ? Is he explaining the meaning of the word ' intelligence ' to someone who does not know it ? Is he explaining how he himself proposes to use the word in future ? Or is he offering a ' real ' definition in one or more of Robinson's twelve different senses, and, if so, in which sense ?

Despite the absence of any explicit answer to these questions, some of Wechsler's intentions can be understood from the context. Clearly he is not content merely to offer his own stipulative definition. This can be inferred from the fact that he is concerned to answer the plain man's question, " Do your tests really test intelligence ? " He must therefore be concerned, at any rate among other things, with the plain man's use of the word. If this is all, however, nothing very exciting follows *whatever* answer he gives. " Do your tests really test intelligence ? " if re-phrased with more precision appears to mean, " Do those who score highly on your tests correspond with those whom we should call ' intelligent ' in normal speech ? " But if this is how the plain man's question should be understood (and it is hard to see what other interpretation is possible) nothing very helpful is being asked. In the first place the list of exemplaries carried by the word ' intelligent ' in ordinary speech is ' open '—in other words there are many different grounds for saying of a person that he is intelligent. Only if there were a clearly specified list of exemplaries would it be possible to tell whether these exemplaries tended to be satisfied significantly more often among high test-scorers than among low test-scorers. As ordinary speech gives *no* clearly specified list of exemplaries, the question " Do your tests really test intelligence ? " allows at best for only an approximate answer. This, of course, is not due to any human failing nor to the presence of any overwhelming mystery, but arises simply as a result of the imprecision of ordinary speech—an imprecision that for everyday purposes is altogether useful. Secondly, even if it were agreed that those who scored highly on the tests were *not* those who could appropriately be labelled ' intelligent,' still nothing of importance would follow. It might be misleading to label the tests ' intelligence 'tests, but they could quite well be given another name.

It follows, if the above argument is right, that Wechsler cannot be (or perhaps should not be) interpreted as attempting a simple lexical definition of intelligence—an account of how the plain man uses the word. Indeed, I think he would be somewhat surprised if someone hearing his definition for the first time replied, " Yes, I agree ; that is just what the plain man *does* mean," or " No, you are wrong ; people have used the word differently." What Wechsler says should be regarded rather as a key for understanding something. It is as though he said, " An important key for understanding people can be obtained by determining if they have an aggregate or global capacity to think purposefully . . . etc." The conclusion to be drawn is that tests which sample such capacity are to be commended. What Wechsler's definition does in effect is to commend a policy.

Now it is at this point that the crucial decisions really begin. The psychologist has to decide—partly by appeal to evidence, partly by personal

T. R. Miles

' hunch '—whether such a policy is worth following, whether in effect the Wechsler tests (which claim to sample such ability) are good and helpful ones, whether measuring the correlations of test-scores with other personality traits will lead to further important discoveries, and so on. Decisions of this sort, however, are beyond the scope of this paper. All that I have attempted to do is to clear the ground, to leave a straight issue to be decided on its merits. Appeals to the plain man's use of the word ' intelligent ' are liable to confuse the issue, and talk of underlying ' energy ' is liable to confuse it still further. If Wechsler's definition of ' intelligence ' is thought to agree with ordinary usage, it does not follow that his policy is right ; and if it is thought *not* to agree with ordinary usage, it does not follow that his policy is wrong. I have made no attempt to criticise the way in which Wechsler *operates* his policy, but he is not alone among psychologists in being better able to operate a policy than to talk about his operations.

V.—Burt's definition.

Unlike Wechsler, Burt (1955) shows himself extremely sensitive to the sort of problem which I have been discussing in this paper. That being so, my discussion in this section will be mainly a commentary on his article rather than a criticism of it. Even in Burt's case, however, there are certain confusions in his use of the word ' definition ' which seem to me to require to be exposed. Once again, needless to say, I shall not take sides on the more fundamental question of whether the definition is a good one.

Burt's formula is " innate general cognitive ability." What we need to examine, therefore, is the sort of argument which should be taken as relevant if this formula is to be justified.

Let us start by considering his comments on the famous 1921 Symposium. " The editor of an American journal," he writes, " submitted two searching questions about the nature of intelligence to a dozen different psychologists, and received a dozen different replies. But the varying descriptions suggested were not, as Dr. Heim and others have supposed, intended to be ' definitions ' *in the strict logical sense* " (my italics) : " they were, in the language of J. S. Mill, merely ' attempts to explain the thing ' not ' attempts to interpret the word,'." (p. 159). Unfortunately, nowhere in this article does Burt say what he means by " *the* strict logical sense " ; and this, in view of Robinson's distinction between the many different senses of the word ' definition ' is surely a defect. (What, any way, is meant by a ' logical ' sense of the word ' definition ' ? Surely the contrast cannot be with some *illogical* sense ?).

There is an even more puzzling footnote. Burt writes, " In framing his question, the editor specifically asked not how is intelligence to be defined but ' what do you conceive intelligence to be . . . ? ' etc." According to Burt, then, " How is intelligence to be defined ? " and " What do you conceive intelligence to be ? " are to be understood as different questions. This seems to me very unsatisfactory—not, indeed, because I think the questions should be regarded as identical, but because both are so thoroughly ambiguous that there is just no means of knowing if they overlap or not. Robinson's comments* seem appropriate here. " The confusedness of the concept of real definition is an effect of the vagueness of the formula ' What is x ?' For it is the vaguest of all forms of question except an inarticulate grunt. Real definition flourishes because the question-form ' What is x? ' flourishes ; and this question-form flourishes precisely because it is vague. It saves us the trouble of thinking out and saying exactly what we want to know about x . . . We can use this question-

* *Loc. cit.*, p. 190.

On Defining Intelligence

form to express a general desire to be given any useful information about x of any sort." The conclusion to be drawn, as Burt would no doubt agree, is that the editor of the 1921 Symposium asked an ambiguous question ; and it is therefore scarcely surprising that he received a wide range of different answers. Burt's unexplained distinction, however, between " What do you conceive intelligence to be ? " and " How is intelligence to be defined ? " seems to me to confuse his main argument rather than add to its effectiveness.

Burt himself claims to be asking two questions : " . . . (i) how precisely should the term (intelligence) be defined, and (ii) what evidence is there for believing that something really exists corresponding to the definition proposed ? "

In what sense of ' definition,' then, is the formula " innate general cognitive ability " intended to be a definition ? How much can we infer from his general argument about what is required of a " definition in the strict logical sense " ?

" How *the term* should be defined." This remark suggests that Burt is concerned on the face of it with words rather than things. This does not, of course, mean that he is concerned *merely* to say that in sentences where the word ' intelligence ' occurs the words " innate general cognitive ability " can be substituted (or should be allowed to be substituted). He assumes that we are already familiar with the words ' innate,' ' general,' ' cognitive,' and ' ability,' and can apply them correctly. His point is that we *need a word* to refer to the ability in question.

" The definition proposed." This suggests a proposal, a stipulation. It is clear, however, that Burt is not offering simply a stipulative definition out of the blue. He backs his proposal by what may be called " the appeal to Cicero." The argument on *p.* 160 of his paper seems to be" Cicero used the Latin word ' intelligentia ' as a technical term. My stipulation involves no radical departure from Cicero's usage. It is not; therefore, a misleading Humpty-Dumpytism, like using ' glory ' to mean ' a nice knock-down argument ' ;* but my definition is in part lexical as well as stipulative."

To assess the merits of a lexical definition we examine its historical accuracy. To assess the merits of a stipulative definition we ask, Is such a stipulation useful ? In the case of Burt's definition we are therefore required to do both.

Although it is outside the scope of this paper to carry out such a programme in detail, one comment may perhaps be made on the lexical side. Burt says on p. 160 that ' intelligence ' is not a " word of popular speech." But this surely does not follow, as Burt seems to suggest, from the fact that Cicero used the Latin word ' intelligentia ' as a technical term. There can be no reasonable doubt that many Englishmen use the word ' intelligence ' without having the least idea how Cicero used it ; some, indeed, may not have heard of Cicero at all. If the argument is to do what Burt wants it to do, he should surely indicate that his definition conforms not with Cicero's usage, but with the usage of a twentieth century English-speaking person. And it is surely precisely because the word ' intelligence ' *is* a word of popular speech (and, therefore, ' open,' imprecise, ambiguous) that an accurate account of its use in popular speech cannot be given. It cannot be given not because none of us is clever enough to find the right formula, but because there is no formula to be found.†

* See *Through the Looking Glass*, Chapter VI : " ' When I use a word,' Humpty Dumpty said in rather a scornful tone, ' it means just what I choose it to mean—neither more nor less '."

† A further criticism of the historical section of Burt's paper should be made in passing, namely his interpretation of the Greek words θυμός and θυμοειδές. Burt suggests that these words have something in common with the English word ' moral ' ; but the interpretation ' moral ' seems to me, not a " rough but inexact equivalent," as Burt says, but a definite blunder.

T. R. MILES

In any case, as has been indicated already, the whole question of whether a definition of intelligence conforms to ordinary usage is unimportant. Ordinary usage may be vaguely suggestive of possible test-items, but there is nothing more to it than that. A person who is dissatisfied with a definition of intelligence on these grounds can always invent a new technical term in its place. Burt, of course, would agree with this. As he makes clear later in his paper, he would be quite prepared to allow that in place of " innate general cognitive ability " some other label could be substituted.

The crucial problem, then, has nothing to do with conformity to ordinary usage. It is rather whether the policy commended by Burt is a helpful one to follow for future research. In a sense, what Burt is offering is a stipulative definition—a proposal how the word ' intelligence ' should be used. But he is doing more than this. He is, I think, offering a definition of intelligence in the two other senses which we mentioned earlier. He is offering (a) description plus naming, and (b) a key for understanding a wide range of subject matter. As regards (a), Robinson puts the matter in general form by saying " The character yz occurs, and I call this character (or it is commonly called) by the name x." Applied to this case, the formula becomes " Innate general cognitive ability occurs, and I give it the name ' intelligence '." As for (b), the key, according to Burt, is that we should *look for* an innate general cognitive ability. Later in his paper he is even more specific ; he has in mind a characteristic transmitted by the genes. The psychologist who studies intelligence must, in other words, become a geneticist ; and, if we direct our research in this direction, then according to Burt, we are likely to produce worthwhile results. Such claims, it should be added, are seldom decisively confirmed or refuted. Either they turn out to be fruitful and win general acceptance, or they gradually fall into oblivion.

Thus, (i) it would be no argument against Burt's policy to accuse him of " measuring something called ' intelligence ' without knowing what that something is or how it is defined " (Richmond, quoted by Burt, *loc. cit.*, p. 158). Burt makes quite explicit both what his policy is and what he is trying to measure. (ii) It is no argument against Burt that a person who does not know what ' intelligence ' means would be even less likely to know the meaning of " innate general cognitive ability," for he is not attempting to explain the meaning of the word to someone who does not know it already. (iii) For the same reason, it serves little purpose to discuss whether or not his definition conforms to ordinary usage—whether, for instance, in ordinary usage the word ' intelligence ' is taken as referring to something innate.

On the other hand it *would* be an argument against Burt's definition if all discoverable tests consistently failed to produce appropriate distributions—i.e., distributions that would be expected on the assumption that what is being measured is something transmitted by the genes. Thus, if identical twins reared apart regularly produced widely different scores, if changes in environment were regularly followed by large-scale differences in score, the notion of an *innate* ability would become progressively more uncomfortable. Again, if reduction of emotional tension (e.g., by psycho-analysis or some other method) regularly resulted in improved performance, the whole distinction between the ' cognitive ' and the ' affective ' sides of human nature might seem to be an unhelpful one, and the idea of a specifically ' cognitive ' ability just no use.* Burt's definition

* This statement requires qualification. Correlation coefficients can be worked out between as many different abilities (or ' substrates ') as we please ; but no figures, whether high or low, can lead us to abandon a substrate which we are sure is helpful or accept one which we are sure is unhelpful. To work out correlation coefficients is to *operate* our hypothesis, not to *test* that hypothesis. Whether we are ' getting anywhere ' with our hypothesis has to be settled rather by the general ' feel ' of the research undertaken.

On Defining Intelligence

would then be useless in much the same way as it would be useless having a word—say ' hexothippus '—meaning " a horse with six ears." It is not that ' hexothippus ' does *not* mean " horse with six ears " if we choose to make it mean that ; it is simply that we do not need the word. We do not need it for the obvious reason that horses do not have six ears. Thus it is crucial for Burt's argument, as he himself realises, to establish that " something really exists corresponding to the definition proposed " (p. 159).

This brings us to a problem that is central in any theoretical study of intelligence—the problem of how to establish assertions of the form " There really exists an x " when ' x' is not a straightforward concrete noun. Whatever the practical difficulties, we all know how to set about establishing the existence or non-existence of giraffes, dodos, fairies, etc. ; but whether a particular sort of *ability* exists is clearly a very different question from whether a particular sort of giraffe exists ; and it is this that constitutes the central problem. Part of the proof of the ' real existence ' of intelligence in Burt's sense depends on factorial analysis ; and the question which this technique forces upon us is, What conditions must be satisfied if factorial analysis is to justify statements of the form " There really exists an ability (or a factor) so and so " ? This question can, I think, be satisfactorily answered as follows. It is not a sufficient condition for asserting the real existence of a factor that correlation coefficients between tests should form this or that pattern. A factor has a ' real existence ' only when it becomes identified—that is, when the results which produced the particular pattern of correlation coefficients can be linked with independently discoverable events. Spearman (1927) has a chapter entitled " Proof that g and s exist "—his ' proof ' being to show that, under suitable conditions, the surprising result of vanishing tetrads can be obtained. This is a misleading use of the word ' exist '. According to the usage which I would commend, " vanishing tetrads occur " is *not* a sufficient condition for asserting " g and s exist " ; some independent attempt to identify g is also required. In this respect Spearman's suggested identification of g with ' mental energy ' seems scientifically useless, since it suggests no independently discoverable events beyond those which in fact *did* produce the vanishing tetrads. In contrast, the factors of both Burt and Thomson (1950) have at least a chance of having a ' real existence,' for there is a suggested link between the test-behaviour which produced particular correlation coefficients and the independently discoverable behaviour of genes or neurones. There is a further possible justification for speaking of the ' reality ' of factors. A factor is real, it might be said, if from behaviour at one test successful prediction is regularly made about behaviour at another test allegedly saturated with the same factor. This, however, opens the door to the postulation of a host of useless factors. We can be most sure of progress when links are found, not between one test and another, but between a person's test behaviour and the behaviour of genes and neurones. Genes and neurones, be it noted, are parts of the *body* ; and, to put the matter epigrammatically, we could perhaps say that factors have a real existence, not when they are " factors of the mind " (whatever that means), but when they are *factors of the body*. Burt's definition involves the hope that the postulation of such genes will lead to a wide range of important findings. If this hope is fulfilled, his definition will have justified itself ; otherwise not.

VI.—References.

BRIDGMAN, P. W. (1927). *The Logic of Modern Physics*. Macmillan.
BURT, C. L. (1947). *Mental and Scholastic Tests*. Staples.

T. R. MILES

BURT, C. L. (1955). The evidence for the concept of intelligence. *Brit. J. Educ. Psychol.*, 25, 158-177.

HEIM, A. (1954). *The Appraisal of Intelligence*. Methuen.

PIAGET, J. (1950). *The Psychology of Intelligence*. Routledge and Kegan Paul.

ROBINSON, R. (1950). *Definition*. Oxford University Press.

RYLE, G. (1949). *The Concept of Mind*. Hutchinson.

SPEARMAN, C. (1927). *The Abilities of Man*. Macmillan.

THOMSON, G. H. (1950). *Factorial Analysis of Human Ability*. University of London Press.

WECHSLER, D. (1944). *The Measurement of Adult Intelligence*. Baltimore: Williams and Wilkins.

(Manuscript received 2nd July, 1956.)

PART II

MEASUREMENT AND THE PROBLEM OF UNITS

Scaling, Zero Point and Distribution of the IQ

This section is concerned with certain important psychometric properties of the IQ. A scale of measurement should have a proper zero point; does intelligence have such a zero point? The answer was given by Thurstone in his famous 1928 paper, here reprinted; it depends on his method of "absolute scaling" which he developed in his 1925 paper, and which for space reasons is not here reproduced. An attempt will instead be made to explain this method briefly in this introduction. Another important question regarding any quantity is its distribution. Most textbooks state that intelligence is normally distributed, i.e. in terms of the Gaussian curve; does this statement have any meaning (i.e. is it anything more than a consequence of the mode of construction of the tests most widely used) and, more important, is it true? Burt suggests that the statement is meaningful, but untrue, except to a very rough approximation; this estimation is probably correct, as is his further suggestion that the proper curve to apply is a Pearson Type IV curve. This may seem a rather unimportant departure from normality (the two curves are not very dissimilar), but as he points out, at the extremes there are marked differences, and from the social point of view these may be very important indeed.

As regards "absolute scaling," consider Figure 1, which is taken from Thurstone's paper (1925). It represents two normal distributions for two groups of children of adjacent age levels. M_1 and M_2 denote their average scores, and σ_1 and σ_2 denote their S.D.'s (assumed to be unequal). The base line represents achievement, or relative difficulty of test questions, while the ordinates represent relative frequencies of children at each degree of achievement. "Let the small circle represent any particular test question. The shaded area in the B surface represents the proportion of the older age group who can answer the question correctly. The remaining unshaded part of the distribution represents the proportion who fail on that question. The same reasoning applies to the A distribution. There is a larger proportion of the older children who can answer the question, and that is reasonable because B represents children older than A. If we know the percentage of children of different ages who can answer each question, it is possible to locate the questions on an absolute scale, and it is also possible to locate the means of the successive age groups on the same absolute scale, and to determine the standard deviations of the successive ages on the same scale. The present method assumes that the distribution of abilities is normal, but it does not assume that the standard deviations of the successive age or grade groups are the same." Algebraically, let X indicate the position of a certain test item on the scale (i.e. the small circle in Figure 1); X_1 denotes the deviation from M_1, and X_2 denotes the deviation of the same test item from M_2. These values are derived from P_1 and P_2, the proportions of the individuals in groups A and B who pass this item, represented by the shaded areas under the two curves. Now clearly $M_1 + X_1\sigma_1 = M_2 + X_2\sigma_2$; dividing through by σ_2 and solving for X_2, we get

$$X_1 = X_1\left(\frac{\sigma_1}{\sigma_2}\right) + \left(\frac{M_1 - M_2}{\sigma_2}\right)$$

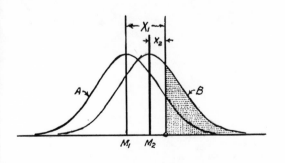

Fig. 1

which is the equation of a straight line with a slope of σ_1/σ_2 and an X_2 intercept of $(M_1—M_2)/\sigma_2$. Granted that we know the values involved, all of which are readily available, we can translate the scale values of an item from one distribution into the terms of another. Figure 2, also taken from Thurstone (1925) shows a plot of paired X_1 and X_2 values taken from the two adjacent groups "and it is immediately apparent that the relation is linear."

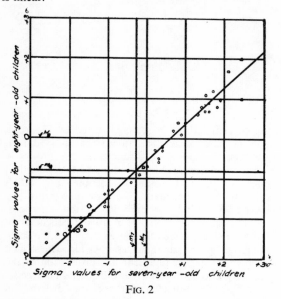

FIG. 2

This method of scaling has many important advantages. As will be seen in the Thurstone paper reprinted in this section, it enables us to discover a proper zero point for intelligence. It also enables us to obtain a better notion of the growth curve for intelligence (Thurstone, L. L. and Ackerson, L., 1929). Last but not least, it makes it possible to obtain scale values for each test question. These are valuable gains if our aim is to make the measurement of intelligence more quantitative, and hence more scientific. It is curious that in spite of their great value these methods have not been as widely used as one might have expected; test construction is still not geared to a routine inclusion of Thurstone's methods.

REFERENCES

THURSTONE, L. L. A method of scaling psychological and educational tests. *J. Educ. Psychol.*, 1925, *16*, 433–451.

THURSTONE L. L. & ACKERMAN, L. The mental curve for the Binet tests. *J. Educ. Psychol.*, 1929, *20*, 569–583.

From L. L. Thurstone, Psychological Review, *35, 175–197.*
Copyright (1928), by kind permission of the American Psychological Association

THE PSYCHOLOGICAL REVIEW

THE ABSOLUTE ZERO IN INTELLIGENCE MEASUREMENT

BY L. L. THURSTONE
The University of Chicago

The object of this paper is to describe a discovery concerning the variability of intelligence by which it is possible to locate its absolute zero. The discovery will be described with four implications, namely, (1) two laws of variability of intelligence, (2) determination of the absolute zero of test intelligence, (3) the construction of a true mental growth curve which has not hitherto been possible, and (4) determination of the age at which test intelligence begins.

The discovery was made by studying a variety of data by means of absolute scaling.[1] The details of this method have been previously described[2] so that it will suffice here to review merely the underlying idea in absolute scale construction. We are here primarily concerned with several of its applications.

The provocation for the absolute scaling method lies in the two most fundamental limitations of intelligence measurement, namely, (1) that we have had no satisfactory unit of measurement for it, and (2) that we have had no origin of measurement except the arbitrary zero score of each

---

[1] The writer wishes to acknowledge the statistical assistance of Miss Annette McBroom who has carried out most of the calculations for this study.

[2] THURSTONE, L. L., 'A Method of Scaling Psychological and Educational Tests,' *J. Educ. Psychol.*, 1925, 16, pp. 433–451. Cyril Burt's data on the Binet tests were used to illustrate the method. An application to educational scale construction is shown in 'The Unit of Measurement in Educational Scales' by L. L. THURSTONE, *J. Educ. Psychol.*, Nov., 1927. A refinement in statistical procedure for the method is described in 'Scale Construction with Weighted Observations' by L. L. THURSTONE, also to be published in the same journal.

educational and psychological test. The whole study of intelligence measurement can hardly have two more fundamental difficulties than the lack of a unit of measurement and the lack of an origin from which to measure!

If an intelligence test such as the National is given to a large sample of eight-year-old children, we find of course that some of them attain scores much higher than others. In so far as the test is regarded as an adequate index of the function to be measured, we are justified in arranging the children in *rank order* for the trait in question. But measurement implies more. We have no direct means of knowing that the difference in ability represented by the raw scores of 10 and 20, for example, is the same as that between the raw scores of 90 and 100. If the frequency distribution of raw scores is normal *and if we assume that the 'actual' distribution of the trait in question is also normal*, then the difference 20–10 in raw score represents the same increment of ability as the difference 100–90. But, strictly speaking, there is no 'actual' distribution to which we can refer for a final verdict. All that we can ask is that the unit be consistent with a constant meaning throughout the scale. The increments provided by the raw scores do not necessarily satisfy this criterion, because they represent different tasks of different degrees of difficulty.

Another way of stating the insecurity of the raw score unit is that if we were to select a group of children so as to have intentionally a skewed distribution of intelligence, by general impression or otherwise, we could readily select the elements for a test in such a way that the final distribution of scores for this group of children would be normal. Hence the normality of the distribution of raw scores simply proves that the test has been so constructed that the distribution will be normal! It proves nothing regarding the shape of the 'true' distribution, which is in any case indeterminate.

ABSOLUTE SCALE CONSTRUCTION

Absolute scale construction consists first of a statistical criterion to determine whether two adjacent age groups can be represented as normal distributions on the same base line. If this criterion is not satisfied, it is impossible to construct a scale so that the overlapping distributions will both be normal on the same scale. Any function of the raw scores that gives a normal distribution for one of these two groups will then necessarily give a skewed distribution for the other. If the criterion is satisfied, then it is possible to find such a function of the raw score that both of the overlapping distributions become normal. This is the manner in which the absolute scale is defined, although the same logic may be applied to try frequency distributions of any form. In absolute scale construction the only necessary assumption is that the distributions of ability in the successive age or grade groups have *the same form*. It is not necessarily assumed that they are normal.

The result of absolute scaling, applicable only when the data satisfy the criterion, is a series of overlapping normal curves on the same base line. These curves represent the distributions of ability in the overlapping age or grade groups. Two constants are determined for each curve, namely, its mean and its standard deviation. The mean ability of one of the groups is arbitrarily chosen as an assumed origin, and its standard deviation on the absolute scale is chosen as a unit of measurement for the whole scale.

The final test of the validity of the construction is as follows. Calculate the scale value of any raw score, or of any test element, with the above unit and origin, and locate it on the scale. Draw a vertical line through this point. Now the proportion of each distribution that lies above this point should agree with the experimentally determined proportion of children in each age group who actually exceed that score or who actually pass that test element. If this final criterion is satisfied throughout the whole range of the scale, then we have a scale construction which is internally consistent with the data throughout the whole range. I have shown elsewhere [3] that this unit of measurement gives results consistent with both psychological and educational test data and that

[3] THURSTONE, L. L., *operibus citatis*.

the generalized 'p.e.' unit which is now in common use gives results that are grossly inconsistent with the data. In the absolute scaling method we have a consistent unit of measurement but the measurement is made from the mean ability of one of the overlapping groups as an assumed origin. Our present problem concerns the discovery of the absolute zero for mental measurement.

LINEAR RELATION BETWEEN VARIABILITY AND MEAN TEST PERFORMANCE

The discovery is that *a linear relation exists between the standard deviation (σ) and the mean test performance (M) for the several age groups.* This law holds for a number of psychological tests when their frequency distributions are restated in terms of absolute scaling. It is not universally true for raw scores because of the fact, previously noted, that the raw scoring unit cannot be relied upon to represent a constant increment of ability throughout the whole range.

The generalization made above must be stated with one condition, however, which is implied in the test data from which it is derived, namely, that the social and intellectual factors of selection must operate more or less uniformly for the several age groups. This can be seen if we consider an extreme case. Suppose that we were to select one thousand children of each age for purposes of standardization and that we selected the fifteen year olds exclusively from the eighth grade, while the fourteen year olds were selected from all grades and from the high school. Naturally our norms for the fifteen year olds would not include the brightest children of this age who have already passed the eighth grade nor would we have the dullest children of this age who have not reached the eighth grade. The result would show the variability of the fifteen year olds to be too small in comparison with that of the fourteen year olds even though their respective means were approximately correct. Hence, since the mean and the variability of successive age groups are markedly affected by the conditions of selection of each age group, we must insert the condition of uniform selection on our generalization. The discovery, so stated, then takes the following form. *With uniform conditions of selection there is a linear relation between the absolute variability and the mean test performance of successive age groups.* This statement refers of course to absolute scaling and not to raw scores.

The above law has been demonstrated for the following tests: National Intelligence Tests; Merrill-Palmer (Stutsman) tests for preschool children; Illinois General Scale; Dearborn Test, Series I; Dearborn Series II; Otis Advanced Intelligence Test; Binet tests (Cyril Burt standardization). The available data for all seven of these tests show a linear relation between absolute variability and mean test performance.

Table I is a summary of the absolute variability and the mean test performance of each age group for each of the seven psychological tests. The National test [4] is represented graphically in Fig. I where σ is plotted against M. Note the linearity of this graph. Even a physicist could hardly ask for a clearer case of linearity. The Stutsman tests [5] are represented in Fig. 2 in the same manner. Here the errors of measurement are greater because her tests were standardized on only fifty children of each age group, but the linearity is rather clearly indicated. In Fig. 3 the Illinois General Scale [6] has been shown in the same manner, and the linearity is here also pretty clear. The Dearborn tests,[7] Series I and II, are shown in Figs. 4 and 5 in the same manner indicating very clearly a linear relation between variability and mean performance. The Otis Advanced test [8] is represented in Fig. 6 with the same kind of plot. Here it would

[4] 'The National Intelligence Tests,' A manual of directions, published 1924 by the World Book Company. The absolute scaling was done by C. L. Odom for a master's thesis, not yet published.

[5] Data for the Stutsman Test were obtained from Miss Stutsman. They will be published in her doctor's thesis.

[6] Data for the Illinois General Scale were obtained from C. L. Odom's master's thesis, not yet published.

[7] Data for the two Dearborn tests, Series I and II were obtained from C. L. Odom's master's thesis, not yet published.

[8] 'Otis Intelligence Scale,' a manual of directions published by the World Book Company. The absolute scaling was done by C. L. Odom for a master's thesis, not yet published.

L. L. THURSTONE

be possible to interpret the diagram either as linear or as slightly positively accelerated but Otis himself discards his data for the lowest and for the highest age groups and gives estimated norms for the age groups at both ends of his age range. I have included here only those distributions which he himself uses in establishing age norms for his test. The plot is easily interpreted as linear. In Fig. 7 a similar diagram has been drawn for the Binet test [9] according to the data of Cyril Burt.

The law can be stated in simple algebraic form as follows:

$$\sigma = s \cdot M + K,$$

in which σ is the absolute standard deviation of ability in any age group in terms of the standard deviation of one of the age groups chosen as a base; M is the mean test performance of the same age group, measured in terms of the above unit and from the mean performance of the basic age group as an origin; s is the slope of the graph and K is the intercept on the σ-axis. These two constants will be used for the calculation of absolute zero of test intelligence.

The tests here represented all support the generalization that with uniform conditions of selecting the successive age groups there is a linear relation between the variability of test performance and the mean performance. When the relation of σ and M is plotted for successive *grade* groups, the generalization does not necessarily hold. This is probably because of the progressive selective factors which sometimes govern grade classification.

THE ABSOLUTE ZERO

Perhaps the most interesting application of the linearity just noted is the possibility of locating the absolute zero of test intelligence. Consider first the increase in mean raw score for increasing age. When the mean score is tabulated for each age group we find of course that the mean increases with age at least up to the adolescent years. But the zero score of any one of these tests, the National for example, is

[9] THURSTONE, L. L., *operibus citatis*.

not intended to represent zero intelligence. A child may be too young to attain any score above zero on this test but we do not therefore say that its intelligence is actually zero. The zero score in every psychological and educational test is an assumed or arbitrary origin. If we could imagine the scale continuing downward to negative values the very young child might be represented with a certain negative score which would however represent some mental development above the absolute zero intelligence of an inanimate object.

For some time I have considered this problem of an absolute zero as insoluble because no matter how far down we go on the scale of negative scores there seemed to be no *a priori* reason why some organism might not be found with even less intelligence. As long as we deal with raw scores or immediate derivatives of raw scores we really cannot talk about negative values because the scale of raw scores may have no meaning for negative values. As long as the scoring unit is the number of questions correctly answered, or some function of it, the unit is not so defined that any interpretation can be given to negative values. What might be the interpretation of the ability to solve 'minus fifty of these questions'?

Having a unit of measurement the consistency of which can be experimentally checked throughout the whole range of ability we discover the linear relation which has been described. We can now locate the absolute zero indirectly. We have seen that as long as we follow the scale of raw scores downward there is no certain meaning to negative raw scores. If we follow the mean performances, M, on the absolute scale below our assumed origin, there seems to be no direct way of identifying the absolute zero for, here again, how can we know but that some organism might be found whose intelligence would be represented at a point on the absolute scale lower than any point that we might choose?

We arrive at the absolute zero by an indirect route. *The absolute variability of test intelligence must be zero when the mean test performance is absolute zero because, in the nature of the case, the variability cannot be negative.* The procedure of

L. L. THURSTONE

locating absolute zero consists merely in extrapolating the linear relation of σ and M to ascertain the numerical value of the mean test performance at which the variability vanishes. That value of M will necessarily be the absolute zero.

My original plan was to express variability, σ, as a function of mean test performance, M, and then to find by extrapolation the mean test performance at which the variability vanishes. Much to my surprize I discovered that this relation of σ to M is linear. The only exception that I have so far discovered is the situation in which the variability, when plotted against age, is so erratic that no function can be made out at all.[10]

The linearity of the relation σ and M simplifies our problem of locating the absolute zero because extrapolation of a linear function is easy. We simply continue the linear graph so as to determine the value of M at which the variability vanishes and we have at that value of M the absolute zero that we are seeking. Absolute scale values below that point would require negative variability if the linearity of the function can be assumed to continue throughout the whole range of the scale. Since negative variability would be meaningless we assume that the absolute zero of the scale has been found. We shall present a rather convincing check on this calculation because we may determine by extrapolation of the mental growth curve the age at which test intelligence has a value of absolute zero, and it will be found that this age turns out to be approximately at birth or shortly before.

We may now determine the numerical value of the absolute zero for each of the tests that we have considered. In Fig. 1 we have the linear plot σ against M for the National Intelligence Test. It should be noted that the method of least squares is not applicable to this linear plot because this method, in its usual form, assumes that all of the errors of measurement are in the dependent variable and that the

[10] Such a case is the series of age norms for the Army Alpha test, published by the Bureau of Educational Measurements and Standards, Kansas State Teachers College, Emporia, Kansas, Feb. 1, 1926.

independent variable can be regarded as free from such errors. But here we have errors of measurement in both σ and M. Hence the line was fitted by the two conditions (1) that it should pass through the center of gravity of the plot, and (2) that the slope should be the ratio of the dispersions of σ and of M. I have elsewhere described this procedure of fitting a straight line on psychological data so that its detail will not here be repeated.[11] The points were given equal weight in this study, although in a very refined procedure they can be weighted. By means of the equation

$$\sigma = .2006M + 1.034$$

we determine the value of M for which σ vanishes. It is

$$\text{Absolute zero} = -5.15\sigma_8.$$

In other words, the absolute zero of the ability measured by the National Intelligence Test is about $5\sigma_8$ below the mean

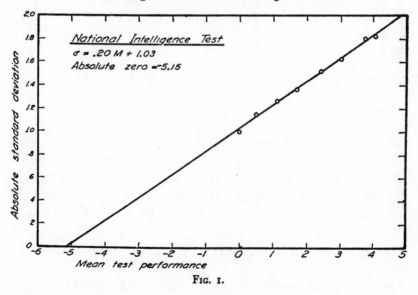

FIG. 1.

performance of the eight-year-old children where σ_8 is the absolute standard deviation of the distribution of this ability in eight-year-old children. If we should represent this fact

[11] THURSTONE, L. L., *operibus citatis.*

L. L. THURSTONE

graphically we should plot a single normal frequency distribution for the National Intelligence Test to represent eight-year-old children and we should locate the absolute zero at the point — 5σ on that diagram.

But here another interesting generalization appears. By Fig. 1 it appears that the absolute standard deviation is directly proportional to the mean performance when the

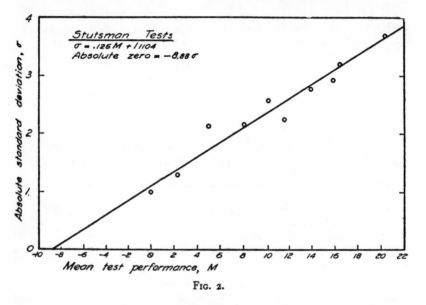

FIG. 2.

latter is measured from the absolute zero instead of from the assumed origin at the mean of the eight-year-old children. Hence we can generalize the above statement by saying that the absolute zero of any age group, n, on the National Intelligence Test is about $5\sigma_n$ below the mean of that age group, or simply,

$$\text{Absolute zero} = -5.15\sigma_n.$$

The higher the mean test performance the greater is the absolute variability of the group and hence the above equation locates the absolute zero as a scale distance below the mean of the group in terms of the dispersion of the age group.

ABSOLUTE ZERO IN INTELLIGENCE

The same analysis is shown for the other tests in the several diagrams. The absolute zero for the Stutsman test

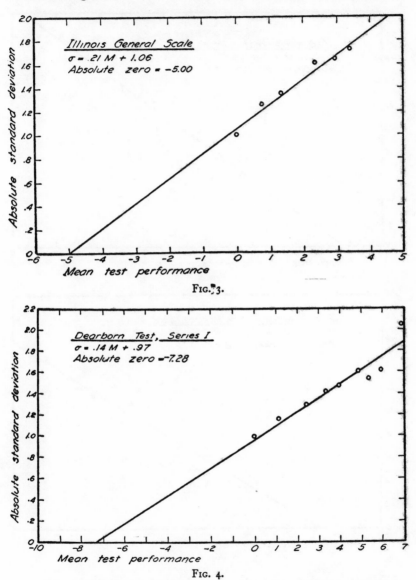

Fig. 3.

Fig. 4.

is shown in Fig. 2, for the Illinois General Intelligence Test in Fig. 3, for the Dearborn Series I and Series II in Figs. 4

and 5 respectively, for the Otis Advanced Examination in Fig. 6, and for the Binet Test (Cyril Burt) in Fig. 7. In each

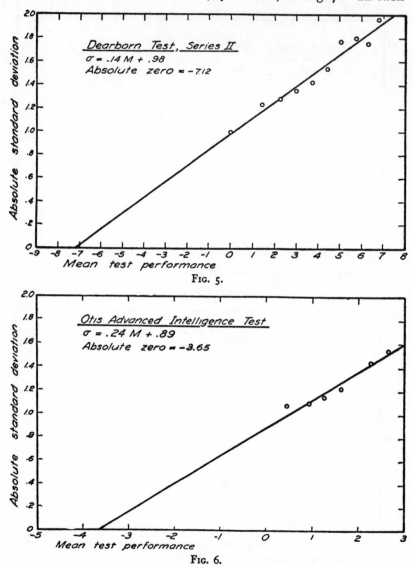

Dearborn Test, Series II
$\sigma = .14\,M + .98$
Absolute zero $= -7.12$

FIG. 5.

Otis Advanced Intelligence Test
$\sigma = .24\,M + .89$
Absolute zero $= -3.65$

FIG. 6.

of these diagrams inspection first showed the plot to be linear, the equation was then calculated, and the absolute zero determined.

ABSOLUTE ZERO IN INTELLIGENCE

The absolute zero may also be located in terms of the raw score of a test if one is willing to allow an imaginal extension of the raw scores downward into negative values. This may be logically a questionable procedure because there is usually a slightly curvilinear relation between raw scores and absolute

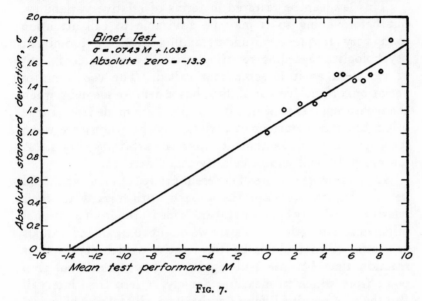

FIG. 7.

scale values. If the relation is plotted and some function established empirically, and if we are willing to assume a fictitious scale of negative raw scores, then it is possible to calculate that negative raw score which corresponds to the absolute zero. Such a procedure is at best rather far-fetched and it will therefore be best to locate the absolute zero as an absolute scale distance below the mean ability of any given age group in terms of the standard deviation of that group as a unit of measurement.

A LAW OF VARIABILITY

Another result of the linearity of the function σ against M is that if we measure M, the mean test performance, from its absolute zero we find that the dispersion is directly proportional to the absolute mean performance. This leads to the formulation of the following law: *With uniform conditions of selection, the absolute variability in the test intelligence of different age groups is proportional to their absolute mean test intelligence.* This is apparent in all the diagrams where σ is plotted against M for different age groups.

This law can be restated in terms of relative variability, but before doing so it may be advisable to call attention to a very frequent misunderstanding even by prominent psychologists regarding relative variability or the coefficient of variation as it is sometimes called. The coefficient of variation, or relative variability, has a definite meaning when the measurements to which it is applied are made from a true origin but the coefficient of variation is sheer nonsense when it is applied to measurements from an arbitrary origin. A few examples will serve to clarify this difference.

If we measure stature of different groups of men, we should be justified to compare the groups with regard to their relative variability because stature is measured from a rational origin of zero length. Similarly we might compare individuals or groups of individuals by the relative variability in their reaction time because here again we have a rational zero point from which to measure, namely, a zero time interval. But the case is quite different with practically all psychological and educational tests which are scored from an arbitrary zero point. Suppose that two groups A and B have the following constants for their raw scores.

	A	B
Mean Score	50	100
σ	10	20
coef. var.	.20	.20

Here the naïve calculation of the coefficient of variation would show the relative variability to be the same for the two groups. Let the test items be graded in difficulty in this test. We may then assume that both groups passed successfully the five or ten easiest items in the test. The test would differentiate the two groups equally well if these easiest ten items were eliminated or, for that matter, if the author had happened to begin even farther down with ten items still easier. Now notice that if the author had happened to start the test farther down so that the gross score averages had been, say, 70 and 120, the variability probably would not have been affected because of the addition of twenty very easy questions. But now the coefficients of variation 10/70 and 20/120 would no longer be the same. In other words, the coefficient of variation is affected by the degree of difficulty at which the test itself begins and that is not what we are after when we want to compare the variabilities of two groups. We might just as well compare the relative variabilities of two groups of men as to stature by measuring their heights from a point one foot above the floor! The absolute variabilities of the two groups would remain unaffected but the coefficients of variation would fluctuate depending on where the measurements begin.

In order for the coefficient of variation (relative variability) to have any meaning we must have our measurements from a true or rational origin. The frequent use of the coefficient of variation on psychological test data in terms of raw scores is meaningless. It seems strange that so absurd a procedure can be so common. The absurdity has been well stated by Franzen [12] with special reference to psychological test data.

Since we are here dealing with an absolute zero we are justified in stating the above law of variability in relative terms. The law then takes the following form: *With uniform conditions of selection, the relative variability of absolute test intelligence of different age groups is constant.* It should be evident that this law does not concern the variability of raw scores.

The Mental Growth Curve

In previous articles [13] I have described the possibility of drawing a mental growth curve. At that time I had a rational unit by means of absolute scaling but I did not have an absolute origin. I used as an assumed origin the mean Binet test performance of three year old children. Since we

[12] Franzen, R., 'Statistical Issues,' *J. Educ. Psychol.*, 1924, **15**, pp. 367–382.
[13] Thurstone, L. L., *operibus citatis.*

L. L. THURSTONE

now have not only a rational unit of measurement but also an absolute origin it becomes possible to draw a bona fide mental growth curve. The only representation of mental growth that has so far been possible is the curve of progressive increase in raw score with increase in age. Such curves are of course in common use as norms of performance. It has not been possible to study the function because of two defects, namely, (1) that the unit of raw score gives no assurance of representing equal increments of mental development in different parts of the scale and (2) that there has not been available a true origin from which to measure. Of these two defects the first is by far the more serious, because the nature of a function can be determined even though the origin of measurement be arbitrary, but the nature of the function is itself lost if the unit of measurement is subject to progressive variation of unknown nature.

The mental growth curve which I drew for the Binet test was a legitimate mental growth curve even though the origin was arbitrary, but the function can now be drawn more satisfactorily since we can show it in its true elevation above absolute zero. This has been shown in Fig. 11.

At What Age Does Test Intelligence Begin?

Since we have discovered a method of determining the absolute zero of test intelligence and since we have a consistent unit of measurement for test performance, it becomes possible to draw a mental growth curve, and the question naturally arises as to whether this mental growth curve passes through absolute zero at or near birth. It should be noted that in determining the absolute zero we have not made use of chronological age measurement. If it should turn out that the absolute mental growth curve passes through the absolute zero at some preposterous age such as minus five years or plus several years, then we should be suspicious of the method by which the absolute zero was determined. It is just this sort of common sense check to which we can submit the location of absolute zero. We should expect the mental growth curve to pass through the absolute zero at or near birth, or not more than nine months before.

ABSOLUTE ZERO IN INTELLIGENCE

For the purpose of this practical check we shall use four tests, namely the National, the Stutsman, the Otis Advanced and the Binet as standardized by Cyril Burt in London. We shall use the Stutsman test for preschool children although standardized on small groups because her norms extend down to the age of 21 months and consequently the extrapolation for that test covers a relatively short age range. This is a decided advantage because if the norms begin at eight years it is necessary to extrapolate the mental growth curve over an age range practically equal to the range of the whole standardization from 8 to 16 and this introduces of necessity a possible error of several months in the age at which the growth curve passes through absolute zero. This error is relatively smaller when the extrapolation covers only a short age range such as eighteen months.

We shall start with the National Intelligence Test. In Fig. 8 the mean test performance is plotted against chronological age with data obtained directly from Table 1. The growth curve seems to be linear over the age range studied. This may be due to intrinsic linearity of the mental growth curve, but it is more likely that a progressive selective factor is superimposed on the natural negative acceleration of the mental growth curve so as to give it the appearance of linearity. However, since the data show the curve to be linear we shall treat it that way. We draw a horizontal line at the level of absolute zero which has been determined in Fig. 1. The linear growth curve is extended downward until it intersects the level of absolute zero. We then find that the age at which the mental growth curve passes through absolute zero is zero age, namely at birth! This determination is accurate at least within several months if the continued linearity of the growth curve can be assumed.

At this point a word should be said regarding the probable shape of the mental growth curve near its origin. It is hardly likely that the growth curve starts with a negative acceleration. It is more likely, and in fact more natural, to expect it to begin with a positive acceleration and to change gradually to a negative acceleration which continues toward maturity.

L. L. THURSTONE

TABLE I

Mean age in yrs.	Binet (Burt's Data)		National In-telligence Test		Dearborn Series I		Dearborn Series II		Illinois General		Otis Advanced		Mean age in mos.	Stutsman Test	
	M	σ	M	σ	M	σ	M	σ	M	σ	M	σ		M	σ
3.5	0.000	1.000											21 mos.	0.0000	1.0000
4.5	1.231	1.191											27	2.2222	1.3072
5.5	2.336	1.255											33	4.9858	2.1363
6.5	3.372	1.255			0.000	1.000							39	8.0386	2.1642
7.5	4.061	1.333	0.000	1.000	1.072	1.165	0.000	1.000					45	10.1406	2.5770
8.5	4.875	1.496	0.512	1.162	2.394	1.292	1.369	1.231					51	11.5982	2.2283
9.5	5.433	1.500	1.082	1.269	3.315	1.415	2.241	1.276	0.000	1.000			57	13.9082	2.7822
10.5	6.190	1.453	1.711	1.371	3.955	1.485	2.990	1.357	0.737	1.258	0.440	1.068	63	15.7360	2.9286
11.5	6.776	1.446	2.418	1.533	4.849	1.606	3.748	1.425	1.315	1.362	0.941	1.092	69	16.3761	3.2007
12.5	7.314	1.503	3.028	1.633	5.321	1.554	4.402	1.553	2.368	1.621	1.236	1.154	75	20.3180	3.6947
13.5	8.040	1.532	3.761	1.806	5.944	1.622	5.062	1.774	2.929	1.645	1.666	1.222			
14.5	8.684	1.792	4.040	1.818	6.890	2.050	5.734	1.798	3.382	1.728	2.240	1.441			
15.5							6.329	1.757			2.627	1.552			
16.5							6.767	1.959							

ABSOLUTE ZERO IN INTELLIGENCE

It is probable that the mental growth curve should be represented as theoretically asymptotic to the level of absolute zero so that the sperm and the ovum would represent not zero but infinitesimal amounts of the process which matures into measurable intelligence. The mental growth curve may ultimately be shown to have the characteristics of Raymond Pearl's generalized population growth curve.[14]

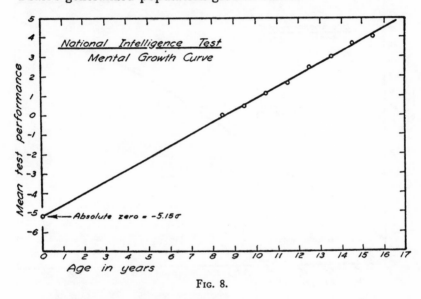

Fig. 8.

The continuity of the growth curve in Fig. 8 through the absolute zero at birth and the mean performances at the several age levels is very striking. The linear growth curve of Fig. 8 as determined by the eight means from the data can be projected downwards until it reaches zero age and the value of the mean at that point agrees with the absolute zero as determined by the variability diagram of Fig. 1. This is a common sense test of the reasonableness of our determination of absolute zero.

The growth curve for the Stutsman test is shown in Fig. 9.

[14] This reasoning is in agreement with Professor Culler's analysis of the learning function. For another discussion of initial positive acceleration of the learning function, see my monograph 'The Learning Curve Equation,' PSYCHOL. MONOG., 1919, 26 (No. 114), pp. 51.

The ten mean performances were first plotted from Table 1. The absolute zero was determined in Fig. 2. Now when the growth curve of Fig. 9 is projected downward it is found that it reaches the level of absolute zero at birth. This is again rather striking evidence of the reasonableness of the determination of absolute zero. The graph in Fig. 9 could be

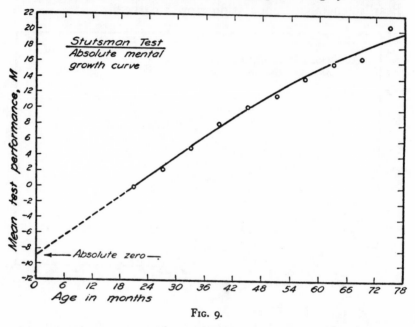

FIG. 9.

represented as a straight line. That has been done and the equation calculated as previously described. Such a line reaches the level of absolute zero at an age of about minus three months, *i.e.* about three months before birth. It is probable that absolute scaling of the developmental reflexes in young infants would reveal a growth curve of positive acceleration which begins with the early development of the foetus. The choice between a straight line and a line of slight curvature as shown in Fig. 9 is not here of primary importance because in either case the growth curve is at the level of absolute zero at or slightly before birth.

The mental growth curve for the Otis Advanced examination is shown in Fig. 10. It was plotted from the data of

ABSOLUTE ZERO IN INTELLIGENCE

Table 1. The relation seems to be linear and when it is extended it reaches the level of absolute zero at birth. The fact that these mental growth curves when extrapolated pass through absolute zero at birth is rather convincing evidence that the mental functions which are operative in the adult intelligence tests begin their development at birth even though these functions cannot be measured at a very early age. It might possibly seem as though the functions that are operative in taking the paper-pencil tests in group form begin to develop at the time when the writing coördination

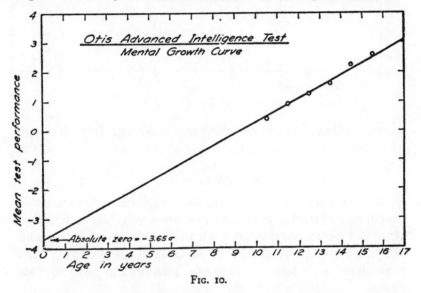

FIG. 10.

is begun, but these results show rather definitely that whatever it is that is measured by the group intelligence tests, it begins its development at birth or shortly before. This is a psychological finding of no mean interest.

The mental growth curve for the Binet test is shown in Fig. 11. The twelve points on this curve are again plotted from Table 1. It appears immediately that this growth curve is not linear. It has a negative acceleration and it can readily be thought of as continuous with the absolute zero of performance at birth. The continuity of this function is rather striking. Owing to the curvature of this function the

L. L. THURSTONE

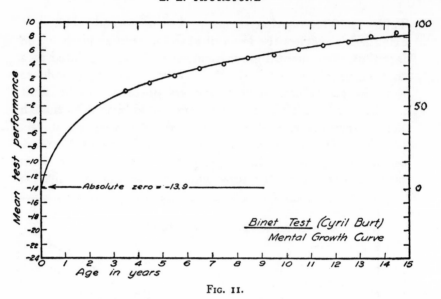

Fig. 11.

determination of age at absolute zero is not nearly so accurate as in the other three tests for which mental growth curves are shown.

SUMMARY

1. The discovery which has been verified so far on seven psychological tests is that with uniform conditions of selection there is a linear relation between the absolute variability and the mean test performance of successive age groups. This generalization refers to absolute scaling and not to raw scores.

2. The absolute zero is located indirectly. The absolute variability of test intelligence must be zero when the mean test performance is absolute zero because, in the nature of the case, the variability cannot be negative. The absolute zero is located by extrapolating the above linear relation to ascertain the scale value of the mean performance at which the variability vanishes. That scale value is the absolute zero. It is defined as a distance below the mean performance of any age group in terms of its own standard deviation.

3. Having found the linear relation above described and having located the absolute zero, the following law of vari-

ability is a necessary inference: With uniform conditions of selection, the absolute variability in the test intelligence of different age groups is proportional to their absolute mean test intelligence. This law can be stated in terms of relative variability as follows: With uniform conditions of selection, the relative variability of absolute test intelligence of different age groups is constant. These laws refer to absolute scaling and not in any sense to raw scores.

4. By means of the unit of measurement provided by absolute scaling and the absolute zero it becomes possible to construct a true mental growth curve for a specified mental test. It has not hitherto been possible to study the function of mental growth because of the lack of a unit and an origin.

5. The validity of the determination of absolute zero is subjected to a practical test by determining the age at which the mental growth curve passes through absolute zero. It is found that this happens at birth or shortly before.

6. The fact that the mental growth curve passes through absolute zero at or before birth constitutes statistical evidence that test intelligence begins its development at this early age even though it is not then directly accessible for measurement.

[MS. received November 25, 1927].

From C. Burt (1963). Brit. J. Statist. Psychol., *16*, 175–190; *by kind permission of the author and the British Psychological Association*

IS INTELLIGENCE DISTRIBUTED NORMALLY?

By Cyril Burt

University College, London

Frequency distributions obtained on applying intelligence tests to large samples of the school population are analysed, and compared with those given by the formulae for the commoner types of frequency curve. It is noted that the distributions actually observed are more asymmetrical and have longer tails than that described by the normal curve. The best fit is given by a curve of Type IV: this is in fact the type of distribution we should expect if (as has been argued in earlier papers) individual differences in general ability are determined partly by multifactorial and partly by unifactorial inheritance. It follows that the usual assumption of normality leads to a gross underestimate of the number of highly gifted individuals. The conclusions thus drawn are confirmed by a study of data from other sources; and various practical corollaries are deduced.

I. Problem

In recent controversies about the abilities both of schoolchildren and of adults a number of questions have repeatedly been raised, some theoretical, others eminently practical, which cannot be answered without some fairly precise knowledge of the way in which individual differences in such abilities are distributed. Hitherto most psychologists and educationists have assumed that the distribution of abilities conforms to the so-called ' normal curve of chance '. In the case of ' general intelligence ' this alleged normality has often been cited as evidence in favour of some particular hypothesis about the nature or origin of the individual differences observed: on the other hand, several critics have maintained that the apparent normality is merely an artificial consequence of the way mental tests are standardized, and can therefore have no such implications.

Nevertheless, it has become increasingly clear that deductions based on the assumptions of normality may at times be highly questionable. In discussing what is called ' the pool of intelligence ' educationists have varied widely in their estimates of the number of ' potential geniuses ' available in the child population—potential geniuses being defined for such purposes as ' those with I.Q.s of 175 or upwards '. Not many months ago, in reply to a question put to him in Parliament, the Minister of Education gave an estimate of ' little more than one or two in a million '. The assessment, like others of its type, was obtained by employing the normal distribution with a conventional I.Q. scale and a standard deviation of 15 points. But, as the correspondence that followed quickly showed, the figure cited was considered much too low by many headmasters and

Cyril Burt

educational psychologists, who found it quite out of keeping with the number of pupils with high I.Q.s who passed through their hands.[1]

The general acceptance of the theory that individual differences in ability are distributed in strict accordance with the Gaussian curve seems largely due to the advocacy of Thorndike, the acknowledged leader during the earlier decades of the century in the field of educational measurement. In his book, *The Measurement of Intelligence*, he devotes a chapter and a long appendix to demonstrating the conclusion that, providing the amount of intelligence is measured on a scale of ' truly equal units ', the distribution should be exactly normal. On applying the chi-squared test to his own measurements he reaches values for P ranging from 0·99 to 0·999,999. Now we used to be warned that " a value of P very near to unity should lead the investigator to suspect his hypothesis quite as much as very small values: such very close correspondences are too good to be true " ([19], p. 423). But in any case the argument in practice tends to become circular: Thorndike's followers, at least in this country, were very prone to declare that, if the distribution did not conform to the normal curve, that showed that the units were not ' truly equal '.

Subsequent work in genetics has since furnished strong theoretical grounds for believing that innate mental abilities are not distributed in exact conformity with the normal curve. So far as they are inborn, individual differences in general intelligence are apparently due to a large number of genes of varying influence. Were inheritance solely ' multifactorial ', i.e., if the genes consisted solely of numerous 'polygenes', each giving rise only to a very small deviation one way or another, then we might reasonably expect the resulting distribution to conform with the ' normal curve of chance '. But there can be little doubt that some of the genes are responsible for comparatively large deviations; and if their effects were sometimes favourable, sometimes unfavourable, the net result would be to enlarge the tails of the distribution in both an upward and a downward direction. However, since the genetic constitution of man is so delicately balanced and adjusted, the effects of these exceptional genes, or of the mutations that produce them, are more likely to be unfavourable than favourable. Hence, the final outcome will be a distribution that is more or less skewed, the longer tail being in the downward direction.

Since these exceptional genes are, by hypothesis, comparatively rare, it would seem to follow that, so long as we are concerned with small samples or with the general run of the population, a normal curve might still be trusted to yield a plausible fit. But when we are concerned with the more extreme type of deviation—the exceptionally bright and the exceptionally dull, cases which are

---

[1] See more especially *The Times Educational Supplement*, March 9 and 16, 1962. According to the report of the Parliamentary debates the estimate was said to have emanated from the National Foundation for Educational Research. In a personal communication, however, the Director, Dr. Wall, tells me that he has in point of fact never been " asked directly how many children there might be with I.Q.s over 175 ". He adds ," I myself would come to a very similar conclusion to the one stated in your paper: it is even possible that my estimate would be higher still ".

so infrequent that they are only found in investigations covering very large groups—then the predictions deduced from the normal curve may easily prove mistaken. But—and this is a point which I wish most emphatically to stress—the nature of the distribution is not a matter to be decided (as is so commonly supposed) by mere ' assumptions ', or even by deductive inference from general principles. It is an issue which can only be settled by an empirical investigation—that is to say, by an *ad hoc* analysis of data collected from actual surveys.

Oddly enough, nearly all of those who have joined in these discussions, whether as critics of the normality hypothesis or as supporters, seem to have missed the real reason for its popularity. It springs not so much from theoretical as from practical considerations. The ordinates and the areas of the curve were long ago calculated and tabulated once for all by Dr. Sheppard, later H.M. Inspector of Schools [15], and are now readily accessible in most popular textbooks on mental measurement. If on the other hand some other type of curve is assumed, the frequencies would have to be calculated *de novo* by each investigator for every fresh research. In the following analysis the chief novelty is the detailed comparison of the frequencies actually observed with theoretical values specially computed from the formulae for a curve of Type IV. Indeed, the primary object of the paper is not so much to supply better estimates for the number of children possessing this or that grade of intelligence, but rather to illustrate the practicability of more adequate methods of statistical analysis.

II. Data and Methods

The earliest of the statistical analyses which were carried out to gain light on the foregoing problems seemed plainly to indicate that the distributions of ability among school children by no means conformed to a strictly normal distribution (Burt, 1917, p. 34; esp. footnote 2, 1921, pp. 160f.). The two anomalous characteristics which might be expected to result from a combination of ' multifactorial ' with ' unifactorial ' inheritance—the elongated tails and the downward asymmetry—were already discernible in the frequency curves then obtained. The chi-squared test was regularly applied; and, wherever the samples were sufficiently large, the divergences from strict normality proved to be statistically significant. However, these initial surveys were merely experimental. The types of test used for such purposes—the original Binet–Simon scale and the earliest group tests—were predominantly verbal, and, as was to be anticipated, could claim no very high reliability or validity. On the whole and in this country the most efficient procedures now available for the purpose would appear to be the later British adaptations of the Stanford–Binet scales. Accordingly in what follows I shall confine myself mainly to data procured by this means.

In a previous publication [4] I have already reported results obtained during investigations undertaken to secure material for an English standardization of the original Stanford–Binet scale. It was then shown, not only that the discrepancies

Cyril Burt

were statistically significant, but also that the values for the usual criteria (the so-called beta coefficients) indicated that the distribution should be regarded as belonging to Pearson's Type IV. Further results have since become available during investigations with the 'new revised Stanford–Binet tests' [16]. The total number of children assessed in the course of all these surveys amounts to 4,665. Their distribution is shown in the first column of Table I. It is plainly skewed, with a prolonged lower tail. Of the entire group more than 10 per cent have I.Q.s under 80; only 7·7 per cent have I.Q.s over 120.

TABLE I. OBSERVED AND THEORETICAL DISTRIBUTIONS
Frequencies in Percentages

I.Q.	Observed			Theoretical	
	Before Screening	After Screening	Normal	Type IV	Type VII
Below 30	0·11	0·02	—	0·03	0·01
30–	0·06	0·02	—	0·03	0·01
35–	0·09	0·04	—	0·05	0·03
40–	0·21	0·11	0·01	0·09	0·05
45–	0·23	0·16	0·03	0·14	0·09
50–	0·39	0·27	0·10	0·27	0·17
55–	0·62	0·46	0·26	0·43	0·33
60–	0·77	0·64	0·62	0·74	0·62
65–	1·35	1·24	1·32	1·30	1·71
70–	2·34	2·08	2·54	2·28	2·16
75–	3·97	3·40	4·37	3·71	3·77
80–	6·41	5·70	6·75	5·86	6·16
85–	9·01	9·07	9·37	8·78	9·18
90–	11·60	11·96	11·61	11·47	12·13
95–	13·01	13·42	12·94	13·79	14·02
100–	13·42	13·84	13·01	14·11	14·09
105–	12·67	13·07	11·66	12·57	12·18
110–	10·01	10·33	9·41	9·66	9·22
115–	6·00	6·19	6·76	6·38	6·18
120–	3·45	3·56	4·38	3·92	3·79
125–	1·97	2·03	2·54	2·15	2·16
130–	1·20	1·24	1·32	1·12	1·17
135–	0·60	0·62	0·62	0·57	0·62
140–	0·28	0·29	0·26	0·28	0·33
145–	0·11	0·11	0·10	0·13	0·17
150–	0·06	0·07	0·03	0·06	0·09
155–	0·04	0·04	0·01	0·04	0·05
Above 160	0·02	0·02	—	0·04	0·05
Total	100·00	100·00	100·00	100·00	100·00

However, with each of the component batches we have endeavoured to eliminate all those cases in which there was the smallest reason to believe that the low I.Q. was mainly or largely due to non-genetic causes, either environmental,

Is Intelligence Distributed Normally?

pathological, or accidental (e.g. caused by injury at birth).[1] The number remaining[2] after these eliminations were made was 4,523. The data for this composite group have now been analysed by Miss Baker along the lines which I adopted in reporting the separate surveys. To conform to the conventional scale now in current use all the I.Q.s have been restandardized so as to yield a standard deviation of 15 points.[3]

---

[1] One critic asks for a brief explanation of our use of the word 'pathological'. In previous reports we followed Dr. Lewis's terminology (adopted in the Wood Report), and used the word to designate those cases that are apparently due to non-genetic or post-conceptual disturbances. Some writers, however, have included under the term cases showing clinical symptoms that result, not only from environmental causes, but also from rare recessive or dominant genes. For this mixed group Penrose's term 'clinical' seems more suitable ([11], pp. 46f.). His data and that of other investigators suggest that something like three-quarters of the certifiable defectives are of a mixed 'clinical' type; the other quarter—the so-called 'residual' cases—may be regarded as almost wholly genetic. Among the 'clinical' cases the defect in about one-third of the total number seems attributable, partly at any rate, to genetic causes. The rest form the group we have called 'pathological'. However, the real difficulty is to classify those cases—perhaps the most numerous of all—in which both types of factor operate and in which environmental factors tend to aggravate and often to obscure factors that are essentially genetic. Sometimes it is possible to allow for the joint causation by raising the observed I.Q. by 10 to 20 points; but any such classification (as was emphasized above) is bound to be somewhat speculative. In our own assessments we have sought to err on the side of eliminating too many rather than too few.

[2] This total is made up of three main batches. (i) A set of 433 children tested during the course of a preliminary study of the Stanford–Binet scale: for these, in the original L.C.C. report, 1925, Terman's age-allocations were adopted, but the I.Q.s have now been restandardized. (ii) A set of 2,835 children, tested in the course of a joint research planned to secure data for an English re-standardization of the Stanford–Binet scale ([3], p. 348). The distribution of these first two batches combined into a single group, is shown in [9], p. 56 and Figure 1. (iii) The latest batch consists of 1,255 children tested with the 'new revised tests', i.e. the so-called Terman–Merrill scale. The restandardization of the Terman–Merrill revision was undertaken by a small committee originally formed under the chairmanship of Professor Hamley, with Miss Baker as secretary. We should like once again to express our indebtedness to all those who assisted in the work or allowed us to carry out tests in their schools.

The shortcomings of such a composite sample are obvious. In the London surveys those who co-operated in the testing usually had received a training in such work, and were given personal instructions; the results could be referred to the children's teachers, and where necessary checked by further study or by different types of test; in particular, the majority of the subnormal children in the area belonging to the age-group (including defectives not attending school) were tested and included in the survey. With the surveys carried out in other areas all this was seldom possible. In these the number of subnormal children is probably disproportionately small, especially as we were anxious that if errors were made, they should be made on the safe side—i.e. by excluding too many genetic cases and not by including non-genetic cases: otherwise it might be argued that the gravest cases of subnormality were pathological.

[3] We have kept to measurements expressed in terms of the I.Q. in order that the results may be intelligible to the general reader and comparable with those obtained in other investigations. Such a unit is not without its drawbacks. For example, if we reintroduced all the cases of subnormality, and re-calculated the standard deviation, it would turn out to be much larger. Some may argue that this is the standard deviation we ought to take as our unit, since it is based on the entire population. But in another educational area the entire population would probably yield yet another value. And in any case most investigations exclude the more extreme cases of mental deficiency from their calculations. As I have argued elsewhere the whole problem of a suitable mental unit calls urgently for reconsideration; but that is a side-issue which cannot be examined here and does not affect our present problem.

Cyril Burt

The distribution of the group, after this preliminary screening had been carried out, is shown in the second column of Table I. In I.Q. points the mean is almost exactly 100, and the standard deviation almost exactly 15 (calculated to two decimal places they are 100·07 and 15·09 respectively). These values of course are the results of the standardization. The amount of individual variation, however, differs in the two different directions: in the upper half of the curve it corresponds to a standard deviation of only 14·8, and in the lower half to one of 15·4.

Column 3 in the table shows the theoretical distribution calculated from the usual tables for the normal curve and based on the calculated mean and standard deviation given above. It is at once obvious that the frequencies found in the survey rise in the centre to too sharp a peak and exhibit tails that are far too widely and unequally spread out for the observed distribution to be regarded as typically normal. On applying the usual test for goodness of fit, we find $\chi^2 = 107·3$, and consequently, if the distribution in the general population were strictly normal, it would be well over a million to one against discrepancies so large as those observed occurring as a result of the mere chances of random samples. At the same time it will be noted that, with a much smaller sample (e.g., one which only justified us in calculating the percentages to one decimal place and contained no individuals with an I.Q. over 150 or under 60—as indeed is the case with many of the frequency tables published for surveys), the normal curve would provide a very plausible fit. (See Figure 1, which shows

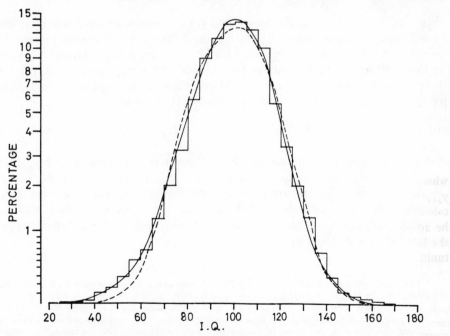

FIGURE 1. Observed and theoretical distributions. (Type IV continuous line; Normal Curve dotted line.)

Is Intelligence Distributed Normally?

the observed frequencies after the doubtful cases have been eliminated by screening, and the best-fitting curves of the ' normal ' type and of type IV.)

In order to discover to what class of curve the distribution belongs, we have here followed the same procedure as before. Using the notation suggested by Karl Pearson we find β_1 (the criterion for skewness) $= 0\cdot048$, and β_2 (the criterion for kurtosis) $= 3\cdot918$. This suggests that the curve is either Type VII or Type IV. Taking Fisher's forms of the criteria, we obtain $g_1 = -0\cdot219 \pm 0\cdot036$ and $g_2 = 0\cdot918 \pm 0\cdot073$, and from these values or from the betas we obtain[1] $\kappa = 0\cdot007$. Curves for which the criterion κ lies between 0 and 1 are classified by Pearson as belonging to Type IV. This is the only type in his series which is (i) of unlimited range in both directions and at the same time (ii) asymmetrical and (iii) leptokurtic, i.e., peaked.

To determine how closely a hypothetical curve of this type will fit the actual data it will be necessary to compute the theoretical frequencies. The method adopted is virtually that which I described and used in my previous reports, and is based (with minor modifications) on the second of the two working procedures discussed by Palin Elderton ([6], pp. 67f). Instead of the simpler formula which he uses we have preferred the slightly more complicated expression in which the deviates to which the frequencies refer are deviates from the mean instead of from the arbitrary origin, namely,

$$y = y_0 \left\{ 1 + \left(\frac{x}{a} - \frac{v}{r} \right)^2 \right\}^{-m} \exp \left\{ - v \tan^{-1}(x/a - v/r) \right\} \qquad . (1)$$

where y_0 is the ordinate at the mean, and r, m, v, and a are constants computed from β_1 and β_2, and a varies with the standard deviation. With the present data the values are $r = 10\cdot184$, $m = 6\cdot092$, $v = 1\cdot527$, and $a = 9\cdot501$. This yields values for the ordinates at mid-points of the successive intervals into which the total range is subdivided. To effect a valid comparison we need areas rather than ordinates; and for this purpose we have applied the formula

$$\int_{-\frac{1}{2}}^{+\frac{1}{2}} y_x \, dx = \frac{1}{24} (y_{x-1} + 22y_x + y_{x+1}) \qquad (2)$$

where y_x denotes the ordinate at the mid-point of the interval and y_{x-1} and y_{x+1} the ordinates next below and next above. Elderton observes that the calculation of the values relating to this curve " needs considerable care: it is ", he adds, " the most difficult of all the Pearson-type curves ". We have found the labour lengthy rather than difficult; but admittedly there are ample opportunities for slips and mistakes.

---

[1] The small size of κ is due to the small degree of asymmetry combined with the high degree of lepto-kurtosis. In the London sample, where special efforts were made to locate all the low-grade cases (including defectives not in attendance at a school) the values for β_1 (0·035) and κ (0·04) were appreciably larger, and the asymmetry was far more conspicuous. Readers unfamiliar with Pearson's criteria and his scheme for classifying frequency curves may refer to the *Note* on the subject recently published in this *Journal* (XV, 1962, pp. 80f., especially Figure 1, p. 86).

Cyril Burt

III. Results

Let us now glance at the results and conclusions reached on adopting these somewhat novel formulae. The detailed frequencies computed by the foregoing equations are shown in the fourth column of Table I. χ^2 is now only 18·2; $P=0·57$. The fit is perhaps not quite so close as that obtained by Karl Pearson for distributions derived from physical measurements. But it is clear that the discrepancies between the theoretical values and the values observed may now quite well be due to the chances of sampling, and that the agreement is far better than that commonly obtained in cases of mental measurement.

To estimate the proportional number of individuals having I.Q.s above any borderline which lies outside the range of Table I—e.g., the borderline of 175 I.Q. mentioned in the question put to the Minister of Education—we must undertake some kind of extrapolation. With the aid of the formula we can extend the theoretical calculations beyond the limits reached by our sample and sum the areas. Table II shows the chief results. Here the figures in column ii represent the cumulative frequencies thus obtained, i.e., the proportional numbers reaching or exceeding the I.Q. specified in the left hand margin. Column i gives the proportions deduced from Pearson's tables for the normal curve, assuming as before a standard deviation of approximately 15 I.Q. It will be seen that according to our estimates the number having I.Q.s of over 160 is more than ten times the number deduced from the normal curve, and that, instead of the proportion of those with I.Q.s of 175 or over being only 3 or 4 per million, it rises to nearly 77 per million. At the present day the male school population in England and Wales amounts to rather over 4 millions. That would yield more than 300 boys of school age with I.Q.s over 175. Among the female population, just as the number of defectives is smaller than that obtaining among the males, so apparently is the number of geniuses. But in any case, the total number of children reaching the high level specified cannot be far short of five or six hundred.

TABLE II. The Estimated Proportions of the Population Reaching or Exceeding the Borderline Specified

Borderline	Number per million	
	(i) Normal Distribution	(ii) Type IV Distribution
160	31·7	342·3
175	3·3	76·8
190	0·1	19·4
200	<0·001	6·2

It is however of interest to consider whether a simpler formula might not furnish a reasonable fit. We have seen that, when pathological cases are eliminated, the degree of asymmetry becomes comparatively slight; both β_1 and κ have decidedly low values. Accordingly let us ask what type of curve would give the closest fit if we assumed that the apparent asymmetry resulted

Is Intelligence Distributed Normally?

solely from errors of sampling. This would imply that the true value of β_1 and κ is zero. In that case the constant ν, which is based on β_1, would likewise be zero. The exponential factor in eqn. (1) then becomes unity, and the equation reduces to the extremely simple form

$$y/y_0 = \left(1 + \frac{x^2}{a^2}\right)^{-m} \tag{3}$$

—the formula for a curve of Type VII. The equations for the two constants are correspondingly simplified. Substituting the numerical values for β and σ (the standard deviation) we now obtain

$$a^2 = \frac{2\beta_2}{\beta_2 - 3}\,\sigma^2 = 77\cdot876 \tag{4}$$

and

$$m = \frac{5\beta_2 - 9}{2(\beta_2 - 3)} = 5\cdot770. \tag{5}$$

With the aid of a table of logarithms the theoretical frequencies can be readily computed. The figures obtained are shown in column 5 of Table I. Applying the usual test we have $\chi^2 = 23$, and $P = 0\cdot28$. The fit is decidedly better than that given by the normal curve. If therefore the distribution in the general population was in fact a distribution of Type VII, the probability that discrepancies as large as this or larger would occur as a result of random sampling would be just under 1 in 3.

The well-known relation between the very simple formula thus reached (eqn. 3) and the more familiar formula for the normal curve is worth a passing comment for the benefit of training college lecturers and others concerned with elementary courses on statistical psychology. The relation turns on the fact that, as n increases indefinitely, the limit of $(1 + 1/n)^n$ is the number e, the base of the natural logarithms, and the limit of $(1 - z/n)^n$ is e^{-z}. Now let us write eqn. (4) in the form $a^2 = -\sigma^2 k^2$, then eqn. (5) gives $m = -\frac{1}{4}k^2\,(5 - 9/\beta_2)$; so that, as β_2 approaches 3, m approaches $-\frac{1}{2}k^2$, and k^2 increases indefinitely. In that case eqn. (3) will take the form

$$y/y_0 = \left(1 - \frac{x^2}{\sigma^2 k^2}\right)^{\frac{1}{2}k^2},$$

or, putting $z = x^2/2\sigma^2$ and $n = \frac{1}{2}k^2$

$$y/y_0 = e^{-x^2/2\sigma^2}$$

when k^2 becomes indefinitely large.

Moreover, it will be noted that, if in eqn. (3) we put $a^2 = n$ and $m = \frac{1}{2}(n+1)$, we obtain the equation which expresses the distribution of Student's t. Suppose we take m as approximately 6; then n will be 11; and, on referring to the table for t given in Yule and Kendall ([19], p. 537), it will be seen that with a standard deviation of $t = 11$, the values in the column for $n = 11$ yield on subtraction proportionate frequencies which are not unlike those in column 4 of Table I, and so offer a rough fit to data such as the present.

Cyril Burt

IV. Supplementary Evidence

Critics who still wish to defend the hypothesis of strict normality may perhaps be inclined to suggest that, since our list of observed frequencies has been obtained from a composite sample, the two peculiarities we have noted—the asymmetry and the elongated tails—might well be just the incidental consequences of the ways in which the constituent groups have been selected and combined. In reply may I point out that each of the constituent groups themselves showed the same features, and in particular, with the largest group of all—based on a survey in which we sought to include the entire child population between the ages of 6·0 and 11·0 residing in a representative electoral division of London—the calculated values for the beta coefficients indicated, even more clearly, a curve of Type IV (cf. [4], p. 170)?

It is instructive to compare the results obtained in these and later surveys with those found by the American investigators while standardizing the latest revision of the Stanford–Binet tests, i.e., the so-called Terman–Merrill scale ([10], pp. 21–23). For this purpose a group of just under three thousand children was tested with the two alternative forms of the scale—L and M. With form L, the I.Q. ranged from 35 to 170, with form M from 35 to 165. The average of the whole group, however, was appreciably higher than ours— 104·0 I.Q. with form L and 104·4 with form M. This means that the range runs from 70 points below the average to 60 or 65 points above—limits which are not very different from our own. On applying the chi-squared test for agreement with normality, McNemar found, for form L, $P = 0·03$ and for form M, $P = 0·005$. Thus, particularly in the latter case, the divergences from the normal curve are fully significant. The discrepancies of the fit, though numerically large, are by no means obvious to the eye when inspecting the various graphs that show for each scale the observed frequencies superimposed on the best-fitting normal curve: (*op. cit.*, figs. 1 and 2, p. 19). The relevant constants are as follows. For form L, $g_1 = 0·028 \pm 0·045$, and for form M, $0·029 \pm 0·045$; for form L, g_2 is $0·346 \pm 0·090$ and for form M, $0·298 \pm 0·090$. Thus both frequency distributions are significantly leptokurtic as the diagrams certainly suggest on a closer examination: both seem too sharply peaked to be regarded as normal, and the frequencies at the end of either tail extend too far. On the other hand, the criterion of skewness is in both cases non-significant. However, as McNemar points out, there were several unavoidable defects in the sampling. The distribution, we are told ([17], pp. 15f.), contained an unduly small proportion of children from the lowest occupational groups: indeed, to judge by the table (*loc. cit.*, p. 14) the percentage in the lower group (unskilled day-labourers) was apparently only one-third of what it should have been. Moreover, since the sample was restricted to schools—and indeed to what are described as ' average schools '—and therefore did not include subnormal children living at home or in institutions, the number of defective as well as of dull and backward pupils must have been disproportionately small. Had they been included, the downward asymmetry, which appears in 4 out of the 6 constituent groups, would be much more clearly marked. McNemar himself makes no attempt to identify the

Is Intelligence Distributed Normally?

type of distribution shown. He expressly refrains from drawing any conclusions from these data concerning the probable distribution of intelligence, and merely observes that "the I.Q.s are *approximately* normal in distribution". And of course, so long as we are dealing with the ordinary run of children in the primary and secondary schools, the assumption is not likely to lead us far astray.[1]

However, scattered throughout the relevant literature there is a good deal of additional evidence which strongly suggests that for those who are definitely subnormal the relative frequencies deduced from the normal curve are far too low. In his discussion of the "medical grouping of institutional cases" Penrose, for instance ([11], p. 45), points out that "far too many individuals exist, whose abilities are more than 3 or 4 times the standard deviation below the normal mean, to be fitted under a Gaussian curve: on that assumption only about 1 idiot among 10,000 and 1 imbecile among 6 could belong to a normal population with a standard deviation of 15 I.Q. points": with his classification, as his table shows, the 'observed percentages' are 0·04 and 0·24 respectively, whereas a normal distribution would predict only 0·000,004 and 0·06. Unfortunately in official reports on mental deficiency the figures commonly given have been collected for administrative purposes, and relate only to those defectives who have been formally 'ascertained'. Nearly always they are expressed as fractions of the total population not of the relevant age groups; nor do they, as a rule, attempt to distinguish between the cases that are undoubtedly pathological and those that are presumed to be wholly or partly of genetic origin. Moreover, owing to the variation in the standard deviation and the inadequacy of the tests employed, the I.Q.s used in defining the border-lines are by no means equivalent to the I.Q.s on the conventional scale that is now in use among psychologists.[2] When a reasonable allowance is made for these disturbing factors, the estimates for the incidence of subnormality, as shown in nearly all the published surveys, both British and American, nearly always suggest proportional numbers far

---

[1] Unfortunately the data from the two Scottish surveys throw little light on the problem. In the first survey the group tests produced "a very skewed distribution"; but this the investigators ascribe to the "ceiling of the test" which tended to curtail the upper end ([14], p. 108); for the Binet tests no special schools were included, and consequently the frequency curve drops abruptly at about 70 I.Q. ([14], pp. 91f.). In the second survey special schools and institutions were visited, but "testing was undertaken only when the pupils' handicaps would not invalidate the test" ([15], pp. 9 and 57): with the Terman–Merrill tests, which were applied to over 1,300 pupils, more than 10 per cent had I.Q.s above 160 and nearly 1 per cent I.Q.s of 170 or more. Thus the figures obtained lend no support to the assumption of normality. But it could be argued that quite possibly much of the discrepancy was due to the peculiarities of the tests and samples rather than to the actual distribution of the general population.

[2] Let me repeat that those who think of comparing the frequencies reported in this section with those obtained in their own inquiries should bear in mind that the I.Q.s referred to are not the raw quotients calculated by dividing mental age by chronological age—a method which yields standard deviations anywhere between 13 and 17 I.Q. points or more according to the set of tests employed. As explained above, the performances of the children tested were first re-scaled—a point which critics of my previous papers seem to have overlooked. And yet, as we have seen, even in the present inquiry the standard deviation of the *composite* group turned out to be a fraction over that 15 points. Thus I.Q.s of 70 and 130 represent not ±2 S.D. exactly, but only ±1·988 S.D.; and this is the value adopted in deducing the theoretical frequencies given in the text.

Cyril Burt

higher than those which would be deduced from a distribution that was strictly normal (see [5] and refs.)

This point, however, has been sufficiently stressed in earlier publications. The exact determination of assessments for supernormal ability has received far less consideration from previous investigators. In recent discussions about the ' national pool of ability ' and the ' need for more adequate methods of selecting and training the undiscovered reserves of ability ' attention has been chiefly concentrated, both in this journal and in the popular press, on the numbers at the higher end of the scale—more especially the number of potential entrants to the grammar schools and to the universities, i.e., of those whose abilities rise above levels of about 110 and 130 I.Q. Here I should like to insert a special plea for a more adequate recognition of the needs and the numbers of those I have called the ' *exceptionally* gifted '. They form a group who constitute one of the nation's most valuable assets, and whose special educational requirements have hitherto been grossly neglected. The average I.Q. of pupils with I.Q.s over 160 (about 170 I.Q.) must be as far above the average I.Q. of the general mass of grammar school children (about 122 I.Q.) as the average of these selected children is above that of the educationally subnormal (i.e., pupils with I.Q.s below 85, whose average would be about 77 I.Q.). Such highly gifted individuals must therefore feel as much out of place in the ordinary grammar school as the grammar pupils would in a class of dull and backward youngsters; and this is fully borne out by evidence gathered from such youngsters while still at school, or later on when, as adults, they have reported or recorded their school experiences.

Let us therefore glance first of all at one of the very few factual inquiries relating to these exceptionally gifted children. In Terman's investigation the initial aim was to select and study those whose I.Q.s would place them " well within the top 1 per cent of the school population ". The working borderline was fixed at 140 I.Q. Of those selected the number with I.Q.s of 170 or over amounted to 6·7 per cent, i.e., between 300 and 600 per million in the general population according as we interpret " well within 1 per cent ". The proportion, as several reviewers pointed out at the time, was unexpectedly high; and perhaps some allowance should be made for the fact that the average level of the population in the cities of California was said to be 4 or 5 points above the general average of the U.S. population, while the standard deviation (with Terman's age-allocations) was nearer 16 points than 15 ([17], pp. 19, 44f). In a later search for exceptionally gifted pupils in New York City—a search described as by no means ' exhaustive '—Dr. Leta Hollingworth found at least a dozen with I.Q.s over 180, i.e. a proportion of about 20 per million. Deviations of this size, she tells us, would be expected " only once in more than a million times if the distribution corresponds to Quetelet's curve of probability "; but, she adds, " it seems more likely from existing data, that children who test above 180 I.Q. are present in greater frequency " ([8], pp. xiii, 23f). Still more recently the Counseling Centre of New York University reported a follow-up study of a batch of children

Is Intelligence Distributed Normally?

who at the time of testing (approximately age 5) had I.Q.s of 170 or more; and in that inquiry over a hundred cases were discovered.

In this country the figures I and my co-workers have obtained in the course of various surveys have varied widely from one area to another. In my earliest inquiries, carried out with the assistance of the Department for the Training of Teachers at Oxford, I found, in a single age-group (aged $9\frac{1}{2}$ to $10\frac{1}{2}$) numbering approximately 1,600 children in all, six children with test-scores equivalent to an I.Q. of 175 or above, nearly 0·4 per cent; nearly all of them came from one particular preparatory school which catered specially for the children of dons. On the other hand, in Liverpool, within a group of the same age but nearly eight times as large and consisting solely of pupils attending public elementary schools, not a single child of this high level was discovered; outside the elementary schools, however, a number of such cases were located, and we estimated that their proportional frequency amounted to just under 30 per million. In my first survey of Council schools in London I found 3·24 and 0·45 per cent with deviations exceeding twice and three times the standard deviation respectively, i.e., with I.Q.s of 130 and 145, instead of 2·27 and 0·13 per cent as we should expect with a strictly normal distribution ([2], pp. 161, 174f.; 4th ed., pp. 199, 218f.); the London child whom we discovered with an I.Q. of 190 (the case cited by Dr. Hollingworth in the discussion just mentioned) was encountered in a private school. However, at the time of the earliest L.C.C. surveys comparatively few parents belonging to the professional classes sent their children to the public elementary schools, and the test then used—which consisted either of those forming the original Binet–Simon scale or those adopted in our first attempts at group testing—scarcely did justice to children who were exceptionally bright. At a later date, when carrying out inquiries for the Consultative Committee of the Board of Education, we found at what were then called ' secondary schools ' 23 boys between the ages of 11 and 16 with I.Q.s of 175 or over—most of them attending ' Headmasters' Conference Schools '. But the parents of two of these ' exceptionally gifted ' children lived outside London, and three others had come to London specifically for the sake of the child's education, which reduces the number of genuine Londoners to 18. In the County of London the male population between those ages then amounted to just over 200,000 which would suggest a proportion of about 90 per million.[1]

Finally, for the benefit of readers who may feel doubtful about a purely statistical approach we may try an alternative method of estimation by following the lines adopted by Galton in his early study of genius ([7], p. 34). With this aim in view let us consider a single generation—that of men born in the

---

[1] Since the above was written, Mr. G. C. Robb, Educational Psychologist for the Lincoln and Lindsey Education Authorities, tells me that, out of 1,085 children who took the 11-plus examination in Lincoln City last year, 29 scored an I.Q. over 130 with the Moray House Test. On examining them individually with the Terman–Merrill scale (Form L) he found 7 who scored more than 170 I.Q. However, Terman himself gives the standard deviation at 11 and 12 or 18 and 20 I.Q. points. Hence on the scale we ourselves have used Mr. Robb's figure of 170 would at this age probably be equivalent to about 160 or less.

Cyril Burt

British Isles during the first 30 years of the 19th century. I choose this period rather than any other, first because with any later period it would be hard to compile an agreed list of the most eminent persons, and secondly because during an earlier period it is highly likely that many geniuses of humble origin, such as Faraday and Dickens, might have failed to develop or manifest their true powers; nor would it be easy to secure satisfactory evidence for assessing their I.Q.s.

Since few eminent people succeed in demonstrating their claim to the title of genius before they reach middle life (say 45), we must confine ourselves to those males who survived to at least that age; and for simplicity of calculation let us keep to round figures. The total number in the generation selected would be about two and a half millions. Now in the case of five men of eminence born within the period chosen—John Stuart Mill, Sir William Rowan Hamilton, Lord Macaulay, Lord Kelvin, and Sir Francis Galton—we have detailed records of their early childhood sufficient to indicate that their I.Q.s must have been approximately 200. This is already a proportion of about 2 per million. But many other equally famous names will spring to mind—men born within the same dates who reached the same level of eminence, but for whom the records of childhood are less informative. Looking through the *Dictionary of National Biography*, we find that, roughly speaking, there were well over a dozen in each of the following categories: (1) men of letters (poets, novelists, essayists, historians, etc.), (2) classical scholars and philosophers, (3) mathematicians and scientists, (4) men of eminence in industry or commerce, and rather less than a dozen (5) politicians and lawyers, and (6) men of eminence in other fields—engineers, architects, painters, musicians, explorers, military commanders, etc. This makes about 75 in all out of 2,500,000, or almost 30 per million. We are, however, frequently assured, that, owing to the handicaps of poverty and social class, there must have been in the 'under-privileged' groups quite as many 'mute inglorious Miltons' who had no opportunity to develop their latent abilities, and so died with all their music in them. To make allowance for these unknown abortive geniuses we ought at least to double the figures. We should then reach a proportion of about 60 per million.

However, a critic may object that we have hit on an unusually productive era.[1] I myself should be inclined to agree that, owing to the diminished birth-rate among the professional and upper classes and the mortality during the first world war, the proportion of those with I.Q.s of 200 or more would today very probably be smaller. Accordingly let us meet this criticism by lowering the borderline rather than the per-millionage. We might still reasonably maintain that the proportion with I.Q.s over 175 would reach, and in all likelihood exceed, the figures just cited. Thus the estimate reached by these broader considerations

---

[1] Galton's own estimate of the proportional number of 'geniuses' at the time when he was writing (1865) was 250 per million: indeed, he adopted this figure as his definition of genius. However, on scrutinizing the names in his list, it seems clear that only a small proportion of these could have had I.Q.s of over 180, and many probably had I.Q.s nearer 160. He himself assumed a normal distribution. But a careful study of his data and his analyses shows clearly that the number of those with I.Q.s over 175 is far above the figure we should deduce from a normal distribution.

would seem to be quite in keeping with that which we deduced from our Type IV curve—viz. somewhere between 60 and 80 per million.

V. Summary and Conclusions

1. A detailed analysis of test results obtained from a large sample of English children (4,665 in all), supplemented by a study of the meagre data already available, demonstrates beyond reasonable doubt that the distribution of individual differences in general intelligence by no means conforms with strict exactitude to the so-called normal curve. In the present inquiry an endeavour has been made to exclude all cases where non-genetic factors appeared to play an important part; and, in doing so, in order to forestall any suspicion as to a preconceived bias, we have always sought, wherever any doubt arose, to deal quite ruthlessly with any cases which might tend to impair the requirements of a normal distribution. When this is done, the discrepancies remaining are admittedly by no means large. Nevertheless, they appear to be fully significant statistically.

2. The main divergences are due to an elongation of the tails in both directions and to a marked tendency towards negative asymmetry. These are in fact the divergences we should expect if, as I have argued elsewhere, unifactorial as well as multifactorial modes of inheritance are the basic causes of the individual differences so found. The calculated constants suggest that the distribution actually obtained can be fitted much more appropriately with a curve belonging to Pearson's Type IV. The discrepancies between the actual frequencies and the theoretical frequencies calculated on this assumption prove to be statistically non-significant. Type IV is the type we should expect from the combined operation of the two modes of inheritance; it is also the type that yields the closest fit to the majority of distributions reported for biological data generally.

3. For many practical purposes, particularly when dealing with small samples and with children falling within a fairly limited range, the tabulated values for the normal curve will give a reasonable approximation. But they furnish very misleading assessments for the number of individuals showing an extreme deviation in either direction from the general mean. The fact that the number of *subnormal* individuals is far larger than that which would be expected from a strictly Gaussian distribution has long been suspected by various writers, both on genetic and on statistical grounds. What seems hitherto to have escaped general notice is the fact that the number of *supernormal* individuals also shows a similar though slightly smaller excess. And the evidence here summarized indicates that the current assumption of normality has led to a gross underestimate of the number of highly gifted children in the school population. Thus the proportion of those with I.Q.s over 160 proves to be more than 12 times as that deduced from the normal curve, and the proportion of those with I.Q.s over 175, instead of being only about 3 or 4 per million (assumed in several official or semi-official statements), must be at least 70 per million, probably more.

Cyril Burt

4. The data on which we have chiefly relied were for the most part obtained from investigations concerned with the standardization of the tests employed; and it is always somewhat precarious to answer questions about one set of problems from information collected primarily to answer a different set. For the more general conclusions the evidence appears fairly convincing. But the detailed figures, both for the statistical constants and for the various frequencies, may possibly need some degree of modification. In particular, for the reasons stated in paragraph 1 above it seems likely that the figures here reached may actually underrate the discrepancies between the actual distribution and that which would be inferred from the assumption of strict normality.

5. In view of the practical importance of the issues thus raised it is to be hoped that one or more of the larger educational authorities will in the near future plan and carry out a systematic survey with the express purpose of securing more exact and trustworthy specifications.

REFERENCES

[1] BURT, C. (1917). *The Distribution and Relations of Educational Abilities.* London: P. S. King.

[2] BURT, C. (1921). *Mental and Scholastic Tests.* London: P. S. King. 4th ed. (1962), Staples Press.

[3] BURT, C. (1935). *The Subnormal Mind.* London: Oxford Univ. Press.

[4] BURT, C. (1957). The distribution of intelligence. *Brit. J. Psychol.*, XLVIII, 161–175.

[5] CLARKE, A. M. and A. D. B. (1958). *Mental Deficiency.* London: Methuen.

[6] ELDERTON, W. P. (1938). *Frequency Curves and Correlation.* Cambridge: At the University Press.

[7] GALTON, F. (1869). *Hereditary Genius.* London: Macmillan.

[8] HOLLINGWORTH, L. S. (1942). *Children Above 180 I.Q.* New York: World Book Company.

[9] MAYER-GROSS, W., SLATER, E., and ROTH, M. (1954). *Clinical Psychiatry.* London: Cassell.

[10] McNEMAR, Q. (1942). *The Revision of the Stanford–Binet Scale.* New York: Houghton Mifflin.

[11] PENROSE, L. S. (1954). *The Biology of Mental Defect.* London: Sidgwick & Jackson.

[12] *Report of the Mental Deficiency Committee* (1929). London: H.M. Stationary Office.

[13] Scottish Council for Research in Education (1933). *The Intelligence of Scottish Children.* London: University of London Press.

[14] Scottish Council for Research in Education (1949). *The Trend of Scottish Intelligence.* London: University of London Press.

[15] SHEPPARD, W. F. (1903). New Tables of the probability integral. *Biometrika*, II, 174–190.

[16] TERMAN, L. M. (1925). *Mental and Physical Traits of a Thousand Gifted Children.* Stanford: Stanford. Univ. Press.

[17] TERMAN, L. M. and MERRILL, M. A. (1937). *Measuring Intelligence.* London: Harrap.

[18] THORNDIKE, E. L. *et al.* (1927). *Measurement of Intelligence.* New York: Teachers' College, Columbia University.

[19] YULE, G. U. and KENDALL, M. G. (1937). *An Introduction to the Theory of Statistics.* London: Griffin.

PART III

DEVELOPMENT AND CONSTANCY OF THE IQ

A concept like the IQ is only useful, scientifically and socially, if it remains relatively constant under considerable variation of external circumstances; clearly, if a child had an IQ of 80 today and one of 150 tomorrow, or if an adult changed from 120 to 50 without incurring some sort of brain damage, or senile decay, we would not be able to use a person's IQ for any predictive purpose whatever—unless, of course, we could link the change with some form of environmental interference, planned or unplanned. The constancy of the IQ has therefore become a problem of considerable interest, but the answer to the question posed is not a simple one, such as: "The IQ is constant," or: "The IQ is not constant." The facts are very complex, and subject to many qualifications. The most important point to be remembered is, of course, that the IQ is remarkably constant after adolescence, and until senescence. During this time, crystallized intelligence remains at the same level, or even rises gently; fluid intelligence declines gently, to fall more drastically with the arrival of senescence. But the relative standing of individuals remains quite constant; there are few if any marked changes in IQ. Thus for adults (i.e. persons over 17 years of age, for the purpose of this comparison) it may with justice be said that the IQ is constant. To say this does not mean to imply that this constancy is due entirely or mainly to congenital causes; most people have finished their schooling at 17, and little further learning takes place in their lives which might alter their relative standing (except that many of the brightest go to University, or have some form of further education). Thus both the hereditary and the environmental hypothesis would predict relative constancy of mental level after the completion of schooling; specially designed experiments are required to answer the nature-nurture question.

Prior to the age of 17, however, we encounter a much more complex problem, and the three papers here reprinted may serve as an introduction and a summary to the problems and solutions encountered. There are several excellent follow-up studies, in which children have been tested repeatedly over the years; these furnish us with the information on which any descriptive hypothesis must be based. Anderson's "overlap" theory, described in detail in his paper, and discussed and criticized by Thorndike in the following one, has been widely accepted. This hypothesis is discussed in detail by Bloom (1965); essentially it deals with the relationship between the first measurement (in point of time) of a given variable, such as height or IQ; the second measurement of the same variable on the same sample of subjects after a lapse of time t; and the difference (or gains) from the first to the second measurement. If the relationship between first measurement and difference (gains) is zero, the correlation will be equal to the ratio of the two standard deviations ($\sigma X_1/\sigma X_2$). "Although all longitudinal data do not show this zero relationship between initial measurement and gains ($rX_1 (X_2-X_1)$), many of the studies do show relationships which approximate zero." (Bloom, 1965, pp. 27). Anderson hypothesized that the correlations in longitudinal data are a direct function of the percent of the development at one age which has been attained at an earlier age. His formulation of the Overlap Hypothesis assumes an absolute scale with equal units and a defined zero; it presents an obvious development of Thurstone's pioneering approaches to scaling, or those of Thorndike (1927) and Heinis (1924).

Actual studies of children come up against one difficult hurdle which must be understood before the actual data can be judged. Tests covering the first 18 months are largely concerned with motor and physical development skills (Maurer, 1946; Hofstaetter, 1954). Tests after the age of 4 are highly saturated with cognitive skills and verbal ability. The tests used for children between 18 months and 3 years are often combinations of these two types of ability. Furthermore, tests for very young children are usually very unreliable, particularly when only administered once. When these difficulties are overcome by statistical means (correction for attenuation; use of motor test scores as suppressor variables) the following relationships emerge (Bloom, 1965, Pp. 61). Terminal intelligence correlates with IQ at the age of 3 to the extent of about .65; with IQ at the age of 5 to the extent of about .80; and with IQ at the age of 8 to the extent of about .90. "After age 8, the correlations between repeated tests of general intelligence should be between $+.90$ and unity." (Remember that these values apply to correlations corrected for attenuation). Bloom uses absolute scaling methods applied to empirical data, and concludes that "the absolute scales for the development of intelligence when related to Anderson's Overlap Hypothesis do account for the increasing correlations between intelligence test scores as the measurements approach a terminal or critical age" (p. 65). He concludes that, in terms of terminal IQ (at age 17), "at least 20% is developed by age 1, 50% by about age 4, 80% by about age 8 and about 92% by age 13. Put in terms of intelligence measured by age 17, from conception to 4, the individual develops 50% of his mature intelligence, from ages 4 to 8 he develops another 30% and from ages 8 to 17 the remaining 20%. This differentially accelerated growth is very similar to the phenomenon we have noted . . . with regard to height growth."[*] Pointing out the very rapid growth of intelligence in the early years, Bloom mentions the "possible great influence of the early environment on this development. . . . We would expect the variations in the environments to have relatively little effect on the IQ after age 8, but would expect such variation to have marked effect on the IQ before that age, with the greatest effect likely to take place between the ages of about 1 to 5."

The figures quoted by Bloom do not actually support the view of great environmental effectiveness before the age of 5, even if they could be accepted as they stand, and in spite of the criticisms made by Thorndike in the paper here reprinted. They are equally compatible with a genetic maturation hypothesis, according to which most maturation takes place before the age of 5. What Bloom would be entitled to say would be that if there were any independent evidence that environmental influences determine individual differences in adult IQ to any large extent, then these influences are most likely to be effective at a very early (pre-school) age. Such a formulation leaves open the question of nature and nurture, which, as stated before, requires quite different types of empirical and experimental investigations for a proper answer. Longitudinal experiments are very important in their own right; they cannot in the nature

of the case answer questions they were not designed to answer.

We can now, however, answer the question of the constancy of the IQ. Up to the age of 5 or 6, prediction of terminal IQ is decidedly hazardous; by the age of 8, prediction is reasonably accurate for most scientific and social purposes. The precise answer to the question of the age at which prediction is sufficiently accurate depends of course on the problem in question; the figures quoted will serve as a sufficient guide. In terms of the general question posed, we may say that the IQ is not constant at early ages of childhood, becomes more constant as the child grows up, and achieves a satisfactory degree of constancy after the age of 8. Lack of constancy at an early age does not mean that terminal IQ is not predetermined in some sense; it simply means that it cannot be predicted from knowledge of the IQ measures at the early age. Better prediction can be made by special selection of test items (Maurer, 1946), or by using a regression formula on parental IQs. This dependence of terminal IQ on parental IQ is interesting, but again should not be interpreted in terms of either an environmental or a genetic hypothesis concerning the determination of individual differences in intelligence; both these theories, as well as any form of interaction hypothesis, could account for the facts. A later section will deal with the facts of familial correlations, and the deductions which may be made from these.

As we shall see in the next section, there are several primary mental ability factors in addition to general intelligence, and it is of interest to ask whether these grow in much the same way as g. Thurstone (1955) has used cross-sectional data for large groups of children (ages 5 to 19) in order to derive an absolute scale for the tests in his Primary Mental Abilities series. Gompertz equations were fitted to three parameters based on these data: (1) the adult level, which is the asymptote which the average performance approaches with increasing age; (2) the zero point, i.e. the point on the scale at which the dispersion of performance reaches zero; (3) the relative rate at which the asymptote is approached. Using 80% of adult performance as his index for comparing different abilities, Thurstone finds that the Perceptual Speed factor reaches this level at age 12; Space and Reasoning do so at 14; Number and Memory at 16, and Verbal Comprehension at 18; Word Fluency does not do so until after the age of 20. These values are suggestive, but of course require checking by proper longitudinal studies. As they stand the results suggest quite clearly that different mental abilities develop at different rates from each other, and from g.

The paper by Thorndike which concludes this section makes some cogent criticisms of the overlap hypothesis. It may be useful to state an alternative hypothesis recently put forward by Jensen (1973). Starting from the usual pattern of correlation coefficients between individuals tested at different ages in a longitudinal study, in which the size of the correlations is largest near the

---

[*] These conclusions, based as they are on correlations, must be regarded with some caution. If we applied the argument on which they are based to Bloom's own figures for height, then we would conclude for the data given for height at the age of 4 that adults would grow to be 6 ft. 7 ins., which even a casual look around will render unlikely as a true description of reality.

leading diagonal and decreases more or less regularly the further away they are from the diagonal, he points out that this corresponds to Guttman's *simplex* model. The theory of the simplex is rather well understood, and Jensen asks what kind of model will produce a simplex in this situation. As he points out, "only two basic elements are required: (1) a rate of *consolidation* factor, C, on which individuals maintain their relative positions in the population over the course of development, and (2) a random increment or gain, G, from time x to time $x+1$ (t_x to t_{x+1}). An individual's status, S, at any given time consists of the sum of $C \times G$ over all previous time plus the G of the immediate past. In effect, the consolidation factor C is a positive constant for a given individual; the gain factor G is a positive random variable in each time interval $t_x — t_{x+1}$. An individual's growth curve can then be presented as follows:

$t_1 : G_1$ (Gain since t_0)

$t_2 : CG_1 = S_2$ (Consolidated gain from time 1 to time 2 plus unconsolidated gain at time 2 = status at time 2.

$t_3 : CG_1 + CG_2 + G_3 = S_3$
$t_4 : CG_1 + CG_2 + CG_3 + G_4 = S_4$
$t_n : C(G_1 + G_2 + G_3 + G_4 + \ldots + G_{n-1}) + G_n = S_n$

Actually, only one element is needed for a simplex, the random G element in the following model (as would be the case if $C=1$ or was the same constant value for every member of the population). But this one-element model, consisting of cumulating random increments, as we shall see, would be too simple to reproduce all the essential characteristics of the growth curves and intercorrelations actually found in such characteristics as intelligence, stature, and achievement, e.g., the predictability or predetermination of the individual growth curves' asympotic values implied by the substantial heritability of these characteristics.

Can we make a reasonable psychological interpretation of this model? The S values, of course, are no problem; they are simply the achievement measurements taken at different times. They are composed of consolidated gains, CG, plus unconsolidated gains, G, plus random errors of measurement, e.

The consolidation factor, C, is a variable which is more or less intrinsic to the individual; it is that aspect of individual differences in S values in the population at any cross section of development which may be attributed to genetic and constitutional factors (which are not distinguishable in this model per se). The term consolidation as used here does not refer to the consolidation of short-term memory traces into long-term storage, but to the assimilation of experience (i.e., learning) into cognitive structures which organize what has been learned in easy stages that subsequently permit quick and adequate retrieval and broad transfer of the learning in new relevant situations. Stated in simplest terms, C is the process of understanding what

one has learned. It is "getting the idea," "catching on," having the 'Aha'!" experience that may accompany or follow experiencing or learning something, and the relating of new learning to past learning and vice versa. When learning takes place without C acting upon it, it is less retrievable and much less transferable for use in solving problems that are more or less remote from the original learning situation. C is what is generally meant by the term *intelligence*, but it can be manifested, observed, and measured only through its interaction with experience or learning. There can be learning without intelligence (i.e., without C) but intelligence cannot be manifested without learning. In our simple model we have represented the capacity for consolidation as a constant value for each individual; this is not an essential feature, although a more or less constant rank order of individuals' C values is essential. On the average, over the life span the C value probably increases up to maturity, levels off at maturity, and gradually declines in old age. Our concept of C comes very close to R. B. Cattell's concept of *fluid intelligence*. All intelligence tests measure S, but some tests reflect more of the C component (which Cattell would call tests of fluid intelligence) and some reflect more of the G component (which Cattell would call tests of crystalized intelligence).

The gain factor, G, consists of experience or learning and unconsolidated (or rote) memory of such learning. But is G properly represented as a random variable in our model? Consider the following quite well established empirical findings. Learning abilities (which do not involve problem solving) have been found to show quite low, often negligible, correlations with intelligence. (For an excellent review, see Zeaman and House, 1967). Moreover, a general factor of learning ability has not been found. There is a great deal of situation specific or task specific variance in learning, making for very low or even zero correlations among various kinds of learning. Therefore, learning *per se* in the vast variety of conditions under which it occurs in real life, cannot show much correlation, if any, with relatively stable individual difference variables such as intelligence.

Furthermore, consider the relative unpredictability or randomness of the individual's day-to-day experiences or opportunities for learning this or that, and the poorly correlated other variables, such as attention, motivation, and persistence, that can affect learning at any given moment. All these factors within a given interval of time, add up in effect to a more or less random variable. It should be understood that random does not mean uncaused. A child may come down with measles and have to stay out of school for 10 days and so miss out on a good many school learning experiences. Another child may miss out for a few weeks because his family moves to another city. Another child may learn a great deal for a period when the teacher is presenting something that especially interests him. And so on. The gains (or lack of gains) in any short period, though caused by a multitude of factors, appear in effect to be more or less random in the school population."

On Jensen's model, then, intelligence can be thought of psychologically as that aspect of mental ability which *consolidates* learning and experience in an integrated, organized way, relating it to past learning and encoding it in ways that permit its retrieval in relevant new situations. The products of learning become an aspect of intelligence (or are correlates of intelligence) only when they are organized and retrievable, generalizable and transferable to new problem situations. The G component is on this account largely a function of environmental influences, interests, motivation, and the like, acting at any given time; C, on the other hand, is genetically and constitutionally determined. The evidence that G is more related to environmental factors while C is genetically determined, has been well reviewed by Bloom (1964, 113–119). This accounts for the fact that accelerated achievement gains brought about by an enriched and intensified instructional program generally "fade out" in a few months to a year; without a strong C factor, accelerated gains are not maintained without constant rehearsal of the acquired knowledge or skill. Other deductions from his hypothesis are made by Jensen, and the largely confirmatory evidence reviewed. It seems to fit the facts better than the overlap hypothesis, and is likely to take its place in the near future.

REFERENCES

BLOOM, B. S. *Stability and change in human characteristics.* London: Wiley, 1965.

HEINIS, H. La loi du developpement mental. *Arch. de Psychol.* 1924, *74*, 97–128.

HOFSTAETTER, P. R. The changing composition of "intelligence": a study in T-technique. *J. gene). Psychol.*, 1954, *85*, 159–164.

JENSEN, S. R. *Educability and group differences.* London: Methuen, 1973.

MAURER, K. M. *Intellectual status of maturity as a criterion for selecting items in pre-school tests.* Minneapolis: Univ. of Minnesota Press, 1946.

THORNDIKE, E. L. *The mesurement of intelligence.* New York: Teachers College, Columbia Univ., 1927.

THURSTONE, L. L. The differential growth of mental abilities. Chapel Hill, N.C.: Univ. of North Carolina Psychometrics Laboratory, No. 14. 1955.

ZEAMAN, D. & HAUSE, B. J. The relation of IQ and learning. In: R. M. Gage (Ed.) *Learning and individual differences.* Columbus: Bobbs Merrill, 1967.

From R. L. Thorndike (1933). J. Educ. Psychol., *24*, 543–549. *Copyright* (1933), *by kind permission of the author and the American Psychological Association*

THE EFFECT OF THE INTERVAL BETWEEN TEST AND RETEST ON THE CONSTANCY OF THE IQ

ROBERT L. THORNDIKE

Columbia University

There are reported, in the psychological literature, a number of experiments in which a group of individuals, generally children, were tested with the Binet intelligence test and then retested after an interval. Commonly, coefficients of correlation have been computed between the IQ's on test and retest. These correlations vary widely, as do also the intervals between test and retest. The purpose of this paper is to bring together the results of these various experimenters and, by the method of least squares, determine how the coefficient of correlation varies with the interval between test and retest.

Rather than fit a curve to the obtained values of r, whose sampling distribution is badly skewed in the high values that we are considering, and whose standard error depends upon the value of the true correlation in the population, we have converted all our r's to z's, as defined by R. A. Fisher, and fitted our curves to the z's. The conversion equation is

$$z = \tfrac{1}{2}\{\log (1 + r) - \log (1 - r)\}. \qquad (1)$$

z has the advantages (1) that its sampling distribution approaches the normal for the size samples that we have to consider and (2) that its standard error is independent of the value of the true correlation in the population. When N is the number of individuals in the sample, the standard error of z is

$$\sigma_z = \frac{1}{\sqrt{N - 3}}. \qquad (2)$$

In fitting our curves by least squares, it was necessary to assume that the time interval between test and retest was known accurately. This was not the case. In some samples the interval was the same for all individuals and was known with a high degree of accuracy, while in others it varied for different individuals over a rather wide range. The original experimenter would say that "the children were tested and then retested after an interval of from twelve to twenty-four months." It would perhaps have been desirable to fit a curve by making the sum of the perpendicular distances from the points to the line (after both the time and z had been divided by their variances) a minimum. But as the variance in each direction was different for each point, it was not

The Journal of Educational Psychology

possible to apply this method with the knowledge at hand. The only alternative seemed to be to assume that the time interval between test and retest was definitely known, not using those results in which the range of times included in a given correlation was too great.

Experimenter	N	t, months	r	z
Cuneo and Terman	25	0	.95	1.832
Lincoln	30	0	.95	1.832
Brown	221	0–12	.91	1.528
Cuneo and Terman	21	5–7	.942	1.755
Randall	103	0–18	.798	1.093
Rosenow	69	7½ or 11 (Mn. 10.25)	.82	1.153
Berry	351	6–18 (Mn. 11)	.74	.950
Baldwin	173	12	.901	1.475
Garrison	298	12	.88	1.376
Garrison and Robinson	131	12	.88	1.376
Garrison and Robinson	131	12	.92	1.589
Gray and Marsden	100	12	.883	1.389
Gray and Marsden	42	12	.834	1.201
Rugg and Colloton	137	10–16	.84	1.221
Brown	149	14 (Av.)	.87	1.333
Brown	320	12–24	.87	1.333
Cuneo and Terman	31	20–24	.852	1.263
Berry	273	19–30 (Mn. 23)	.67	.811
Baldwin	139	24	.817	1.147
Garrison	127	24	.91	1.528
Garrison and Robinson	131	24	.91	1.528
Gray and Marsden	42	24	.839	1.218
Randall	37	19–30	.699	.866
Brown	149	29 (Av.)	.70	.867
Brown	99	24–36	.88	1.376
Gordon	44	30.7 (Av.)	.84	1.221
Berry	82	31–48 (Av. 35)	.56	.633
Baldwin	105	36	.797	1.091
Gray and Marsden	42	36	.843	1.231
Randall	6	31–42	.793	1.079
Madsen	34	41	.85	1.256
Brown	41	36–48	.87	1.333
Baldwin	71	48	.786	1.062
Garrison	43	48	.83	1.188
Randall	6	43–66	.801	1.101
Baldwin	37	60	.812	1.133

We finally included the results of thirteen experimenters in our work, and fitted curves to thirty-six correlations which they give.

Effect of Interval between Tests and Retests

We list below the data to which our curves were fitted. Column I gives the name of the experimenter; Column II lists the number in each sample; Column III gives the available information about the interval between test and retest; Column IV gives the value of r obtained; Column V gives the value of z.

In the remainder of this paper, t will be understood to mean the interval between test and retest in months. w signifies the weight applied to a given point. Each point was weighted by the reciprocal of its variance, that is, by $(N - 3)$.

We first fitted a straight line to the data. The equation is of he form $z = A + Bt$, where A and B are determined from the equations

$$A \Sigma w + B \Sigma wt = \Sigma wz$$
$$A \Sigma wt + B \Sigma wt^2 = \Sigma wtz \tag{3}$$

Substituting numerical values, we get

$$3732A + 71{,}080B = 4{,}624.76$$
$$71{,}080A + 1{,}795{,}298B = 84{,}038.26$$
$$A = 1.415, \; B = -.00916 \tag{4}$$

The best-fitting straight line is

$$z = 1.415 - .00916t \tag{5}$$

The theoretical variance from the trend line of a point of unit weight is unity. The observed variance from the trend line of a point of unit weight is given by the equation

$$s^2 = \frac{\sum_{i=0}^{n} v_i^2 (N_i - 3)}{n - 2} \tag{6}$$

where v is the difference between the observed z and the z determined by the equation and n is the number of points from which the trend line was determined. s^2 is found to be 6.1845. The agreement between the observed and theoretical variances may be tested by the fact that

$$\frac{(n - 2)}{\sigma^2} s^2 = \chi^2 \tag{7}$$

with $(n - 2)$ degrees of freedom. As $n - 2 = 34$, we must test the agreement by making use of the fact that $\sqrt{2\chi^2} - \sqrt{2(n - 2) - 1}$ is normally distributed with mean at zero and standard error of unity for samples of this size. In this case, $\sqrt{2\chi^2} - \sqrt{2(n - 2) - 1}$ comes out to be 12.33. This value could practically never arise by chance, so we may feel sure that our observed variance is significantly greater than is to be expected from theoretical considerations.

This great excess of observed over theoretical variance may be open to a variety of explanations. In the first place, a straight line may not adequately fit the data at hand. That this is not one of the more important causes of the excess variance is shown by the fact that (as we shall see) a second degree curve does not reduce the variance of the residuals greatly. We believe the chief causes of the unduly large variance to be (1) variation in the adequacy of testing and retesting from experimenter to experimenter and (2) different ranges of ability among the different groups examined.

Knowing the variance of a point of unit weight, it is possible to compute the variances and standard errors of the coefficients A and B in equation (5). Consider the determinant

$$\begin{vmatrix} \Sigma w & \Sigma wt \\ \Sigma wt & \Sigma wt^2 \end{vmatrix}$$

Let us call this determinant Δ. It can readily be shown that

$$\sigma_A{}^2 = \sigma_z{}^2 \frac{\Delta_{11}}{\Delta} \qquad \sigma_B{}^2 = \sigma_z{}^2 \frac{\Delta_{22}}{\Delta} \tag{8}$$

These variances are correlated with one another, so the ordinary tests of significance do not hold, but a comparison of the values of the coefficients with their standard errors gives us some information about the importance to be attached to the coefficients. The standard errors of the coefficients as found to be

$$\sigma_A = .082 \qquad \sigma_B = .0015$$

Inasmuch as the coefficient of the linear term is six times its standard error, we may feel reasonably sure that there is a real drop in the value of z as t increases.

We then fitted a second degree curve to the data by the equations

$$A\Sigma w + B\Sigma wt + C\Sigma wt^2 = \Sigma wz$$
$$A\Sigma wt + B\Sigma wt^2 + C\Sigma wt^3 = \Sigma wtz$$
$$A\Sigma wt^2 + B\Sigma wt^3 + C\Sigma wt^4 = \Sigma wtz^2 \tag{9}$$

These become

$$3{,}732A + 71{,}080B + 1{,}795{,}298C = 4{,}624.76$$
$$71{,}080A + 1{,}795{,}298B + 56{,}796{,}141C = 84{,}038.26$$
$$1{,}795{,}298A + 56{,}796{,}141B + 2{,}125{,}501{,}513C = 2{,}060{,}510.93$$
$$A = 1.616, \qquad B = -.0301, \qquad C = .000409 \tag{10}$$

Effect of Interval between Tests and Retests

The equation is

$$z = 1.616 - .0301t + .000409t^2 \tag{11}$$

The variance of a point of unit weight is now given by the formula

$$s^2 = \frac{\sum\limits_{i=0}^{n} v_i^2(N_i - 3)}{n - 3} \tag{12}$$

and is found to be 6.0497. This is such a slight reduction from the variance from the straight line that it seems doubtful whether the second degree equation is much of an improvement over the straight line. When we compute the standard errors of the coefficients A, B, and C we get

$$\sigma_A = .148, \qquad \sigma_B = .0132, \qquad \sigma_C = .000248$$

Again the values of the standard errors are correlated with one another, so we do not know exactly what they signify, but the fact that the quadratic term is only 1.65 times its standard error suggests that this quadratic term is not of very great importance.

It is possible to convert either the linear or the quadratic equation back into an equation in r, to show how r decreases with an increase in t. We convert the linear equation as follows:

$$z = \tfrac{1}{2}\{\log(1 + r) - \log(1 + r)\}_i^j$$
$$e^{2z} = \frac{1 + r}{1 - r}$$
$$r = \frac{e^{2z} - 1}{e^{2z} + 1}$$
$$r = \frac{e^{2.830 - .01832t} - 1}{e^{2.830 - .01832t} + 1}$$
$$r = \frac{16.96e^{-.01832t} - 1}{16.96e^{-.01832t} + 1}$$

The values of r for different values of t can be shown in tabular form as given below.

t	r
0	.889
10	.868
20	.843
30	.814
40	.781
50	.743
60	.698

The Journal of Educational Psychology

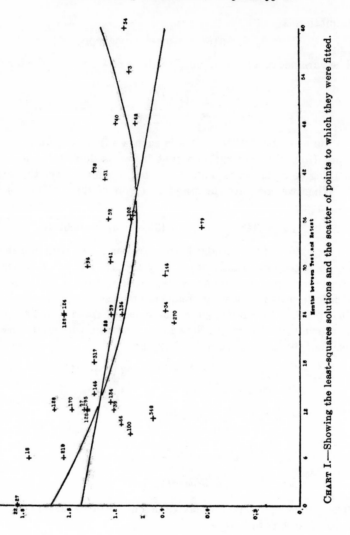

CHART I.—Showing the least-squares solutions and the scatter of points to which they were fitted.

Effect of Interval between Tests and Retests

In Chart I we show graphically the scatter of points to which the curves were fitted (each point is marked with its own weight), and the linear and quadratic curves which were determined as fitting the points.

In conclusion, we can say that the correlation between Binet test and retest falls off as the interval between tests is increased. As far as we have been able to determine, a linear equation expresses the relationship between t and z adequately. Our least squares solution for this line is

$$z = 1.415 - .00916t.$$

BIBLIOGRAPHY

Baldwin, B. T. and L. I. Stecher: Additional Data from Consecutive Stanford-Binet Tests. *Iowa Univ. Studies*, Vol. II.

Berry, C. S.: The Intelligence Quotients of Mentally Retarded School Children. *School & Soc.*, Vol. XVII, pp. 723–729.

Brown, A. W.: The Change in Intelligence Quotients in Behavior Problem Children. *J. Ed. Psychol.*, Vol. XXI, pp. 341ff.

Cuneo, I. and L. M. Terman: Stanford Binet Tests of One Hundred Twelve Kindergarten Children, and Seventy-seven Repeated Tests. *Ped. Sem.*, Vol. XXV, pp. 414–428.

Garrison, S. C.: Additional Retests by Means of the Stanford Revision of the Binet-Simon Tests. *J. Ed. Psychol.*, Vol. XIII, pp. 307–312.

Garrison, S. C. and M. S. Robinson: A Study of Re-tests. *J. Ed. Research*, Vol. XI, pp. 190–196.

Gordon, K.: Some Retests with the Stanford-Binet Scale. *J. Ed. Psychol.*, Vol. XIII, pp. 363–365.

Gray, P. L. and R. E. Marsden: The Constancy of the Intelligence Quotient—Further Results. *Brit. Jour. Psychol.*, Vol. XV, pp. 169ff.

Lincoln, E. A.: The Reliability of the Stanford-Binet Scale and the Constancy of the Intelligence Quotient. *J. Ed. Psychol.*, Vol. XVIII, pp. 621–626.

Madsen, I. N.: Some Results with the Stanford Revision of the Binet-Simon Tests. *School & Soc.*, Vol. XIX, pp. 559–562.

Rosenow, C.: The Stability of the Intelligence Quotient. *J. of Delinquency*, Vol. V, pp. 160–173.

Randall, F. B.: A Study on the Constancy of the IQ. *School & Soc.*, Vol. XXVI, pp. 311–312.

Rugg, H. and C. Colloton: Constancy of the Stanford-Binet IQ as Shown by Retests. *J. Ed. Psychol.*, Vol. XII, pp. 315–322.

From J. E. Anderson (1939). J. Psychol., Fig. 8, 351–379, by kind permission of The Journal Press, Massachusetts

THE LIMITATIONS OF INFANT AND PRESCHOOL TESTS IN THE MEASUREMENT OF INTELLIGENCE[*][1]

Institute of Child Welfare, University of Minnesota

JOHN E. ANDERSON

The practical application of intelligence tests and the scientific and theoretical problems opened up by them, have been so valuable that they constitute one of the greatest achievements in the modern study of man. Recently, however, some of the assumptions of modern test theory have been called into question. Wellman (23, 24, 25, 26), Skeels (15, 16, 17, 18), and Skodak (19, 20), in a series of articles, state that scores on intelligence tests are determined by environmental opportunities and imply that inherited factors are of little or no weight. Children, with nursery school experience, made better scores on subsequent intelligence tests than did children without such experience. Foster children, tested in infancy, increased in test score when placed in good homes. Children in a good orphanage environment increased in test score over those in a poor orphanage environment. These results, all of which are based on infant or preschool tests as origins, are interpreted to show that a favorable environment produces great changes upward and an unfavorable environment great changes downward in *true* intelligence. It is not the purpose of this paper to analyze these studies in detail, but to concern itself with certain problems of theory which raise the question as to the reliance to be placed upon infant and preschool tests as measures of the function later known as intelligence.

In my opinion the projection of these Iowa results into the heredity-environment controversy is most unfortunate. The interpretation of test results obtained on young children presents basic methodological problems that have as yet been only partially attacked and which render hasty generalization dangerous. This is true even if we accept the Iowa results as presented, independent of the interpreta-

---

[*]Received in the Editorial Office on June 14, 1939, and published immediately at Provincetown, Massachusetts. Copyright by The Journal Press.
[1]Assistance in the preparation of these materials was furnished by the personnel of Works Progress Administration Official Project No. 665-71-3-69.

tion put upon them. Because early tests may measure different functions than do those given later in the developmental sequence, it is possible that the prediction from early scores of both terminal status and the final series of interrelations with other factors, is hazardous. If to this hazard there is added that of constant errors arising out of the emotional reactions of the child, the prediction of ultimate interrelations becomes doubly hazardous.

The traditional criteria for the standardization of intelligence tests have been: first, increase in score with chronological age; second, the correlation of test performance with ratings of brightness; third, the correlation of test performance with composite academic achievement; and fourth, the correlation of items with total score, i.e., internal consistency. Of these, the first and the second were used by Binet, and the third and fourth by subsequent investigators. In the derivation of intelligence test scales for young children, only one of these criteria—that of progression with chronological age— has been consistently used.

THE CRITERION OF TERMINAL STATUS

Because of the use of the criterion of age progression, infant scales consist very largely of motor items. It has long been known that the total scores based on infant scales show zero or very low positive correlations with intelligence test scores at later ages (2, 6). Recently Richards and Nelson (10, 11, 13) found that the items in infant scales correlate in different degrees with total intelligence test scores at 2 and 3 years and suggest that by item analysis and weighting through partial correlation the correlations of infant scales with later measures may be raised. Unfortunately, their reported increases could not be checked on a separate group from that on which the validation was done, and so few items were available that a final answer on the possibilities of weighting and item selection could not be obtained. In any event, however, their results suggest the possibility of developing infant scales of greater predictive value, if the techniques of item analysis are applied to the selection of individual items, and if performance at later age levels can be used as a criterion against which to check items at earlier levels. The criterion suggested in this paper, then, is that of evaluating items in terms of a later or final mental status.

In spite of the Wellman and Skeels results, intelligence tests

JOHN E. ANDERSON

will continue to be used for practical and predictive purposes. What is it that we wish to measure? Is it present standing or the level that will be reached when development is complete? Strong arguments could be made for either position. *This paper, however, assumes that in making the best possible prediction of terminal status, we will also make the best measurement of present status, in so far as our concern is with potentiality rather than achievement.* When tests are used in clinic or court, interest is in terminal status, i.e., at the age of 9 years, we wish to forecast status at 12 or 16 years. If this reasoning is sound, measuring instruments should be developed for the highest possible prediction of final standing and, in addition to the criteria ordinarily used, items should be selected in terms of their correlation with final status. With the use of this criterion, some of the items now included in our scales might be eliminated, and others now on the borderline with respect to present criteria might be included.

The use of this criterion would impose upon a series of subtests and items a selective device related in some respects to the criterion of internal consistency. It should result in tests that are more homogeneous in terms of content and underlying psychological functions and in a clear delimitation of that which is now defined as intelligence. So far as our present infant and preschool tests are concerned, it would involve a thorough reworking of the field. The problems here raised grow out of longitudinal studies, and would not have arisen in that period when cross-section studies held the stage.

Correlations with Initial and Terminal Status

A number of investigators have commented on the decrease in the correlations of successive measures with an initial measure. It is especially evident in the Bayley (2) studies of growth in mental functions. Robert Thorndike (21) has fitted curves to the earlier data obtained from intelligence tests at older age levels, but did not then have the data on the earlier age levels now available and in which the phenomenon is particularly striking.

Honzik (9) made a very interesting analysis of the relation between mental test constancy and the interval between tests. She obtained an age ratio by dividing chronological age on the first test by chronological age on the second test and then correlated this ratio with the correlation coefficients obtained between the tests. She finds

JOURNAL OF PSYCHOLOGY

the correlation between 22 age ratios and the corresponding r's for *Cal*. I to be $+.92\pm.02$. For *Cal*. II, the figure is $.78\pm.06$. Thus higher correlations are found between tests that are closer together in time and lower correlations between those separated by longer intervals.

Honzik also finds that a test at 21 months gives a negligible prediction of success on the Stanford-Binet at 6 or 7 years, and that later tests are increasingly predictive of such success. She interprets her results as suggesting the impossibility of making an accurate prognosis of the future ability of a child on a single mental test before the age of two. Her data are so important that a detailed analysis of them is made later by means of the methods developed in this article. Although somewhat less attention has been paid to the increase in the correlation of successive measures with terminal status, it is an equally marked phenomenon in longitudinal studies.

In the Bayley (2) study, the correlations of mental tests at successive periods from 1 to 36 months show a striking decrease (from .57 to —.09) as we move away from initial status and a striking increase (from —.09 to .80) as we move toward terminal status (Table 1).

TABLE 1

BAYLEY RESULTS

Age	With initial status 1, 2, and 3 mos.	With final status 27, 30, and 36 mos.
1, 2, and 3 mos.		—.09
4, 5, and 6 mos.	.57	.10
7, 8, and 9 mos.	.42	.22
10, 11, and 12 mos.	.28	.45
13, 14, and 15 mos.	.10	.54
18, 21, and 24 mos.	—.04	.80
27, 30, and 36 mos.	—.09	

In Table 2 similar coefficients from the Honzik (9) study are presented. In this study the Stanford-Binet results at 6 and 7 years are also available as measures of final status.

Here again the phenomenon of progressive decrease in correlations with initial status and progressive increase in correlations with terminal status are apparent.

I was unable to find longitudinal studies on older children which presented correlations at successive ages with initial and terminal status. However, Hirsch (8) presents the intelligence quotients for each child in his study for six successive retests at yearly intervals,

JOHN E. ANDERSON

TABLE 2

HONZIK RESULTS

Age	Relia-bility	Guidance		Control		Cal. I		Cal. II	
		Initial 1.90	Final 7.00	Initial 1.90	Final 7.00	Initial 1.90	Final 7.00	Initial 1.90	Final 7.00
1.9	.83		.42		.19		.30		.26
2.0	.80	.68	.46			.74			
2.6	.89	.59	.38			.65			
3.0	.84	.47	.56	.59	.54	.58	.57	.46	.54
3.6	.92	.50	.63	.47	.59	.59	.59	.35	.58
4.0	.94	.46	.66	.33	.53	.41	.59	.34	.58
5.0	.95	.32	.73	.43	.72	.39	.69	.42	.76
S-B									
6.0		.30	.81	.30	.83	.32		.17	
7.0			.42		.19		.30		.26

starting with a group that originally was between 6 and 8 years of age. The correlations obtained from reworking his data and including only the 150 cases that had the entire six tests are presented in Table 3. It should be noted that the span covered at each suc-

TABLE 3

RECALCULATED DATA FROM HIRSCH STUDY

Age	Mean	σ	With first test 6-8 yrs.	With final test 11-133 yrs.
6- 8 yrs.	102.91	13.55		.800
7- 9 yrs.	106.74	12.95	.868	.770
8-10 yrs.	106.75	14.39	.824	.773
9-11 yrs.	107.01	16.46	.787	.828
10-12 yrs.	107.79	19.00	.839	.902
11-13 yrs.	111.46	19.51	.800	

cessive yearly measurement is 3 years of chronological age, rather than one year or less, as is true of the other data in this paper.

In this table the correlations of intelligence quotient with initial status decrease from .868 to .80, while those with final status increase from .800 to .902 over a five-year span.

From the data of the Harvard Growth study (4), I selected 135 boys and 130 girls, on whom 10-year records were complete and calculated the correlation coefficients for mental age at each year level, with the mental age at 7 years as initial status and mental age at 16 years as terminal status. Unfortunately, the children in this study were not given the same mental tests year after year. This operates to reduce the correlations by decreasing their reliability and

JOURNAL OF PSYCHOLOGY

makes the data much more unsatisfactory for our purposes than would be data obtained throughout from the same test scales. In spite of this deficiency a trend is clear which justifies further analysis. The results are presented in Tables 4 and 5.

TABLE 4

CALCULATED DATA ON 135 BOYS FROM HARVARD GROWTH STUDY

Mean chrono-logical age	Mean mental age	*SD* mental age	Proportion initial of later meas-urements	Proportion earlier of terminal measurement	Corre-lation with initial status	Corre-lation with terminal status
7.44	90.98	14.88		46.2		.582
8.43	103.39	16.98	88.0	52.5	.735	.641
9.42	113.11	19.45	80.4	57.4	.697	.581
10.43	128.79	23.56	70.6	65.4	.726	.744
11.42	146.69	24.87	62.0	74.5	.670	.752
12.42	159.36	23.26	57.1	80.9	.642	.790
13.41	163.81	20.52	55.5	83.1	.659	.778
14.41	169.33	22.62	53.7	86.0	.653	.829
15.42	185.13	28.65	49.1	94.0	.606	.901
16.42	197.02	31.03	46.2		.582	

TABLE 5

CALCULATED DATA ON 130 GIRLS FROM HARVARD GROWTH STUDY

Mean chrono-logical age	Mean mental age	*SD* mental age	Proportion initial of later meas-urements	Proportion earlier of terminal measurement	Corre-lation with initial status	Corre-lation with terminal status
7.41	94.74	12.07		45.7		.542
8.40	108.35	16.41	87.4	52.3	.651	.584
9.40	117.98	18.01	80.3	56.9	.604	.533
10.40	133.95	20.15	70.7	64.6	.719	.700
11.40	148.75	22.29	63.7	71.8	.668	.728
12.39	161.56	22.92	58.6	78.0	.655	.776
13.39	166.98	19.21	56.7	80.6	.642	.812
14.39	175.08	20.78	54.1	84.5	.632	.822
15.39	194.37	28.58	48.7	93.8	.569	.906
16.39	207.22	29.63	45.7		.542	

For the boys the correlations with initial status decrease from .735 to .582, while those for the girls decrease from .651 to .542. For the boys the correlations with terminal status increase from .582 to .901, while those for the girls increase from .542 to .906. In connection with these tables it should be noted that a mental

JOHN E. ANDERSON

age standardization forces the results into a linear framework[2] with equivalent increments of mean mental age and standard deviation for each chronological year. Examination of the columns in Tables 4 and 5, presenting the means and standard deviations of mental age at each year level, reveals this to be approximately the case though the increments from year to year vary enough to indicate some inaccuracy in standardization. They are probably more irregular than they would have been, had the same scale been used throughout.

TABLE 6
CORRELATIONS WITH INITIAL STATUS AT DIFFERENT AGE LEVELS

| Honzik | | Harvard | | |
With 1.9 years age		With 7 years age	Boys	Girls
2 yrs.	.68	8 yrs.	.735	.651
3 yrs.	.47	9 yrs.	.697	.604
4 yrs.	.46	10 yrs.	.726	.719
5 yrs.	.32	11 yrs.	.670	.668
6 yrs.	.30	12 yrs.	.642	.655

In Table 6 the correlations from the Honzik data and the Harvard Growth study are compared over a six-year span; the correlations for initial status being with 1.9 and 7 years, respectively.

In Table 7 similar data for terminal status are presented, the correlations being with 7 and 16 years, respectively. Although the

---

[2]The linearity imposed by mental age scaling becomes of some importance for the subsequent discussion, since it proved difficult to interpret the correlations which were also calculated with initial and terminal measurements for height and weight at successive year levels. The facts that the growth curves for height and weight are sigmoid in character and that different individuals reach their final heights at different ages result in increments at some levels that are negatively correlated with previous status. Hence the curves for the relation between successive correlations with initial and terminal status for height and weight at different levels and the proportion of growth attained calculated directly from the measurements, possess peculiar characteristics which deserve more extensive analysis and treatment in another article. But the coefficients do decrease away from initial status and increase toward terminal status. Thus for the boys the correlations for height with initial status at 7 years decreased from .982 to .876, while those for the girls decreased from .988 to .799. For the boys the correlations for height with terminal status at 16 increased from .876 to .967, and for girls the increase is from .799 to .994. For boys' weight the correlations with initial status decrease from .906 to .740, and for girls' weight decrease from .923 to .734. For boys' weight the correlations with terminal status increase from .740 to .921, while for girls' weight the increase is from .734 to .956.

JOURNAL OF PSYCHOLOGY

TABLE 7
CORRELATIONS WITH TERMINAL STATUS AT DIFFERENT AGE LEVELS

Honzik With 7 years age		Harvard With 16 years age		
			Boys	Girls
2 yrs.	.46	11 yrs.	.752	.728
3 yrs.	.56	12 yrs.	.790	.776
4 yrs.	.66	13 yrs.	.778	.812
5 yrs.	.73	14 yrs.	.829	.822
6 yrs.	.81	15 yrs.	.901	.906

data are not as perfect or as comparable as one would wish, nevertheless it is clear that the coefficients obtained later in the developmental course are significantly higher than those obtained earlier and that the correlations with initial status drop much more rapidly in the earlier ages. Correlations with terminal status build up more rapidly in the earlier ages, but do not reach as high a level within a comparable span. It is unfortunate that a complete series from 2 to 16 years on the same children is not available. Such a series would make possible a much more adequate check of the principle involved.

THE CONCEPT OF OVERLAP

Obviously we deal here with a phenomenon in which we are basing our prediction of final status upon a larger and larger proportion of that which is included in the total, i.e., scores at 10 years include a larger proportion of that which is present at 16 years, than do scores at 3 years. We can then inquire into the nature of the relation between an earlier and a later measure when successive measurements include a larger and larger part of that which makes up final status and a smaller and smaller part of that which makes up initial status. In order to arrive at the determining principle, two packs of playing cards from which the Kings had been removed were thoroughly shuffled. The numbers on the face of the cards were then recorded at face value, calling the Jacks elevens and the Queens twelves. The cards were again shuffled and the figures obtained added in succession to the results of the first shuffle, then the cards were again shuffled and the results obtained added to the sum of the previous two shuffles, and so on for 16 shuffles. This procedure gave scores for 96 cases, which cumulated from the first to the sixteenth shuffle. The cumulated scores at each shuffle were then correlated successively with initial score and with final score. A similar procedure was followed using the Tippett (22) tables of random numbers to make up a series of 300 scores, cumulated from the first score to the sixteenth.

The characteristic of each series is determined by the fact that the increments were uncorrelated and have a uniform mean and standard deviation. As a result the means at successive levels resulting from the cumulation of the increments increase by a constant amount, while the standard deviations increase in systematic fashion. By obtaining the ratio of the means at each successive level to the initial mean and terminal mean, the proportionate amount of overlap can be obtained, and the correlations obtained can be plotted against these percentages or proportions.

The formula for handling the problem of overlapping is found in the coefficients of determination and non-determination, which measure the amount of association between two measures, or the extent to which the variance in one variable is determined by that in the other variable (5, 7, 12). Since $r^2 + k^2 = 1$, r^2 becomes a coefficient of determination and k^2 a coefficient of non-determination. The per cent of overlapping is given by:

$$r^2 = \text{per cent overlap or } r = \sqrt{\text{per cent overlap.}}$$
$$k^2 = \text{per cent non-overlap or } k = \sqrt{\text{per cent non-overlap.}}$$

In Figure 1, the curve obtained by plotting the formula with the correlation coefficient as the ordinate and the fraction of overlap with the initial measure as the abscissa is presented, together with the results obtained from the playing card series and the random number series of cumulations. Note that the abscissa is in terms of fractions rather than percentages. In this respect Figure 1 differs from the curves presented later.

In Figure 2, the curve obtained by plotting the correlation of each successive measure with the terminal measure against per cent of overlap is presented, together with the data obtained in the playing card and Tippett number series. With a one-half or 50 per cent overlap, r is the square root of .50 or .707, with a one-fourth overlap r is the square root of .25 or .50, etc. It is clear that the results obtained with the playing card series and the random numbers fit the formula. The cumulation, however, fits least well as

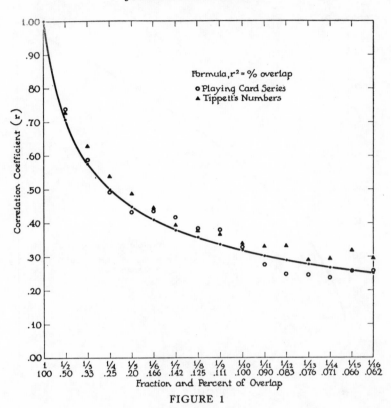

FIGURE 1

we move farthest from the initial measure in Figure 1 and as we move farthest from the terminal measure in Figure 2. Obviously the chance variation between single sortings of cards or single series of random numbers is greater than between cumulations. Thus a chance variation in the initial sorting will affect earlier measures in the descending series less when they are a larger part of the total, than later measures when they are a much smaller part of the total. For the ascending series the reverse relation is true: i.e., the relation between the first sorting and the cumulation of 16 sortings is less stable than the relation between the cumulation of 15 sortings and the cumulation of 16 sortings.

We may then suggest the principle that the earlier in a develop-

JOHN E. ANDERSON

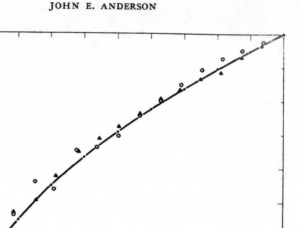

FIGURE 2

mental series a measurement is taken the less predictive it will be of final status and the later it is taken the more predictive it will be, and inquire as to the conditions under which the principle will hold. It may hold only if the increments, as in the playing card series or random number series, are uncorrelated, or if the increments correlate with previous position in varying but moderate degrees. If the increments are perfectly uniform, it will not hold because the relative positions at successive periods will be unchanged as a constant will be added uniformly to each score. It will not hold if the increments are differential with respect to original scores and always perfectly correlated with them, because only a fanning out of the individual growth curves will result. If, then, correlations

JOURNAL OF PSYCHOLOGY

with terminal and initial status for mental test data show the characteristics of the curves obtained from the use of playing cards and random numbers, it would appear that the process of mental growth is one in which the increments either are not exactly constant or proportional to the original measures from which they start, or one in which that which is measured at different periods is composed of different elements or functions which overlap the initial and the terminal measures in content and function to different degrees. It is likely that both of these alternatives are characteristic to some extent of mental growth as measured by intelligence tests.

If now we ask what a measurement of a living organism, such as one of height, is, we see that it is a composite, i.e., total body length includes leg, trunk, and head length, each of which proceeds at a different rate and reaches its points of flexion and terminus at different times. The head grows rapidly in infancy and slowly in adolescence, legs grow slowly at first and more rapidly later. Weight is again a composite made up of the weights of skeleton, muscle, body organs, etc., each with its own characteristic growth pattern. If we think of intelligence in somewhat similar terms, we see it likewise as a composite of many different functions, each with its own characteristic growth pattern. It is unfortunate that, because we lack the means of measuring in absolute units these functions and their total, we must throw our measurements into a mental age standardization with its framework of linearity. Nevertheless we are led to a concept of the prediction of final status in terms of overlapping elements in earlier measures, and of a progressive differentiation of the structures and functions which go to make up the composite whole. We deal ultimately then not with increments of a single function, but with the resultant or combination of a series of increments spread over a variety of changing and growing functions. In this sense, the intelligence quotient as a measure of rate is an abstraction, which in so far as it shows constancy measures elements that are common to a number of functions. Moreover, at any particular level the intelligence quotient measures present status, and gains its predictive value only from the fact that positive and high correlations have been shown to hold for successive determinations.

We may now ask whether or not the coefficients obtained for mental test results at successive periods in longitudinal studies fit the formula given for determining overlap. In the nature of the

JOHN E. ANDERSON

case, this is a difficult question to answer, because of the fact that intelligence te:t scores are far from being perfect measures of whatever they measure. Not only are different tests used at different levels in the data which we have available, but also whatever tests are used, the problem of the reliability of the measures arises. The two sets of data analyzed in this study are the Honzik data, obtained in the early years, for which reliability coefficients are available, and the Harvard Growth data at the later age levels for which reliability coefficients are not available.

In Figure 3, the curves for the decrease in coefficients[3] with successive measurements are plotted in terms of the proportion the initial measure is of later measures. For the Harvard Growth study data these proportions could be calculated directly from the material presented in Tables 5 and 6. For the Honzik material, since the actual results are not available, the mean mental age at any level was assumed to correspond to the chronological age, and the chronological age at the time of the first measurement was divided by the chronological age at later levels of measurement. This is the same ratio that Honzik herself used, and is probably not as accurate for the problem of this paper as actual mental age figures would be. I suspect that the curve for the Honzik data lies too far to the left, and that the fit would be closer had the actual mean mental ages been available. The Honzik data has been corrected for attenuation, using the reliability figures given in Column 1 of Table 2. The coefficients from the guidance group presented in Table 2 were used.

For the Harvard Growth data, the original coefficients from Tables 5 and 6 were used, together with the same series of coefficients corrected for attenuation, by assuming the reliability[4] at age 7 to be .85, age 8 .86, and so on, adding .01 to the reliability with each year of age. This makes the assumed reliability at the terminal measure .94. The resulting curves are plotted in Figure 3.

---

[3]In examining Figures 3 and 4, the reader should keep in mind that the initial measurement for the Honzik data is at 1.9 years and the terminal measure at 7 years, while the initial measure for the Harvard data is at 7 years and the terminal measure at 16 years.

[4]I also corrected the coefficients of the Harvard data for attenuation by assuming reliabilities of .95, .90, and .85 throughout the whole age span. The effect of correcting for attenuation is to move the curves upward, nearer the curve given by the formula. On the whole, the best assumption seemed to be that of a slight increase in reliability with increase in age. Except for raising the whole level of the curves, the effect of correction upon the form of the curve is negligible.

JOURNAL OF PSYCHOLOGY

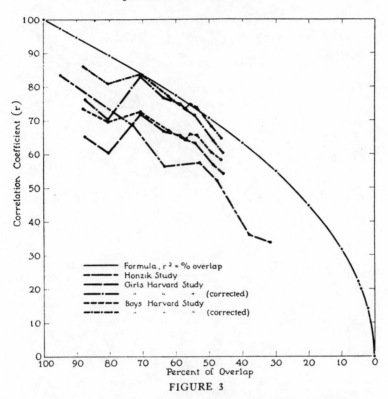

FIGURE 3

It is clear from Figure 3 that in general form the curves obtained approximate the curve for the formula, but that they lie under it. The Harvard Growth curves are approximately 10 points of r under the curve, the Honzik data approximately 15 points of r under it. With corrections for attenuation the Harvard data from the 9-year level on, come close to the formula. The data in the Harvard series for the 7- and 8-year measurements, when the Dearborn group Test A was used, are erratic in both curves and tables.

In Figure 4 the curves for correlation with terminal status are presented. These curves are subject to the same limitations as the data on which Figure 3 is based. When corrections for reliability are made, the curves are raised but never come quite up to the formula curve.

JOHN E. ANDERSON

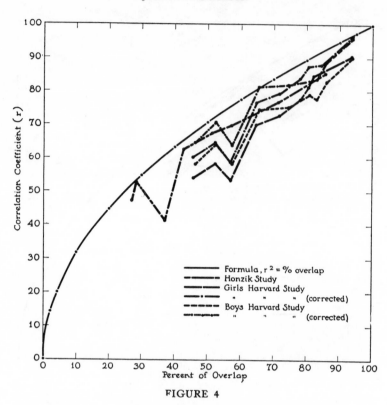

FIGURE 4

Whatever question may be raised with reference to the accuracy with which the data obtained fits the formula, it is clear that the phenomenon of the increase and decrease of correlation coefficients as we move toward terminal status or away from initial status is one that is related to the per cent of overlap between the measures.[5]

_____

[5]It is possible that by reversing the formula for overlap we might use it as a device for measuring the amount of mental growth completed at any particular age level in relation to the final level achieved, i.e., a correlation, corrected for attenuation, of .707 between a measure at 10 years and a terminal measure at 16 years, might be interpreted as indicating that 50 per cent of the elements that go to make up the final constellation, intelligence, had been achieved by that age. Before, however, any such use can be made, the correlations between each successive measurement and the terminal measure should be maximized through item analysis and the

JOURNAL OF PSYCHOLOGY

Since the formula gives the curves for this relation when increments are uncorrelated, the question why the curves for the obtained data fall below rather than above the formula curve can well be raised. At the present time this cannot be answered. If there were consistent increments from age to age, plus commonalty of factors in the tests, the coefficients would tend to lie above the formula curve. If the increments were uncorrelated with previous status, but were of the same order from year to year, i.e., possessed identical means and standard deviations, the situation that exists in the playing card series and the random number series would hold and there should be close approximation. Since the curves lie under the expected curve the factors that are to be sought are (*a*) unreliability of the measures, which we know if corrected, brings the curves nearer expectancy; (*b*) differences or variations in the content of the tests from year to year, which would serve to reduce the intercorrelations; (*c*) small variations in the means and standard deviations of the increments which are apparent if one goes back to Tables 4 and 5, and which may result from poor standardization of the original tests, and (*d*) negative correlations of increments with previous status. If the latter holds it would give some weight to the view that the concept of the constancy of the intelligence quotient is of more significance for grouped measures than for individual cases. In this connection it should be pointed out that mental growth seems not a matter of increments that are proportionate to the original measures in the sense that increments occur in the functions described in physics or mechanics, but is rather one of increments that are differential with respect to both the stage of growth reached and the unique pattern of variation in the individual.

Moreover, it is clear that the constancy of the intelligence quotient is in large measure a matter of the part-whole or overlap relation, since the growing individual does not lose what he already has attained. The farther he is along in the growth process, the smaller proportionate part are the increments which are added. Thus with linear age scaling, an increment of one year at 10 years is one-tenth of what has been attained, while an increment of one year at 3 years

selection of test components, and every precaution taken to see that the test is an adequate and accurate measure of the function involved. Since this paper is not concerned with this possible use of the formula, it is only mentioned.

JOHN E. ANDERSON

is one-third of what has been attained. If the true form of the mental growth curve is a parabola, as some writers maintain, this phenomenon is even more striking. After 10 cumulations in the playing card and random series, the correlations are .80 or above—figures comparable to those for mental tests—but produced entirely by uncorrelated increments.

Certainly these data suggest the desirability of a re-examination of the whole problem of individual increments in intelligence quotient in longitudinal series, using accurately standardized tests and the best possible conditions of testing. If this paper leads those who have or are in a position to secure extensive longitudinal series of data on children to a re-examination of the problem of constancy in the light of the concept of overlap, and age increments, it will have fulfilled its purpose.

RELATION TO OUTSIDE FACTORS

The relation between a measure of intelligence and measures of any other functions at successive intervals, may change in accordance with the principle of overlap. Thus a relation may be high in the early years and decrease, or be low early and increase with development. Successive measures, then, can be viewed as indicators of more or less of that which is associated with the outside variable. A striking example is furnished in the study by Bayley and Jones (3), in which scores on mental tests at successive age levels were correlated with measures of parental and socio-economic status. Table 8 presents in shortened form several series of the relations they report.

TABLE 8

MENTAL SCORE WITH DIFFERENT MEASURES: BAYLEY AND JONES

Age in months	Mother's education	Father's education	Father's occupation	Total SE scale
1 + 2 + 3	—.15	—.07	—.12	.12
4, 5, 6	—.23	—.26	—.26	—.10
7, 8, 9	—.01	—.09	—.05	—.04
10, 11, 12	.06	—.06	.01	.05
13, 14, 15	.03	—.11	—.09	—.10
18	.12	—.10	—.06	—.10
21	.37	.19	.16	.15
24	.52	.39	.35	.34
36	.46	.28	.23	.04
48	.50	.37	.31	.22
60	.48	.53	.43	.36
72	.58	.50	.38	.41

The correlations of mental test score with mother's education, father's education, father's occupation, and standing on the socio-economic scale are predominantly zero or negative up to the age of 21 months and then become positive and increase in size until a maximum seems to be reached. The tests seem to measure more and more a factor which is associated with these other variables. How are these results to be interpreted?

In the Skeels' (15, 16) studies, the low correlations ($+.04$ to $+.12$) between the mental test scores of children tested at a median age of 18.8 months and measures of the true parents are interpreted as indicating a lack of relationship between the intelligence of the child and that of the parents. In view of the extensive literature on parent-child resemblances, this absence of relationship might well be viewed with suspicion and a question as to what the tests measure raised. But Skeels assumes that the tests are true measures of intelligence and goes on to make generalizations about the effects of environment upon intelligence that are opposed to the findings of many other investigators. Likewise the zero or negative coefficients between the infants' scores and the education of their foster parents ($-.05$ to $+.10$), are also suspicious in view of the positive coefficients of the order of .20 so commonly reported in the literature as the result of selective placement. If the principle put forth in this paper is correct, it is dangerous to interpret low coefficients of resemblance between parent and child based on infant tests as meaning that a parent-child relation in ability does not exist. Rather should we ask the question whether the tests which show such a lack of relationship are measuring the same configurations of ability that tests of older children measure.

Bayley and Jones (3) clearly recognize this problem when they say:

> From previous work, the hypothesis has emerged that test performance during the first 18 months is not diagnostic of intellectual ability. This is based partly on the greater community of function found between motor and mental scores in infancy (correlations are of the order of .5 during the first 15 months, after which age the relationship drops markedly). More directly pertinent is the fact that early mental test performance is uncorrelated with mental scores made after two years, even when a selection of the most "intellectual" items is used for comparisons. This emphasizes the fact that the

JOHN E. ANDERSON

increasing correspondence between mental score and environmental variables is not necessarily attributable to the influence
of the environment; it may equally well be a phenomenon
of infant development, that inherited parent-child resemblances
become evident only after a certain stage in the process
of maturation has been reached. Evidence can be adduced
in favor of each of these interpretations; the probability is that
each has some validity, and that the growth of children involves both an increasing assimilation of environmental pressures and an increasing manifestation of complex hereditary
potentialities. The extent to which these factors interpene-
trate, and their relative importance, cannot be stated in general
terms, since the answer must vary according to the function
involved, the age level, and the central tendency and variability of each set of impinging factors.

The Use of an Early Score as an Origin

We may regard *true* intelligence as a parameter of which the
actually measured intelligence in terms of a particular test at any
particular time is an approximation. The problem of the age level
at which this approximation is the most accurate indication of *true*
intelligence then arises. But this is a double problem. First, does
true intelligence change with age and, second, do tests given at
particular age levels approximate more or less the parameter intelligence than do tests given at other ages of developmental periods?

To the first of these questions there is no clear answer at the
present time. That there is absolute growth in intelligence cannot
be doubted. But is this growth an increase in level, i.e., quantitative
or is it both an increase in level and a change in kind, i.e., qualitative
as well as quantitative? Thurstone's attempt to determine primary
mental abilities and to study their age relations may make a significant contribution. To the second of these questions the answer
given by this paper is that measurement later in the developmental
sequence gives a closer approximation than does an earlier determination. This is precisely the opposite of the assumption made by
Wellman and Skeels, who match children with respect to intelligence on the basis of early tests, and, second, consistently use test
results obtained in infancy or early childhood as the origin from
which to make calculations of increments and gains. While it may
be said that this is the only possible procedure that can be followed

JOURNAL OF PSYCHOLOGY

in a longitudinal study, nevertheless *the adequacy with which a particular test measures what it purports to measure, has to be determined in terms of its correlation with tests at later ages before it can be used as an origin, in those instances in which an attempt is made to measure a particular function, and it is assumed that the changes that occur take place only in that function.* A low correlation between the initial test and the terminal test in a series would tend to make both unsatisfactory as origins, whereas a high correlation would make both satisfactory. To some extent the case that Wellman and Skeels make for gains breaks down if the principle is accepted that the earlier a measurement is made the less predictive it is of final status and the more it is subject to both constant and random errors and it is assumed that the same function is tested throughout. Because of the extraordinary importance of the first measurement when it is used as an origin in a series, every precaution should be taken to insure its validity and reliability and the avoidance of constant errors. The latter would involve the use of several tests or forms rather than one or the repetition of the test after a short interval of time, discounting any gains made during that interval.

In this connection it may be said that workers in the mental test field have always placed different valuations upon particular types of tests. Thus performance tests are given when verbal tests cannot be used because of a handicap or deficiency in training. Beta was used for illiterates in the Army, when Alpha could not be used. It may well be that tests given prior to three years are to be regarded in much the same light as substitutes for better measures which cannot be used because of age limitations. But if this is the case every precaution should be taken to maximize their correlations with measures of intelligence at a later level when we know it is well measured, just as we standardize performance tests by reference to standard tests of a verbal or symbolic character.

The problem of the use of early tests as origins from which to calculate gains or losses is closely related to the problem of whether or not they are adequate measures for attacking the heredity-environment problem. If correlations with later tests are of the zero order and if correlations with measurements of the true mother or with secondary measures such as mother's education or father's occupational status known to be of some size later on, are of zero order,

JOHN E. ANDERSON

the question of the validity of an early test as an origin from which to calculate gains or as a device to measure the inheritance of intelligence must be met, since the zero order relations may result from deficiencies in the measuring instrument itself.

THE PROBLEM OF PAIRING AT EARLY AGES

Suppose that two groups of children are paired on the basis of infant or preschool test performance and that these scores show decreasing correlations with subsequent test performances. What are the chances that the two groups will be equivalent at subsequent periods? This is an important question in the set-up of a longitudinal experiment. If other factors, such as the hereditary factors, have not been controlled in the sampling, they may operate in successively greater amounts to produce differentiation between the groups, i.e., it is perfectly possible that there may be a spurious matching of the groups and that later on they may diverge quite widely irrespective of the type of training received. Thus, if we suppose two groups matched at the age of one year with the coefficients with initial status decreasing by 10 points each year, the amount of overlap may be indicated by the formula for determination as follows:

	2 Yrs.	3 Yrs.	4 Yrs.	5 Yrs.	6 Yrs.	7 Yrs.	8 Yrs.
Correlation		90	.80	70	.60	.50	40
Per cent overlap	100	81	64	49	36	25	16

There would seem to be no guarantee that the groups matched at 3 years will still be matched at 6 or 7. Thus it is quite possible that matching children on the basis of an initial score will not produce matching at any subsequent period for characteristics or traits that are subsequently differentiated on the basis of maturation.

If the principles brought out in this paper hold, it should be possible to do a much more effective job of matching from the measurements of children's intelligence at 7 or 8 years, when the correlation coefficients with final status are of the order of 60 or more, than from measurements prior to 3 years when the coefficients with a measure of terminal status, such as that at 7 years, are around .40, or below (see Tables 2 and 4). The value of the matching procedure will increase as the measurements are taken later in the age sequence and the more effectively the infant and preschool tests predict final status. Further, if correlations with initial status decrease, it will always be possible to select a number of striking individual cases which will show consistent gains or losses from an early determination as a base, and in extreme cases, gains and losses of very large amounts.

It is also likely that the results obtained from the use of matching or control group techniques in which other variables, such as mother's education or mother's intelligence quotient, are used for selecting the groups will be affected. Thus, if one were to select a group of mothers of low intelligence quotients, and a group of mothers of average intelligence quotients, and measure the mental level of their children at successive ages, the phenomenon described in this paper would result in a series of decreasing intelligence quotients for the children of the mothers with low intelligence quotients, while the intelligence quotients of the children from mothers of average intelligence quotient would show little or no change with age. On the basis of regression the mental level of the children of the mothers of low intelligence quotient would fall halfway between the mean mental level of the mothers and that of the general population. But if the original tests measure little of that which is finally measured in an intelligence test, the earliest measures of the children from the mothers of low mental level would tend to fall about the mean of the population, and then as intelligence is measured more and more accurately, to move from that position to the true intermediate position. Irrespective of other factors, this trend would appear. This downward trend is quite apparent in Figure 1 of Skodak's study (20, p. 307) or Figure 12 (19, p. 90). Likewise, children from an hereditary background of high level would fall near the mean of the population on early tests and show a marked upward trend as intelligence was measured more and more accurately. Perhaps also this phenomenon explains why early training *seems* to be so much more important in producing the desirable effects found in the Iowa studies than is late training.

The Effect of Constant Errors

Throughout this paper the early tests in a series have been assumed to be reliable. When reliability coefficients were available, it was found that by correcting for attenuation there was closer approxima-

JOHN E. ANDERSON

tion to the formula for overlap or determination. When, however, a factor is present which produces large errors and these errors are in a constant direction, the correlations with both terminal and initial status and with any outside measure would be seriously affected. While no data is available which enables me to evaluate such errors in terms of initial and final status, many investigators have raised the question as to the effects of resistance or negativism upon the determination of the intelligence quotient of young children. Resistance is a much greater problem at the preschool than the older age levels. Modern scales have taken some account of this factor by eliminating those items and tests which children often refuse and substituting those which have more intrinsic interest. The Merrill-Palmer Scale includes a method of correcting for refusals which clearly recognizes the existence of this factor. One of the most interesting investigations of the phenomenon was made by Rust (14), who gave 3-year-old children both Kuhlman-Binet and Merrill-Palmer tests, repeating those tests which were refused (not those failed) on successive days a second, a third, and a fourth time, etc., until the children either definitely passed or failed them. The results from this study, as presented in Table 9, indicate significant changes

TABLE 9

INCREASE IN INTELLIGENCE QUOTIENT FROM FIRST TO FINAL PRESENTATION
Rust (14)

Points	Kuhlman-Binet	Merrill-Palmer I*	Merrill-Palmer +
25-35	7	2	0
15-24	18	3	0
5-14	26	38	3
1- 4	14	14	26
Unchanged	31	42	70
Total	96	99	99

*Not corrected for refusals.
+Corrected for refusals.

in intelligence quotient level, as a result of recording on the basis of ultimate success or failure on the items.

On the Kuhlman-Binet only 31 out of 96 intelligence quotients were unchanged, and in 51 out of 96 cases the change upward in the intelligence quotient ranged from 5 to 35 points. Somewhat similar, but not as striking results were obtained for the Merrill-Palmer, when the scores were not corrected for refusals. When corrected for refusals the changes were slight, as shown by the last column in the table.

On the basis of this study negativism seems to result in a constant error in the direction of lowering the intelligence quotient. If such a factor is present the relations of preschool tests to terminal mental level will be seriously affected. In formulating criteria for the selection of tests and test items, then, some account must be taken of the emotional reactions elicited by the tests. It is likely that many items in which this factor is pronounced would be automatically eliminated by the application of the criterion of relation to terminal status, because of the low relationships that will inevitably result. But despite this, in preparing and standardizing tests for young children, it would seem to be both profitable and necessary to subject items to rather rigorous selection in terms of the emotional reactions and resistance they elicit. However perfectly this is done, there would still be somewhat greater likelihood of variation in rapport for younger children. And it may be pointed out that we must be very careful in interpreting the results of examinations which were given many years ago when tests were markedly subject to this constant error, *which seems always to be in the direction of a lowered score.*

If the constant errors arising out of test refusals and negativism are in the direction of a lowered score and the regression effect (becoming more and more apparent with age as the measurements increase in their capacity to measure the underlying functions) is for the low intelligence quotient group to be in the direction of a spuriously high score, as suggested in the previous section, the interpretation of the trends in curves showing change in mental level with age, becomes difficult. For here are two phenomena which may mask one another, or so distort the relations found in any particular study that any correct determination of the inter-relationships of factors cannot be made, without extensive statistical analysis and further experimentation and refinement of tests.

The Effect of Item Analysis

L. Dewey Anderson (1) has been kind enough to make available some of the results of a study he has made of the relation between early achievement on infant test items and Stanford-Binet intelligence quotients at 5 years of age. One hundred children followed in a longitudinal study from 3 months to 5 years were given from 85 to 183 test items at each of the following ages: 3, 6, 9, 12, 18, and 24 months. The items were selected from the Gesell, Linfert and Hierholzer, and Buhler scales. Dichotomous groups of 15 cases, each differing widely in intelligence quotient at 5 years, were set up and an item analysis made on the basis of which a selection was made and a new scoring done. The number of items which have significance is low at the early years, but increases at 18 and 24 months. While it was impossible for him to set up an independent group on which to validate the increases in correlation with subsequent status, he did recalculate the coefficients after item analysis and selection both for the total group and for the intermediate group of 70 cases with the cases in the dichotomous groups excluded.

Table 10 compares the predictive value of a point summation of

TABLE 10
CORRELATIONS OF INFANT TESTS WITH STANFORD-BINET AT 5 YEARS

Age	Including validation group		Eliminating validation group	
	Before analysis	After analysis	Before analysis	After analysis
3 mos.	.086	.315	.016	.144
6 mos.	.042	.413	.021	.148
9 mos.	.087	.202	.072	.178
12 mos.	.085	.200	.061	.108
18 mos.	.231	.365	.126	.179
24 mos.	.523	.550	.250	.309
N	100	100	70	70

all the items before analysis, and the predictive value after items had been selected to maximize predictive value and reliability.

After analysis there is a significant increase in correlation with Stanford-Binet results at 5 years. The results at the early levels are somewhat inconsistent when the dichotomous validation groups are included, but are quite consistent when they are not. These results suggest that item analysis and selection will produce significant increases in the predictive value of an early test for a later or terminal score.

Table 11 compares the correlation coefficients of the score of the successive tests after item selection with measures of initial and terminal status.

From these results it is clear, first, that the correlations of infant

JOURNAL OF PSYCHOLOGY

TABLE 11

CORRELATIONS WITH INITIAL AND TERMINAL STATUS AFTER ITEM SELECTION

Age	Initial 3 months	Terminal 24 months
3 mos.		.341
6 mos.	.592	.303
9 mos.	.378	.363
12 mos.	.206	.469
18 mos.	.241	.484
24 mos.	.341	
5 yrs. Stanford-Binet	.315	.550

and preschool tests with subsequent measures of intelligence can be appreciably raised and, second, that after so raising the coefficients the principle of decreasing correlation with final status still holds.

PRECAUTIONS IN THE USE AND INTERPRETATION OF EARLY TESTS

From the principles brought out in this paper several general precautions to be observed in the practical or theoretical use of measurements can be formulated. These are:

1. The earlier in the developmental course measurements are made, the less reliance can be placed on a single measurement or observation, if that measurement or observation is used for predicting subsequent development.

2. The earlier in the developmental course measurements are made, the greater care should be taken to secure accuracy of observation and record and to follow standardized procedures.

3. The earlier in the developmental course measurements are made, the more account should be taken of the possibility of disturbing factors, such as negativism and refusals, which operate as constant errors to reduce score. On young children, in particular, two tests separated in time are superior to a single test for determining status.

4. Since development is a timed series of relations or sequences, there are for many functions periods below which only a small portion of the function can be measured and above which a progressively larger portion can be measured. Hence, the possibilities of prediction are limited and progression with age is not an infallible indicator of the value of a measurement. Every effort should then be expended to secure the most accurate and predictive tests by standardizing tests against multiple rather than single criteria.

JOHN E. ANDERSON

CONCLUSION

The problem put by this paper is one that is concerned not so much with the effects of training in the early years upon mental age scores and intelligence quotients as now measured as with a return of emphasis to the selection of test materials in order that there will be present in the tests available the highest amount of the stable factor which we call intelligence, as distinct from the more unstable factor which we call achievement. Modern testing literature recognizes the existence in all measuring devices of factors that do not change greatly with experience—measurement of nature—and of factors which do so change—measurement of nurture. For practical and theoretical purposes, we need both types of measures. The effectiveness of each increases as it becomes a purified measure of what it seeks to measure. To say that it is impossible to develop such measures is to fly into the face of a very substantial literature that is in many respects the outstanding contribution of scientific psychology. The outright admission that present measures are inadequate, particularly at certain developmental levels, will facilitate scientific progress and center our attention upon the improvement of our instruments. The bald statement that intelligence is determined by environment alone, denies the possibility of any psychological measurement of innate factors or of the constitution of the human being. From Binet's time on any well-trained psychologist, knowing the basic criteria, has been able to produce a reasonably good intelligence test with high reliability in a relatively short period of time. But no psychologist, despite the expenditure of much time, effort, and money, has been able to produce a scale for measuring motor or mechanical ability or personality or character, that compares with our intelligence scales, so far as generality, coherence, or consistency is concerned. Some psychological functions do not hang together because they are markedly affected by the environment; measures of intelligence when selected in accordance with rigidly applied criteria hang together, because they seem to tap to a greater degree an inherent organization of abilities. This organization is probably not static but is achieved over a period of years.

Infant tests, as at present constituted, measure very little, if at all, the function which is called intelligence at later ages. Preschool intelligence tests, while they are instruments of some value and usefulness, measure only a portion of that function. Whether it would be possible to develop tests at these levels which measure more of that function, remains to be seen. But it is unfortunate that workers in the preschool period have used age progression as virtually the only criterion for validating their tests. With a clearer recognition of the importance of other criteria, and particularly of the necessity of maximizing correlations with terminal measures, it may be possible to develop tests of high predictive value and usefulness. But until these methodological problems are clarified, it seems futile to make sweeping generalizations with respect to the nature of intelligence on the basis of present measures in the preschool period, and especially so on the basis of present measures obtained in infancy.

REFERENCES

1. ANDERSON, L. D. Brush Foundation, Western Reserve University, Cleveland, Ohio. Article in preparation on the correlation of infant test scores with Stanford-Binet *IQ* at 5 years.
2. BAYLEY, N. Mental growth during the first three years: An experimental study of sixty-one children by repeated tests. *Genet. Psychol. Monog.*, 1933, **14**, 1-92.
3. BAYLEY, NANCY, & JONES, H. E. Environmental correlates of mental and motor development: A cumulative study from infancy to six years. *Child Devel.*, 1937, **4**, 329-341.
4. DEARBORN, W. F., ROTHNEY, J. W. M., & SHUTTLEWORTH, F. K. Data on the growth of public school children from the materials of the Harvard Growth study. *Monog. Soc. Res. Child Devel.*, 1938, **3**, No. 1, 1-136.
5. EZEKIEL, M. Methods of Correlation Analysis. New York: Wiley, 1930. Pp. xxv+429. (Pp. 117-120.)
6. FURFEY, P. H., & MUEHLENBEIN, J. The validity of infant intelligence tests. *J. Genet. Psychol.*, 1932, **40**, 219-223.
7. GUILFORD, J. P. Psychometric Methods. New York: McGraw-Hill, 1936. Pp. xvi+566. (Pp. 361-366.)
8. HIRSCH, N. D. M. An experimental study upon three hundred school children over a six-year period. *Genet. Psychol. Monog.*, 1930, **7**, 487-548.
9. HONZIK, MARJORIE P. The constancy of mental test performance during the preschool periods. *J. Genet. Psychol.*, 1938, **52**, 285-302.
10. NELSON, VIRGINIA L., & RICHARDS, T. W. Studies in mental development: I. Performance on Gesell items at six months and its predictive value for performance on mental tests at two and three years. *J. Genet. Psychol.*, 1938, **52**, 303-325.

JOHN E. ANDERSON

11. ————. Studies in mental development: III. Performance of twelve months' old children on the Gesell Schedule, and its predictive value for mental status at two and three years. *J. Genet. Psychol.*, 1939, **54**, 181-191.

12. NYGAARD, P. H. A percentage equivalent for the coefficient of correlation. *J. Educ. Psychol.*, 1926, **17**, 86-92.

13. RICHARDS, T. W., & NELSON, VIRGINIA L. Studies in mental development: II. Analysis of abilities tested at the age of six months by the Gesell Schedule. *J. Genet. Psychol.*, 1938, **52**, 327-331.

14. RUST, METTA M. The effect of resistance on intelligence scores of young children. *Child Devel. Monog.*, 1931, No. 6. Pp. xi+80.

15. SKEELS, H. M . Mental development of children in foster homes. *J. Genet. Psychol.*, 1936, **49**, 91-106.

16. ————. Mental development of children in foster homes. *J. Consult. Psychol.*, 1938, **2**, 33-43.

17. SKEELS, H. M., & FILLMORE, E. A. The mental development of children from underprivileged homes. *J. Genet. Psychol.*, 1937, **50**, 427-439.

18. SKEELS, H. M., UPDEGRAFF, R., WILLIAMS, H. M., & WELLMAN, B. L. A study in environmental stimulation. *Univ. Iowa Stud. Child Wel.*, 1938, **15**, 191.

19. SKODAK, MARIE. Children in foster homes. *Univ. Iowa Stud. Child Wel.*, 1939, **16**, 1-155.

20. ————. The mental development of adopted children whose true mothers are feebleminded. *Child Devel.*, 1938, **9**, 303-308.

21. THORNDIKE, R. L. The effect of the interval between test and re-test on the constancy of the *IQ*. *J. Educ. Psychol.*, 1933, **24**, 543-549.

22. TIPPETT, L. H. C. Random sampling numbers. *Tracts for computers, No. 15.* London: Univ. London, 1927. Pp. 55.

23. WELLMAN, BETH L. Growth in intelligence under differing school environments. *J. Exper. Educ.*, 1934, **3**, 59-83.

24. ————. Mental growth from preschool to college. *J. Exper. Educ.*, 1937, **6**, 127-138.

25. ————. Some new bases for interpretation of the *IQ*. *J. Genet. Psychol.*, 1932, **41**, 116-126.

26. ————. The effect of preschool attendance upon the *IQ*. *J. Exper. Educ.*, 1932, **1**, 48-69.

Institute of Child Welfare
University of Minnesota
Minneapolis, Minnesota

From R. L. Thorndike, J. Educ. Psychol., 57, 121–127. *Copyright* (1966) *by kind permission of the author and the American Psychological Association*

INTELLECTUAL STATUS AND INTELLECTUAL GROWTH[1]

ROBERT L. THORNDIKE

Teachers College, Columbia University

Studying growth in ability is made difficult by (a) unreliability of measures, (b) inequality of units in which measures are expressed, and (c) nonequivalence in what is measured by different instruments and at different levels. These problems are illustrated in analyses of Harvard Growth Study data, where 2 intelligence tests were given to each of 593 pupils each yr. for 6 yrs. The maximum reliability of intellectual growth appears to be about .25 or .30. An unbiased estimate of the obtained correlation of status with gain appears about .10, but this correlation has apparently been reduced by inequalities in the units of measure between (and within) instruments, and by the fact that different tests measure somewhat different functions.

Ever since psychologists began investigating individual differences, they have been interested in determining the extent to which differences in intellectual growth patterns are orderly and predictable from something that can be known about the individual relatively early in life, to what extent these differences are under the control of ascertainable and describable environmental conditions, and to what extent they are inherently erratic and unpredictable.

Much of the use of tests in education is based on the premise of stability—that the bright child at Age 8 will continue to be a bright child at Age 10 or 12. And there is abundant evidence that, within limits, this is the case. But this is stability of status —that he *is* still bright, not necessarily that he has continued to grow rapidly. As Anderson pointed out as early as 1939, a good deal of stability of intellectual *status* can be accounted for by a model that says that ability at a later date consists of ability at an earlier date plus a growth

increment that is completely uncorrelated with the earlier level of ability. Bloom (1964) has developed this theme at some length in his recent book, *Stability and Change in Human Characteristics.*

What *are* the substantive findings with respect to increments in intellectual ability? Do these increments represent an extrapolation of growth trends established at an early age? Or do they represent the addition of a random increment—random in the sense that it is completely uncorrelated with intellectual status at the beginning of the period in question?

Unfortunately, it is very hard to say. The study of change is one of the trickiest areas in which to work if one must use the fallible instruments that are the psychometrician's tools. The questions asked are simple ones: To what extent are the children who show rapid intellectual growth over one period of time the same children who had a prior history of rapid intellectual growth? To what extent are individual differences in rate of intellectual growth over an earlier period of time related to individual differences in growth rate over some later period? To simple questions we would like simple answers, and that

[1] This paper was presented in a slightly different version as a presidential address before the American Psychological Association's Division of Educational Psychology (Division 15), Chicago, 1965.

might be possible if three conditions could be met: having completely error-free measures, having measures expressed in meaningfully equal units, and having at all ages measures referring to identically the same attribute of the individual. Then gains could be correlated with initial status, and it would be possible to see to what extent initial status is related to gain or gain over one period is related to gain over another period. In the best of physical measures—that is, measures of height or weight—these conditions are approached, but when we deal with mental tests, we are distressingly far away from meeting the specifications.

Three problem areas will be examined in turn—reliability of measurement, equality of units, and comparability of function—to see how serious they turn out to be, and what the implications are for inquiry.

RELIABILITY OF MEASUREMENT

Much of this presentation will be based on some reanalyses of Harvard Growth Study data. In terms of extensiveness and continuity of testing these data are in many respects unique, but they were gathered when computing facilities were neolithic by present-day standards, and it is the author's impression that they have never been fully analyzed.

In the Harvard Growth Study that Dearborn initiated in the early 1920's, over 3,000 pupils in public schools near Boston were studied from the time they entered the first grade until they left the school system—either by dropping out, moving away, or completing the twelfth grade (Dearborn, Rothney, & Shuttleworth, 1938). A great many different anatomical and physical measures were obtained, but interest here is limited to the group-intelligence-test results, which

were obtained by first one and then two different tests each year throughout the duration of the experiment.

The present analysis is limited to the 593 cases out of the total of some 3,000 for whom complete records were available on one intelligence test at Age 8, and on two tests at each age from 9 through 14. These are, of course, group tests—the tests that were available for use in the 1920's—with whatever limitations attach to them. In all, 13 test scores expressed in mental-age units were available, spread over a 6-year period. The matrix of correlations was computed not only among the 13 status scores but also among all the difference scores generated by taking the tests in pairs. Thus the correlation of Test 9_1 with Test 10_1 and the correlation of 9_2 with 10_2 is available, together with the correlation of the difference between 9_1 and 10_1—the gain as measured by this one pair of tests—with the difference between 9_2 and 10_2—the gain as measured by another pair of tests.

With these data in hand, the problems arising from errors of measurement will first be examined. Psychologists are all quite conscious of the fact that intelligence tests fall well short of being perfectly reliable. When it is thought of at all, a correlation coefficient of .85 or .90, or, most optimistically, .95, is conceived as representing the reliability for a group homogeneous with respect to age or grade. And psychologists are all vaguely aware that change scores are less reliable than status scores. It is recognized that much of what is measured at any one point in time is common to what is measured at another point in time, and that this common component disappears when gain scores rather than status scores are used. But how *much* less reliable are the gain scores? What *is* the residual reliability of a set of change scores?

To answer this question empirically, there is within the Harvard Growth Study data a whole set of correlations between *two* gain scores, each covering the same span in the child's life, but each being based on a separate pair of tests. That is, gain based on Tests 9_1 and 10_1 can actually be correlated with gain based on 9_2 and 10_2. Some of these gains cover only a span of 1 year—9–10, 10–11, 11–12. Some cover 2 years, some 3, some 4, and one pair of correlations is for gains over 5 years. The actual average correlations are as follows: 1-year interval, .101; 2-year interval, .240; 3-year interval, .266; 4-year interval, .188; 5-year interval, .265.

It appears, then, that the ceiling for the reliability of a measure of intellectual growth based upon the administration of two group-intelligence tests, even with an interval of several years between them, is somewhere around .25 or .30. The result for individual tests might be somewhat higher, but probably not much, since the data being examined involve children 9 or 10 years old at the earlier testing. In any study involving gain scores, it must be recognized that the datum is really fragile, with a reliability that appears to lie in the range from .1–.3, depending upon the tests and the interval, and research must be planned and evaluated accordingly.

As has been repeatedly pointed out by previous critics of growth studies, the substantial amount of error variance in test scores leads to especially misleading conclusions if one attempts to correlate gains with initial status, using the same testing to provide both the initial-status score and the subtrahend in the gain score. The reason, of course, is that the error of measurement in this common test appears in the status score with a positive sign and in the gain score with a negative sign, and so generates a spurious tendency towards negative correlation based on the reversed error component. That is, if status is represented by Test A, and gain by B minus A, a positive measurement error in A results in a falsely high A score, but a falsely low gain.

The present data provide an excellent opportunity to demonstrate this effect empirically and to get some idea of its size. It is possible to do this by comparing two sets of correlations between initial status and subsequent gain. In one set, the same testing is used both to define status and to calculate gain; in the other set gains are calculated from the second set of measures. That is, if status is defined by Test 9_1, in the first case gain is defined as 10_1 minus 9_1, while in the second case gain is defined as 10_2 minus 9_2. These two types of correlations are shown in Table 1.

The average value varies somewhat with the time interval, but a roughly representative figure might be −.20 when the same test is used to define both status and gain and .10 when different tests are used in the two cases. Thus, the difference between −.20 and .10 is the magnitude of the spurious effect generated by lack of experimental independence in the data and the incorporation of a common measurement error with opposite sign in each variable.

TABLE 1

CORRELATION OF INITIAL STATUS WITH GAIN

Based on common test		Based on experimentally independent tests	
Intervals (in yrs.)		Intervals (in yrs.)	
1	−.273	1	.045
2	−.287	2	.006
3	−.283	3	.031
4	−.194	4	.139
5	−.053	5	.329

The experimentally independent correlations just cited, for which the typical value is perhaps .10, provide the best estimate of the correct and unbiased correlation between initial status and subsequent gain. It is a pretty minute correlation, but considering what has just been seen about the reliability of gain measures, its small size is not too surprising. A rough estimate can be made of what it would become if it were corrected for the unreliability of both status measure and gain measure. Using .85 and .25 as working estimates of the two reliabilities, the corrected correlation becomes about .22—still pretty unimpressive.

In the light of the results to this point, two conclusions seem reasonable. The first is that rate of gain in intelligence-test score over the school years is in large part inherently unpredictable because of the extremely low reliability of the measures of individual differences in gain. The second conclusion, which becomes rather tentative because of the situation implied by the first conclusion, is that the nonchance component in gain score is positively related, but only slightly positively related to initial status. In considerable part, the factors that produce gains during a specified time span appear to be different from those that produced the level of competence exhibited at the beginning of the period.

EQUALITY OF UNITS OF MEASURE

But it will be remembered that three requirements were stated for meaningful studies of individual differences in mental growth. So far only the effects of violation of the first condition have been considered —error-free measures. What about equality of units and homogeneity of the function being measured?

Whenever correlational techniques are applied to psychological data, it is assumed that the numerals in which the variables are expressed represent equal increments in some attribute. It is also recognized that this assumption is usually not well supported. But for "rough and ready" studies of relationship, the violation of the assumption usually does not hurt much. However, when starting to deal with something as fragile as a change score, the violation of this basic assumption becomes a good deal more critical. The variance of change scores is in some cases no more than one-fourth the size of the variance of status scores. With two measures contributing to the gain score, any variance arising from irregularity in the two tests' converted score will tend to bulk 8 times as large as a fraction of the gain-score variance.

Furthermore, any systematic shift in the size of the units, such as that produced by a test ceiling too low to permit full expression of the abilities of those tested, may produce a systematic distortion of the relationship between status and gain. With such a ceiling effect those initially highest will not be fully measured by the test at the later ages, and will necessarily show smaller increments. Thus, in the Harvard Growth Study all test results were presented in mental-age units. However, for the older groups of pupils—13- and 14-year-olds—the mental-age equivalents for the brighter fraction were necessarily extrapolated values, based on whatever type of assumption may have seemed reasonable to the test makers of the 1920's. (The test manuals are notably terse on the procedures used to set up the scale of mental-age equivalents.) If the extrapolations were made somewhat conservative, so as not to overstate a level of ability that was arbitrary and not empirically based on the age schema then in favor, the effect would be to underestimate the scale values for able pupils at the higher ages, with the result that gain scores for these pupils would be depressed. Even a small systematic depression could substantially reduce or even eliminate the necessarily small correlation between initial status and the highly unreliable gain score.

Some evidence from the present data bearing on the reality of the problem of unit of measure comes from the comparison of means and standard deviations (expressed as mental ages) of the two tests given in the same year. These are shown in Table 2. Differences in parameters for these nearly simultaneous tests cannot be attributed to growth or environmental impact or anything but the characteristics of the tests themselves. Thus, it is found that the two 9-year test means of 9-10 and 10-0, respectively, agree quite well; but for the corresponding standard deviations of 20 and 13 months, one surpasses the other by 50%. For the 10-year tests the standard deviations agree well—both are 23 months—but the two means are 11-5 and 10-3, a difference of 14 months. At 11 there is a 6-month difference between the two means and a 5-month difference in the two standard deviations. Similar, though less dramatic, differences are found at 12, 13, and 14. Clearly, the units of the *different* tests are not equivalent. One suspects that the same can be said for different segments of the score scale for a single test.

The changing standard deviation for different variables makes for quite erratic correlations between status and gain. Simple algebra reveals the fact that the sign and the size of the correlation of Status Score A with gain from Score B to Score C depends upon the relative

TABLE 2

MEANS AND STANDARD DEVIATIONS OF PAIRS OF TESTS GIVEN IN THE SAME YEAR

Ss	Test No. 1		Test No. 2	
	M	SD	M	SD
9-year-olds	118.0	19.9	119.7	13.3
10-year-olds	137.4	23.0	123.2	22.7
11-year-olds	153.6	24.4	148.1	29.4
12-year-olds	164.6	22.9	164.5	26.3
13-year-olds	167.7	22.0	176.1	24.7
14-year-olds	178.1	23.9	181.4	23.0

size of $s_C r_{AC}$ and $s_B r_{AB}$. The formula is as follows:

$$r_{A(C-B)} = \frac{r_{AC}s_C - r_{AB}s_B}{\sqrt{s_C{}^2 + s_B{}^2 - 2r_{BC}s_B s_C}}.$$

Thus a change in scale unit, resulting in a change in standard deviation, can wreak havoc upon one's results. This appeared, in our data, in the wide range of values that were obtained for the correlation of status with gain. Though a value of .10 has been suggested as best representing the relationship, this average value is based on a range of correlations from .64 to −.43 for different specific combinations of initial test and subsequent test to define gain. This variation illustrates the point that the result obtained is spectacularly responsive to distortions of the unit of measure as between the initial and final test.

One particularly misleading pastime that is sometimes engaged in, even by those who should know better, is to study the relationship between an initial IQ and the change in IQ during some subsequent period. The absurdities of this procedure become clearer if the IQ is thought of as a standard score keeping the same mean and standard deviation at each age—a characteristic that is explicitly true of recently developed tests and approximately true of those developed in an earlier day.

When the standard deviations of two sets of scores at different points in time, B and C, are forced to be equal, and the correlation of a third score, A, with the difference between the two is studied, the sign of the resulting correlation depends solely on the relative size of the two correlations r_{AB} and r_{AC}. Thus, if it is desired to study the correlation between IQ on Test A at Age 8 and change in IQ from 9–12, the only way that the correlation *can* be positive is for the 8-year-old test to correlate more highly with the 12-year-old test than with the 9-year-old test —a fairly improbable and unnatural situation. If the correlation with the later test is lower, correlation with the change score will necessarily be negative.

By eliminating from the score scale the differences in standard deviation at different ages, that which is the essence of growth is eliminated— the greater variability of specimens as they mature. Imagine a group of adults whose heights and weights showed no greater standard deviations than those of newborn babies! And a statistical treatment that automatically excludes greater variability in intellect as we go from birth to maturity is equally absurd. Thus, any studies of intellectual growth that use as a score scale an IQ with a uniform standard deviation from age to age are, by that very fact, meaningless for any analytical study of the growth process. The constraint that has been put on the score scale assures distorted results.

UNIFORMITY OF FUNCTION MEASURED

A basic assumption, if growth is to be studied, is that the same function is being measured throughout the range of ages being studied. But when intellectual performance over a range of ages is studied, it is quite usual for the particular test to change as we go from an earlier to a later age. The change in test is likely to be accompanied by some change in the functions measured by the test, depressing the consistency between early and late performance, with a resulting depression of the relationship between a status measure based on Test A and a gain measure based on Tests B and C.

The Growth Study data permit a look at this problem because there were several age spans during which the same test was used in successive years. In all, six comparisons were possible between the correlation of some test, A, used in one year with Test A in the following year and its correlation with a different test, B, the following year. In the same way, six comparisons were possible of correlations of some test, A, in a given year with Tests A and B in the preceding year. The same-test correlations with a 1-year interval averaged to exactly .80, the correlations with another test in the following year to .75, and with another test in the prior year, .73, or a pooled average of .74 for the correlation between different tests.

This means that, while identical tests showed 64% of common variance from one year to the next, with a change in test the common variance was only 55%, or only 86% as great. Nine percent of the total variance and 14% of the stably measured variance was unique to the specific test.

If this change in function measured was cumulative, so that each time a new test was introduced 14% of what was measured by the prior test was replaced with new variance unique to the new test, it would take only seven shifts before measures of completely unrelated functions were obtained. Of course, this is not the way things operate. As we go from Test A to B to C, it is likely that part of what is unique to Test C so far as Test B is concerned is shared in common with Test A. It is unlikely that a clear picture of further drop in correlation with a successive shift will be found. Thus, in the Harvard data, Dearborn C at Age 11 correlates .808 with Dearborn C at Age 12 and only .760 with Haggerty Delta 2 at Age 12; .693 with Haggerty Delta 2 at Age 13, but .685 with Terman Group at Age 13, and .736 with Terman Group at Age 14. There is no evidence of further drop as we move on to the third test, in this case the Terman Group Test.

The reduction in correlation from .80 to .74 that has just been seen in comparing same with different tests does not seem like very much, but once again reference to the formula for correlation between one status score and another change measure shows that anything that introduces even a small extraneous reduction in the size of the correlation between status and the terminal measure of the change sequence can extinguish or even reverse the sign of the correlation between status and change. Thus, though the lower correlation between different tests looks pretty unimportant as we look at the reasonably robust test scores, it becomes very significant when we are dealing with the very fragile change scores. A drop from .80 to .74 in intercorrelation could reduce the correlation between status and gain from .20 to .10, cutting it in half, or from .10 to 0, extinguishing it completely.

CONCLUSION

Thus it has been seen that change scores are very sensitive creatures, very responsive to changes in score scale and to changes in the function being measured. So perhaps we need to modify the earlier conclusion that seemed appropriate from the Harvard Growth Study data—the conclusion that only a small fraction of the gain in later competence can be thought of as arising from a continuation of early growth trends. Perhaps it must be concluded that, unless and until scales are developed that are truly homogeneous in the functions that they tap at all levels and are truly expressed in equal units, we will have to forego serious attempts to give a quantitative answer to the simple but tantalizing question: To what extent will the children who have grown rapidly in intellect up to the present moment continue to grow rapidly in the future?

REFERENCES

ANDERSON, J. E. The limitation of infant and preschool tests in the measurement of intelligence. *Journal of Psychology,* 1939, **8,** 351–379.

BLOOM, B. S. *Stability and change in human characteristics.* New York: Wiley, 1964.

DEARBORN, W. F., ROTHNEY, J. W. M., & SHUTTLEWORTH, F. K. Data on the growth of public school children. *Monographs of the Society for Research in Child Development,* 1938, No. 14.

(Received September 13, 1965)

PART IV

TYPES OF INTELLIGENCE

The assumption is sometimes made that the term intelligence, in order to be meaningful, has to be inviolate; the recognition of several different factors of ability has seemed fatal to its scientific survival. It is not clear why that should be so. The atom was originally thought to be incapable of subdivision; the fact that we now have a host of elementary particles which go to make up the atom has not destroyed the usefulness or meaningfulness of the atomic concept. The belief that "intelligence" must be unitary or "univocal" in order to survive seems itself a survival of an early historical phase in which Spearman (1927) was thought to have put forward a simple, clear-cut two-factor theory, in which only g (general intelligence) and a number of s (specific) factors identical with the number of tests included in the analysis were recognized. Similarly, Thurstone (1938) was believed to have put forward a view which excluded g completely, and centred entirely on a variety of primary mental abilities. These notions are at best a caricature of the real views of these men, and in some ways are quite erroneous. Spearman acknowledged the existence of such group factors (to use Burt's term) as verbal ability and fluency (a factor which many years later was revived under the title of "originality" or "divergent ability"), and Thurstone, once he broadened his work to include a more representative sample of the population than high-level University students, acknowledged the existence of a general factor, derived from the intercorrelations between his primaries (Thurstone & Thurstone, 1941). Both, in fact, came close to the position held since the publication of his 1911 paper by Burt, who advocated a hierarchical structure in which g and primary abilities (group factors) played an important part. Even Thurstone's original 1938 paper contains evidence to support such a hierarchical scheme, as the reanalysis of his matrix of intercorrelations reprinted here makes clear. There is still a difference in emphasis between the British and the American schools, with the former preferring to extract g first, and restrict themselves to just a few of the most important primaries,

while the latter prefer to extract the primaries first, and then go on to the extraction of higher order factors from the matrices of intercorrelations between the primaries. But no difference in principle is involved in all this.

Those who have criticized Spearman have often failed to pay attention to the conditions he laid down for the discovery of g. He specified that there should not be undue similarity between the tests used, as such similarity would lead to overlap of functions (s's) causing correlation over and above that due to g, and he specified that tests should be administered to representative samples of the population. Thurstone's first paper violated both conditions, and is consequently not relevant to a consideration of Spearman's theory. Clearly, if we reduce the differences in g within our population by only testing very bright University students, we do not give g a proper chance to emerge. It is as if we measured the body build of a sample made up of English policemen, all of whom must be at least 6 feet tall; this so much reduces differences in height that it is doubtful if a factor of height would emerge—as it does from less selected samples. When Thurstone and Thurstone (1941) studied school children, this was forcibly brought home to them; the problem which faced them was then, in mathematical terms, the following. Thurstone had laid down two main rules for his rotation of axes: orthogonality and simple structure. With his population of students he found that he could find a solution which satisfied both conditions more or less; with the school children he found that this was impossible, and that he had to give up one condition or the other. He decided to retain simple structure, and let the axes go oblique; this of course led to the postulation of higher order factors whose position was determined by the obliqueness of the primaries. Nearly all psychometrists have followed his example, and there is probably no doubt that this decision was correct. Only one man has made the opposite decision; Guilford (1967) has retained orthogonality, and in fact thrown simple structure overboard. This has led to certain developments which require discussion.

Guilford has published a theoretical conception of the structure of the intellect (SI), in which he postulates three major dimensions along which mental tests can differ: Operation (evaluation, convergent production, divergent production, memory, cognition), Product (units, classes, relations, systems, transformations, implications), and Content (figural, symbolic, semantic, behavioural). The $5 \times 6 \times 4 = 120$ cells in the SI model are each supposed to give rise to a factor, and in their recent book Guilford & Hoepfner (1971) have claimed the identification of 84 ability factors occupying 79 of the cells, with a few cells having two or more factors. These are by definition orthogonal, as Guilford only admits orthogonal rotations; that means that the results cannot be determined by the requirements of simple structure. What is done is as follows. Guilford first uses a principal-factor technique, with iterated communalities; he then rotates to an orthogonal matrix that best fits a "target factor matrix" in which postulated factor loadings have been inserted to conform to simple structure, positive manifold requirements, and hypotheses derived from the SI model. The target matrices for this "Procrustes" method are not in fact given in the book, but in any case their inclusion would not rescue the method from a degree of subjectivity which is not acceptable to anyone who does not on a priori grounds accept the SI model as it stands. Horn (1967) has clearly demonstrated that Procrustes rotations of complex data matrices can be manipulated to fit in with almost any theory whatever. Clearly a worker who prescribes in great detail the nature of the solution and ensures that the calculations give the closest possible fit to that solution cannot claim that the data support that solution; it would be necessary to test the data against alternative hypotheses, such as the Burtian schema, or else to reanalyse them by more objective methods, as had been done by Haynes (1970) and by Harris and Harris (1971), with results which do not support Guilford any more strongly than they would some form of Thurstonian scheme. (Horn and Knapp, 1973).

Guilford's scheme has been widely accepted because of its neatness, and because of the tremendous amount of empirical work that has gone into it; it is unfortunate that it is not really acceptable on psychometric grounds. Reanalysis of the main body of results by properly objective, non-prescriptive methods may give some qualified support to Guilford's claims, but it seems more likely that the data will support at least equally strongly the traditional paradigm. Vernon's paper, reprinted in this section, describes his version of this paradigm; there is nothing in Guilford's published work that would make this approach obsolete. The traditional primary factors emphasize what Guilford calls "operations" (memory, reasoning) and "contents" (perceptual, verbal, numerical), and these are more easily discoverable in re-analyses of Guilfords data than are "pro-

ducts". It does not seem unreasonable, as Vernon emphasizes, that operations and content should in part determine the efficacy with which g should get to work on different kinds of cognitive material; for the products one would want rather stronger evidence than exists at the moment.

Critics sometimes seem to think that such problems as whether intelligence is one single concept, or rather a group of distinct ones, are peculiar to psychology. This is of course not so. Less than 150 years ago, the question of whether electricity was one single type of power, or whether it could be broken down into quite distinct and separate powers, such as static and Voltaic, was very much to the fore. In 1832 the idea of the identity of all electricities was strongly challenged in the Philosophical Transactions; thus Ritchie (1832) wrote: "Common electricity is diffused over the surface of the metal;— voltaic electricity exists within the metal. Free electricity is conducted over the surface of the thinnest goldleaf, as effectively as over a mass of metal having the same surface;—voltaic electricity requires thickness of metal for its conduction." Faraday opposed these divisive beliefs, but was hard put to it to provide the experimental evidence which finally settled the question—still leaving different "group factors" showing at least partial differences in certain respects. Williams (1966) gives a good account of the whole episode, which in some ways resembles quite strikingly the sort of arguments still heard in psychology. The evidence for a *general* factor of intelligence is by now reasonably strong, provided we recognize also the existence of additional group factors, or of primaries which are linked together by the overwhelmingly strong general factor.*

---

* As we shall see in later sections, general intelligence ("g") is strongly determined by genetic factors; are primary factors independently determined to any extent by genetic factors? The only available study which really gives us reliable evidence on this point has been published by Partanen et al. (1966); they used 135 pairs of MZ twins and 164 pairs of DZ twins, and administered 8 tests of what might be considered to be 4 primary abilities. It requires at least 4 tests to define a primary properly; hence the use of only 2 tests for each primary underdetermines the solution drastically. Extracting canonical variables on the basis of within-pair covariance matrices they found four independent factors each of which showed significant genetic determination. "It would be tempting to claim that these correspond exactly to the four special abilities, Verbal, Space, Number, and Memory, which our tests were designed to measure. However, examination of the loadings indicates that the pattern is rather irregular." The authors raise the possibility of rotation; when this was done in our statistical laboratory, results, though still not too clear, seemed rather more in line with psychological expectation. The first factor, as in the original solution, is a general factor with a heritability of ·72. The second factor has high positive loadings on the spatial tests and high negative loadings on the numerical ones; the heritability is ·49. The third factor has high loadings only on

The development of primary mental abilities, as Thurstone calls them, or of group factors, as Burt does, is one way of emphasizing that intelligence, like the atom, can be split; there are two other ways of carrying out this split. The first of these, which makes the distinction between fluid and crystallized ability, has already been alluded to, and is here dealt with in the paper by Horn; the other, which analyzes test performance into experimentally discriminable components of mental speed, continuance or persistence, and error checking, will be dealt with in the next section. The terms "fluid" and "crystallized" intelligence were coined by Cattell (1963), but the notions underlying these terms go back at least as far as Thorndike's (1927) distinction between altitude and width of intellect. "Being able to do harder things than some one else can do" is his informal definition of altitude; it clearly involves the notion of difficulty scaling of problems. "Knowing more things than someone else, and being able to do more things than someone else" is his informal definition of width; it clearly involves the prior application of mental ability which is now crystallized into knowledge or skill. "The two things have been somewhat confused in general discussions and in the construction of measuring instruments because, by and large, a person increases the number of things he can do in large part by adding on harder ones, and also because the person who can do the harder ones can on the average learn those which the duller person can learn more quickly than he, and so learns more of them. Consequently what we may call the *level* or *height* or *altitude* of intellect and what we may call its *extent* or *range* or *area at the same level* are correlated and either one is an indicator of the other. It will be best, however, to keep them separate in our thinking." (p. 24).

Thorndike at first assumed that altitude would be more readily determined by nature, width by nurture. "According to the orthodox views of what original nature is likely to contribute and what the environment is likely to contribute, it would be reasonable to choose the altitude of intellect and the width . . . as the two extremes, the area . . . being intermediate in its causation. It seems, at least, much easier for a good home or school to increase the number of easy things which a child can do than to enable him to do harder things than he has ever done. . . . A favourable opportunity and

assiduity seem to be all that are needed to teach anybody twice as many thousand easy accomplishments as he has acquired with meagre opportunity and less study." Thorndike goes on to say that this is almost axiomatic; "we were almost convinced of it until we investigated the actual relations between altitude, width and area of Intellect CAVD and between the higher selective and organizing abilities and the lower or associative. The correlations are such as to cast doubt upon the doctrine that the number of easy intellectual accomplishments which a person learns depends chiefly, or even largely, on the stimulus of the environment. On the contrary, the number which a person can learn seems to be limited by his nature almost as much as is the degree of difficulty which he can master. . . . As things are, the competent intellects learn approximately all the easy things which the incompetent intellects learn, plus a large balance of harder things." (1958).

Cattell (1963) made precisely the same prediction which Thorndike called "almost axiomatic", but finally rejected; he says that "for any same-age group the nature-nurture variance ratio will be much higher for g_f than g_c on the hypothesis that g_f is directly physiologically determined whereas g_c is a produce of environmentally varying, experientially determined investments of g_f." (p. 4). (The subscripts c and f stand for crystallized and fluid ability). The facts apparently bear out Thorndike's view rather than Cattell's. Shields (1962) studied the performance of monozygotic twins, brought up apart and brought up together, and of dizygotic twins on tests of fluid ability (Dominoes) and of crystallized ability (Vocabulary); he found hardly any difference between the two kinds of intelligence. For MZ twins brought up together, the intraclass correlations were ·71 and ·74; for MZ twins brought up separate, they were ·76 and ·74. For DZ twins, intraclass correlations were − ·05 and ·38; this correlation is odd because of the negative value of the Dominoes test, and cannot be taken too seriously. If accepted as it stands, it would suggest that DZ twins, in spite of 50% identical heredity, are completely unlike each other on a good measure of fluid intelligence! At most, the available data (discussed in a later section) might be compatible with a slightly greater heritability index for fluid intelligence tests, but whether this is so or not is by no means clear at the moment; certainly any large difference is ruled out completely.*

The notion of "fluid intelligence" is based on the absence of specially learned skills and information (beyond such universally available acquired abilities as holding a pencil, making marks on paper, etc.), and is intimately tied up with the notion of "culture-free" or "culture-fair" intelligence tests. The difference between

---

W (word fluency), with a heritability of ·41. The fourth factor opposes verbal comprehension (V) and the two memory tests; its heritability is ·51. The bipolar nature of these three factors makes interpretation difficult; it is a direct consequence of the underdetermination resulting from having too few tests. Nevertheless, the results indicate unequivocally that primaries are determined by genetic factors independently of g; the nature of the process of extraction and rotation of factors guarantees their independence. This is an important conclusion; it will require extensive work with larger numbers of tests to put this conclusion on a firmer basis.

* Jinks and Fulker (1970) used the Shields data for a thorough-going genetical analysis; they concluded that the broad heritability for the Dominoes test is 71%, for the Vocabulary 73%; this difference is negligible, and goes in the opposite direction to that predicted by Cattell.

such tests and the more usual type of IQ test is of course not absolute, just as the difference between crystallized and fluid ability is not absolute; even the most "culture-fair" test is not really culture-free, but only relatively so. Nevertheless, the construction of such tests, following the theoretical advances of Spearman's laws of neo-genesis, has given us very useful tools for investigating many problems which previously presented great difficulties. A brief history of the concepts involved, and the efforts made by many psychologists to construe such tests, is given in the final paper in this section, in which Cattell outlines the principles along which his own test was constructed.

It may be useful to discuss briefly an objection often made against the term "culture-fair" in connection with such tests. It is found that working-class children as compared with middle-class children, and coloured children as compared with white or oriental children, are still poorer at doing these tests; this is interpreted by some psychologists as proof that cultural, educational and other environmental influences are still effective in pushing the scores of such children below the level at which they would equal those of white, middle-class children. Such an argument of course only has force if it can be shown that there are not in fact genetic differences between the groups which are being compared; such an assumption requires proof, and cannot be accepted as obviously true. This, in turn, means that we must turn to properly designed studies which attempt directly to deal with the relative contribution of heredity and environment, nature and nurture, to the production of individual differences in intellectual ability. It seems very unlikely that any scale will ever eliminate observed differences between members of different social classes; even direct attempts to base scales on items selected in such a way as to eliminate class differences (e.g. the Davis-Eells Test of General Intelligence or Problem-Solving Ability) have proved unable to provide equal scores for middle- and working-class children (Angelino & Shedd, 1955; Geist, 1954; Haggard, 1954; Rosenblum, Keller, & Paponia, 1955). Such failure is very important; it suggests that those who suggest that IQ tests are a repository of middle-class values, or are simply a mirror of white supremacy, are incorrect in their statements; it seems physically impossible to construct tests even remotely resembling measures of intellectual functions which do not demonstrate differences between classes very much like the traditional IQ tests. Certainly the onus of demonstrating the validity of such claims would now be on such critics.

A last, very short paper deals with an important problem which has not received anything like the attention it deserves. Factory-analysts usually assume that factors derived from one sample of the population will be very much the same as factors derived from another, and that factor structure is independent of choice of sample (except perhaps when sampling involved restriction of range). This may not be so, however, and the paper here reprinted presents some evidence that when a sample of stable children is compared with a sample of unstable children (all within the non-pathological range, of course) then a more stable structure of abilities is found in the more stable group. Too little is known as to how general such a finding might be; all one can say is that factor analysts ought to pay more attention to the problem, and not assume what remains to be proved. It seems likely that we could learn much of interest about the structure of intelligence if we analysed different samples selected on the basis of various personality traits.

REFERENCES

ANGELINO, H. & SHEILD, C. L. An initial report of a validation study of the Davis-Eells Test of General Intelligence or Problem-Solving Ability. *J. Psychol.*, 1955, *40*, 35–38.

CATTELL, R. B. Theory of fluid and crystallized intelligence: a critical experiment. *J. educ. Psychol.*, 1963, *54*, 1–22.

GEIST, H. Evaluation of culture-free intelligence. *Calif. J. Educ.*, 1954, *5*, 209–214.

GUILFORD, J. P. *The nature of human intelligence.* New York: McGraw-Hill, 1967.

GUILFORD, J. P. & HOEPFNER, R. *The analysis of intelligence.* New York: McGraw-Hill, 1971.

HAGGARD, E. A. Social-status and intelligence: an experimental study of certain cultural determinants of measured intelligence. *Genet. Psychol. Monogr.*, 1954, *49*, 141–186.

HARRIS, M. L. & HARRIS, C. W. A factor analytic interpretation strategy. *Educ. & psychol. Measurement*, 1971, *31*, 589–606.

HAYNES, J. R. Hierarchical analysis of factors in cognition. *Amer. Educ. Res., J.*, 1970, *7*, 55–68.

HORN, J. L. On subjectivity in factor analysis. *Educ. & Psychol. Measurement*, 1967, *27*, 811–820.

HORN, J. L. & KNAPP, J. R. On the subjective character of the empirical base of the structure of intellect model. *Psychol. Bull.*, 1973, to appear.

JINKS, J. L. & FULKER, D. W. Comparison of the biometrical genetical, MAVA, and classical approaches to the analysis of human behavior. *Psychol. Bull.*, 1970, *73*, 311–349.

PARTANEN, J., BRUUN, K. & MARKKANEN, T. Inheritance of drinking behaviour. Helsinki: Finnish Foundation of Alcohol studies, Vol. 14, 1966.

RITCHIE, W. Experimental researches in Voltaic electricity and electro-magnetism. *Philos. Treas.*, 1832, *Part II*, 279–352.

ROSENBLUM, S., KELLER, J. E. & PAPONIA, V. Davis-Eells ("culture-fair") test performance of lower class retarded children. *J. consult. Psychol.*, 1955, *19*, 51–59.

SHIELDS, J. *Monozygotic twins.* Oxford: University Press, 1962.

SPEARMAN, C. *Abilities of Man.* London: Methuen, 1927.

THORNDIKE, E. L. *The measurement of intelligence.* New York: Teacher's College, Columbia University, 1927.

THURSTONE, L. L. *Primary mental abilities.* Chicago: Chicago University Press, 1938.

THURSTONE, L. L. & THURSTONE, T. G. Factorial studies of intelligence. Psychometric Monogr., No. 2, Chicago: University of Chicago Press, 1941.

WILLIAMS, L. P. *Michael Faraday.* London: Chapman & Hall, 1965.

From Brit. J. Educ. Psychol. (1939) *Vol IX part III*, 270–265, *by kind permission of Scottish Academic Press*

PRIMARY MENTAL ABILITIES.

(PSYCHOMETRIC MONOGRAPHS No. 1.)

By L. L. THURSTONE. (Chicago: University of Chicago Press, pp. x+121. 9s.)

THIS publication is the opening number of a series which the Psychometric Society proposes to issue. It reports the first large experimental inquiry, carried out by the methods of factor analysis described by Thurstone in *The Vectors of the Mind*[1]. The work was made possible by financial grants from the Social Science Research Committee of the University of Chicago, the American Council of Education, and the Carnegie Corporation of New York. The results are eminently worthy of the assistance so generously accorded. Thurstone's previous theoretical account, lucid and comprehensive as it is, is intelligible only to those who have a knowledge of matrix algebra. Hence his methods have become known to British educationists chiefly from the monograph published by W. P. Alexander[8]. This enquiry has provoked a good deal of criticism, particularly from Professor Spearman's school; and differs, as a matter of fact, from Thurstone's later expositions. Hence it is of the greatest value to have a full and simple illustration of his methods, based on a concrete inquiry, from Professor Thurstone himself.

Fifty-six tests, selected according to a provisional classification of cognitive factors, were applied to 240 volunteers. The correlations between the tests were then estimated by means of the charts for tetrachoric correlation previously published by Thurstone and his colleagues.[2] The huge table of correlations has been factorized by the so-called centroid method; and twelve factors extracted. All except the first are bipolar, i.e., have negative as well as positive saturations. It is then assumed that "primary factors act positively unless they are absent from a performance." Hence the co-ordinate axes, representing the factors, are rotated, two at a time, until the negative saturations are virtually obliterated, and the number of zero saturations maximized. For this purpose thirty diagrams have been plotted, and fresh axes fitted by eye.

It is stated that "the graphical method of rotating in one plane at a time is probably the best single method; but the graphical method is not ideal." Although the principles involved have been briefly explained in *The Vectors of the Mind* and elsewhere, hitherto, as Professor Thurstone points out, "there has not been published any adequate description of the method as applied to an actual problem." This,

H. J. Eysenck

therefore, is in some ways the most interesting section of the report. The final upshot is thirteen fresh factors, of which nine can readily be given a psychological meaning. In the main, though not in every detail, the interpretations correspond with the categories which the tests were originally selected to represent.

When the editor of this *Journal* first suggested a review of Professor Thurstone's new report, it appeared that the large collection of data contained in its tables would offer an admirable opportunity for testing recent statements about the mode of factor analysis, statements for the most part reached *a priori* and never yet verified by any concrete comparison. How, for example, do Thurstone's methods and results compare with earlier methods and results put forward by workers in this country ?

In his 1935 Memorandum ([3], page 306) Burt has pointed out that there are in theory two general ways of factorizing a table of correlations between tests : (*a*) with the first method—a ' submatrix ' or ' group factor ' method—we may look for relatively specific factors whose influence is solely positive ; (*b*) with the second method—a ' general factor ' method—we may look for common factors which will be bipolar and therefore have both positive and negative saturations. Where, as in Thurstone's present research, the selection of tests is to a large extent abruptly discontinuous, the former method is evidently the more appropriate. It was, for example, used by Burt and his co-workers nearly twenty years ago in several studies of educational tests, where the subjects tested fall into obviously discontinuous groups. In these early researches the centroid formula (as it is now called) was employed for the first time ; and factors very similar to those now reached by Professor Thurstone were elicited ([4], Tables XVIII–XXIV).

The categories which Thurstone's tests were selected to represent are described as follows : (i) Abstraction (Tests 4–8) ; (ii) Verbal (9–16, to which should obviously be added 56–60 from the ' unclassified ') ; (iii) Space (17–25) ; (iv) Number (30–35) ; (v) Numerical reasoning (36–39) ; (vi) Verbal reasoning (40–42) ; (vii) Spatial reasoning (43–45) ; (viii) Rote-learning (46–51) ; (ix) Unclassified, including spelling, grammar and vocabulary (52–60). Thurstone's own grouping thus shows how discontinuous his categories are. To a large extent they coincide with well-established group factors. There can, therefore, be little question that the group-factor method is the natural procedure.

Accordingly, it seemed eminently desirable to test this view by applying the group factor method to Thurstone's table of correlations. The formula used is a modification of the simple summation formula (viz., [5], p. 359, equation iv). After eliminating the general factor the remaining

Primary Mental Abilities

factors are derived from the smaller submatrices of residuals. The only point of difficulty is to determine in advance the lines of division between the several submatrices or clusters, so as to base the general factor on correlations uninfluenced by the one and same group factor. Where the grouping of tests is itself a subject of investigation, we cannot adopt the categories by which the original selection of tests was made ; for this would obviously beg the question at issue. The criterion proposed is the dégree of resemblance between the various columns of correlations. To study these resemblances we may either calculate the unadjusted inter-columnar correlation or make graphs of the coefficients and judge the resemblances between the contours (cf. 4, fig. 9). Where the correlations between the correlations are non-linear, the latter seems the more reliable as well as the speedier method.

The saturation coefficients obtained by this method are shown in Table I. The first or general factor is responsible for 31 per cent of the variance. On eliminating its effects, there are six submatrices containing significant positive residuals. The group factors derived from these contribute about 2 to 6 per cent of the total variance only. Thus, the general factor is five times as significant as any other.

Professor Spearman, in a paper read at the recent Reading con-ference, has maintained that Thurstone's table could be fitted by a two-factor analysis and that this procedure would reveal a single general factor. Thurstone, on the other hand, declares : " We cannot report any general common factor in Spearman's sense in the 56 tests that have been analyzed." This is rather surprising, since, in selecting the tests, " special emphasis was laid on those tests which are used as measures of intelligence." Now his Table III does, as a matter of fact, show a ' general common factor in Spearman's sense ', i.e., a column of saturation coefficients, all positive, and larger than those in any other column ; and its subsequent disappearance is plainly an inevitable result of his method of rotation : this aims, not only at abolishing negative saturations, but also at maximizing the zeros *in every column*, even where the satura-tions are large and positive throughout. No general factor could survive such a procedure. An analysis by Burt's procedure appears to reconcile the two conclusions : for, with Spearman, we discover a general factor, accountable for more of the total variance than any other, and with Thurstone we discover a number of group-factors having a clear psycho-logical meaning.

In their general nature the group-factors shown in Table I agree almost entirely with those of Professor Thurstone. They prove, indeed, to be much the same as those noted in the earlier researches of Burt and

H. J. EYSENCK

TABLE I. FACTOR SATURATIONS BY GROUP-FACTOR METHOD.

Test.	G	V	L	A	S	C	M	R	Z
4	·554	·483	—	—	—	—	—	—	—
5	·662	·525	—	—	—	—	—	—	—
9	·293	·531	—	—	—	—	—	—	—
10	·649	·511	—	—	—	—	—	—	—
11	·669	·492	—	—	—	—	—	—	—
16	·611	·437	—	—	—	—	—	—	—
52	·533	·496	—	—	—	—	—	—	—
56	·497	·404	—	—	—	—	—	—	—
58	·398	·832	—	—	—	—	—	—	—
59	·237	·265	—	—	—	—	—	—	—
60	·741	·465	—	—	—	—	—	—	—
12	·605	—	·351	—	—	—	—	—	—
13	·537	—	·548	—	—	—	—	—	—
15	·437	—	·628	—	—	—	—	—	—
57	·688	—	·351	—	—	—	—	—	—
30	·678	—	—	·448	—	—	—	—	—
31	·302	—	—	·649	—	—	—	—	—
32	·395	—	—	·575	—	—	—	—	—
33	·349	—	—	·743	—	—	—	—	—
34	·461	—	—	·641	—	—	—	—	—
35	·565	—	—	·444	—	—	—	—	—
37	·627	—	—	·313	—	—	—	—	—
38	·483	—	—	·465	—	—	—	—	—
39	·683	—	—	·446	—	—	—	—	—
8	·444	—	—	—	·424	—	—	—	—
17	·389	—	—	—	·589	—	—	—	—
18	·495	—	—	—	·606	—	—	—	—
19	·520	—	—	—	·512	—	—	—	—
20	·340	—	—	—	·750	—	—	—	—
21	·670	—	—	—	·489	—	—	—	—
22	·504	—	—	—	·622	—	—	—	—
23	·510	—	—	—	·497	—	—	—	—
24	·565	—	—	—	·453	—	—	—	—
27	·367	—	—	—	·555	—	—	—	—
28	·575	—	—	—	·382	—	—	—	—
29	·561	—	—	—	·336	—	—	—	—
36	·304	—	—	—	·214	—	—	—	—
45	·696	—	—	—	·325	—	—	—	—
53	·299	—	—	—	·525	—	—	—	—
6	·814	—	—	—	—	·436	—	—	—
7	·684	—	—	—	—	·364	—	—	—
14	·657	—	—	—	—	·427	—	—	—
26	·418	—	—	—	—	·549	—	—	—
51	·309	—	—	—	—	·445	—	—	—
46	·361	—	—	—	—	—	·499	—	—
47	·527	—	—	—	—	—	·569	—	—
48	·420	—	—	—	—	—	·457	—	—
49	·472	—	—	—	—	—	·404	—	—
50	·370	—	—	—	—	—	·495	—	—
40	·688	—	—	—	—	—	—	[·575]	—
42	·653	—	—	—	—	—	—	[·575]	—
54	·409	—	—	—	—	—	—	—	[·520]
55	·707	—	—	—	—	—	—	—	[·520]
25	·584	—	—	—	—	—	—	—	—
41	·824	—	—	—	—	—	—	—	—
43	·868	—	—	—	—	—	—	—	—
44	·772	—	—	—	—	—	—	—	—
Per cent Variance	30·80	5·00	1·65	4·58	6·61	1·74	1·79	[1·16]	[·097]

Factor V—Verbal-Literary.
Factor L—Verbal-Linguistic.
Factor A—Arithmetical.
Factor S—Visuo-Spatial.
Factor C—Classification.
Factor M—Memory.
Factor R—Relational.
Factor Z—Audio-Rhythmic.
Factor G—General Factor of Mental Ability.

Primary Mental Abilities

his co-workers on London school children : there he found, in addition
to the general factor, more or less identifiable with ' intelligence ', two
verbal, one arithmetical, a manual, and (in tests more purely psychological) a factor for memory and a factor or factors for sensory perception.
Here no manual factor is discovered : but that is presumably because in a
collection of tests to be given by the group procedure Thurstone was
unable to include any tests of manual dexterity or skill ; the place of the
manual or mechanical factor seems largely taken by the spatial factor.
But perhaps the most interesting point of agreement between the present
table and the earlier results is the presence of *two* distinguishable verbal
factors : this moreover accords, not only with the conclusions drawn in the
London work ([4], p. 59), but also, it would seem, with Thurstone's own
conclusion. The only important discrepancy between Thurstone's list
and ours is that he distinguishes three types of relational or rational
factors, whereas we find hardly any significant evidence for one. The
reason is clear. If (as Burt has maintained) intelligence is manifested
most fully and most clearly in ' activities involving reasoning, i.e., the
use of logical relations ' ([7], p. 12), then Thurstone's ' logical factors '
are mainly a special manifestation of our general factor. Thurstone
does not refer to Alexander's work ([8] ; cf. 9, pp. 365–71) : but it may be
noted that Alexander, who used a similar method of rotation, also
confirmed the existence of a general, a verbal, an arithmetical, and a
practical factor, and endeavoured to demonstrate their importance for
educational and vocational practice.[1]

Perhaps, however, the most interesting result of our analysis is this.
By the use of a very simple procedure we are able to demonstrate and
calculate much the same factors as are demonstrated and calculated by
Thurstone. Thurstone's own analysis depends first on making an
elaborate formal analysis by the centroid method and then rotating the

[1] Since the foregoing analysis was undertaken, we have learnt that Professor
Holzinger has also made an analysis of Thurstone's data on somewhat similar lines[9].
The volume of *Psychometrika*[9] containing this study was not received by our Department until late in the year ; hence our investigation was taken in complete independence of Holzinger's. As has elsewhere been pointed out ([5], p. 361), Holzinger's
new method of bi-factor analysis (not his original method) is in general principle
largely identical with Burt's earlier group-factor method. The chief differences
are, first, that Holzinger allocates the tests on the basis of what he calls a beta-
coefficient, and, secondly, that his method of deducing the general factor saturations
would appear to depend on a multiplication formula rather than on a summation
formula. Neither in his *Student Manual* nor in his previous Reports of the Spearman-
Holzinger Trait Committee does he express his method in terms of an actual formula ;
but the method as described would appear to imply the use of Burt's equation vi
instead of his equation iv ([5], p. 355). In spite of these slight divergences in procedure, our results appear to be closely similar. In each group, however (except
those for arithmetic and memory), our own table shows one or two minor additions
and one or two omissions as compared with Holzinger's. It may be added that our
method, with 9 factors, accounts for more of the total variance than Holzinger's with
10.

H. J. EYSENCK

axes thus found by a somewhat prolonged and admittedly precarious graphical procedure. The submatrix method reaches the same results directly with one set of simple calculations. Since we have relied on fewer factors, our figures do not fit the observed correlations quite so well as Thurstone's. But of the residuals remaining from our analysis only 2 out of 1,596 are over 0·3. When, as here, the probable errors are high (±0·07 according to Thurstone), residuals of this size can have no statistical significance, particularly in so huge a table. If a more complete set of saturations were required, giving a slightly closer fit, it could be obtained by carrying the calculation a stage further according to the method described and illustrated in a previous number of this *Journal* ([6], p. 55).

To educationists one of the most interesting chapters in the monograph is the last. This deals with the uses of mental ' profiles ' based on the factor measurements, and suggests the possibility of picking out those individuals who are marked by exceptionally high or exceptionally low performance in some particular factor and therefore might be said to belong to the ' type ' which that factor designates. In particular, it is found that many of the individual profiles show an instructive relation to the vocational interests and wishes of the persons they represent : thus the two youths having profiles with the highest relative scores in the factor of verbal relations (what we have called the verbal literary factor) desire to be teachers ; others, who have high scores in the visiospatial factor, wish to be engineers or geologists.

In conclusion we must express our admiration for the great care and thoroughness which has evidently been expended upon this research. It is, indeed, one of the most valuable educational experiments of its kind hitherto carried out. It provides a mass of figures for those who wish to test alternative methods of analysis ; and anyone who wishes to be acquainted with the factorial technique in educational research will find this book a most lucid and instructive introduction.

H. J. EYSENCK.

REFERENCES.

[1] THURSTONE, L. L. (1935). *The Vectors of the Mind.*—University of Chicago Press.
[2] —— CHESIRE, L., and SAFFIR, M. (1933) : *Computing Diagrams for the Tetrachoric Correlation Coefficient.*—University of Chicago Bookstore.
[3] HARTOG, P., RHODES, E. C., and BURT, C. (1936) : *Marks of Examiners.*—London : Macmillan and Co.
[4] BURT, C. (1917) : *Distribution and Relations of Educational Abilities.*—London : P. S. King and Sons.
[5] —— (1938).—*Journal of Psychology*, VI, 339–375.
[6] —— (1939).—This *Journal*, IX, i, 45–71.
[7] —— (1911).—*Journal Exper. Pedagogy*, 1, 93–112.
[8] ALEXANDER, W. P. (1935) : *Brit. J. Psych. Mon. Suppl.*, XIX.—London : Cambridge University Press.
[9] HOLZINGER, K. J., and HARMAN, H. H. (1938).—*Psychometrika*, III, i, 45–60.

From J. L. Horn, Psychological Review, 75, 242–259. *Copyright (1968), by kind permission of the author and the American Psychological Association*

ORGANIZATION OF ABILITIES AND THE DEVELOPMENT OF INTELLIGENCE

JOHN L. HORN [1]

University of Denver

Performances which are accepted as indicators of intelligence are interrelated in ways which indicate 2 broad factors. Each factor represents a kind of intelligence. The 1st, called crystallized intelligence, indicates the extent of acculturation as it determines human abilities. The other, called fluid intelligence, indicates a pattern of neural-physiological and incidental learning influences. The 2 become independent as development proceeds from infancy to adulthood. Measures of fluid intelligence are the more sensitive indicators of brain malfunction; fluid intelligence declines with brain damage and aging in adulthood. Performances on ability tests involve processes in addition to those of intelligence. These are associated with sensory modality functions (visual, auditory, tactile processes), perhaps indicate endocrine functions (in speediness), represent "strategies or styles of performance (carefulness, speediness), and relate to motivation (need for achievement). Results in support of the theory are presented and evaluated. Some needed research is indicated.

At the APA Convention of 1941 R. B. Cattell (1941) and D. O. Hebb (1941) presented papers based upon separate arguments but converging towards very similar conclusions; both concluded that two distinct concepts of intelligence should be recognized. In Hebb's theory the central ideas were expressed in the concept of an intelligence A, representing potential, and an intelligence B, representing realized intelligence. In Cattell's developments the somewhat similar ideas were represented in the concepts of fluid intelligence and crystallized intelligence. These papers aroused considerable discussion and debate. Yet surprisingly little has been done to bring the implications of the two statements into focus within general developmental and personality theory. The present paper is an attempt to rectify this (as the

writer perceives it) unfortunate turn of events and thus to point the way toward more meaningful research on human intelligence.

The theory developed here will build primarily upon the Cattellian concepts of fluid and crystallized intelligence (abbreviated Gf and Gc respectively), rather than upon the Hebbian notions. There are several reasons for this. A major argument is that the Gf-Gc formulation is preferable to the Hebbian cenceptualization because the principal concepts in this theory have specifiable and measurable behavioral referents, whereas in Hebb's theory intelligence A does not refer to measurable behavior but to neurological potential. It is desirable for the behavioral scientist (in contrast, perhaps, to the physiologist, biochemist, etc.) to define intelligence in terms of observable, measurable behavior, whence it may become possible to relate this variable to important variables of neurology, sociology, etc.

A major theme in this refinement of

---

[1] This paper was first written during the tenure of a visiting appointment at the University of California at Berkeley. The author thanks Kenneth B. Little for helpful comments and criticisms on an early draft of this paper.

JOHN L. HORN

the theory of fluid and crystallized intelligence concerns the *development of abilities* and, more particularly, the development of a distinction between the broad patterns of abilities, Gf and Gc. It is hoped that this treatment of the topic will go some way toward achieving rapprochement between factor-analytic research on human abilities and research and theory which has proceeded largely without benefit of factor-analytic findings.

DEVELOPMENT OF FLUID AND CRYSTALLIZED INTELLIGENCE

In the earliest period of development no distinction can be drawn between fluid intelligence and crystallized intelligence. Indeed, one can seriously question the contention that intelligence (conceived of as a behavioral variable) is measured by tests developed for use in the first few years of life. The infant tests thus far developed seem to measure mainly a kind of sensory motor alertness which bears little relationship to that which is identified as intelligence at later stages of development (Bayley, 1949, 1955, 1965; Hofstaetter, 1954; Hofstaetter & O'Connor, 1956). It can be argued that while such sensory-motor alertness sets limits on the rate at which intelligence can become manifest in behavior, it is not an integral part of intelligence, per se.

However, granting that at least a small proportion of the variance on infant scales does represent measurement of intelligence as it is defined at later stages of development, the present theory argues that the relationship between early and later measurements of intelligence *cannot* be large for two principal reasons:

(*a*) early in development intelligence is manifested in only one kind of behavioral function—what is called *anlage* function—whereas at later stages of development it is manifested not only in anlage function but also in functions which are referred to as *concept formation* and *attainment* (Bruner, Goodnow, & Austin, 1956) and the use of *generalized solution instruments* or *aids* (Cattell, 1963; Ferguson, 1954, 1956). Although these kinds of function interact to some extent, one kind is not perfectly predictable from either or both of the other kinds and thus it is not possible for measurements which involve only one kind of function (namely, infant tests) to correlate highly with measurements which involve all three kinds of function (namely, childhood and adult tests).

(*b*) The influences of acculturation, maturation, and damage to the physiological structures which support development of intelligence operate somewhat independently throughout development and with respect to the above-mentioned functions to produce distinct, measurably separate patterns of those abilities which, putatively, are said to indicate intelligence: The two principal patterns which emerge in this process are referred to as fluid intelligence and crystallized intelligence. But since the influences which produce these operate after the time that measurements on infants would have occurred and since many of these influences (excluding maturational influences more than the others) could not *in principle* be predicted from infant-scale measurements, the latter cannot be expected to correlate highly with childhood or adulthood measurements of either fluid or crystallized intelligence (much less a conglomerate of the two).

To clarify these points it will be necessary to more fully define the above-mentioned functions and to indicate the supposed process whereby fluid and crystallized intelligence become distinct.

Anlage Function

This represents very elementary capacities in perception, retention, and expression, as these govern intellectual performance. For example, span of apprehension—the number of distinct elements which a person can maintain in immediate awareness—is an elementary capacity and yet one which determines, in part, the complexity with which one can successfully cope in an intellectual task. It would seem that such capacities are not much affected by learning—anlage functioning is closely associated with neural-physiological structure and process—but that such functions operate to some extent in all intellectual performances and thus produce variance in all ability measurements.

The effects of anlage functioning can be felt in basically two ways in observed performances: (*a*) through a history of learning, which learning is then assessed in actual test performance, and (*b*) through demands imposed by the immediate task, per se, with little reference to previous learning. For example, a memory span test requires span of apprehension in the immediate testing situation more or less irrespective of prior learning, whereas a vocabulary test measures span less directly in outcomes which are results of this functioning over extended periods of learning.

In Hoffstaetter's (1954) work a factor was defined primarily by test performances of the first 2 years of life. This could involve anlage function. However, anlage function is not to be equated with sensorimotor alertness. The latter refers to peripheral neural-effector-affector organizations which, although they may be important precursors of intellectual development, are not to be identified with it. Anlage function, on the other hand, involves central neural organizations which are integral to intellectual performances.

Generalized Solution Instruments: "Aids"

An aid is a technique which may be used to compensate for limitations in anlage capacities. For example, although most adults can retain no more than about seven distinct elements in the span of immediate awareness, they can nevertheless organize elements in such a way that they can effectively use considerably more than seven distinct elements in solving problems. Most of us remember a telephone number, for example, by coding the seven- or ten-digit number into sets of three and four digits, which sets are then called sequentially into immediate awareness. The formal rules of algebra are aids in this sense, as are many other problem-solving techniques. Algebra represents a collection of aids which have been developed by many people, over a long course of human history, and deposited in what can be called the intelligence of a culture.

Concepts

The term concept, as used in the present theory, is in many respects similar to an aid. However, a concept is regarded as a category for classification of phenomena, whereas an aid is defined as a technique or method. In the formation of concepts one must perceive essential relations among phenomena and, on some basis of similarity, dissimilarity, etc., categorize different things as the "same." For example, things which are perceived as similar with respect to "leafiness," "barkiness," etc., may be classified as "trees" in distinction from other things which are classified as, say, "poles."

A concept is not to be equated with a verbal representation of the concept. At any stage in development a concept may be known only idiosyncratically and not be represented in conventional language. A child may be aware of a distinction between trees and poles but have no conventional words with which to represent this awareness. However, idiosyncratic representations of concepts tend to become associated with conventional signs, such as the word "tree." When this occurs, it becomes possible to indirectly measure

John L. Horn

capacity for forming concepts by assessing ability to respond to conventional signs. This is the rationale upon which many items in intelligence tests are based. However, it must be recognized that one can be aware of more categories of phenomena than he is able to associate with conventional signs and that familiarity with such signs may not always indicate clarity of perception of the relations defining a concept. Indirect measures are bound to be somewhat invalid indications of capacity for forming concepts.

The Accretion-Transfer Model

We need to conceive of how anlage functions, aids, and concepts become welded together in the abilities which we measure and accept as indications of intelligence. J. E. Anderson (1939, 1940) has presented an accretion model which seems to account for some of the relevant facts. According to this, broad intellectual abilities are outcomes of an adding together (in development) of a series of specific abilities. In Anderson's mathematical representation of this idea each specific-ability accretion to the expanding store of skills is assumed to be independent of all others and no elements are lost as the process continues. If the development of an ability proceeds in this manner, one result will be a simplex matrix (Guttman, 1954) of intercorrelations among test-retest measurements of the ability in question, as Humphreys (1960) has pointed out. Rather surprisingly, in view of the restrictiveness of the assumptions, this model has been found to work rather well to describe test-retest intercorrelations deriving from repeated measurements of intellectual abilities (Anderson, 1939; Humphreys, 1960; Roff, 1941). Hoffstaetter and O'Connor (1956) have shown that by removing

Anderson's second assumption, thereby allowing for the possibility that some additions in an early period could drop out in later measurements, the degree of congruence between predictions from the theory and test-retest intercorrelation data can be improved.

Ferguson (1954, 1956) has shown how principles of learning—in particular, transfer—can be utilized to help explain the way rather specific skills can be added together to form broad abilities. He points out that what is learned at one stage in development will tend to facilitate learning at later stages in development: The learning of one skill will tend to promote the learning of other similar skills and thus advanced learning in a particular area will be built upon less advanced learning. The end result will be a pattern of interdependent skills. But since this process would proceed in a somewhat different way for every individual, and it would proceed further for some than for others, the skills which enter into such a mutually-facilitating pattern will correlate less than perfectly (even after eliminating error of measurement). Factors identified by means of factor analysis with ability-test performances represent such patterns of positively but imperfectly correlated skills. Thus the Ferguson theory provides an indication of the learning processes which operate to produce the well-replicated results of factor-analytic studies of human abilities (as summarized by French, 1951; French, Ekstrom, & Price, 1963; Guilford, 1967; Vernon, 1961). The Fleishman-Hempel (1954, 1955) studies (which Ferguson cites), and, more recently, the study of Duncanson (1964), illustrate how this kind of process operates over short periods of learning.

Several influences in addition to positive transfer in learning would operate in development to produce interdependence among skills and thus lead to the formation of the ability patterns identified by means of factor analysis. Skills learned under the aegis of a particular institution—a school, for example—would tend to be positively intercorrelated relative to skills learned in another setting—in a church, say—even in the absence of positive transfer. Similarly learned avoidance of particular educational situations and such influences as are represented by the promotion systems of schools and other institutions would tend to produce positive intercorrelation among skills which were not related by means of positive transfer. These processes are described in some detail by Horn (1965, 1967).

Separation of Gf and Gc through Development

Any measured ability involves anlage function in the immediate situation and is a product of such functioning over the period of development which has preceded measurement. It would seem, in fact, that some primary-level ability factors, such as Memory Span (Ms [2]), represent anlage function in fairly pure form. However, most primary-level factors (as established by the replicated research reviewed by French et al., 1963, and Guilford, 1967) would appear to be compounds of anlage functions, concepts, and aids welded together by the kind of developmental influences mentioned in the last section: Surely the more general ability patterns, such as those indicated at the second order among primary-level factors or in the hierarchical bifactor (centroid) analyses described by Burt (1955) and Vernon

(1961), are such compounds. This implies that a replicated ability factor, established at a primary or higher-order level,[8] is an outcome of an orderly pattern of developmental influences operating in interaction with anlage functions. Such factors would thus be expected to appear only after a requisite period of development: Vernon (1961) and Guilford (1967) have pointed out that ability factors do not become distinct until relatively late in childhood. Also, some such factors would be expected to be relatively specific and cohesive, as, for example, many of those identified in the extensive research of Guilford and his co-workers, and others would be expected to be broad and diffuse, as in the case of the higher order factors said to represent fluid and crystallized intelligence. The question now before us is: What is the general nature of the orderly patterns of influence which produce Gf and Gc?

Acculturation constitutes a more or less orderly pattern of influences. These shape a crystallized intelligence factor. Of the myriad concepts and aids developed within a culture a relatively small number are seen to be sufficiently useful and/or interesting to pass from one generation to the next. These constitute what might be called the "intelligence of the culture." The major educational institutions of a society (including the home and its substitutes) are directed at instilling this intelligence in the persons (i.e., the young) who are expected to maintain the culture. The anlage capacities of individuals are thus harnessed, as it were, by the dominant culture for the purpose of maintaining and extend-

[2] The abbreviations used for primary-level factors are those suggested by French (1951), French et al. (1963), or Guilford (1967).

[8] As in the studies of Botzum (1951), Cattell (1963, 1967), Horn (1965, 1966), Horn and Bramble (1967), Horn and Cattell (1966b), Martin and Adkins (1954), Rimoldi (1948) and others.

ing the "intelligence of the culture." This process is architectonic, building from a base of prerequisite concepts and aids to a superstructure of complex and esoteric concepts and aids by means of a promotion system which systemically increases the extent of acculturation of some and systemically reduces this for others. Thus, as development proceeds, individual differences in extent of acculturation will increase. Since many of the concepts and aids acquired under this pattern of influence are of a kind which, putatively, are said to indicate intelligence, the factor which results from this pattern of influence can be identified as a kind of intelligence. This is the factor representing crystallized intelligence.

However, it must be recognized that some of the learning which underlies expression of intellectual abilities and some of the basic processes involved in this expression, such as anlage function, are not very closely related to acculturation. For example, Piaget's (1947, 1952; Hunt, 1961) work indicates that the young child develops concepts and aids as a result of manipulations and experiments which are *not* arranged by those who would educate the child. Such incidental learning occurs throughout development. Although acculturation will depend upon this to some extent, the learning itself is not a product of acculturation and this latter is determined by many factors which are quite independent of the incidental learning.[4] Similarly, to the extent that all persons in a so-

ciety are exposed to comparable conditions for learning, individual differences in that which is learned need not be a product of acculturation. In these cases individual differences in learned abilities will be rather directly related to individual differences in the physiological structures which support intellectual functioning. It is apparent that influences which affect these structures occur largely independently of acculturation. Injuries to the brain are not determined by prior learning and although the effects produced by such injuries often will be felt in subsequent learning, they do not necessarily result in cessation of courses of learning already set in action, nor do they necessarily eliminate skills already learned (as Hebb demonstrated in 1941). The influences of heredity and maturation are likewise independent, to a considerable extent, of acculturation. Thus, to the extent that measured intellectual abilities involve primarily only anlage functions or aids and concepts which are products of incidental learning, the abilities will have been formed under a unitary set of influences affecting physiological functioning. If these abilities are of the kind which, putatively, are said to indicate intelligence, then the broad factor which involves them can be said to be a kind of intelligence—namely what, in this theory, is called fluid intelligence.

NEUROLOGICAL COUNTERPARTS OF FLUID AND CRYSTALLIZED INTELLIGENCE

Both Gf and Gc reflect neural-physiological-heredity influences and both involve learned abilities. The essential difference is that a relatively large proportion of the reliable variance in fluid intelligence reflects a pattern of physiological influences and a relatively small proportion of this vari-

[4] That is, the extent of one's exposure to acculturational influences is partly a function of such factors as area of residency, occupation of father, stimulation by peers, etc., factors which although they can be correlated with attributes of individuals, need not result from anything an individual does and thus can come about quite independently of the behavioral attributes of that individual.

ance reflects acculturation, whereas the opposite emphasis occurs for crystallized intelligence.

Behaviorally, an intellectual ability is a compound of anlage functions, aids, and concepts. Such a compound is represented in physiological function principally as a pattern of neurons which fire together (cf. Hebb, 1949). The firing of one neuron (or a small number of neurons) in such a pattern will tend to activate the entire pattern. Such patterns may be highly over-determined, as when a great number of neurons are linked together in mutually-facilitating networks, or they may be relatively "under-determined"— that is, involve only a few neurons the firing of which is not over-determined by the firing of any one of many other neurons. The loss (as by brain damage) of a small number of neurons in a highly over-determined pattern may have virtually no influence on the overall functioning of the pattern, since the firing in the network is determined by the vast number of neurons still remaining. In an "under-determined" pattern, on the other hand, the loss of a few neurons can result in loss of functioning of the entire pattern.

The behavioral counterpart of an over-determined neural pattern is a set of mutually supportive skills linked together through positive transfer. Crystallized intelligence is comprised of such sets of skills. The abilities of this factor should therefore not be greatly affected by brain damage and similar loss of efficiency of neurological function, provided, of course, that the damage or loss of efficiency is not extensive. The neurological counterpart of anlage function is a "built in" network of neurons, probably not over-determined in the above-mentioned sense. Similarly, the patterns of skills acquired by incidental learning generally would be smaller and more isolated, neurologically speaking,

than would the patterns of skills constructed through the architectonic process of acculturation. On this basis it is predicted that fluid intelligence will be more sensitive to changes in efficiency of neurological functioning than will crystallized intelligence.

SOME CONSEQUENCES AND EVIDENCE

A basic hypothesis deriving from this theory stipulates that if the interrelationships among a wide variety of intellectual performances are analysed by means of covariational procedures such as factor analysis, there should be found two broad patterns, one involving performances which rather clearly indicate advanced knowledge of the culture and one in which this is not the case but which in other respects clearly indicates intelligence.

Extensive but rather tangential evidence relating to this hypothesis has been collected by Horn (1965). Studies designed specifically for the purpose of exploring implications of the hypothesis have been reported by Cattell (1963, 1967), Horn (1965, 1966), Horn and Bramble (1967), and Horn and Cattell (1966b). Humphreys (1967) has presented a critique of the Cattell (1963) study along with re-analysis of the data of this and the Horn-Cattell (1966b) studies. The general conclusion to be drawn from these investigations is to the effect that, indeed, two broad factors having the properties specified by the Gf-Gc theory are found among ability test performances. The specific nature of these factors is indicated in the summary of Table 1.

The factors of Table 1 are somewhat cooperative—that is, they involve some of the same tests. Each has about the same relationship to General Reasoning, for example. The factors are positively correlated. But it is clear that, in heterogeneous samples of older chil-

JOHN L. HORN

dren and adults, the two patterns are distinct. Humphreys (1967) criticized Cattell's (1963) study on almost every count, and he found several points to question in the Horn-Cattell (1966b) study, but he concluded that the evidence indicated two broad patterns of the kind stipulated in the Gf-Gc theory.

Each factor in Table 1 contains tests which are accepted as measures of aspects of intelligence. The performances assessed by these tests can be seen to involve processes—of reasoning, perception of relations, eduction of correlates, abstraction, problem solving, etc.—which are widely recognized as integral to intelligence. Each factor thus indicates intelligence in an acceptable sense of this term.

But while both patterns indicate intelligence, they differ in noteworthy ways. The tests which are most char-

TABLE 1

SUMMARY OF SOME RESULTS FROM STUDIES IN WHICH GF AND GC FACTORS HAVE BEEN IDENTIFIED

Symbol	Behavioral indicant[a]	Approximate factor coefficient[b]		Symbol	Behavioral indicant[a]	Approximate factor coefficient[b]	
		Gf	Gc			Gf	Gc
CFR	Figural Relations. Eduction of a relation when this is shown among common figures, as in a matrices test.	.57	.01	Rs	Formal Reasoning. Arriving at a conclusion in accordance with a formal reasoning process, as in a Syllogistic Reasoning test.	.31	.41
Ms	Memory Span. Reproduction of several numbers or letters presented briefly either visually or orally.	.50	.00	N	Number Facility. Quick and accurate use of arithmetical operations, such as addition, subtraction, multiplication, etc.	.21	.29
I	Induction. Eduction of a correlate from relations shown in a series of letters numbers or figures, as in a Letter Series test.	.41	.06	EMS	Experiential Evaluation. Solving problems involving protocol and requiring diplomacy, as in a Social Relations tests.	−.08	.43
R	General Reasoning. Solving problems of area, rate, finance, etc., as in an Arithmetic Reasoning test.	.31	.34	V	Verbal Comprehension. Advanced understanding of language, as measured in a Vocabulary or Reading test.	.08	.68
CMR	Semantic Relations. Eduction of a relation when this is shown among words, as in an Analogies test.	.37	.43				

Note.—After Cattell, 1963, 1967; Horn, 1965, 1966; Horn and Bramble, 1967; Horn and Cattell, 1967a.
[a] The referents here are primary factors, the names and symbols for which have been taken from French (1951), French, Ekstrom, and Price (1963) and Guilford (1967).
[b] These are rough averages computed over the several studies in which the primary factor was used.

acteristic of Gf are relatively culture fair in one of two senses: either the test materials are about equally common to all persons tested or else they are about equally novel. For example, the figural materials of the Matrices test are about as novel for college professors as for untutored laborers and the order of the English alphabet, as involved in the Letter Series test, is about as much over-learned by well-educated as by poorly-educated adults. In contrast, the vocabulary required in tests of verbal comprehension typically is that of a rather literate adult. Performance on such tests rather clearly indicates degree of acculturation. We cannot expect that any test will be perfectly culture fair or a perfect indicator of acculturation, but insofar as tests can be seen to involve one or the other of these emphases in measurement, they fall into the distinct patterns identified as Gf and Gc.

If anlage functioning is supported by relatively simple neural patterns and if abilities based upon incidental learning are supported by less complex cell assemblies than abilities based upon intensive acculturation, then fluid intelligence can be expected to show more impairment with loss of neurons than crystallized intelligence. If there are short-period, reversible fluctuations in the efficiency of neural functioning, producing an effect analogous to loss of neurons, fluid intelligence can be expected to show greater within-person variability over short periods of time than will crystallized intelligence. If aging in adulthood is associated with loss of neurons, either because of accumulation of brain injuries or because of inherent degenerative processes, then the trend of change with age in adulthood for fluid intelligence will tend to be downward relative to the change with age for crystallized intelligence. It is on this basis that evidence on

short-period fluctuations in abilities, changes accompanying brain injury, and changes associated with aging can all be said to pertain to the construct validity of the general Gf-Gc theory.

The test performances which Hebb (1949) found to be most severely affected by brain injuries are of the kind which characterize the fluid intelligence, whereas the performances which he found to be least affected by neural damage are characteristic of crystallized intelligence. In the studies of Horn (1965) and Horn and Cattell (1966a, 1967), the age differences in the Gf and Gc factors, and in the separate tests which defined these, were found to be in accordance with the theory. That is, Gf was found to decline with age in adulthood, Gc was found to increase, and omnibus measures, involving about equal parts of the Gf and Gc functions, neither declined nor improved.

In the Horn (1966) study, the Gf and Gc patterns were identified in terms of variations *within* persons, as well as by the more usual *R*-technique correlational procedures. This is an important kind of evidence, for it indicates that not only do the various behaviors which define the Gf and Gc factors covary to distinguish one person from another, they also covary in a reliable manner within a person over short periods of time. Cattell (1957) has pointed out that this kind of evidence is necessary to establish that an observed phenomenon represents a *functional unity*—that is, a process within the person—but there have been relatively few studies designed to show this kind of evidence, and none in the area of human abilities. More pointedly, the evidence of this study suggested that of the reliable variance available in Gf and Gc a larger proportion of that for Gf pertained to short-period fluctuations within persons.

These studies thus suggest that sev-

JOHN L. HORN

eral aspects of the Gf-Gc theory are in contact with reality. However, there are several points of controversy and several refinements of the theory which should be considered in the design of further research in this area.

COMPARISON WITH HIERARCHICAL THEORIES

Humphreys (1962, 1967) has pointed out that in many respects the Gf-Gc theory is congruent with hierarchical, group-factor theories put forth (mainly in Britain) by investigators such as Vernon (1961), Burt (1949, 1955), and Moursey (1952). In Vernon's work, for example, a distinction is drawn between a broad "abstract" verbal-numerical-educational factor (abbreviated V:ed), having properties similar to Gc, and an equally broad "practical" mechanical-spatial-physical factor (referred to as k:m), which is somewhat similar to Gf. But while this theory is, in its broad aspects, similar to the Gf-Gc theory, it is different in the following rather important respects:

1. In the V:ed-k:m theory mechanical abilities are regarded as "practical" and thus integral to k:m, whereas in the Gc-Gf theory these abilities are regarded as very possibly an outcome of intensive acculturation and thus likely to fall into Gc, rather than Gf.

2. In the most recent refinements of the Gc-Gf theory (as outlined below) a broad visualization function is regarded as distinct from Gf, whereas in the V:ed-k:m theory several tests involving visualization to a very considerable extent enter prominently in the definition of k:m.

3. The operational definitions of Gf and Gc derive from factor analyses based upon the principle of simple structure (Thurstone, 1947) objectively determined (as specified by Horn, 1967), whereas the V:ed and

k:m dimensions are defined by factoring procedures in some of which (bifactor procedures) the investigator makes subjective decisions concerning which variable goes into which factor and in all of which the principle of simple structure is not employed.

4. Although it is mainly only a matter of semantics, not a crucial point in theory, it is perhaps worth noting that the "abstract" versus "practical" distinction which is drawn to characterize the difference between V:ed and k:m is not used and is not appropriate for distinguishing between Gc and Gf: Performance on the Advanced Matrices test demands a very high level of abstraction and this helps to define Gf, whereas performance on such tests as Associational Fluency requires a lower level of abstraction and such tests help to define Gc, but in both factors there are tasks involving rather high-level and rather low-level abstractions (cf. Hayakawa, 1949).

In his critique of the Horn-Cattell (1966b) work Humphreys (1967) pointed out that the answer to the question concerning the separation of visualization and fluid intelligence may depend rather crucially upon the answer to the (as yet) unsolved question of the number of factors which can be reliably determined in a factor analysis. In his reanalysis Humphreys found a distinction between the Gf dimension and a broad visualization factor, but only when he estimated five factors, not when he estimated a smaller number of factors. Perhaps this issue should be considered from a pragmatic point of view: "Is it useful to maintain a distinction between visualization and fluid intelligence?"

As for the question about where the mechanical abilities fall in the higher-order relationships among all abilities, the existing evidence lends some support for both of the contending theories, as Humphreys (1967) pointed out. In the simple structure factor-analytic solutions which Horn (1965) reviewed, the mechanical abilities had noteworthy relationships with both the Gf and the Gc abilities and this was also a finding in the Horn-Cattell (1966b) study. This indicates that Procrustean procedures are not required to get the mechanical abilities into a k:m-like dimension. However, it also indicates that these abilities involve components of crystallized intelligence. It would seem that the purely reasoning aspects of mechanical abilities may permit the use of fluid intelligence but that a substantial proportion of the observed variability in these skills must relate to the same kinds of intensive educational influences as determine other aspects of crystallized intelligence.

FURTHER REFINEMENTS

Sensory Modality Factors

Visual processes are instrumental in much of the learning upon which the development of intelligence is based. To a large extent, such processes govern the immediate expression of abilities, particularly in tests. If vision is lacking, (as in the apes of Riesen's (1947, 1951) studies of early deprivation of sensory stimulation) some of the concepts and aids which otherwise might be developed simply cannot be developed. Insofar as these are skills which enable persons to behave intelligently, the blind individual inevitably will lack this aspect of intelligence. Moreover, the figures, small printing, etc., which constitute the basic materials of tests are often such that if one is somewhat deficient in visualization, test performance can be expected to be impaired.

But visualization processes can be distinguished from central intellective functions. The ability to scan a visual display quickly is not to be equated

with the ability to solve problems utilizing the information obtained from such scanning. Hence, while visualization will enter to some extent in the performances indicating both fluid and crystallized intelligence, it is possible that a visualization function can be distinguished from these intellective functions.

Although most current ability tests involve visualization to some extent, several involve this more than others. In particular, the tests of the primary factors known as Vz (Visualization), S (Spatial Orientation), Cs (Speed of Closure), Cf (Flexibility of Closure) explicitly require a subject to visualize movements of objects in space, find particular configurations imbedded within other configurations, bring about closure among disparate parts of a configuration, quickly scan configurations, etc. A central process seemingly involved in many of these tasks is one of visualizing in some sense of this term. Hence, if a broad visualization function pervades performance on many ability tasks but the above-mentioned primaries represent this to a greater degree than do other primaries, then a factor identified by these primaries can be expected to appear in a well-designed factor-analytic study. The factor identified as Gv, visualization, in the analyses of Horn (1965, 1966), Horn and Bramble (1967), and Horn and Cattell (1966b) is interpreted on this basis (see also Smith, 1965).

The finding of a broad visualization influence pervading performances in ability tasks provokes the idea that analogous functions should exist to represent the influences of other sensory modalities, as, for example, audition and tactility. Such functions could not have been identified in the research thus far completed simply because the performances studied in this research were not of a kind that could be expected to involve systematic variance due to these factors. Holmes and Singer (1966) have found, however, that audition plays a rather important role in the learning of such crystallized skills as reading comprehension and that the influences represented by audition are somewhat independent of those represented by visualization. Similarly, Jones and Wepman (1961) have shown that sensory modality influences produce independent dimensions of variance in measurements of aphasia. If new tests were constructed which were otherwise like existing tests but involved auditory or tactile processes, rather than visual processes, then in factor analyses involving these and a broad sample of primary ability tests auditory and tactile factors might be identified and be shown to have variance in existing intellectual tests. If such functions were found to account for substantial portions of the variance in putative tests of intelligence, then it would be implied that truly balanced measures of intelligence (as Horn and Cattell, 1965, have discussed "balanced") should contain items emphasizing use of audition and tactility, as well as visualization.

Speediness-Carefulness Factors

Questions about speed of performance, as it relates to intellectual functioning and speededness of test administration, have a long and complex history (cf. Morrison, 1960). It is not proposed that these questions be gone into in detail here. However, some of these questions have already come up in consideration of results obtained in previous research (Horn, 1965, 1966; Horn & Cattell, 1966b) and so must be recognized in the general theory.

Two broad factors identified in previous studies involved tasks wherein speed of performance was emphasized: These were labeled Gs (Speediness)

and F (Fluency). One factor identified in previous work indicated a kind of opposite of speediness: This was labeled C (Carefulness). It will be worthwhile to consider these separately.

The Gs function was defined primarily by relatively simple tests in which virtually all subjects would get all problems correct if the test were not speeded. Tasks such as canceling, copying (backward as well as forward), and simple numerical operations produced the principal variance in this factor. There is thus some suggestion that the speediness function is more closely related to temperament and/or effortfulness in the immediate testing situation than to a capacity to think quickly. However, the question implied here cannot be answered on the basis of existing evidence. More research is needed to clarify the possible distinction between involuntary and voluntary speediness and between speediness pertaining to central intellective functions and that associated with peripheral functions.

The broad fluency factor mentioned above was defined by the primaries Fa (Associative Fluency) and Fi (Ideational Fluency), but the factor also had variance in such tests as Vocabulary and Verbal Analogies. On logical and psychological grounds it might be expected that the fluency tests would correlate with speediness measures to represent a truly general speed-of-thinking function, but Gs and F were found to be largely independent. In the Horn (1965) study Furneaux's (1956) tests of intellectual speed had no appreciable correlation with F.

The F factor is not broad enough to represent intellectual speed, per se. Instead it seems to represent speediness only in tasks wherein it is necessary to bring concept labels (that is, words) from a long-term storage center into immediate awareness. As Christensen and Guilford (1963) point out, such a function might relate to size of store of labeled concepts and/or to quickness in finding those concept labels which are stored, regardless of number.

That the latter accounts for some of the observed variance in the fluency function is indicated by the results from Horn's (1966) study of short-period fluctuations in abilities. One of the factors accounting for a substantial proportion of the reliable variability within persons over occasions was defined by associational and ideational fluency. This factor had a substantial *negative* correlation with fluent production of irrelevant associations, a variable which had substantial *positive* correlation with the F factor when this was identified among correlations based upon variation between people. Taken together, these results suggest that fluency may mainly represent an anlage function of ease of finding concept labels.

It should be noted, too, that the ideational and associational fluency primary factors which determine the second-order fluency factor are among those which currently are being discussed as indicative of creativity (cf. Getzels & Jackson, 1962; Guilford, 1962; Taylor, 1964). Moreover, some of this discussion seems to imply that creative ability—to be distinguished, theoretically, from motivation to create and creative temperament—may be functionally independent of intelligence. Thus it is possible that the factor identified as "general fluency" is, in fact, a shadowy indication of a broad creativity function.

This hypothesis is made somewhat suspect, however, by results from recent research. The primary factor known as Figural Adaptive Flexibility (DFT), and sometimes discussed as indicative of creativity, was included in the Horn-Cattell (1966a) study, but it did not fall into the broad fluency factor and, in fact, had relatively little variance in common with associational and ideational fluency. In the Horn (1966) and Horn-Bramble (1967) studies, Mednick's (1962) Remote Association Test (RAT) was included. This is often referred to as a measure of creativity and is very similar to the tests which identify the factor O, Originality, also usually mentioned as indicating creativity (Guilford, 1962). Yet RAT did not come into the factor involving the fluency variables and, in fact, had relatively little variance in common with these. Instead the variance for this variable went into the Gc factor, suggesting that the "originality" seen in remote associations may represent, primarily, crystallized intelligence. In any case, this evidence does *not* provide support for a hypothesis stipulating that the primary factors and variables said to be indicative of creativity do, in fact, indicate a unitary influence. It must be noted, however, that one of the areas most neglected in the sampling of factors in previous studies on the higher-order structure of abilities has been in this area which contains the primaries that are said to be indicative of creativity.

Carefulness in an intellectual test is measured by subtracting the number of incorrect or irrelevant responses from a constant (the same constant being used for all subjects, of course), rather than by recording the number of correct responses, as is more usual (cf. Fruchter, 1950, 1953). If a test is speeded, so that not all people will attempt all items, the correlation between the carefulness score and the number-correct score can be less than 1.0. On first consideration, it might seem that carefulness in ability performances is merely the obverse of speediness. But the evidence does not support this notion. Speediness and carefulness in timed ability tests appear to be independent functions, although the correlation between them is slightly negative (−.26 in the Horn-Cattell, 1966b, results). The finding of a carefulness factor indicates that unwillingness to give incorrect answers is a fairly general characteristic, pervading a variety of intellectual tasks. This is one possible meaning of the concept of "style" or "strategy" in ability performances (cf. Bruner, Goodnow, & Austin, 1956; Sigel, 1963).

When a test is scored by the constant-minus-wrongs procedure, the person who adopts a strategy of avoiding errors has the advantage; when the same test is scored by the usual number-correct procedure, the person who adopts a strategy of getting as many right as possible—even if this entails making a few errors—has the advantage. An interesting finding of the Horn-Bramble study was that if all of a set of primary factor variables are obtained in the first-mentioned way, the structure indicated by factoring the intercorrelations among these variables is very similar to that found by factoring among primaries measured by the usual number-correct procedure. This suggests that the same ability processes are mirrored in performances involving both careful and "sloppy" strategies. Yet the Horn-Bramble results indicated that persons who score high on a factor when it is measured in a way which penalizes carefulness may score relatively low (as indicated by correlations of about .5) in a factor involving the same tests scored in a way which penalizes "sloppiness." Some interesting practical and theoretical questions are provoked by these results.

A hypothesis in the Horn-Cattell (1966b) study was to the effect that carefulness represents a kind of cautiousness such as might be determined by superego or self pride; but the evidence of this study provided little support for this hypothesis. It could be argued (after the fact) that really good measures of superego and self pride were not included in this study. In future studies it will be desirable to try out some new measurements of this kind, such as those identified (Cattell & Horn, 1963, 1964; Cattell, Horn & Butcher, 1962) among attitude variables as representing superego and self-sentiment functions.

It would seem that some of the observed variability in speediness and carefulness factors may stem from differences in motivation to achieve—that is, the kind of attribute which McClelland (1950, 1953) and his co-workers have described as need for achievement (n Ach). Similarly, it would seem that some of the variance in these factors might stem from an attribute similar to that which Atkinson (1958) has rather fully described as fear-of-failure (f-fail). It could be, too, that such n Ach and f-fail influences could represent states, not traits (cf. Horn, 1963, 1966; Horn & Little, 1966), engendered by situational factors. On a priori grounds it is reasonable to suppose that either the speediness, fluency or carefulness factor—or any two or all three—may represent variability which distinguishes individuals on a given occasion but is not a stable characteristic of any particular individual.

SOME GENERAL IMPLICATIONS

It is well known that even in rather homogeneous samples of subjects most tests which are accepted as measuring the intellectual abilities of humans have positive intercorrelations. Primary mental ability factors usually are found to be positively intercorrelated. The functions described in previous sections were positively intercorrelated in the studies cited. This well-documented finding of generally positive intercorrelations—a positive manifold—among intellectual abilities has been accepted widely as evidence in support of a hypothesis of a general intelligence factor underlying observed performances. While this evidence cannot be discounted and there is a sense in which it indicates a general intelligence, too much should not be inferred from it. Positive manifold is not equivalent to hierarchical order among intercorrelations (Spearman, 1927), although this seems to be assumed in some discussions of the concept of general intelligence. Hierarchical order may be interpreted parsimoniously as indicating one and *only* one influence, but positive manifold permits the possibility of many influences only loosely interrelated.

It is worth observing in this respect that not only do ability performances intercorrelate positively, but also many nonintellectual personality factors fall into this same positive manifold. When anxiety tests are scored in the non-anxious direction, for example, they have generally positive correlations with ability measurements. Similarly, the self-sentiment and superego factors among attitude variables (Cattell & Horn, 1963, 1964; Cattell, Horn, & Butcher, 1962) have generally positive correlations with ability tests. And, of course, social status and education are in the positive manifold. While it is reasonable to suppose that these several kinds of variables are mutually interdependent in rather complex ways, there is little to suggest that they all represent the operation of a single kind of influence. It is this kind of proviso which needs to be kept clearly in mind when interpreting the fact of positive intercorrelations among ability performances.

A practical implication of the theory and findings reviewed in this paper is that in educational and clinical settings we should move away from the idea of using a single ability test for the purposes of counseling, selection, diagnosis, and prognosis. This does not mean that we should move to the other extreme of separately measuring every aspect of human intellectual ability, as seems to be implied by Guilford's theory. Nor does it mean that ability distinctions defined purely, or mainly, on the basis of logic alone—such as the verbal-quantitative distinction which McNemar (1964) seems to favor—should constitute a basis for applied use or theoretical formulation. Broad constructs of intellect should be based upon empirically-established patterns of correlation in performance. Granted that the linear patterns established by linear factor-analytic procedures are not ideal and are somewhat Procrustean, still they constitute reasonable first approximations of the more nearly ideal patterns and thus represent a useful first step toward accomplishing a truly adequate description of human abilities. In several ways, then, the position put here is a compromise of opposing positions currently extant in the field of human abilities.

A more argumentative implication of this review is that more future research should be directed toward bringing together results from studies pertaining to process and development, on the one hand, and results on structure (or correlational patterns) among performances in ability tests, on the other hand. For too long there have been too many invidious comparisons of work stemming from these sources, the implication sometimes being that one approach had the inside road to truth while the other was patent nonsense. When stated thus bluntly, of course, such extreme positions can be rejected rather easily. Nevertheless, there has been precious little cross-reference in the two major streams of research here indicated. Fortunately, many signs point toward removing communication barriers between these two. In this sense the Gf-Gc theory, with its emphasis on bringing factor-analytic research on abilities into the context of developmental and process theories, is just one among several aspects of a Zeitgeist.

REFERENCES

Anderson, J. E. The limitations of infant and preschool tests in the measurement of intelligence. *Journal of Psychology,* 1939, **8,** 351–379.

Anderson, J. E. The prediction of terminal intelligence from infant and preschool tests. *39th Yearbook of National Society for Studies in Education,* 1940, **1,** 385–403.

Atkinson, J. W. *Motives in fantasy, action and society.* New York: Van Nostrand, 1958.

Bayley, N. Consistency and variability in the growth of intelligence from birth to eighteen years. *Journal of Genetic Psychology,* 1949, **75,** 165–196.

Bayley, N. On the growth of intelligence. *American Psychologist,* 1955, **10,** 805–818.

Bayley, N. Comparisons of mental and motor test scores for ages 1–15 months by sex, birth order, race, geographical location and education of parents. *Child Development,* 1965, **36,** 379–411.

Botzum, W. A factorial study of reasoning and closure factors. *Psychometrika,* 1951, **16,** 361–386.

Bruner, J. S., Goodnow, J. J., & Austin, G. A. A study of thinking. New York: Wiley, 1956.

Burt, C. Subdivided factors. *British Journal of Statistical Psychology,* 1949, **19,** 176–199.

Burt, C. The evidence for the concept of intelligence. *British Journal of Educational Psychology,* 1955, **25,** 158–177.

Cattell, R. B. Some theoretical issues in adult intelligence testing. *Psychological Bulletin,* 1941, **38,** 592. (Abstract)

Cattell, R. B. *Personality and motivation structure and measurement.* Yonkers-on-Hudson, N. Y.: World Book, 1957. Pp. 1–20, 871–880.

Cattell, R. B. Theory of fluid and crystallized intelligence: A critical experiment. *Journal of Educational Psychology,* 1963, **54,** 1–22.

Cattell, R. B. The theory of fluid and crystallized general intelligence checked at the 5–6 year-old level. *British Journal of Educational Psychology,* 1967, **37,** 209–224.

Cattell, R. B., & Horn, J. L. An integrative study of the factor structure of adult attitude-interests. *Genetic Psychology Monographs,* 1963, **67,** 89–149.

Cattell, R. B., & Horn, J. L. *The handbook for the MAT.* Champaign, Ill.: Institute for Personality and Ability Testing, 1964.

Cattell, R. B., Horn, J. L., & Butcher, J. The dynamic structure of attitudes in adults. *British Journal of Psychology,* 1962, **53,** 57–69.

Christensen, P. R., & Guilford, J. P. An experimental study of verbal fluency factors. *British Journal of Mathematical and Statistical Psychology,* 1963, **16,** 1–26.

Duncanson, J. P. Intelligence and the ability to learn. (Research Bulletin RB-64-29.) Princeton: Educational Testing Service, 1964.

Ferguson, G. A. On learning and human ability. *Canadian Journal of Psychology,* 1954, **8,** 95–112.

Ferguson, G. A. On transfer and the abilities of man. *Canadian Journal of Psychology,* 1956, **10,** 121–131.

Fleishman, E. A., & Hempel, W. E. Changes in factor structure of complex psychomotor tests as a function of practice. *Psychometrika,* 1954, **19,** 239–252.

Fleishman, E. A., & Hempel, W. E. The relation between abilities and improvement with practice in a visual discrimination reaction task. *Journal of Experimental Psychology,* 1955, **49,** 301–310.

French, J. W. The description of aptitude and achievement tests in terms of rotated factors. *Psychometric Monographs,* No. 5, 1951.

French, J. W., Ekstrom, R. B., & Price, I. A. Manual for kit of reference tests for cognitive factors. Princeton: Educational Testing Service, 1963.

Fruchter, B. Error scores as a measure of carefulness. *Journal of Educational Psychology,* 1950, **41,** 279–291.

Fruchter, B. Differences in factor content of rights and wrongs scores. *Psychometrika,* 1953, **18,** 257–265.

Furneaux, W. D. *The Nufferno manual of speed and level tests.* London: National Foundation of Educational Research, 1956.

Getzels, J. W., & Jackson, P. W. *Creativity and intelligence.* New York: Wiley, 1962.

Guilford, J. P. Creativity: Its measurement and development. In S. Parnes & H. Harding (Eds.), *A source book for creative thinking.* New York: Scribner, 1962.

GUILFORD, J. P. The nature of human intelligence. New York: McGraw-Hill, 1967.

GUTTMAN, L. A new approach to factor analysis: The Radex. In P. F. Lazarsfeld (Ed.), *Mathematical thinking in the social sciences.* Glencoe, Ill.: Free Press, 1954. Pp. 216–348.

HAYAKAWA, S. I. *Language in thought and action.* New York: Harcourt-Brace, 1949.

HEBB, D. O. Clinical evidence concerning the nature of normal adult test performance. *Psychological Bulletin,* 1941, **38,** 593. (Abstract)

HEBB, D. O. *The organization of behavior.* New York: Wiley, 1949.

HOFSTAETTER, P. R. The changing composition of intelligence. *Journal of Genetic Psychology,* 1954, **85,** 159–164.

HOFSTAETTER, P. R., & O'CONNOR, G. P. Anderson's overlap hypothesis and the discontinuities of growth. *Journal of Genetic Psychology,* 1956, **88,** 95–106.

HOLMES, J. A., & SINGER, H. *Speed and power of reading in high school.* Washington, D. C.: United States Government Printing Office, 1966.

HORN, J. L. The discovery of personality traits. *Journal of Experimental Research,* 1963, **56,** 460–465.

HORN, J. L. Fluid and crystallized intelligence: A factor analytic and developmental study of structure among primary mental abilities. Unpublished doctoral dissertation, University of Illinois, 1965.

HORN, J. L. Short-period changes in human abilities. (National Aeronautics and Space Administration Report-618.) Denver, Colorado: Denver Research Institute, 1966.

HORN, J. L. Intelligence—Why it grows, why it declines. *Transaction,* 1967, **4,** 23–31.

HORN, J. L. On subjectivity in factor analysis. *Educational and Psychological Measurement,* 1967, **27,** 811–820.

HORN, J. L., & BRAMBLE, W. J. Second-order ability structure revealed in rights and wrongs scores. *Journal of Educational Psychology,* 1967, **58,** 115–122.

HORN, J. L., & CATTELL, R. B. Vehicles, ipsatization and the multiple-method measurement of motivation. *Canadian Journal of Psychology,* 1965, **19,** 265–279.

HORN, J. L., & CATTELL, R. B. Age differences in primary mental abilities. *Journal of Gerontology,* 1966, **21,** 210–220. (a)

HORN, J. L., & CATTELL, R. B. Refinement and test of the theory of fluid and crystallized intelligences. *Journal of Educational Psychology,* 1966, **57,** 253–270. (b)

HORN, J. L., & CATTELL, R. B. Age differences in fluid and crystallized intelligence. *Acta Psychologica,* 1967, **26,** 1–23.

HORN, J. L., & LITTLE, K. B. Methods for isolating change and invariance in patterns of behavior. *Multivariate Behavioral Research,* 1965, **1,** 219–229.

HUMPHREYS, L. G. Investigations of the simplex. *Psychometrika,* 1960, **25,** 313–323.

HUMPHREYS, L. G. The organization of human abilities. *American Psychologist,* 1962, **17,** 475–483.

HUMPHREYS, L. G. Critique of Cattell's "Theory of fluid and crystallized intelligence: A critical experiment." *Journal of Educational Psychology,* 1967, **58,** 120–136.

HUNT, J. McV. *Intelligence and experience.* New York: Ronald Press, 1961.

JONES, L. V., & WEPMAN, J. M. Dimensions of language performance in aphasia. *Journal Speech and Hearing Research,* 1961, **4,** 220–232.

MARTIN, L., & ADKINS, D. C. A second-order analysis of reasoning abilities. *Psychometrika,* 1954, **19,** 71–78.

MEDNICK, S. A. The associative basis of the creative process. *Psychological Review,* 1962, **69,** 220–232.

McCLELLAND, D. C. *Personality.* New York: McGraw-Hill, 1950.

McCLELLAND, D. C. *The achievement motive.* New York: Appleton-Century-Crofts, 1953.

McNEMAR, Q. Lost: Our intelligence. Why? *American Psychologist,* 1964, **19,** 871–882.

MORRISON, J. R. Effects of time limits on the efficiency and factorial composition of reasoning measures. Unpublished doctoral dissertation, University of Illinois, 1960.

MOURSEY, E. N. The hierarchical organization of cognitive levels. *British Journal of Statistical Psychology,* 1952, **3,** 151.

PIAGET, J. *The origins of intelligence in children.* (Trans. by M. Cook.) New York: International University Press, 1952.

PIAGET, J. *The psychology of intelligence.* (Trans. by M. Piercy & D. E. Berlyne.) London: Routledge & Kegan Paul, 1947.

RIESEN, A. H. The development of visual perception in man and chimpanzee. *Science,* 1947, **106,** 107–108.

Riesen, A. H. Post-partum development of behavior. *Chicago Medical School Quarterly*, 1951, **13**, 17–24.

Rimoldi, H. J. Study of some factors related to intelligence. *Psychometrika*, 1948, **13**, 27–46.

Roff, M. A statistical study of the development of intelligence test performance. *Journal of Psychology*, 1941, **11**, 371–386.

Sigel, I. E. How intelligence tests restrict our concept of intelligence. *Merrill-Palmer Quarterly*, 1963, **9**, 39–56.

Smith, I. M. *Spatial ability: Its educational and social significance.* San Diego: Knapp, 1965.

Spearman, C. *The abilities of man.* New York: Macmillan, 1927.

Taylor, C. W. *Creativity: Progress and potential.* New York: McGraw-Hill, 1964.

Thurstone, L. L. *Multiple-factor analysis.* Chicago: University of Chicago Press, 1947.

Vernon, P. E. *The structure of human abilities.* (2nd ed.) London: Methuen, 1961.

Vernon, P. E. Environmental handicaps and intellectual development. Parts I and II. *British Journal of Educational Psychology*, 1965, **35**, 1–22.

(Received May 11, 1967)

155

THE JOURNAL OF
EDUCATIONAL PSYCHOLOGY

Volume XXXI	March. 1940	Number 3

A CULTURE-FREE INTELLIGENCE TEST I

RAYMOND B. CATTELL

Clark University

SOME CONSEQUENCES OF DEFECTIVE INTELLIGENCE THEORY

Psychologists dealing with the application of intelligence tests seem to pass through alternating phases of uncritical overconfidence and cynical despair with regard to the validity of their measurements. To judge by recent utterances the fashionable phase at the moment is disillusionment; the tests do not measure any constant characteristic of the individual, and no two tests measure the same thing.[1]

The paralyzing effect of such antics upon steady investigation and constructive theory is most apparent in social psychology, where some far-reaching causative relations are just becoming apparent between the dynamics of population, the dynamics of socio-political ideas, and the static resistances arising from the distribution of intelligence quotients.[2,3] Justifiable limitations to the interpretation of tests are indicated by Neff when he says, "Most authorities are now agreed that a test standardized on one racial or national group cannot be applied to a group of differing culture and background"; but he joins absurdly in the current panic stampede from a sense of perspective when he concludes, "All of the twenty point mean differences in IQ

---

[1] Most of the current statements about IQ's are really statements about special environment skills, functional fluctuation, experimental error, etc. in unassigned degrees, as may be represented by the following equation.

$$\text{IQ (apparent)} = \text{IQ (real)} + s + f + e + p,$$

where s is a large special factor of knowledge or skill.

    f is the functional fluctuation of the individual's intelligence, diurnally etc.

    e is experimental error of measurement.

    p is a factor of intelligence test sophistication.

[2] Lorimer, F. and Osborn, F.: *Dynamics of Population.* 1934.

[3] Cattell, Raymond B.: "Some Changes in Social Life in a Community with a Falling Intelligence Quotient." *The British Journal of Psychology*, Vol. xxviii, 1938, pp. 430–450.

The Journal of Educational Psychology

found to exist between children of the lowest and highest social status may be accounted for entirely in environmental terms."[1]

That such capricious doubts can be thrown on the whole of the closely dovetailed superstructure of educational and social research data and theory is possible only because of years of neglect in regard to the real foundations of intelligence testing. It represents the cost of precipitate, incontinent, and complacent multiplication of intelligence tests without sound research and theory concerning the nature of intelligence. True, in the last eight years there has been a more widespread tendency for research workers to examine their tests more carefully in the light of general principles; but the crop of results in educational and social research available today springs from tests designed before this period. Consequently discussion gets nowhere; and it is logically possible for Neff,[2] for example, to argue that there are no social status differences in innate intelligence, or for Klineberg[3] to argue that even the most biologically distant racial groups do not differ in average native ability, in face of the general sense of all the direct and indirect evidence to the contrary.

In the unfortunate medley of tests employed we find only this much in common: that they measure a good deal of obviously acquired knowledge and skill, and that they are heavily weighted with scoring on special abilities distinct from intelligence. The meaning of the measurements used in these researches will probably remain forever obscure. There has been much painstaking work on the theme around which most of the applied problems cluster; namely, the nature-nurture issue, but their expenditure is rendered null and void in most instances because the experimenters argue in a circle, first putting environmental skills in their tests and then proving that environment effects "intelligence"—obtaining various results according to the amount of contamination of the instrument. One might as well wipe the slate clean of these earlier results—and especially those at the nursery school age—and begin afresh with sounder tests.

A COMMON SOURCE OF ERROR

Instead of bringing a charge seemingly at random it would be best to pillory one of the leading offenders, the Binet test, on which a

---

[1] Neff, W. S.: "Socio-economic Status and Intelligence: a Critical Survey." *Psychological Bulletin*, Vol. xxxv, No. 10, 1938.

[2] *Ibid.*

[3] Klineberg, O.: *Race Differences.*

A Culture-free Intelligence Test

surprising amount of the nature-nurture evidence is allowed to depend. Some time ago I dealt with the objections to this test,[1,2] which I will only summarize briefly here.

(1) The component items are frequently tests of scholastic attainment and life experience rather than "*G*."

(2) The test items are too few in number (over any limited age range) for good consistency or validity.

(3) The higher mental ages are not catered for.

(4) Certain special group factors play a large part, notably "*V*" or the verbal factor; the "practical ability" found by Alexander,[3] El Koussy,[4] and in the Chicago research,[5] and almost certainly the "*F*" factor of "fluency of association" which is a matter of temperament rather than of cognitive ability.[6,7]

(5) If, as most clinical psychologists concede, the test is not concerned with any one ability, the use of a single quantitative value for the hodgepodge is meaningless.

(6) In consequence of dilution of the "*G*" measurement with scholastic attainment and life experience, which is less scattered than "*G*" (*e.g.*, the old dull child has more experience than the young bright) the Binet does not give a standard deviation of intelligence quotients as wide as that which actually exists.

(7) The personal situation in this form of individual testing is not an unmixed blessing, producing possible embarrassment in the subject and subjectivity of scoring in the examiner.

The gravamen of these objections applies as much to the revisions of the Binet as to the original. As I have remarked elsewhere, a person of Binet's lively mind would be the last to be using the Binet test in the present stage of advance, and "the prolonged worship of the Binet scale has left us with an encumbering heritage of erroneous

---

[1] Cattell, Raymond B.: "Measurement Versus Intuition in Applied Psychology." *Character and Personality*, Vol. VL, 1937.

[2] Cattell, Raymond B.: *A Guide to Mental Testing*, 1936.

[3] Alexander, W. P.: "Intelligence, Concrete and Abstract." *Brit. Journ. Psych. Monograph Supplement*, No. 19, 1936.

[4] El Koussy, A. A. H.: "The Visual Perception of Space." *Brit. Journ. Psych. Monograph Supplement*, No. 20, 1937.

[5] Reports 1–9 of the Spearman-Holzinger Unitary Trait Study. Psychology Department, University of Chicago, 1935.

[6] Cattell, R. B.: "Temperament Tests. II Tests." *Brit. Journ. Psych.*, Vol. XXIV, 1933.

[7] Cattell, R. B.: *A Guide to Mental Testing*, 1936.

conceptions, especially in matters concerning the distribution of intelligence and its rôle to society." This remark is quoted by Burt in a recent article[1] in which he continues to defend the Binet test, but yet definitely admits that "The ideal plan would be to take each separate test problem and examine its special value in a criterion of intelligence. Curiously enough, this has rarely been attempted."[2]

Bristol and the present writer in 1932 evaluated the "*G*" saturations of seven of the Binet subtests in the course of producing from eighteen types of test the best test for children of four to eight years of age.[3] Four of the seven came in the five lowest tests on the list of eighteen, their mean intercorrelations averaging less than 0.30. As regards the alternative basis of evaluation—that actually used in the Binet revisions—which considers increase of score with age to be the criterion of intelligence, Spearman[4] has well said that it would lead to measuring the child's intelligence by counting his teeth.

Evidence of the unusual heavy weighting with acquired skills is found in such researches as that in which Freeman[5] correlated scores on intelligence tests with the estimated difference of educational background among identical twins reared apart, with the following result:

Binet IQ difference with education difference................ .791
Otis IQ difference with education difference................ .547

Since the Otis itself cannot be considered entirely free from pedagogical effects the Binet is evidently heavily weighted in this respect. Nor is this surprising when one reflects on such typical items as that in which the child is asked to define a "guitar," "treasury," "milksop," etc.

But the final reduction to absurdity of that hasty test construction which has neither relation eduction nor "*G*" saturation as its guiding

---

[1] Burt, C.: "The Latest Revision of the Binet Intelligence Test." *Eugenics Review*, Vol. xxx, No. 4, 1939.

[2] With the same frankness as to the untenability of his position, Burt admits that no two editors of the Binet agree about the order of mental age items. He continues, "The second 'Paper Cutting Test,' which Terman assigns to the third or highest level of 'Superior Adults' we find can be done at age fourteen" whilst "Giving similarities between three things" is at the eleventh and fourteenth-year-old levels in America and Britain respectively.

[3] Cattell, R. B. and Bristol, H.: "Intelligence Tests for Mental Ages of Four to Eight Years." *Brit. Journ. Ed. Psych.*, Vol. iii, No. II, 1933.

[4] Spearman, C.: "The New Stanford Revision of the Binet." *The Human Factor*, Vol. xi, 1937.

[5] Freeman, F. N., Holzinger, K. J., and Newman, H. H.: *Twins: A Study of Heredity and Environment*, 1937.

A Culture-free Intelligence Test

principle, appears when some of these "tests" are intercorrelated. Thus Furfey and Muhlenbein,[1] taking one of the most popular of the numerous recent infant test scales, found that the order of seventy-one children had no correlation with the order on later testings by the Stanford Binet.[2]

The Binet test is discussed more fully, not because it is most open to criticism, but because it is most frequently used. To escape from such a test into performance tests is to go from the frying pan into the fire; for in avoiding knowledge and verbal skills we lose intelligence itself, many performance tests being largely a measure of manual dexterity.[3]

"GREATEST COMMON KNOWLEDGE" AMONG DIVERSE CULTURES

In spite of the fervour with which some psychologists foster the impotent attitude that differences of intelligence with social status, race, or nature-nurture factors must remain permanently uninvestigated, the viewpoint cannot and need not be accepted. The possibility of finding among different culture groups a common ground of knowledge, on which operations of reasoning could be performed, is not chimerical. The following list of objects common to the observations of men wherever and however they live is given as an illustration of a possible nucleus, upon which careful investigation of primitive and civilized cultures might build a far longer and more detailed matrix of items for intelligence tests:

Common objects:

The human body and its parts.
Footprints, etc.
Trees (schematic and unspecific) (except for Eskimos!).
Four-legged animals (schematic and unspecific).
Earth and sky.
Clouds, sun, moon, stars, lightning.
Fire and smoke.
Water and its transformations.
Parents and children (growth) and simple family relationships (except in special tribes).

---

[1] Furfey, P. H., and Muhlenbeim, J.: "The Validity of Infant Intelligence Tests." *Journ. Genetic Psych.*, Vol. XL, 1932, pp. 219–223.

[2] Yet this test happens to be the basis for a widely repeated conclusion that the "intelligence" of nursery-school children has no relation to the intelligence or social status of the parents.

[3] Cox, J. W.: *Manual Dexterity*, 1935.

Common processes:

    Breathing, choking, coughing, sneezing.
    Eating, drinking, defaecating, urinating.
    Sleeping.
    Birth and death.
    Running, walking, climbing, jumping.
    Striking, stroking.
    Sensing—seeing, hearing, smelling, tasting, etc.
    Emotional experiences, anger, grief, etc.

If even this bare nuclear list does not provide a sufficiently rich variety of fundaments between which relations for intelligence tests can be built up, it is a reflection on the ingenuity of the psychologist. Of course the fundaments would have to be given in pictorial or verbal form and therein occurs the difficulty that words which translate with different connotations would have to be avoided. More serious is the objection that the same objects are themselves invested with different meanings by different cultures; but this is an objection to the intelligence tests suggested by the anthropologist rather than to those of the psychologist; for, as we shall see later, the latter can choose his relationships in such a way that only perceptual knowledge of the objects is involved.

Field anthropologists, whom the present writer has consulted as to subjects which have sufficiently strong interest, familiarity, and universality to make a basis for reasoning tests among primitive peoples, generally suggest such material as is involved in hunting and fishing, tracking, tribal law, and case histories, genealogies and family relationships. These provide complete fields in which the primitive shows highly agile reasoning powers.

They indicate tests in the form of "following directions," and "riddles," which have a play value for the native. This is a possible line of approach but is rendered difficult by the specificity of many of the knowledge items to particular cultures and climatic regions; we shall desert it in favor of an entirely new technique. Something midway between this purely anthropological approach and the test using abstract relations between common objects has, however, been exploited with remarkable skill and success by Porteus, who has shown in practical fashions the relative independence of environment which such tests achieve.[1,2] From such field work it seems clear that suitable

[1] Porteus, S. D.: *The Psychology of a Primitive People*, 1930.
[2] ———: *Primitive Intelligence and Environment*, 1937.

A Culture-free Intelligence Test

tests could be built on a properly investigated "greatest common knowledge" basis.

THE ORIGINS OF THE PERCEPTUAL INTELLIGENCE TEST

Nevertheless we need not follow that difficult path, for recent work has revealed a new approach. As early as 1926 Davey[1] had shown that pictorial "tests of intelligence" involved the same "*G*" factor as current intelligence tests. In 1931 Line,[2] while investigating visual perception in children, discovered that a certain test involving the eduction of relations between simple geometrical (*i.e.* less than pictorial) shapes were highly saturated with "*G*." Almost simultaneously Fortes[3] brought evidence towards the conclusion that valid "*G*" tests could be made from relation eduction in simple non-connotative visual material.

As Davey's, Forte's, and Line's work had only been on small populations of one hundred, Stephenson undertook a very thorough research and mathematical analysis on ten hundred thirty-seven subjects. He confirmed that the same "*G*" factor ran through verbal and non-verbal tests[4] and proved what till then had only been suspected: that a group factor of "verbal skill" ran through all verbal tests.[5]

With this assurance Spearman published his visual perception test with pantomime directions[6] in which the items had only their "perceptual" meaning and did not depend on "apperceptial associations," *i.e.*, were geometrical rather than pictorial. Arsenian,[7] Lorge,[8] and Zubin investigated the test in this country and the first showed that it

---

[1] Davey, C. M.: "A Comparison of Group Verbal and Pictorial Tests of Intelligence." *Brit. Journ. Psych.*, Vol. XVII, 1926.

[2] Line, W.: "The Growth of Visual Perception in Children." *Brit. Journ. Psych. Monograph Supplement*, No. 15, 1931.

[3] Fortes, M.: *A New Application of the Theory of Noegenesis to the Problem of Mental Testing.* Ph. D. Thesis, Univ. of London Library.

[4] Stephenson, W.: "Tetrad Differences for Non-verbal Subtests." *Journ. Educ. Psych.*, Vol. XXII, 1931.

[5] ———: "Tetrad Differences for Non-verbal and Verbal Tests." *Journ. Educ. Psych.*, Vol. XXII, 1931.

[6] Spearman, C.: *The Spearman Visual Perception Test*, 1933.

[7] Arsenian, Seth: "The Spearman Visual Perception Test (Part I). With Pantomime Direction." *Brit. Journ. Educ. Psych.*, Vol. VII, 1937, pp. 287–301.

[8] Dorge, I., and Arsenian, S.: "A Comparison of the Scores of the Spearman Visual Perception Test, Part I, Administered by Verbal and Pantomime Directions." *Journ. Educ. Psych.*, 1938, pp. 520–522.

The Journal of Educational Psychology

revealed significant differences between racial groups in situations in which the usual tests would have been ambiguous. He also found the following correlations:

Consistency coefficient.......................... 0.882 ± 0.0062
Correlation with Pintner non-language test....... 0.610
Correlation with C A V D when pantomime directions are used.............................. 0.5808
Correlation with C A V D when verbal directions are used....................................... 0.4795

Finally the test was included in the large scale factor analysis inquiry at Mooseheart, Illinois, under Thurstone and others, where it was again shown to be highly "*G*" saturated and free from any group factor.[1]

Some psychologists are slow to avail themselves of this type of test because its material comes seemingly from a single narrow field of experience, whereas they are used to sampling as widely as possible. We know, however, from the "Principle of Indifference of Indicator"[2] that the general ability factor can be soundly measured by tests from any field however narrow, providing on analysis they prove to have good saturation and to be free from group factor overlap. Incidentally the same principle promises success to culture-free intelligence tests based on even a small nucleus of "greatest common knowledge."

The choice of further forms of perceptual test to make suitable subtests for a culture-free intelligence test can be guided not only by the above specific researches, but also by the commonly accepted observations that in general the kinds of test showing the best "*G*" saturation are those involving relation and correlate education in a high degree and reproduction in the lowest degree. The individual's general ability might, therefore, be defined by the order of complexity of the relations which he is capable of handling. It is regrettable that no one has yet empirically classified common relationships according to complexity, extending from the simplest space or time relation to the most complex relation of evidence. A notable new form based on this principle is the "Progressive Matrix" tried out recently by Penrose and Raven[3] and which we shall describe with added modifications below.

---

[1] Reports 1–9 of the Spearman-Holzinger Unitary Trait Study. Psych. Dept., University of Chicago, 1935.

[2] Spearman, C.: *Abilities of Man*, 1927.

[3] Penrose, L. F., and Raven, J. C.: "A New Series of Perceptual Tests: Preliminary Communication." *Brit. Journ. Medical Psych.*, Vol. xvi, 1938.

A Culture-free Intelligence Test

CONSTRUCTION PRINCIPLES IN A COMPLETE PERCEPTUAL TEST

Aiming at deriving a culture-free intelligence test from this line of research we finally decided on the seven subtests listed below. The use of seven instead of one or two is not through any doubt as to the soundness of the principle of indifference of indicator, but to avoid weighting with one special factor, and, above all, to maintain interest through variety, an important necessity with cultural groups lacking habits of sustained concentration.

Subtests	Number of items	
	Practice part	Main part
Mazes	2	10
Series	5	15
Classification	5	15
Progressive Matrices I relation matrix first order	5	15
Progressive Matrices II relation matrix second order	5	15
Progressive Matrices III sequence matrix	5	15
Mirror images	5	15
Total	32	100

These tests are chosen as having most consistently and in different situations and populations manifested good "G" saturation. Their order is dictated largely by considerations of interest. The maze test has not always shown such good "G" correlation as the others; but as Porteus[1] has shown, it is as intriguing to primitive as to civilized people, and can therefore act here as a good "shock absorber" before the more artificial test forms. Series follows because that also has natural interest and connects with natural happenings, *e.g.*, growth. The mirror image test, which is very simple in form, demanding only short periods of attention, comes last, when fatigue may be present.

With the object of maintaining some direct attractiveness in the test items, as an ancillary to ulterior incentives, the drawings are sometimes representative of real objects (man, animal, tree), but only of such objects as would be common in the above sense; and even then

---

[1] Porteus, S. D.: *Primitive Intelligence and Environment*, 1937, p. 237; "it is also susceptible to practice improvement."

the solution of the item is neither aided nor confused by the pictorial associations, but depends directly on the perceptual evidence.

The subject's conception as to what operation is required of him in each of seven subtests is made to depend more on worked examples than on verbal instructions. The test could, if necessary, be given in pantomime. In the Progressive Matrices this education of the subject to a particular operation and mental set proceeds through carefully graded demonstration items.

Apart from these special considerations the following precautions found in the usual type of intelligence test have been adopted:

(1) There is a sufficient number of pass or fail items for the age range in question: one hundred items (one hundred thirty two including practice) for an age range of "eleven years and upward."

(2) Selective, not inventive, answers are required.

(3) The items have been arranged in order of difficulty by a preliminary research.

(4) A sufficiency of alternatives, of a "near correct" character, is introduced to reduce the proportion of "chance correct" answers to a low figure. It is found that six alternatives can easily be surveyed by the subject in this type of test; where two answers are required this reduces the "chance correct" ratio to 1:15.

(5) The main test is preceded by a "practice" part, with sufficient interval between the practice and the main part to permit some consolidation of notions encountered in the practice part. The results of the practice part are thrown away, whether the subjects have done such a test before or not. Since, as Vernon shows,[1] it is "sophistication" rather than "practice" that accounts for improvement in test scores (largely occurring between the first testing and the repetition), it is hoped that the greater part of test familiarity errors in individual variation measures will be eliminated.

(6) A time limit, of a fairly generous order, seems permissible on grounds of theory,[2,3] and desirable for practical convenience. The time assigned to each test is such that approximately seventy-five per cent of the subjects complete all items, and results in the whole test

---

[1] Vernon, P. E.: "Intelligence Test Sophistication." *Brit. Journ. Educ. Psych.*, Vol. VIII, 1938.

[2] Spearman, C.: *Abilities of Man*, 1927, Chap. XIV.

[3] Thorndike, E. L.: "Tests of Intelligence, Reliability, Significance, Susceptibility to Special Training, and Adaption to the General Nature of the Task," *School and Society*, Vol. IX, 1919.

A Culture-free Intelligence Test

(practice included) taking forty minutes. Because the researches which show that "speed with intention to speed" and "*G*" are not separable, have been based only on civilized populations, we are not entitled to say that the same would be true of mixed populations. Therefore, it has been thought desirable to standardize the test under both conditions: (*a*) timed and (*b*) with unlimited time.

Descriptions of the construction of subtests follow:

1. *Mazes.*—No adequate research exists as to the best design of maze tests, save that they must be seen as a whole, not merely run through, and that they can be scored about equally well by either time or errors.[1] For interest's sake, the present

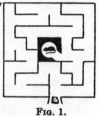

Fig. 1.

mazes were run through from within outwards, to imaginary food, to utilize both the escape drive and the food seeking goal, vicariously. Further, (*a*) the alternative paths were placed early, to force the subject to deliberate on the maze as a whole; and (*b*) the maze was designed to force the same consideration upon the subject if he should try the short cut of running the maze backwards (in imagination). The mazes grade from four passages to ten passages wide. (Fig. 1.)

2. *Series.*—These build up from progressive variations in shape or size to variations, progressive or alternating, in relations between shapes and size. (Fig. 2.)

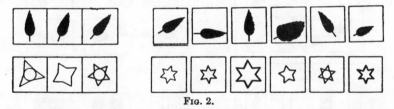

Fig. 2.

3. *Classification.*—The "right type" and "wrong type" method of Line,[2] Spearman,[3] and others has the advantage of being clear and direct, but is too space consuming, and its simplicity is necessary only with younger children. Picking out the odd item, on the other hand, has a certain intrinsic fascination, and resembles operations known to primitives (*e.g.*, picking out the odd animal from the herd). Two odd

---

[1] Porteus, S. D.: *Primitive Intelligence and Environment*, 1937.

[2] Line, W.: "The Growth of Visual Perception in Children." *Brit. Journ. Psych. Monograph Supplement*, No. 15, 1931.

[3] Spearman, C.: *The Spearman Visual Perception Test*, 1933.

The Journal of Educational Psychology

items were required here from six, since the chances of "chance correct" solutions are considerably lowered compared with one odd item. The only other condition specially observed here was that the need of

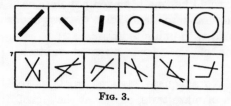

FIG. 3.

"searching around" for the feature on which differentiation is to depend should be cut down to a minimum, by conspicuously balancing

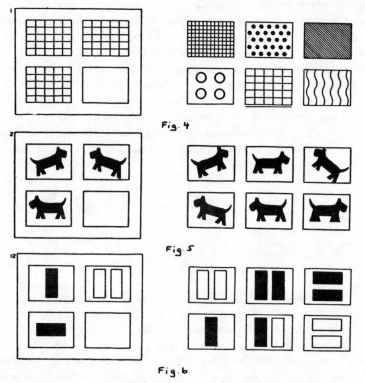

among all items the false irrelevant and partial differentiations. Thus in item 18 there are no two figures having only curved lines or only straight lines, whilst the duality of each figure is immediately conspicuous. (Fig. 3.)

A Culture-free Intelligence Test

4. *Relation Matrices: First Order.*—The subject is required to complete the figure by adding the fourth card, chosen from among the six alternatives at the bottom.

Beginning with a plain matching, Fig. 4; continuing through a bi-laterally symmetrical example, Fig. 5; and so into the main examples, Fig. 6, in which a relationship has to be educed between Figs. 4 and 5 and applied to Fig. 6 to produce a correlate. This correlate can be confirmed by a similar process beginning with the relation between the two left-hand figures. These are really analogies tests, overdetermined, and in perceptual form.

5. *Relation Matrices: Second Order.*—Raven has extended the above type of matrix to include nine figures.[1] The required operation can be gradually inculcated by the steps shown in Figs. 7 and 8. It seems to have been overlooked in designing this matrix type that the second row and the second column are unnecessary in educing the relations which define the missing item. Or, regarded from another angle, the third row and column are unnecessary, providing, as is usually the case, the relation between two and three is the same as between one and two, *i.e.*, if the trend is continuous:

An improvement is, therefore, possible in this matrix design, consisting in requiring the subject to perform a more complex relational operation on the same simple perceptual material. He is now, (after the above introduction), given only the first two figures in the first row and column. (Fig. 9.) From applying the relation between the first and second to the second he arrives at the third figure. From the relation of the first and third figures in the row, now applied to the third in the column, he arrives, as in the first order relation matrix, at the missing item.

6. SEQUENCE MATRICES.—Both Stephenson and Raven have found that the nine items matrix may be used as an intelligence test also when the determination of the missing item depends upon a perception of sequence (conjunction relation) instead of relations of the above kind.

The new subtest is introduced first by horizontal and then by horizontal and vertical "sequences," "rhythms," or "cycles." (Fig. 10.)

Then, first, the horizontal and, secondly, the vertical rhythms may be "staggered" or set in different phases. (Figs. 11 and 12.) Finally

---

[1] Penrose, L. F., and Raven, J. G.: "A New Series of Perceptual Tests: Preliminary Communication." *Brit. Journ. Medical Psych.*, Vol. XVI, 1936.

The Journal of Educational Psychology

the "staggered" sequence relation can be combined with the original straight column sequence and even a second order relation eduction in a dizzy palimpsest of superposed relationships, which may be further complicated by reducing the given figures to four. No research has

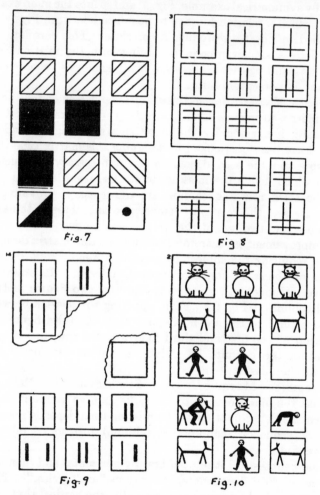

Fig. 7   Fig 8

Fig. 9   Fig. 10

yet shown whether such steps increase the "*G*" saturation, but, since each relationship applies to a different aspect of the figures, it is possible that the gain as an intelligence test, resulting from more complex relation play, is more than compensated for by the introduction of

A Culture-free Intelligence Test

some, presumably temperamental, factor invoked by the greater need to "search around" for the fundaments of the relations. (Figs. 13 and 14.)

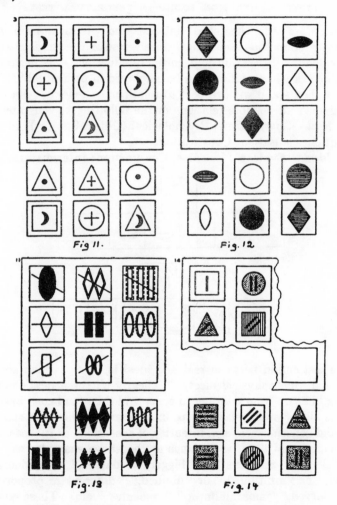

Fig 11.   Fig. 12   Fig. 13   Fig. 14

The variety of forms used in this matrix test, requiring continued re-orientation on the part of the subject, may be helpful in eliminating gain from "test sophistication."

7. MIRROR IMAGES.—The images are mirrored about a horizontal axis, in order that the universal experience of seeing reflections in a

The Journal of Educational Psychology

pool may be utilized in the instructions.   Items are made more difficult by rearranging masses rather than by increasing detail.   (Fig. 15.)

TYPES OF RELATION FOUND IN PERCEPTUAL TESTS

Because of the theoretical interest and practical problems of test construction that associate themselves with the thesis that *"G"* is coincident with relation and correlate eduction, it is desirable to pause and ask what relations can be employed in perceptual *"G"* tests and how they stand with respect to relations in general.   Spearman[1] has classified all possible relations in the following eleven categories:

(1) *Real.*—Space; Time; Psychological (Object-Subject); Identity; Attribution; Causation; Constitution.

(2) *Ideal.*—Evidence; Likeness; Conjunction; Intermixture.

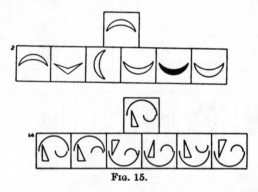

FIG. 15.

The distinction between real and ideal is, as Spearman shows, a traditional "metaphysical nicety."   Clearly all these relations admit of being built up from relations in space and time (and consciousness); they are higher order relationships in a hierarchy which has space and time (and consciousness *e.g.*, intensity of sensation) as its base.

In perceptual tests, as a glance at the above examples will show, we deal with relations of "bigger," "darker," "re-orientated," "added," or "multiplied," or "divided," "different in proportions," "more curved," "more uniform," "truncated," etc.   These relations, Spearman has shown,[2] are resolvable into distance, direction, and likeness, being based on fundaments of blackness and position.   But this overlooks the utilization of shades of greyness (*i.e.*, intensity of

---

[1] Spearman, C.: *Abilities of Man*, 1927.

[2] Spearman, C.: "Intelligence Tests." *Eugenics Review*, Vol. xxx, 1939.

A Culture-free Intelligence Test

sensation) which makes another available fundament.   Valid analogies and series tests have already been made on grey intensities alone.[1]

The fundamental relations possible in perceptual tests of this kind are, therefore, those of space, visually perceived, and visual sensation qualities.   But out of these can be built relations of Similarity, Attribution, Identity, Constitution, Conjunction, Intermixture and, indeed, all higher order relations save those which involve Time and the Psychological relations, *e.g.*, Causality and certain relations of Evidence.

Confining the operations to those that depend on spatial relations does not seem to have reduced the universality of "*G*" in these tests; perhaps because so many higher order relations can be built on those of space; perhaps because most people handle problems in which time is conceptually involved by thinking of it in spatial images, *e.g.*, as in school history charts or in Galton's clock images of time.

It is interesting to note that the perceptual time relation has already been independently used by Porteus[2] in his pragmatic approach to a culture-free intelligence test, in the subtest in which the subjects listened to a sequence of tones on a xylophone.   This is an illustration of the position one can reach on theoretical grounds: that a perceptual intelligence test could be built out of relationships from fundaments in any sense modality, seeing, hearing, tasting, etc.   The extent of the "*G*" factor in Seashore's musical aptitude tests shows that with more attention to higher relations of rhythm, pitch, and intensity, sound fundaments could equally be used for an "intelligence" test.   Because of the weight of apparatus required for experiments with most non-visual senses, and because of the danger that physical sense defects might become important, it seems best to restrict perceptual tests to vision and specifically to non-color vision, in optically groomed populations.   There is considerable opportunity for research, however, into the sensory range in which perceptual tests are practicable and advantageous.

MOTIVATION IN TEST PERFORMANCE

Although the present test is intended primarily for studying intelligence differences in social and cultural divisions of civilized

---

[1] El Koussy, A. H.: "A Note on the Greys Analogy Test."   *Brit. Journ. Educ. Psych.*, Vol. IV, 1938, p. 294.

[2] Porteus, S. D.: *The Psychology of a Primitive People*, 1931.

countries, it should admit of being used also with primitive peoples. *A priori* there would seem to be nothing objectionable for this purpose, in the cognitive material of the perceptual test but its use could perhaps be criticized on orectic grounds, for the interests, habits of attention, and normal speeds of working of primitive peoples are widely different from those assumable in school educated populations.[1]

Apart from introducing intrinsic and "play" interest[2] into the objects to be manipulated, allowing indefinite time and giving variety of subtest, it might appear that nothing has been done here to make the test as universally applicable orectically as cognitively.

Research has shown[3] that increases of motivation beyond a certain minimum level of concentration do not produce increases in intelligence test score. The number of items attempted increases, but so does the number of errors. An army may gain on a narrow salient by concentrating reinforcements but it cannot concentrate on all fronts at once. Similarly effort may improve some narrow specific skill but seems powerless to increase the general mental capacity. Subtests involving certain special factors, notably inferences, require, however, more effort than others, *e.g.*, opposites.[3] There is no reason to suppose that these findings regarding effort need be restricted to civilized people with ready-made attitudes of attention in examination situations. If the individual can be made to attend to a normal extent, by incentives of food, prestige reward, gifts, threats, or any of the numerous possible motivation sources, his intelligence can be measured, and more powerful motivation is not required to increase the accuracy of the measurement.

Further research as to the interchangeability of motives and the effects of varying intensity of motives is required; but the indications from the existing research are that the question of motive is best solved *ad hoc* by the field-worker on the spot, who can best judge what ade-

---

[1] Klineberg, O.: "Racial Differences in Speed and Accuracy." *Journal of Abnormal and Social Psychology*, Vol. XXII, pp. 273–277.

[2] In the research quoted (Cattell and Bristol, "Intelligence Tests for Mental Ages of Four to Eight Years") the writers experimented with food (candy) in puzzle boxes for children of four to eight years. The correlations were no better than for tests done under "please the experimenter" motivation.

[3] Wild, E. H.: "Influence of Conation upon Cognition; Part II." *Brit. Journ. Psych.*, Vol. XVIII, 1927.

A Culture-free Intelligence Test

quate motives he may stimulate in various groups. The work of Porteus shows that the tactful experimenter can induce a proper test attitude in even the most barbarous peoples, by studying their incentive systems. Accurate use of the present test in such situations is intended to be facilitated by the practice test and by administering the test individually.

From P. E. Vernon (1965). American Psychologist, *20*, 723–733. Copyright (1965), by kind permission
of the author and the American Psychological Association

ABILITY FACTORS AND ENVIRONMENTAL INFLUENCES [1]

PHILIP E. VERNON

Institute of Education, University of London

*Walter VanDyke Bingham left with his will a memorandum suggesting that there be established,
under the auspices of the American Psychological Association, an annual lectureship to call attention to the importance of the discovery and development of talented persons. His wishes have
been carried out by Mrs. Walter VanDyke Bingham in her continuing support of the "discovery of
the talented" lectures, of which the following paper was the twelfth. Previous lecturers, and the
institutions at which they spoke, have been:* LEWIS M. TERMAN, *University of California, Berkeley,
1954;* LOUIS L. THURSTONE, *Columbia University, 1955;* DONALD G. PATERSON, *Ohio State University, 1956;* CYRIL BURT, *University of London, 1957;* EDWARD K. STRONG, JR., *University of Minnesota, 1958;* J. P. GUILFORD, *Stanford University 1959;* DAEL WOLFLE, *Columbia University, 1960;*
JOHN M. STALNAKER, *Carnegie Institute of Technology, 1961;* DONALD W. MACKINNON, *Yale University, 1962;* EDWIN E. GHISELLI, *University of Michigan, 1963; and* NORMAN H. MACKWORTH,
Pennsylvania State University, 1964.

*A bibliography of Walter VanDyke Bingham's publications has been prepared and is available
from the American Personnel and Guidance Association, Inc., 1605 New Hampshire Avenue, N.W.,
Washington, D. C. 20009.*

I AM deeply appreciative of the honor of being invited to give this year's Walter VanDyke Bingham Lecture, and would especially like to applaud the initiative of Mrs. Bingham and the American Psychological Association Committee in including some psychologists from outside the United States in their scheme. England indeed has been greatly favored by the selection first of Cyril Burt, then of Norman Mackworth and myself; and I think that this is appropriate, because the Binghams had many friends and were widely respected among British applied psychologists. But might I venture to suggest that the Committee will also sometimes look further afield and consider whether other suitable lecturers might not be found, perhaps from France or Scandinavia, perhaps Canada or Australia? I would like also to take this opportunity to express my thanks to the Local Committee, and particularly to Robert Perloff, for the efficiency and the generosity of their arrangements. It is a special pleasure to visit Purdue University, which has long been associated in my mind with contributions to applied psychology, for example with the work of Joseph Tiffin, Hermann Remmers, and Charles Lawshe.

Although I have not, like some previous lecturers, had the privilege of close professional

contacts with Dr. Bingham, apart from friendly meetings at International Congresses, I have always admired *Aptitudes and Aptitude Testing* (Bingham, 1937) as one of the most sound and comprehensive treatments of the topic. During World War II it was a main textbook for the British military psychologists and personnel selection officers whom we trained for allocation of recruits to suitable trades. Bingham and Moore's (1931) *How to Interview* is likewise still a valuable text for occupational psychologists. And on looking up Dr. Bingham's career, I was delighted to find that his first love was the psychology of music and that he eventually came to vocational and military testing via educational psychology, for these are the areas in which I too have chiefly been interested.

In *Aptitudes and Aptitude Testing*, Walter VanDyke Bingham (1937) clearly attaches major importance to general intelligence, as I wish to do today. But he took no doctrinaire theoretical position on the nature of intelligence, being content to define it as the ability to solve new problems, which he recognized as the product of endowment + growth + opportunity. He admitted, too, that intelligence is complex, that there might be different intelligences for dealing with different kinds of problems, though he did not commit himself as to which main types should be distinguished. He tended rather to classify aptitudes in terms of the

[1] The Walter VanDyke Bingham Lecture given at Purdue University, April 21, 1965.

TABLE 1

DIFFERENTIAL APTITUDE TESTS: MEDIAN CORRELATIONS
WITH SCHOOL GRADES AMONG SEVERAL CLASSES OF
NINTH–TWELFTH-GRADE BOYS

	English	Maths	Science	Social studies
Verbal reasoning	.49	.33	.54	.48
Numerical computation	.48	.47	.52	.46
Abstract reasoning	.32	.32	.42	.32
Space	.26	.26	.34	.24
Mechanical comprehension	.21	.19	.40	.21
Clerical speed and accuracy	.22	.16	.24	.21
Spelling	.44	.28	.36	.36
Sentences (English usage)	.50	.32	.45	.43

Note.—Four highest coefficients in each column are underlined.

main kinds of jobs for which people might be selected.

I want, then, to ask again what are the most useful psychological dimensions or factors under which the vocational psychologist can conceptualize people, and how do these originate? What can research tell us of the environmental influences that chiefly contribute to individual differences in these abilities? I intend to argue the case for a model, or structure, of ability factors which, even 3 years ago, might have been considered by most American psychometrists as hopelessly old-fashioned. This is the model based on g, the general intellectual factor, plus major and minor group factors. Thurstone's scheme of multiple primary abilities is preferred by almost all psychometrists, though apparently it is seldom adopted by counselors or others who use tests for reaching practical decisions. Despite Thurstone's and Guilford's assurance that general intelligence is too vague and heterogeneous a construct to be worth measuring—we should break it down into its components and measure each individual's profile of factors—most practicing psychologists in schools, clinics, and industry happily go on using the familiar group or individual tests of intelligence. The main concessions they make to the factorist are to obtain separate linguistic and quantitative scores in some academic aptitude tests, and separate verbal and performance scores in the Wechsler scales. When I visited some military psychological establishments in 1957, I was told more than once that military psychologists could not ignore g. Try as they would to find differential tests for different army trades, intercorrelations were always so high

that recruits appeared to be differentiated more by all-round level of ability than by type of ability, that is to say, by g rather than by factor profile. Table 1 provides another instance, extracted from the Psychological Corporation's follow-up studies of the Differential Aptitude Tests. True, these are not pure factor tests, but their aim is to give differential predictions for different educational courses or jobs. I have underlined the four highest validity coefficients in each column, and you will see that the pattern of coefficients for different school courses is sickeningly similar. Verbal and Reasoning tests, that is those which are most typical of the conventional general intelligence test, together with the Numerical test, tend to give the best correlations throughout, and only to a limited extent do Space and Mechanical tests add something to the prediction of ability in science courses.

Currently there seems to be greater recognition of the failure of multiple-factor profiles to fulfil their promise, and scepticism over the proliferation of factors. In 1962 Lloyd Humphreys came out in favor of something very similar to the British g + group-factor model, and last year Quinn McNemar (1964) trenchantly criticized the American multiple factorist's "fragmentation of ability, into more and more factors of less and less importance . . . [p. 872]." A general intelligence factor seems unavoidable since substantial positive intercorrelations are found when any cognitive tests are applied to a fairly representative population. But at the same time intelligence has many aspects which can usefully be represented, as Thurstone did, in terms of partially distinct though overlapping primary factors. The trouble arises because any one of these major primaries can be endlessly fractionated, depending simply on the number and variety of different tests in that area which the psychometrist can think up and, I would add, on the homogeneity—the restriction in the range of g—in the tested population. I would entirely agree with Humphreys (1962) that it is useful to superimpose on the hierarchical group-factor model Guttman's notion of facets. Test intercorrelations are affected not only by test content but by the form or technique of the test, its speededness, level of difficulty of the items, whether multiple-choice or creative response, whether analogies, series, or classifications, and so forth. These facets, which are seldom of much diagnostic interest, have been variously referred to as method factors (Campbell & Fiske, 1959), formal factors and work attitudes (Vernon, 1958) instrument factors (Cattell, 1961), and response sets (Cronbach, 1950).

HIERARCHICAL GROUP-FACTOR THEORY

Figure 1 gives the best indication I can manage of the factors that emerge most consistently when large and varied test batteries are applied to representative samples of adolescents or young adults (Vernon, 1961). I admit, of course, that there is no one final structure, since so much depends on the population tested, its heterogeneity and educational background, the particular tests chosen, and the techniques of factorization and rotation employed. I have followed British usage in naming the factors by small letters to differentiate them from the corresponding American primaries from which the *g* element has not been removed.

After removing the general factor (whether by group-factor technique or by rotation of centroid factors), the positive residual correlations always fall into two main groups—the verbal-educational (*v:ed*) group and the spatial-practical-mechanical group. The *v:ed* factor usually yields additional minor fluency and divergent thinking abilities—scholastic and *n* or number subfactors. Likewise the *k:m* complex includes perceptual, physical, and psychomotor, as well as spatial and mechanical factors, which can be further subdivided by more detailed testing. In addition there seem to be various cross-links: For example clerical tests usually combine verbal ability and perceptual speed, *p;* likewise math and science depend both on number and spatial abilities, *n* and *k*. Sometimes an inductive reasoning ability (also very relevant to science) can be distinguished, though most of the common variance of reasoning tests is apt to be absorbed into *g*. At a still lower level in the hierarchy come what are usually referred to as specific factors, though of course any specific can be turned into an additional narrow group factor by devising additional tests.

Now despite certain differences of analytic technique and interpretation of factors, the hierarchical model and the multiple-factor model are fundamentally in agreement. It is just as legitimate to start, as it were, from the bottom upwards—that is to say, to extract the primaries—and from their intercorrelations calculate the second-order factors, and if need be a third-order factor, corresponding to our major group factors and *g*. Bernyer (1958) has shown that the two approaches can yield almost identical results. In actual practice, however, rather few multiple-factor analysts (R. B. Cattell, 1963, is a notable exception) bother to allow for obliquity or go on to calculate the higher-order factor loadings of their tests; and when they

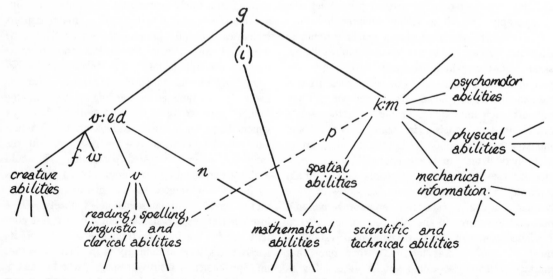

FIG. 1. Diagram of the main general and group factors underlying tests relevant to educational and vocational achievements.

do so the results are apt to be very inconsistent. British *g* factor very regularly shows its largest loadings on tests like Progressive Matrices, Shipley Abstraction and Arithmetic Reasoning, whereas American second-order factors appear to have no stable content. Clearly the main reason why you favor multiple factors is that so much of your work is done with rather homogeneous groups like college students or officers in the armed services, where the range of *g* is so restricted that in effect you only get the group factors which can be rotated to orthogonal simple structure without serious distortion. Several psychometrists, such as Garrett (1946) and Cattell (1963), are inclined to ascribe the lesser prominence of *g* in these older groups to the differentiation of abilities with age, but there is little doubt that in every piece of research claiming to show such differentiation, the older groups are actually more highly selected, less representative. Take, for example, the recent large-scale survey of Grade 9 to 12 students in Project Talent (Flanagan, Davis, Dailey, Shaycoft, Orr, Goldberg, & Neyman, 1964). I picked out seven of the tests which seemed as different as possible from one another, whose intercorrelations would therefore depend mainly on *g*, not on common group factors. These were: Farming Information, Memory for Words, English Expression, Creativity, 3-Dimensional Visualization, Arithmetic Computation, and Clerical Checking. At Grade 9 their average intercorrelation among boys was .280, implying that some 28% of their variance could be ascribed to a general factor. By Grade 12 almost every correlation had decreased and the mean was now .241, i.e., some 24% of general variance. However, one notes that the sample at Grade 9 numbered over 39,000, at Grade 12 only 30,000. Clearly more of the duller students would have dropped out by Grade 12, so that the sample was more homogeneous, and this would more than account for the lowered correlations. In the British Army during World War II, with an almost complete spread of ability, correlations between dissimilar tests were if anything higher than those usually found with fourth- to sixth-grade students (Vernon, 1961).

From the point of view of the practical tester, the hierarchical model seems more logical since, in making educational or vocational decisions, he can cover most of the ground just by applying *g* or *g* + *v* tests, and then supplement by spatial-mechanical, clerical, number, or other group-factor tests where relevant. In other words, measures of factors which are higher in the hierarchy generally have better external validity, or more generalizability (Cronbach, Rajaratnam, & Gleser, 1963) to capacities of everyday life; whereas many of the published primary factors seem to be so narrow, so specific to the particular test material, as to have no practical use. This is true, for example, of Thurstone's and other rote memory factors. The user is tempted, even encouraged, to regard them as measuring memorizing ability which is likely to be highly relevant to school learning. In fact they usually correlate with scholastic achievement only insofar as they have not been purified of *g* and *v*. Similarly a large proportion of Guilford's numerous factors of intellect have failed to show any external validity which could not be accounted for by their *g*, *v*, and space content, though I would agree that some of his originality and creativity factor tests may cover a little fresh ground.

Perhaps the basic source of disagreement is that Thurstone and Guilford regarded primary factors almost as fundamental components or chemical elements of the mind, which in combination go to make up all the important human capacities; whereas Godfrey Thomson (1939), Cyril Burt (1940), and I have always tried to keep in mind that factors are primarily classifications of similar tests. And just because a lot of tests appear to involve memorizing or whatever, and intercorrelate positively, this does not prove that they are good measures of the memorizing that children do in school.

PSYCHOLOGICAL ORIGINS OF FACTORS

At the same time *g* theory has its difficulties, in particular that *g* is not, as Spearman believed, determinate—that is to say, one and the same *g* whatever cognitive tests one likes to apply. Psychologically it is the all-round level of our thinking skills; while statistically it is merely the average of a battery of tests of intellectual capacities which are so diverse that the group factors or facets involved in each separate test mostly cancel one another out. Hence although we know what kinds of tests are most saturated with *g*, it can still vary according to the particular measures the psychologist likes to use. Perhaps, though, this is not a serious disadvantage, since it is what one would expect in the light of the psychological contributions of Hebb (1948) and Piaget (1950), Ferguson (1954) and Hunt (1961).

All of these writers point to the need to get away from the notion of intelligence as a definite entity, an autonomous mental faculty, which simply matures as children grow up. Rather we have to think of it in terms of a cumulative formation of more and more complex and flexible schemata (Piaget's term) or phase sequences (Hebb), or what Miller, Galanter, and Pribram (1960) call plans, which develop through interaction between the growing organism and its environment. They depend both upon environmental stimulation and on active exploration and experiment (Piaget's accommodation and assimilation); i.e., they are formed and organized by use. This implies, to a much greater extent than Piaget seems to have recognized, that they also depend upon personality and motivational factors, organic and social drives, curiosity and interests; and that they are channelled by family, cultural, and educational pressures. Intelligence, then, refers to the totality of concepts and skills, the techniques or plans for coping with problems, which have crystallized out of the child's previous experience. Most representative of these, as Ferguson points out, are the thinking skills which have been overlearned and which are transferable to a wide variety of new situations. Although, of course, each person's accumulation of skills is different, all persons who have been brought up within a fairly homogeneous culture can reasonably be compared at any set of tasks which that culture values and which it likes to include within its conception of intelligence. But obviously, also, the whole structure, from perceptual and linguistic schemata upwards, may differ markedly in other cultures. The group of skills which we refer to as intelligence is a European and American middle-class invention: something which seems to be intimately bound up with puritanical values, with repression of instinctual responses and emphasis on responsibility, initiative, persistence, and efficient workmanship. It is a kind of intelligence which is specially well adapted for scientific analysis, for control and exploitation of the physical world, for large-scale and long-term planning and carrying out of materialistic objectives. It has also led to the growth of complex social institutions such as nations, armies, industrial firms, school systems, and universities, though it has been notably less successful in working out solutions of group rivalries or providing harmonious personal adjustment than have the intelligences of some more primitive cultures. Other cultures have evolved intelligences which are better adapted than ours for coping with problems of agricultural and tribal living. The aboriginal in the Australian desert and the Eskimo in the Far North have many schemata far more efficient than our own. Again subcultures such as our lower working class, or rural groups, develop rather different intelligence.

How about ability factors other than g? It seems entirely plausible that different kinds of skills, or those applied to different kinds of problems, should group together and yield the various group or primary factors that the mental tester discovers. But any reification of such clusters into entities or basic faculties of mind, or what Spearman calls an oligarchic system, is to be deplored. The grouping depends mainly on what cultural and educational pressures dictate. Thus it is very natural, at least in Western cultures, that all the skills bound up with language and school should show a common factor over and above g, and that all contrasted skills of a noneducational type should show a different factor. Likewise we can envisage a whole host of minor group factors arising from the overlapping of schemata involved in similar tasks.

CROSS-CULTURAL TESTING

Let me now turn to the second half of my title—namely, the environmental influences or other causal agencies that underly the development of different patterns of abilities. Here, too, the adoption of the hierarchical model simplifies our problem. It would be extraordinarily difficult to inquire into the agencies associated with a large number of Thurstone's primary factors, with Rote Memory, Induction, Fluency, etc., let alone with Guilford's 60 or more factors, since there would be so much overlapping. It seems more feasible to explore the agencies contributing to general intelligence, and those particularly relevant to verbal-educational and to spatial-practical factors—the group factors that carry a lot of everyday-life variance, and to proceed from there to find out what we can about contributory influences to minor factors of, say, creativity, number, art, music, athletic ability, etc., holding intelligence constant.

I would urge that this is a major responsibility of applied psychology in the second half of the twentieth century. If we are to help the newly developing, nontechnological nations of Africa, Asia, South America, and elsewhere, we must know more about the environmental and other handicaps which retard the development of those abilities that are needed for technological advancement (cf. Schwarz, 1961; Vernon, 1962). We want to assist them in selecting children who will make good professionals, teachers, commercial and political leaders, and technicians, and to tell them what factors of diet and health, cultural tradition and family upbringing, and schooling most require attention if they are to produce sufficient highly skilled personnel.

It is in the controversial area of cross-cultural testing that I am at the moment carrying out a series of small-scale researches, supported by the Association for the Aid of Crippled Children. My wife and I have applied a varied battery of tests, mostly individual, to a reference group of 100 11-year-old boys in England, to 50 boys of the same age in Jamaica, and to 90 Canadian Indians and Eskimos; and I hope to sample some African and other cultural groups later. I am confining myself to boys because, as Schaefer and Bayley (1963) point out, the long-term effects of upbringing are more clear-cut than in girls. Also I am working with groups which, by 11 years of age, have acquired enough English to understand oral instructions. Now I am well aware of the difficulties of cross-cultural testing which Anastasi (1958), for example, has discussed; and indeed it follows from what was said earlier that there is no such thing as a culture-free or culture-fair test. But insofar as the developing nations are aiming to achieve viable technological civilizations, they will need Western-type intelligence. Thus it is entirely legitimate to compare their standing with that of Europeans or Americans on tests which are known to sample abilities relevant to Western-type achievements. Moreover, insofar as the contrasted cultures provide a much wider range of environments than commonly occur within Western societies, their test scores should throw a clearer light on the determinants of abilities.

DETERMINANTS OF TEST PERFORMANCE

Let us broadly distinguish the following classes of determinants: [2]

A. Genetic factors which are nonobservable and nonmeasurable, though we know that they exist since foster children or orphans continue to show some resemblance to their true parents who have had nothing to do with their upbringing. Presumably individuals differ in some quality of the plasticity of the nervous system which makes possible the building up of any schemata or plans; and it may well be that there are genetic differences contributing to linguistic and spatial aptitudes which tend to be sex linked. Certainly there are genetic factors in musical and possibly in mathematical and other talents, however much environment also contributes. One cannot rule out the possibility of genetic differences in aptitudes among ethnic groups or so-called races, but I would agree with the United Nations Educational, Scientific, and Cultural Organization manifesto that we cannot prove them; and they are likely to be small compared with environmentally produced differences.

B. An enormous amount of research, using very varied approaches, has helped to pinpoint the major environmental handicaps to mental development, and I will try to sketch this briefly under nine main headings.

1. Physiological and nutritional factors. These mainly operate during pregnancy and parturition (cf. Stott, 1960); though certain diseases and malnutrition may also be important later insofar as they lower the energy and activity level that the growing child needs to explore his environment and seek out self-stimulating experiences.

2. Perceptual deprivation in the preschool years is suggested by Piaget's and Hebb's work. This may well operate in such situations as Spitz (1945) and Wayne Dennis (1960) describe, but would hardly seem important in most cultural groups where nature provides plenty of sticks, stones, water, and human contacts. I would rather

[2] Note the parallel between this classification and Hebb's Intelligence A and B. Elsewhere (Vernon, 1955), I have coined the term "Intelligence C" to refer to actual test results, i.e., to the particular sampling of Intelligence B which an intelligence test provides. Intelligence C also differs from B on account of the facets or instrument factors mentioned above; in other words it is distorted by the C type of determinant.

emphasize conceptual deprivation during the school years when parents fail to answer questions, encourage curiosity, and provide books, TV, and other types of experience (cf. Bloom, 1964).

3. Repression of independence and constructive play, either through overprotection, arbitrary subjection, or conformity to tribal traditions. This is very noticeable in West Indian and African societies, and seems to be linked particularly with deficit in spatial abilities, in 3-dimensional perception (cf. Hudson, 1962), and in technical skills. My recent studies with Eskimo boys reveal a strong contrast.

4. Family insecurity and lack of planfulness. In families living at the subsistence level, immediate gratification of hunger and sex needs naturally takes precedence over long-term, purposive planning—the Pleasure Principle over the Reality Principle—and discourages the development of internal controls and rational thinking. In our own culture, Schaefer and Bayley (1963) have shown the ill effects of parental anxiety, irritability, punitiveness, and rejection on later intellectual as well as social traits.

5. Female dominance. In many cultures, including the West Indian though not the Canadian Indian or Eskimo, the father may take little part in child rearing, and there is a lack of masculine models with whom the boy can identify. According to Witkin's (Witkin, Dyk, Faterson, Goodenough, & Karp, 1962; Witkin, Lewis, Hertzman, Machover, Meissner, & Wapner, 1954) and some other findings, this may favor verbal at the expense of spatial abilities.

6. Education in the underdeveloped countries is often defective, brief or irregular, starved of materials. Teachers may be poorly qualified and they may follow highly formal and mechanical methods, discouraging any intellectual initiative. Yet at the same time even bad education contributes greatly to the development of nonverbal as well as verbal abilities when the average home provides no intellectual stimulation.

7. Linguistic handicaps are almost universal in these societies. There may be a variety of dialects, or a debased and simplified pidgin or Creole; yet English, or sometimes French, is the main medium of instruction, especially for higher education. Unless the child can acquire complete facility in this second language he is likely to be backward in conceptual development and think-

ing skills, and this too seems to be reflected in nonverbal reasoning as well as in linguistic tests.

8. The conceptual and grammatical structures of the native language may differ markedly from those of English, so that the classifications or relations demanded by a Western-type test may be quite unfamiliar, although the non-Western child can very well classify, relate, and abstract in concrete situations. Again he may never have acquired the ability to interpret pictures as portraying 3-dimensional objects (cf. Biesheuvel, 1952).

9. Adult roles and adolescent aspirations. Here there is little definite evidence. But it is reported of some North American Indian and other cultures that children show fairly normal intellectual development till adolescence, but then, when they realize the depressed status of their minority culture—the absence of opportunity for progress and advancement—apathy sets in. To adapt Gordon Allport's description of personality as "Becoming," intelligence may depend on the future as well as on the past. It is interesting to speculate whether a Western adult does not also cease growing intellectually at 20, 30, 50, or later when he reaches his peak of aspiration and curiosity.

C. This group of determinants obviously overlaps in practice with the B group. But it refers to those characteristics of the test which frequently distort the results of unsophisticated testees, and which could be fairly effectively controlled by appropriate modifications of the form of the test and its administration. Schwarz (1961) has laid down a useful series of principles for getting across Western-type tests to African subjects which, in effect, amounts to teaching them the required mode of response before giving the test. I would still question whether any multiple-choice group test such as Schwarz uses, especially any involving time limits, is suitable for cultures with such different modes of thought and such different attitudes to competition, to working on one's own, or to working at speed.[3] Thus I preferred in my own work to rely more on individual, free-response tests, given like the Terman-Merrill, so that one can expand ex-

[3] It is only fair to point out that Schwarz is not concerned with cross-cultural comparisons, but with devising tests which will give useful predictions within African cultures. Thus a speeded test, say, may actually be more predictive of suitability for technical jobs in a culture where speed plays little part in conventional living.

planations as necessary and try to ensure that motivation is adequate.

While I hope that this summary of determinants and handicaps provides some clarification, the interpretation of cross-cultural data is still extremely tricky, for test results alone tell us little about what determinants are operating in any particular test. Whiting and Whiting (1960) point out that we may be unaware of the crucial parameters in an unfamiliar culture, and Irvine (1965) argues that different sources of variance may be operating: A particular test may be measuring essentially different things in different cultural contexts. For example, amount and quality of schooling may have very little effect on nonverbal tests like Progressive Matrices, Porteus Mazes, or Draw-a-Man in Western cultures, but may have much greater effects in societies where intellectual stimulation by the home is lacking. However one can hope to make some progress:

(a) by contrasting a number of different cultures, (b) by applying factor analysis within each culture to see how the abilities group and what differences occur in factor patterns, (c) by obtaining assessments of major determinants within each culture and observing their correlations with the various test scores or factors.

SOME RESULTS OBTAINED IN ENGLAND AND THE WEST INDIES

Table 2 indicates the main results of group factor analyses among my English and Jamaican subjects; loadings are shown merely by + or ++ signs, as the detailed figures are available elsewhere (Vernon, 1965). It may be seen that the general pattern is similar in the two groups, though there are some differences in the content of particular tests. In the English group there are a large educational and a subsidiary linguistic factor, a large perceptual-spatial factor, and some

TABLE 2

MAIN FACTOR LOADINGS OF TESTS GIVEN TO ENGLISH AND WEST INDIAN ELEVEN-YEAR BOYS

Tests	Mean West Indian deviation quotient	English factors					West Indian factors			
		g	Educational	Verbal	Perceptual	Practical	g	v:ed	Perceptual	Practical ?
Arithmetic Achievement	84	++	+				++	+		
Spelling	94	+	+				+	+		
Memorizing lists of words	91	+	+		+		+	+		
English comprehension, usage, spelling	82	+	+	+			+	+		
Vocabulary, group multiple choice	83	+	+	+			+	+		
Vocabulary, individual Terman-Merrill	72	+	+	+			+	−		
Memorizing oral information	72	+	+				+	+		
Abstraction, verbal induction	?75	++	+							
Piaget, arithmetic-orientational	86	++					+	+	+	
Piaget, visualization-conservation		+			+	+	++			
Matrices, nonverbal induction	75	++					++			
Concept formation, sorting test	90	+		+			++			
Porteus Mazes	91	+					+	+		+
Vernon Formboard	68	+			+	+	+		+	+
Kohs Blocks (WISC-Jahoda)	75	++			+	+	++	+	+	
Goodenough Draw-a-Man	91	+			+	+	+	+	+	
Gottschaldt (Embedded) Figures	88	+			+		+		+	
Reproducing Designs (Bender-Gestalt and Terman-Merrill)	87	+			+		+	+	+	
Picture Recognition, 3-D Perception	?85	+			+		+	+		

Note.— + indicates loadings of psychological interest, almost all statistically significant; ++ represents loadings of .70 or over. In the second column, certain quotients are preceded by "?" where the identical test was not given to the two groups and an approximate estimate was made.

TABLE 3

CORRELATIONS OF ABILITY FACTORS WITH ENVIRONMENTAL VARIABLES AMONG ENGLISH AND
WEST INDIAN ELEVEN-YEAR BOYS

Environmental assessments	English factors					West Indian factors			
	g	Educational	Verbal	Perceptual	Practical	*g*	*v:ed*	Perceptual	Practical?
Length and regularity of schooling	−.15	.31		.21		.23	.19	.26	
Family pattern: unbroken versus broken home	−.11	.30			.14	−.17	.24	.15	+
Stable home background versus frequent shifts						.14	.17		+
Economic: parents' job, housing, equipment	.38	.18	.24			.27	.28		+
Cultural stimulus: books in home, education of relatives, parent interest in education	.56	.29	.16			.33	.46	.25	
Male dominance and identification versus female overprotection or dominance					.39	.25		.27	
Initiative and maturity encouraged in play and household activities	.13			.13		.27	.16		+
Planfulness: rational home climate versus impulsive, emotional, arbitrary	.32	.26				.32			
Linguistic background	.49	.31	.24			.47	.41	.28	
Child's health, physical development, and nourishment							.21	.19.	

Note.—As explained above, no clear practical group factor was established in the West Indian sample. However, Porteus Mazes and Form-board gave substantial positive residual correlations with certain variables, indicated by +.

separation of the more practical performance tests. With the smaller numbers in the Jamaican sample, these subsidiary factors are less clear-cut, and the only sign of a practical factor is in Porteus Mazes and Formboard. The educational factor is definitely more pervasive, entering not only into verbal but also most of the paper-and-pencil perceptual tests. Probably it represents general sophistication in understanding instructions and coping with symbolic material, whether verbal or pictorial. The best general factor tests—Piaget, Matrices, and Concept Formation—are those involving the simplest oral instructions and creative responses.

The median Jamaican performance in each test was expressed as a deviation quotient relative to the English distribution, and it will be seen that these figures range from 94 for Spelling down to 68 for Formboard, i.e., from .4 σ to 2.1 σ below the English mean. Performance is generally best on the more mechanical attainments, though very weak on vocabulary and on information learning which involve verbal comprehension. The quotients for perceptual tests, including Draw-a-Man, are also mainly around 85–90, and the most serious deficits are in verbal and nonverbal induction, Kohs Blocks, and Formboard—that is in g and practical-spatial abilities. This bears out my point that no test can be regarded as culture fair.

Jamaican boys actually score better on conventional verbal intelligence and achievement tests, despite their linguistic handicap, than they do on tests which would appear to be purer measures of g, or of what Cattell (1963) refers to as fluid ability. I suspect that the same result would be found among Negroes in the United States.

Within each group the environmental variables listed in Table 3 were assessed on the basis of semistructured interviews with the boys and reports from the teachers. Time and expense did not permit home interviews, and in any case I was more interested in home and schooling over the past few years than in the kind of details of early upbringing that Sears, Maccoby, and Levin (1957), Prothro (1961), and others have studied. I would certainly not claim high reliability for these assessments, yet they yielded some quite substantial and plausible correlations with the ability factors. The cultural level of the home is clearly the most significant single influence—more important than socioeconomic rating; and in the Jamaican group, but not the English, it affects perceptual as well as general and educational abilities. Linguistic background is similar, and the planfulness or rationality of the home is particularly associated with g factor. Curiously the unbroken home or nuclear family pattern gives slight negative correlations with g in both groups, through positive with other factors.[4] Encouragement of initiative, independence, and maturity seems more important in the Jamaican than the English group though it did not relate, as I had hypothesized, to perceptual-practical ability. But male dominance definitely linked with some aspect of this factor.

During the past 2 months I have been working with groups of boys in Indian reservations in Southern Alberta and Eskimos in the Mackenzie Delta in Arctic Canada. The results are not yet fully scored, let alone analyzed, but they do already bring out one important point—that different groups at similar levels of acculturation, and with similar language difficulties, may show very different patterns of scores. The Eskimos are just about equal to Jamaican standards in written English, though much behind in Arithmetic, probably because less stress is laid in Canadian schools on mechanical drill. The Indian boys do somewhat less well on achievement tests; their linguistic handicap is generally greater since less English is spoken in their homes or at school. Like the Jamaicans they are most retarded in oral understanding and vocabulary.

Both groups score much higher than the Jamaicans on Kohs Blocks and other spatial tests, with a mean quotient of 88 instead of 75; and the Eskimos come up very well also on the inductive reasoning tests—Abstraction and Matrices. Now economic conditions are extremely poor in all three groups, and there is similar family instability and insecurity. Thus it seems reasonable to attribute the better performance of Eskimo and Indian groups to the greater emphasis on resourcefulness in the upbringing of boys, perhaps combined with their strong masculine identification. True, the traditional hunting-trapping life is rapidly disappearing and the majority of parents are wage earning or on relief, but the children are still brought up permissively and encouraged to explore and hunt. Moreover, a subgroup of the Eskimos who came from the most isolated Arctic communities scored better on all three of the tests just mentioned than did those who lived in closer contact with whites and had become more acculturated.

Data such as these do not, of course, necessarily prove causality. Thus the correlation between cultural level of the home and intellectual development in the child might arise because brighter parents, who have brighter children, also provide them with better cultural and educational stimulation. Clearly the cross-sectional survey needs to be complemented by longitudinal and, if possible, direct experimental studies. We are on the verge of extremely exciting advances in the understanding and control of intellectual and personality development through such varied approaches as social learning and reinforcement theory, direct observation and follow-up of children, socioanthropological studies, and work such as I have described with mental tests and factor analysis. But I would not claim to have done more than to have scratched the surface, and to have raised many more problems than I have solved.

---

[4] No explanation can be offered for the slight negative association of schooling with g in the English group. In both groups it appears to contribute to spatial as well as to educational development.

REFERENCES

ANASTASI, A. *Differential psychology*. New York: Macmillan, 1958.

BERNYER, G. Second order factors and the organization of cognitive functions. *British Journal of Statistical Psychology*, 1958, 11, 19–29.

BIESHEUVEL, S. The study of African ability. *African Studies*, 1952, 11, 45–58, 105–117.

BINGHAM, W. VAND. *Aptitudes and aptitude testing*. New York: Harper, 1937.

BINGHAM, W. VAND., & MOORE, B. V. *How to interview*. New York: Harper, 1931.

BLOOM, B. S. *Stability and change in human characteristics*. New York: Wiley, 1964.

BURT, C. *The factors of the mind*. London: Univer. London Press, 1940.

CAMPBELL, D. T., & FISKE, D. W. Convergent and discriminant validation by the multitrait-multimethod matrix. *Psychological Bulletin*, 1959, 56, 81–105.

CATTELL, R. B. Theory of situational, instrument, second order, and refraction factors in personality structure research. *Psychological Bulletin*, 1961, 58, 160–174.

CATTELL, R. B. Theory of fluid and crystallized intelligence: A critical experiment. *Journal of Educational Psychology*, 1963, 54, 1–22.

CRONBACH, L. J. Further evidence on response sets and test design. *Educational and Psychological Measurement*, 1950, 10, 3–31.

CRONBACH, L. J., RAJARATNAM, N., & GLESER, G. C. Theory of generalizability: A liberalization of reliability theory. *British Journal of Statistical Psychology*, 1963, 16, 137–163.

DENNIS, W. Causes of retardation among institutional children: Iran. *Journal of Genetic Psychology*, 1960, 94, 47–59.

FERGUSON, G. A. On learning and human ability. *Canadian Journal of Psychology,* 1954, **8,** 95–112.

FLANAGAN, J. C., DAVIS, F. B., DAILEY, J. T., SHAYCROFT, M. F., OTT, D. B., GOLDBERG, I., & NEYMAN, C. A. Project TALENT: The American high-school student. Final report, 1964, University of Pittsburgh, Cooperative Research Project No. 635, United States Office of Education.

GARRETT, H. E. A developmental theory of intelligence. *American Psychologist,* 1946, **1,** 372–378.

HEBB, D. O. *The organization of behavior.* New York: Wiley, 1948.

HUDSON, W. Pictorial perception and educational adaptation in Africa. *Psychologia Africana,* 1962, **9,** 226–239.

HUMPHREYS, L. G. The organization of human abilities. *American Psychologist,* 1962, **17,** 475–483.

HUNT, J. McV. *Intelligence and experience.* New York: Ronald Press, 1961.

IRVINE, S. H. Testing abilities and attainments in Africa. *British Journal of Educational Psychology,* 1965, **35,** in press.

McNEMAR, Q. Lost: Our intelligence? Why? *American Psychologist,* 1964, **19,** 871–882.

MILLER, G. A., GALANTER, E., & PRIBRAM, K. H. *Plans and the structure of behavior.* New York: Holt, 1960.

PIAGET, J. *The psychology of intelligence.* London: Routledge & Kegan Paul, 1950.

PROTHRO, E. T. *Child-rearing in the Lebanon.* Cambridge: Harvard Univer. Press, 1961.

SCHAEFER, E. S., & BAYLEY, N. Maternal behavior, child behavior and their intercorrelations from infancy through adolescence. *Monographs of the Society for Research in Child Development,* 1963, **28,** No. 87.

SCHWARZ, P. A. *Aptitude tests for use in the developing nations.* Pittsburgh, Pa.: American Institute for Research, 1961.

SEARS, R. R., MACCOBY, E. E., & LEVIN, H. *Patterns of child rearing.* Evanston, Ill.: Row, Peterson, 1957.

SPITZ, R. A. Hospitalism: An inquiry into the genesis of psychiatric conditions in early childhood. *Psychoanalytic Studies of Children,* 1945, **1,** 55–74.

STOTT, D. H. Interaction of heredity and environment in regard to "Measured Intelligence." *British Journal of Educational Psychology,* 1960, **30,** 95–102.

THOMSON, G. H. *The factorial analysis of human ability.* London: Univer. London Press, 1939.

VERNON, P. E. The assessment of children. In University of London Institute of Education, *Studies in education.* Vol. 7. London: Evans, 1955. Pp. 189–215.

VERNON, P. E. Educational testing and test-form factors. (Res. Bull. 58-3) Princeton, N. J.: Educational Testing Service, 1958.

VERNON, P. E. *The structure of human abilities.* (2nd ed.) London: Methuen, 1961.

VERNON, P. E. Intellectual development in non-technological societies. In G. Nielsen (Ed.), *Proceedings of the XIV International Congress of Applied Psychology.* Vol. 3. *Child and education.* Copenhagen: Munksgaard, 1962. Pp. 94–105.

VERNON, P. E. Environmental handicaps and intellectual development. *British Journal of Educational Psychology,* 1965, **35,** in press.

WHITING, J. W. M., & WHITING, B. B. Anthropological study of child rearing. In P. H. Mussen, *Handbook of research methods in child development.* New York: Wiley, 1960. Ch. 27.

WITKIN, H. A., DYK, R. B., FATERSON, H. F., GOODENOUGH, D. R., & KARP, S. A. *Psychological differentiation:· Studies of development.* New York: Wiley, 1962.

WITKIN, H. A., LEWIS, H. B., HERTZMANN, M., MACHOVER, K., MEISSNER, P. B., & WAPNER, S. *Personality through perception.* New York: Harper, 1954.

From H. J. Eysenck and P. O. White (1964). Brit. J. Educ. Psychol., *34*, 197–202, *by kind permission of the authors and Scottish Academic Press*

RESEARCH NOTES

PERSONALITY AND THE MEASUREMENT OF INTELLIGENCE

H. J. EYSENCK AND P. O. WHITE*

(Institute of Psychiatry, University of London.)

SUMMARY. A re-analysis is presented of some data purporting to show that stable children differ from labile ones with respect to the structure of their intellectual abilities. The hypothesis is supported, and additional data are presented tending to show that theories of linear independence between cognitive and non-cognitive areas may have to be supplemented by theories stressing non-linear dependence.

It is usually maintained that intelligence is statistically independent of temperamental factors such as neuroticism and extraversion and the evidence does, indeed, show little cause to doubt lack of correlation between the cognitive and the conative-affective sides of personality. (Cf. Cattell, 1963, for a recent study and discussion). However, it would be unwise to equate *statistical independence* with *lack of interaction* ; most studies reported in the literature have used statistical methods based on product-moment correlations, thus setting orthogonality equal to linear independence, and failing to allow for the possibility of curvilinear regression. This failure to take into account more complex modes of causation may have arisen from the fact that psychometric procedures have been developed very much in isolation, and without connection with the large body of experimental psychology. Eysenck (1957) has argued that the study of temperament and of intelligence can be enriched tremendously by regarding the performance of personality and intelligence tests from the point of view of experimental psychology, considering it as subject to the well known laws of learning theory, and making predictions from these. The usefulness of this approach to the study of personality variables, such as neuroticism and extraversion, has been demonstrated in several publications (Eysenck, 1960, 1964). In this paper, we shall be concerned with a consideration of a similar approach to intelligence test problem solution.

It has been argued (Eysenck, 1957) that the performance of a typical intelligence test may be regarded as an instance of massed practice, in which very similar tasks are attempted repeatedly without the interposition of a programmed rest pause. Under these conditions, we would expect reactive inhibition to build up and interfere with the proper execution of the tasks. We would also expect that extraverted subjects, liable as they are to greater accumulation of inhibition, would show work curves different from those produced by introverted subjects, an expectation shown to be verified by two experimental studies at a high level of significance (Eysenck, 1957, pp. 132-133). In another study, Eysenck (1959) predicted that " in the process of solving the sixty problems of the Morrisby Compound Series Test . . . extraverts would show greater reactive inhibition, and consequently falling off in performance during the last quarter of the test as compared with the first three-quarters." The results showed " that extraverts show greater work decrement . . . by taking longer to obtain correct solutions toward the end of the test, as compared with introverts, and by giving up more easily toward the end " (p. 592). (At the beginning of the work, extraverts were significantly quicker than introverts.)

As regards neuroticism, it has become customary to regard this variable as in some ways being synonymous with drive ; this supposition, taken together with the Yerkes-Dodson Law, may be taken to imply the likelihood of a curvilinear relationship between intelligence and neuroticism, extremely high and extremely low values of N being equally incompatible with high scores on intelligence tests. Lynn and Gordon (1961) have reviewed some of the literature on this point, and they have also

* Supported by the Medical Research Council.

Research Notes

reported an experiment of their own which strikingly (and significantly) supported this prediction, although on only a rather small number of subjects. Their findings on extraversion were indeterminate, probably because they purposely used a very short version of the Matrices test, thus making it impossible for any large amount of inhibition to accumulate. Furneaux (1962) has also shown in connection with the prediction of success of university students that simple linear correlations are much less informative than hypothesis-directed investigations into personality-intelligence relations of a more complex character. We may conclude from this brief review that there is ample evidence to suggest that temperamental and cognitive aspects of personality may not be as unrelated as has often been supposed, and that specific hypotheses about their interrelations can be formulated on the basis of modern learning theory and its extension to personality.

One such extension of the traditional approach may be made in the field of factor analytic determination of personality structure. The problem which arises may perhaps be put as follows : When a factor analysis is carried out of personality inventory scales, a number of factors, such as extraversion, neuroticism, etc., usually results (Eysenck,· 1960) ; similarly, when a factor analysis is carried out of intelligence test scales, a number of factors such as verbal ability, perceptual ability etc., usually result (Vernon, 1958). These factors are independent, in the first case of intelligence, in the second case of neuroticism or extraversion, as long as we preserve the rule that we are only concerned with linear relations. But we may enquire whether similar factors and relations would emerge if we extracted personality factors from populations differing in intelligence level, or intelligence factors from populations differing in degree of neuroticism, say.

A recent study by Shure and Rogers (1963) has attempted to answer the first question. They administered the eighteen scales of the California Psychological Inventory (CPI) to three student groups differing without overlap in I.Q. level, and then intercorrelated and factor analysed the resulting scores for the three groups separately. They found that while there was considerable overall similarity in the solution, the total factor variance associated with their neuroticism factor dropped by over 30 per cent. in going from the high ability group to the low ability group. (The sum of squared loadings is, respectively, 5·18, 4·64 and 3·48 for the three groups.) No such change was observed in their extraversion factor, the sum of squared loadings being 3·46, 3·76 and 3·17, respectively, for the three groups. While confirmation would, of course, be essential before too much credence can be given to this finding, it would appear that factorial studies of personality may not give invariant results under change of ability level.

The other problem raised is perhaps even more important from the educational point of view ; would factorial studies of abilities be invariant under change of personality composition of the groups under analysis ? It is with this question that this paper is particularly concerned.

The only paper concerned specifically with this problem is one recently published by Lienert (1963). His work is based on 1,003 school children with a mean age of between 15 and 16 ; three-fifths of the children were male. These children were administered thirteen intelligence tests of the Thurstone (1938) type, constituting the so-called Leistungsprüfsystem of Horn (1962a). Also administered was a personality questionnaire modelled after Eysenck's (1953) M.M.Q. by Horn (1962b) which gives a measure of neuroticism and also contains a lie scale. Seventy-seven subjects were excluded from the analysis because they had not completed all the tests or because of unusual lie scale scores. Of the remaining subjects, 259 labile and 262 stable children were selected as constituting the 25 per cent. highest scoring and lowest scoring subjects, respectively, on the neuroticism scale. There were no differences between the groups in age but there were more girls in the labile group. However, Lienert was able to show in a preliminary factor analysis that sex had no effect on the factorial structure of the tests. A product moment correlation of the summed standard scores on the thirteen tests with neuroticism gave a value of −0·16 ; while statistically significant because of the large numbers this is for practical purposes equivalent to a finding of orthogonality between the two variables

Research Notes

Separate matrices of intercorrelations were calculated for the labile and stable subjects, respectively, and split-half reliabilities were calculated for all the tests for the two groups. Reliabilities did not differ, but the average intercorrelation of the tests was slightly and significantly higher for the stable group (·33 as opposed to ·27).

TABLE 1

Test :	Stable					Labile			
	I	II	III	h²	Lien-ert	I	II	h²	Lien-ert
1. Discovery of rules (reasoning)	62	·05	18	·63	·67	·25	·58	·47	·54
2. Problems (reasoning) ..	·63	·07	·13	·63	·84	·46	·40	·49	·60
3. Word knowledge (verbal comprehension) ..	·03	·81	·08	·37	·66	·88	−·09	·45	·77
4. Word completion (verbal compr. and closure)	·49	·42	−·03	·57	·69	·27	·13	·22	·14
5. Word fluency (verbal compr. and fluency)	·07	·84	·04	·40	·90	·82	−·02	·45	·78
6. Rotation (spatial orientation)	·18	·06	·43	·39	·45	−·01	·45	·25	·24
7. Brick-counting (spatial orientation)	·07	·00	·76	·43	·63	·07	·71	·44	·53
8. Plane counting (spatial orientation)	·19	·01	·65	·48	·65	−0·2	·53	·29	·32
9. Hidden figures (spatial orientation and clos.)	·56	·06	·21	·60	·69	·32	·38	·39	·36
10. Hidden pictures (closure)	−·03	·27	·40	·27	·62	·04	·47	·29	·30
11. Words (word fluency)..	·24	·38	·02	·36	·56	·56	·05	·34	·42
12. Word beginnings (word fluency and verbal comprehension)	·51	·25	05	·56	56	·62	·15	·44	·48
13. Counting (number) ...	·22	·18	·17	·34	·40	·31	·02	·19	·21
	1·00	·33	·42			1·00	·32		
	·33	1·00	·17			·32	1·00		
	·42	·17	1·00						

Factor loadings of stable and labile groups compared on Promax Solution. Also given are original Lienert communality estimates, and Promax intercorrelations between factors. A brief description of each test is quoted from Lienert, and also the test's suggested factor composition.

Next, Lienert carried out a multiple factor analysis following Thurstone's (1947) procedure. It was found that eight factors could be extracted from the stable group and only four from the labile group. Communalities were lower for the labile than for the stable group and specific factors were more important for the labile than for the stable group. After rotation, it was found that three factors could be interpreted for the labile and six for the stable group ; the latter were said to be closer to Thurstone's primary factors, whereas the former were much more mixed. These figures suggest strongly that children high and low on neuroticism differ very significantly in the way their mental abilities are structured. This conclusion is so important that a thorough critical analysis of the study seems in order.

The first point of criticism is that too little information is given about the analysis to make detailed evaluation possible. The only reference is to Thurstone's book (1947) which contains a number of different methods of analysis, and it is not possible, for instance, to find out just what criteria were used for the extraction of factors or for the interpretability of factors.

Research Notes

Even more disturbing is the failure of the discussion to agree with the results given. Thus, for instance, Lienert says (page 149) that " factor A is a purely verbal factor because it has substantial loadings only in verbal tests." Inspection of Table 5 (b) shows that factor A has the highest loading on a reasoning test, the second highest loading on a word fluency test, the third highest loading on a number test, the fourth highest loading on a space orientation test, and the fifth highest loading on a space orientation test. The sixth highest loading is on a reasoning test. Thus, of the six tests with the highest loading on factor A only one could be interpreted as representing a verbal factor. Factor B is said to be a reasoning factor, having its highest loadings on two tests which, in actual fact, have nearly the lowest loadings on this factor. Altogether, we were unable to make the figures agree with the interpretations, and this must cast doubt on the analysis as a whole, and the conclusions derived by Lienert.

Fortunately, the original matrices were given in the paper, and thus it was possible to carry out a re-calculation based on more modern analytic methods of factor rotation. The method of analysis used by us was Hotelling's principal axes method.

Guttman's (1954) well-known lower bound for the number of common factors indicated the number of factors to be retained. The number is equal to the number of latent roots greater than one in the correlation matrix with unit diagonals. This corresponds identically to Kaiser's (1962) upper-bound for the number of factors with positive generalizability (a term introduced by Cronbach, et al. (1963) for the old notion of internal consistency reliability). Three factors were indicated for the stable group and two factors for the labile group. This is in marked contrast to Lienert's solution in which eight factors are retained for the stable group and four for the labile group. The reason for this discrepancy is difficult to assess since Lienert does not indicate his criteria for this decision. Probably, it is largely due to the inefficiency of the centroid method relative to the principal axes method. But, since we have no indication as to the reflection procedures used in the centroid analyses which Lienert presents, the relative efficiency cannot adequately be assessed.

With the number of factors thus fixed, the communalities were estimated by the now standard procedure of iteration by refactoring (Harman, 1960). The method of principal axes was used and after fifteen cycles, all communalities and converged to three decimal places (though most had converged to four or five places). The final communality estimates are presented in Table 1. For comparison, we also present Lienert's estimates in the same table.

The marked tendency towards very much lower communalities for the labile group which Lienert notes is not so apparent in the present analysis. Since Lienert does not indicate his basis for estimation, the reason for the discrepancy cannot be evaluated.

With the communality estimates thus determined, and the number of factors fixed as before the factor loadings were computed for each matrix by the method of principal axes. Kaiser's (1956, 1958) Varimax procedure for analytical rotation to orthogonal simple structure was applied to the principal axes matrices. The Promax (Hendrickson and White, 1964) procedure for analytic rotation to oblique simple structure was applied to the Varimax solutions. The oblique factor loadings for each matrix appear in Table 1, along with the intercorrelations among the primary factors and the test communalities. The principal axes loadings and the intermediate Varimax loadings are not presented here but all relevant matrices are available at the Institute of Psychiatry.

Upon inspecting the patterns of loadings presented in this table, one is not particularly impressed by the clear and unambiguous interpretability of the resultant factors. Indeed, the crisp, clear simple structure usually associated with P.M.A. material is nowhere to be seen. However, oblique rotation has cleaned up the simple structure considerably and tentative hypotheses may be put forth for at least some of the factors. For convenience of reference, S_1, S_2, and S_3 will indicate the respective factors for the stable group, while L_1, L_2 will indicate those for the labile group.

Research Notes

Factors S_2 and L_1, seem primarily to involve the use of words. In each case, the four tests with highest loadings were postulated as measures of either the Verbal Comprehension factor (V) or the Word Fluency factor (W). Factor S_3 has its three highest loadings on tests postulated as measures of the Spatial Relations (S) factor and no other loadings exceed 0·40. Factors S_1, and L_2 appear to be rather complex. No very simple interpretation is suggested although the pattern of loadings appear to be rather similar for the two factors. Each is loaded by tests hypothesized as measures of Reasoning (R), Spatial Relations (S) and Closure (C). Additionally, S_1 has moderate loadings on putative measures of Verbal Comprehension (V) and Word Fluency.

Our own solution, while differing considerably from Lienert's, does suggest that his main contention is indeed borne out by his data ; the stable group has a more clearly marked structure in the cognitive test field than has the labile group. Three significant factors in the stable group are opposed to two significant factors in the labile group, and as the same standards of selection were employed at all stages, there seems little reason to doubt that these differences are real ones rather than being statistical artefacts. It will, of course, be necessary for this work to be repeated, preferably with a larger selection of tests, before the revolutionary implications of Lienert's work can be accepted ; nevertheless, it would seem likely that personality and intelligence test performance are indeed more closely imbricated than has hitherto been thought likely.

It will have been noted that there is a curious symmetry in the results obtained by Lienert, and those obtained by Shure and Rogers. High ability subjects show higher variance of the N factor than do low ability subjects. High stability subjects show greater organization of abilities than do labile subjects. It would almost appear as if greater stability and ability, respectively, went with greater degrees of organization of ability and stability. It is much too early to speculate about the possible meaning and causes of these relations ; much further research is required before the facts themselves are adequately established to call for explanatory hypotheses. Nevertheless, the theory of linear independence between cognitive and non-cognitive factors may soon have to be supplemented by one stressing non-linear dependence and interrelation.

REFERENCES.

CATTELL, R. B. (1963). The theory of fluid and crystallized intelligence : a crucial experiment. *J. Educ. Psychol.*, 54, 1-22.

CRONBACH, L. J., RAJARATNAM, NAGESWARI, and GLESER, GOLDINE C. (1963). Theory of generalizability : a liberalization of reliability theory. *Brit. J. Stat. Psychol.*, 16, 137-163.

EYSENCK, H. J. (1953). *The Scientific Study of Personality.* London : Routledge and Kegan Paul.

EYSENCK, H. J. (1957). *The Dynamics of Anxiety and Hysteria.* London : Routledge and Kegan Paul.

EYSENCK, H. J. (1959). Personality and problem solving. *Psychol. Rep.*, 5, 592.

EYSENCK, H. J. (1960). *The Structure of Human Personality.* London : Methuen.

EYSENCK, H. J. (Ed.) (1964). *Experiments in Behaviour Therapy.* London : Pergamon Press.

FURNEAUX, W. D. (1962). The psychologist and the university. *Univ. Quart.*, 33-47.

GUTTMAN, L. (1954). Some necessary conditions for common-factor analysis. *Psychometrika*, 19, 149-161.

HARMAN, H. (1960). *Modern Factor Analysis.* Chicago : University of Chicago Press.

HENDRICKSON, A. E., and WHITE, P. O. (1964). Promax : a quick method for rotation to oblique simple structure. *Brit. J. Stat. Psychol.*, 17.

HORN, W. (1962a). *L-P-S Leistungsprüfsystem.* Göttingen : Hogrefe.

HORN, W. (1962b). *S-O-F Stabilitats—und Offenheitsfragebogen.* Göttingen : Hogrefe.

KAISER, H. F. (1956). *The Varimax method of Factor Analysis.* Unpublished Ph.D. dissertation. University of California.

KAISER, H. F. (1958). The Varimax criterion for analytic rotation in factor analysis. *Psychometrika*, 23, 187-200.

KAISER, H. F. (1962). Image analysis. In : *Problems in Measuring Change.* Ed. C. W. Harris. University of Wisconsin Press, Madison.

Research Notes

LIENERT, G. A. (1963). Die Faktorenstruktur der Intelligenz als Funktion des Neuroti-zismus. *Ztschr. f. Exp. Angev. Psychol.*, 10, 140-159.

LYNN, R., and GORDON, I. E. (1961). The relation of neuroticism and extraversion to intelligence and educational attainment. *Brit. J. Educ. Psychol.*, 31, 194-203.

SHURE, G. H., and ROGERS, M. S. (1963). Personality factor stability for three ability levels. *J. Psychol.*, 55, 445-456.

THURSTONE, L. L. (1938). Primary mental abilities. *Psychometric Monogr. No.* 1. Chicago : University of Chicago Press.

THURSTONE, L. L. (1947). *Multiple Factor Analysis.* Chicago : University of Chicago Press.

VERNON, P. E. (1958). *The Structure of Human Abilities.* London : Methuen.

PART V

ANALYSIS OF IQ PERFORMANCE

This section, as pointed out in the Foreword, is concerned with the work of our own Department, and as the product of my own theorising the results and concepts involved may not be treated as critically as those dealt with in other sections. No lengthy introduction will be given because the first reprint in this section was written precisely to discuss in some detail our approach to the problem, and to present some preliminary results. My approach started with the consideration of an extremely important but largely forgotten paragraph in Thorndike's "The Measurement of Intelligence" (1926), one of the most seminal books in this field. This is what Thorndike has to say: "In the instruments that are actually used (i.e. for the measurement of intelligence), it is customary to have the time (for doing a test) a mixture of (1) the time spent in doing some tasks correctly, (2) the time spent in doing other tasks incorrectly and (3) the time spent in inspecting other tasks and deciding not to attempt them. This confusion may be permissible, or even advantageous, in the practical work of obtaining a rough measure of intellect at a small expense of time and labour and skill, but for theory at present and for possible improvement of practice in the future, we need to separate the speed of successes and the speed of failures." (P. 33). Thorndike himself never followed out his own advice, and neither have other psychologists; as will be seen below, we have taken it very much to heart, and believe that our results bear out Thorndike to the full. (In actual fact we made one change in his conception; instead of measuring "the time spent on inspecting other tasks and deciding not to attempt them", we have added to this "the time spent in attempting a task and deciding to give up attempts at solution." In our experience few people "inspect" a task in the way Thorndike describes, but rather try it and then decide to abandon it).

The second paper is a reprint of the general theory, and some experimental evidence relating to it, as worked out by D. Furneaux; it contains details about the division of intelligence test scores into three parts, corresponding roughly to Thorndike's three "times". There is first of all the speed of mental functioning; there is an error checking mechanism; and there is some form of persistence or "continuance". All three can be measured provided we take care to measure the latencies for each individual's solution for each individual problem. This breaking down of "total score" into three component parts, and the provision of scores (latencies) for each separate item, for each individual, constitute the main changes we have introduced into the measurement of intelligence; Thorndike never took these steps, although they are perhaps implicit in his theory. We believe that only by undertaking this more refined analysis of test performance will we obtain the kind of information which is needed in order to replace the rough-and-ready current model with a better one.

It may be asked whether this proposal can be reconciled with the continuation of IQ measurement, and if not how its abandonment can be reconciled with the general position taken in this book that IQ measurement has been extremely successful in providing us with a quantitative paradigm of intellectual functioning. The answer would seem to be that the concept of the atom has continued to play a useful and indeed indispensable part in physics even though the notion that it could not be "split" had to be abandoned. We now have all sorts of elementary particles, baryons, bosons and leptons; we have neutrons, protons, photons, electrons, neutrinos—both in particle and anti-particle form; these all differ in electric charge, in mass, spin, strangeness, mean lifetime, and in disintegration products (Yang, 1962). In the same way it is now suggested that the IQ will remain as an important concept, but that it has been clearly and definitely "split", and that the entities with which we will have to deal in the future will be of the kind suggested above. Detailed analysis is the life-blood of science, and all the research reported in these pages will have to be repeated with close attention paid to the role played by speed, error and continuance. In view of the fact that these are independent (orthogonal) variables—

at least in some populations—it cannot be assumed that what is true of the IQ is necessarily true of all of its three constituents. It is for this reason that it may be possible to claim that the direction of future research seems likely to be determined by the development of these concepts.

The work of Furneaux was followed by that of Iseler (1970), who carried out a concentrated theoretical analysis of the concepts and their relations; unfortunately his monograph runs to over 400 pages, and is not suitable even for partial reproduction. Iseler addresses himself to this problem: definitions of speed of performance based on the joint distributions of time and outcome (e.g. right solution, wrong solution, giving up) get into difficulties because a low probability of giving the right solution up to some time can reflect either a low speed of right solution or a high speed of other outcomes. To meet this difficulty he proposes a model which postulates several stochastically independent processes, each of which is associated with one of its possible outcomes; this model leads to several testable conclusions which are of considerable theoretical and practical interest. Iseler also introduces into his model personality variables, following the general mode of reasoning introduced by Eysenck (1967). Brierley (1961, 1969) has reported some experimental work on neurotic patients which throws much interesting light on this relationship. Thus he found that neurotics have lower values for the speed factor than normals; introverted neurotics were slower than extraverted neurotics, but extraverted neurotics were less accurate (error checking mechanism inferior) than introverted neurotics. (This last difference is significant only at higher difficulty levels of the test items). Continuance was not found to play any part in the observed speed-accuracy differences between extraverts and introverts, nor did it differentiate the two groups.

Our last reprint is an up-to-date report on the state of the art by Owen White, who has developed the Furneaux notions into a psychometrically useful form, and has applied them to various types of performance scores. His work clearly illustrates the great potentialities inherent in the model, but obviously all this is only a beginning. Most of the experimental work to date has dealt with only one type of test material, although this has varied from investigator to investigator. What is needed most now is a comprehensive study using groups of tests differing in mental processes used, and in mental content; each test would then be scored for speed, error and continuance, and these scores for the different tests intercorrelated and factor analyzed. In this way one could discover the degree to which the speed, error and continuance factors were characteristic of individuals over different materials. Data so far available suggest that the results of such an experiment would be positive.

Many other research projects of immediate interest spring to mind. We have discussed in some detail the heritability of the IQ; we know nothing at all about the heritability of mental speed, error checking, or continuance. It is inconceivable that these should not to some degree be characterised by high heritability on a fortiori grounds, but they might differ greatly one from the other in this respect. Nothing is known about the correlation of these factors with evoked potential latency and amplitude which, as we shall see later, correlate quite significantly with IQ; findings along these lines would tell us a great deal about the physical basis of speed, error checking and continuance. Modifiability of intellectual performance is another problem where this new type of analysis could with advantage be attempted; it would seem that continuance, for example, could be modified more easily than speed. Error checking, too, would seem modifiable by special instructions; it has been shown that black children when given special instructions to check their solutions improve their scores significantly more than do white children on an IQ test.

Of particular interest in this connection would seem to be a properly planned study of the influence of motivation on test performance. Burt and Williams (1962) have shown that under conditions of high motivation both children and students improve their IQ score by something like 5 points; they also found that reliability of the tests improved under conditions of high motivation. "In most cases the validity of the tests was also improved; but here the increase was neither so large nor so consistent. The standard deviations increased in those examinations where the motivation was strongest in the case of the brighter candidates, and decreased in the experiment where it was equally strong for the duller examinees." Such results are valuable and of great interest; yet they do not tell us very much about just what precise effect the motivating conditions did in fact have. It would be necessary to know whether motivation affects mental speed, or the error checking mechanism, or rather continuance (as seems perhaps most likely). Such work would seem to have an urgent priority, particularly in view of the often voiced view that "disadvantaged" children are less highly motivated to do well on IQ tests, and that this accounts in part for their low scores.

Altogether, the main burden of this section (and of my own contribution to the measurement of intelligence) may perhaps be summarized by saying that in my view the purely psychometric approach which has characterised so much of the work done in the past half-century is not enough. What is needed is a more experimental approach, strictly in line with the type of work done on conditioning, on perception, or on verbal learning; such experimental laboratory approach has typically been missing from the work of the intelligence tester and the psychometrist. The fact that the complex nature of the IQ was already realized and explicitly stated by Thorndike almost 50 years ago, while intelligence testers have continued to disregard this important contribution, is eloquent testimony to the failure of workers in this field to take seriously their experimental duties. It is of course more difficult to administer tests in such a way that accurate measures of latency are secured for every child, for every problem, and the statistical analysis too becomes very much more complex. One can see that convenience would dictate continuation of the old, simple method of using simply total test scores, often derived from testing carried out under very poorly standardized conditions, by teachers and other not properly qualified for the task. Yet this is not the best way of collecting scientifically valuable results; much of what is printed in educational journals must remain of doubtful status because of the poor conditions under which the material has been collected. No doubt the vocational nature of much clinical and educational testing has contributed largely to this unfortunate state of affairs, yet even here it would seem that educational and clinical description and prediction would be much advanced if attention were paid to the experimental analysis of IQ into its component parts. Clinicians and educationalists often express dissatisfaction about the monolithic IQ which, they say, is not adequate to express the cognitive performance of the child; perhaps

in future they will carry out more analytic tests and report results in terms of a more detailed analysis of the child's performance into mental speed, error checking, and continuance. Brierley's work (1961, 1969) along these lines suggests that much information of great clinical value could be unearthed in this way.

REFERENCES

BRIERLEY, H. The speed and accuracy characteristics of neurotics. *Brit. J. Psychol.*, 1961, *52*, 273–280.

BRIERLEY, H. The intellectual speed and accuracy of psychiatric patients diagnosed as neurotic. Leeds: Unpublished Ph.D. Thesis, 1969.

BURT, C., WILLIAMS, E. L. The influence of motivation on the results of intelligence tests. *Brit. J. stat. Psychol.*, 1962, *15*, 129–136.

EYSENCK, H. J. Intelligence assessment: a theoretical and experimental approach. *Brit. J. educ. Psychol.*, 1967, *37*, 81–89.

ISELER, A. Leistungsgeschwindigkeit und Leistungsgüte. Berlin: J. Betz, 1970.

THORNDIKE, E. L. et al. The measurement of intelligence. New York: Teachers College, Columbia University, 1926.

YANG, Chen Ling. Elementary particles. Princeton: University Press, 1962.

From H. J. Eysenck (1967), Brit. J. Educ. Psychol., *37*, 81–98, *by kind permission of Scottish Academic Press*

INTELLIGENCE ASSESSMENT : A THEORETICAL AND EXPERIMENTAL APPROACH*

By H. J. EYSENCK,

(Institute of Psychiatry, University of London)

I.—DEVELOPMENT OF A CONCEPT.

ATTEMPTS to measure intelligence have passed through several stages since Galton tried to use the measurement of sensory processes to arrive at an estimate of the subject's intellectual level (1883), and McKeen Cattell 1890) employed tests of muscular strength, speed of movement, sensitivity to pain, reaction time and the like for a similar purpose. These largely abortive efforts were followed by the first stage of intelligence measurement properly so called ; it may with truth be labelled the ' g ' phase because both Spearman (1904) and Binet and Simon (1905) stressed the importance of a *general factor of intellectual ability*, Binet contributing mainly by the construction of test items and the invention of the concept of mental age, Spearman contributing mainly by the application of correlational methods and the invention of factor analysis.

The second stage was concerned with the proper definition of intelligence, and theories regarding its nature. Several books concerned themselves with this problem (Thurstone, 1926 ; Spearman, 1923), and a number of symposia were held (*Brit. J. Psychol.*, 1910 ; *J. Educ. Psychol.*, 1921 ; *Internat. Congress of Psychol.*, 1923). Among the theories canvassed were ' mental speed ' hypotheses which placed the burden of intellectual attainment on speed of mental functioning, and ' learning ' hypotheses which protested that the ability to learn new material was fundamental. Both hypotheses faced difficulties ; the fact that reaction times showed no relation to ability tended to discourage believers in the ' speed ' hypothesis, and the negative results of the large-scale work of Woodrow (1946) on the relation between different learning tasks and intelligence discouraged believers in the ' learning ' hypothesis. Psychologists learned to agree to disagree, and to present their work with the dictum that " intelligence is what intelligence tests measure " —a saying less circular than it sounds, but only acceptable if all intelligence tests did, in fact, measure the same thing, which they quite emphatically did not.

We thus reach the third stage, which is essentially a continuation of the early factor analytic approach, but now fortified by recourse to multiple factors and matrix algebra. This phase owes most to Thurstone, but Thomson, Burt, Holzinger, and many others made valiant contributions. In this factorial phase, investigators went back to Binet's idea of different mental faculties making up the complex concept of intelligence, and used factor analysis to sort out these alleged faculties ; they emerged with verbal, numerical, perceptual, memory, visuo-spatial and many other factors. At first, Thurstone and his followers believed that these ' primary factors ' put paid altogether to the notion of intelligence, but when they found the primary factors to be themselves correlated they resurrected the concept of intelligence as a second-order factor, a solution already implicit in the earlier methods and theories of Burt (Eysenck, 1939).

* This paper was originally delivered at a symposium on New Aspects of Intelligence Assessment at the Swansea Meeting of the B.P.S., on 3rd April, 1966. The preparation was assisted by a grant from the M.R.C.

Intelligence Assessment

The fourth stage constitutes essentially an extension of the third, and is associated specifically with J. P. Guilford (1966), whose publication of his " 1965 model of intelligence " provided some of the motivation for this paper. This model, which shows some similarities to one I published in Uses and Abuses of Psychology (1953, p. 38), is illustrated in Fig. 1. Guilford classifies the intellect into *operations* which it can perform, different *contents* of these operations, and different *products* ; by taking all possible interactions we obtain 120 cells corresponding to different mental abilities. Of these Guilford claims to have evidence in actual factorial studies for eighty ; he is optimistic about discovering the remainder. To some critics, this factorial extension of Thurstone's work has appeared almost as a *reductio ad absurdum* of the whole approach. There is a possibility of infinte sub-division inherent in the statistical method employed, and evidence is lacking that further and further sub-factors add anything either to the experimental analysis of intellectual functioning or the practical aim of forecasting success and failure in intellectual pursuits (Vernon, 1965). Worse, the model fails to reproduce the essentially hierarchical nature of the data ; the one outstanding fact which recurs again and again in all analyses is the universality of positive correlations among all relevant tests, and the positive correlations between different factors (McNemar, 1964). By omitting any mention of this central feature of the scene Guilford has truly cut out the Dane from his production of Hamlet. If this is really the best model (1965 style) which psychology can offer of intelligence and intellect, then the time seems to have come to retrace our steps ; something has gone very wrong indeed !

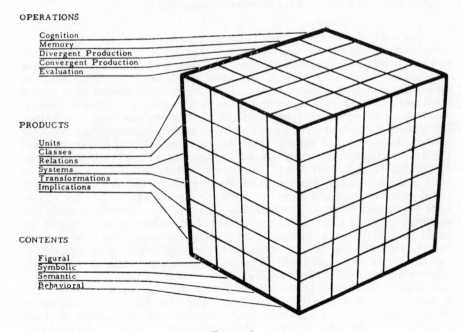

FIGURE 1.

Model of the structure of intellect (Guilford, 1966).

H. J. EYSENCK

II.—LIMITATION OF THE FACTOR ANALYSIS APPROACH.

Zangwill has several times suggested that the whole intelligence testing movement is a technological rather than a scientific one, and in essence my own diagnosis is not too different from his. I would suggest that the psychometric approach has become almost completely divorced from both psychological theory and experiment, and that factor analysis, while an extremely useful tool, cannot by itself bear the whole burden which has been placed upon it. It is the purpose of this paper to raise certain questions in this connection rather than to give definitive answers ; a few empirical results from some of our work will be presented more in order to illustrate an approach than because we believe that these results settle the questions the experiments were designed to investigate.

TABLE 1

FIVE-ITEM INTELLIGENCE TEST, ADMINISTERED TO FIVE CHILDREN ALL HAVING A SCORE OF 2.

	1	2	3	4	5	Total Score
Jones	R	R	N	N	N	2
Charles	W	R	W	R	N	2
Smith	R	A	A	R	A	2
Lucy	R	A	N	N	R	2
Mary	R	W	R	W	W	2

R—Right answer.　W—Wrong answer.　A—Abandoned item.　N—Item not attempted.　(In most tests A and N cannot be distinguished.)

Our work started out with a fundamental criticism of the whole testing movement, directed at the unit of analysis chosen. Nearly all factor analysts and psychometrists correlate test scores and then proceed to work with these correlations ; they thus assume that equal scores are equivalent. Such an assumption is unwarranted in the absence of proof, and consideration of typical intelligence test papers shows that it is, in fact, mistaken. Consider Table 1, which shows the results of giving an imaginary five-item test to five candidates. Let R stand for an item correctly solved, W for an item incorrectly solved, A for an item abandoned, and N for an item not attempted. Let us also assume that the items increase in difficulty. It will be seen that all five children obtain an identical mark of 2 ; but it will also be seen that no two children obtain this mark in the same way. Jones gets the easiest two right, but uses up all his time and does not attempt any more ; he works slowly and carefully. Charles gets some easy items wrong and some difficult ones right ; he works quickly but carelessly. Smith gives up on three items ; had he been more persistent, he might have solved some of them. Lucy is rather selective in the choice of item to be tackled, and Mary fails to check her answers, getting three of them wrong. Can it really be maintained that the mental processes and abilities of these five children are identical, merely because they all obtained the same final mark ? This is the implicit assumption underlying the factor analysis of test scores, and it may be suggested that this assumption requires careful investigation before we can regard it as acceptable. Such investigations are notable by their absence, and factor analysts proceed throughout as if the problem did not exist. This, it may be suggested, is not a proper scientific procedure.

Intelligence Assessment

III.—THE FURNEAUX MODEL.

Our own approach has been to emphasize the point that the fundamental unit of analysis must be the individual test item, and that in addition to determining the category (R, W, A, N) into which it falls for each candidate, it is important to determine the *speed* with which each R item is solved, the length of time devoted to each A item (persistence or continuance), and the number of W items together with the time spent on each. Furneaux (1960) has given a detailed analysis of scores obtained in this fashion, and has suggested on the basis of this evidence that the solution of mental test problems has three main parameters : (1) mental speed, i.e., speed of solution of R items ; (2) Continuance, or persistence in efforts to solve problems the solution to which is not immediately apparent ; and (3) Error Checking Mechanism, i.e., a mental set predisposing the individual to check his solution against the problem instead of writing it down immediately. Two interesting and important consequences follow from this analysis. In the first instance, Furneaux reinstates the mental speed factor to its theoretical pre-eminence as the main cognitive determinant of mental test solving ability, and in the second instance he emphasizes the importance of non-cognitive (personality) factors in determining mental test performance—both persistence and carefulness in checking are personality attributes rather than cognitive abilites. I have attempted to incorporate some elements of this analysis into my own model of intellect (Eysenck, 1953), which is shown in Fig. 2, and which may be compared with Guilford's. What I call ' mental processes ' he calls ' operations ' ; what I call ' test material ' he calls ' contents ' ; so far there is close agreement. But instead of having a third dimension concerned with ' products' (which seems to me a weak and not very important principle of division) I have suggested a dimension rather vaguely labelled ' quality ' into which I wanted to incorporate concepts of mental speed and power, somewhat after the fashion of Thorndike's fundamental contribution (1926). The suggestion is that mental speed and power are fundamental aspects of all mental work, but that they are to some extent qualified by the mental processes involved and the materials used. This seems to me a more realistic concept than Guilford's, as well as having the advantage of retaining the central ' g ' concept in a hierarchical structure in which the

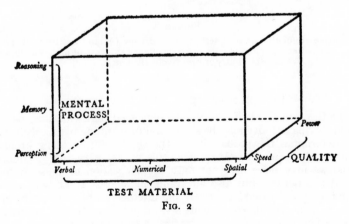

FIGURE 2.

Model of the structure of intellect (Eysenck, 1953).

H. J. EYSENCK

major source of variation is mental speed, averaged over all processes and materials. 'Primary mental abilities,' so called, would then emerge at a lower level of generality, and be related to different processes and different materials used.

Furneaux has demonstrated the fundamental nature of the mental speed function by showing that when an individual's R latencies are plotted against the difficulty level of the items concerned, a negatively accelerated curve is obtained (Fig. 3, A) ; when the time units are then logarithmically transformed *all plots become linear and parallel* (Fig. 3, B). This may be interpreted to mean that the only source of difference in intellectual ability between individuals (in relation to the particular set of test items chosen at least) is the intercept on the abscissa. The increase in log. latency with increase in item difficulty turns out to have the same slope for all individuals tested, and is thus a *constant*, one of the few which exist in psychology. It seems to me that the scientific study of intelligence would gain much by following up the important leads given by Furneaux in this extremely original and path-breaking work.

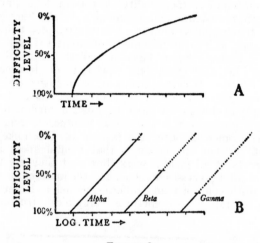

FIGURE 3.

Relation between difficulty level of test items and time (A) and log time (B) needed for solution. Alpha, beta and gamma are three imaginary subjects of high, medium and low mental ability, respectively (Eysenck, 1953).

IV.—MENTAL SPEED AND INTELLIGENCE.

On the theoretical side Furneaux has suggested that what may be involved in problem solving activity may be some kind of scanning mechanism the speed of which determines the probability of the right solution being brought into focus more or less quickly. If we join this notion with that of information processing, we may have here not only the suggestion of a useful theory of intellectual functioning, but also an argument against those who abandoned the whole theory of 'speed' as underlying intelligence because of the failure of reaction time experiments to correlate with intelligence tests. Let us consider the amount of information conveyed by flashing a light and requiring the subject to press a button located underneath the light flashed. When there is only one light/button combination, no information is, in fact, conveyed. As the number

Intelligence Assessment

of combinations increases, the amount of information conveyed increases logarithmically, so that one bit of information is conveyed with two combinations, two bits with four combinations and 3 bits with eight combinations. Response speed has been shown by Hick (1952), Hyman (1953) and Schmidtke (1961), to increase linearly with increasing number of bits of information, as shown in Fig. 4 (Frank, 1963). We have two separate items of information for each subject : one is the raw reaction time, as shown by the intercept on the ordinate, the other is the slope of the regression line, i.e., the rate of increase in reaction time with increasing amount of information processed. If intelligence is conceived of as speed of information processing, then simple reaction time, involving 0 bits of information, should not correlate with intelligence, but the slope of the regression line, showing increase of reaction time with amount of information processed, should correlate (negatively) with intelligence ; in other words, intelligent subjects would show less increase in reaction time with increase in number of light/button combinations than would dull ones (This is a slightly more precise way of phrasing Spearman's first noegenetic law.) Experimentally, the prediction has been tested by Roth (1964) who demonstrated that while as expected simple reaction time was independent of I.Q., speed of information processing (slope) correlated significantly with I.Q., in the predicted direction. Reaction time experiments, properly interpreted, do not appear to contradict a theory of intellectual functioning based on the motion of mental *speed*.

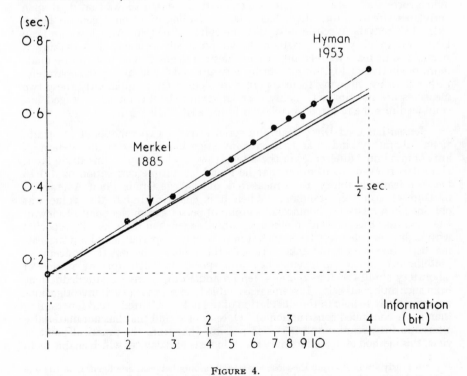

FIGURE 4.

Relation between reaction time in seconds and complexity of task, in bits. Data from Merker (1885) and Hyman (1953). (The Hyman data show results before and after practice.) After Frank (1963).

H. J. Eysenck

V.—Learning and intelligence.

The theory that *learning* is basic to intellectual functioning is not necessarily antagonistic to a theory stressing speed; within the more general speed theory we might expect that speedy learning would be characteristic of the bright, slow learning of the dull. In other words, learning would be one of the 'mental processes' sub-divisions in Fig. 2. The early work of Woodrow (1946) was often considered to have disproved such an hypothesis, but his experiments were too simple altogether to throw much light on the problem; it is not adequate to take subjects who are at different stages of mastery and practice on various types of tasks, who are differentially motivated towards these tasks, and who vary considerably with respect to the abilities involved in these tasks, and then to correlate speed of learning on these tasks with each other and with I.Q. Improved experimental and statistical methods have given more positive results regarding the relationship between I.Q. and learning (Stake, 1961; Duncanson, 1964).*

Another argument has often been presented, e.g., by Wechsler; he has pointed out that a learning task such as 'memory span' correlates poorly with the other tests in the W.A.I.S. and does not predict final total score well. Jensen (1964) has argued that this view is based on a neglect of the low reliability of the test as described by Wechsler; this, in turn, can be raised to any height by simply lengthening the (very short) test, or by improving its design, or both. When correlations are corrected for attenuation, Jensen shows that digit span correlates ·75 with total I.Q., has a factor loading of ·8 on a general factor extracted from the Wechsler tests, is more culture-free than other tests, and can be shown to obey the Spearman-Brown prophecy formula, thus making it possible to increase its relability to any desired degree. The test can be made more predictive of I.Q. by measuring forward and backward span separately, rather than by throwing them together into one score; apparently these two measures are not, in fact, highly correlated and should not be averaged but combined in some multiple correlation formula, if at all.

Jensen has used Digit Span and serial learning experiments of the traditional laboratory kind in an extensive investigation into personality determinants of invididual differences in these tests; we shall return to this study later. Here it is relevant to mention that he found a multiple correlation of +0·76 between learning ability as so measured and college Grade Point Average, a measure of academic standing. When it is considered that this value was obtained in a relatively homogenous group of persons from the point of view of I.Q., and that this correlation is considerably higher than those usually reported with highly regarded I.Q. tests, then it may become apparent why I am suggesting here that we should take seriously the theory relating the concept of 'intelligence' to learning efficiency and speed, and attempt, by means of laboratory studies such as those of Jensen and Roth, to investigate deductions from such an hypothesis. It seems reasonable to expect that such investigations are more likely to help in the elucidation of the nature of intellectual functioning than is the continued construction of I.Q. tests of a kind that has not materially altered in fifty years. And it is also possible that from the practical point of view, this method of procedure may result in tests and devices which enable us to

* An early study showing the close relation obtaining between intelligence, on the one hand, and learning/memory, on the other, was an investigation by Eysenck and Halstead (1945) of fifteen learning/memory tests; these were found to be highly correlated with intelligence. A factorial analysis gave rise to a general factor of intelligence, leaving no residual evidence of any additional contribution by learning or memory.

Intelligence Assessment

give better predictions of school and university success than do existing tests.*

As an example of the much increased possibility of psychological analysis opened by the use of laboratory methods in this field, consider Schonfield's (1965) study of memory changes with age. The general loss of ability of the aged to do I.Q. tests well has been known for a long time, as has their failure to acquire new skills and information, or to retain acquired material. These defects may be due either to a loss of ability to retrieve memories from storage, or to a deficiency in the storage system itself. By comparing recall and recognition scores on a learning task, Schonfield showed that recall was impaired in aged subjects, but recognition was not ; he concluded that it was retrieval from memory storage which was at fault, rather than storage itself, thus suggesting that learning itself might be unimpaired with age. This experiment is cited, not because the results are definitive in any way, but because they illustrate well the approach suggested here ; simple I.Q. testing cannot in the nature of things do any more than reveal the existence of a deficit, but in order to reveal the precise psychological nature of the intellectual deficit in question more experimental methods are required.

VI.—Learning and Personality.

In our discussion of Furneaux's contribution, we found that of his three components of intellectual functioning, only one (speed) was cognitive, while two (persistence and the error-checking mechanism) seemed more orectic in origin, and likely to be related to personality. Most workers in the field of intelligence testing disregard personality factors altogether, but this is almost certainly a mistake. There are several experiments which bring out fairly clearly the importance of personality factors such as neuroticism and extraversion /introversion in the measurement of intelligence, and much of our work has centred on this aspect. Consider first of all the simple learning experiments which we have just discussed ; here one can perhaps expect personality to play little if any role. This, however, is not so, and it may be interesting to speculate about the kind of relation which one might expect to find. We may with advantage begin by considering the well-known experiments of Kleinsmith and Kaplan (1963). These authors argued, briefly, that learning is mediated by a *consolidation process* which takes place after the learned material has been registered, but before it is transferred into permanent memory storage. Consolidation is a function of the state of arousal of the organism ; the greater the arousal, the longer and more efficient the consolidation, so that higher arousal leads to better memory in the long run. However, while consolidation is proceeding, it interferes with recall, so that while the consolidation process is going on the highly aroused organism is at a disadvantage. Kleinsmith and Kaplan tested their theory by measuring the amount of arousal (G.S.R. reaction) produced by different paired stimuli ; for each subject they then picked the most arousing and the least arousing stimulus pairs and had the subject remember the paired stimulus after presentation of the original stimulus.

---

* One interesting possibility which is suggested by Jensen's work relates to his finding that serial learning tasks and paired associate learning tasks both correlate with I.Q., but not with each other. In view of the dependence of paired associate learning on verbal mediation, in contrast to the rote character of serial learning, it seems possible to regard serial learning as the prototype of Cattell's ' fluid ' ability, and paired associates learning as the prototype of his ' crystallized ' ability (1964). If this suggestion has any value, it may show the way to the construction of a battery of tests less dependent on cultural factors and training than are most existing I.Q. tests.

H. J. Eysenck

Recall was arranged at different times after original learning for different groups of subjects, and Fig. 5 shows the results ; it will be seen that as expected high arousal words are poorly remembered immediately after learning, but show very marked reminiscence effects, while low arousal words are well remembered immediately after learning, but fade out quickly. There is little doubt of the reality of this phenomenon, which has since been demonstrated several times.

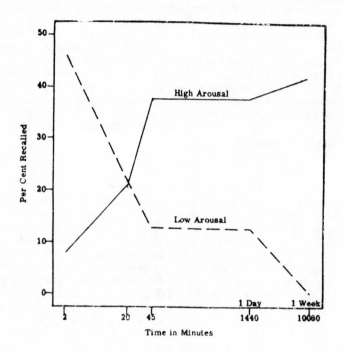

FIGURE 5.

Differential recall of paired associates as a function of arousal level (Kleinsmith and Kaplan, 1963).

In this experiment stimuli were measured and grouped according to their arousing qualities. It is equally possible to group subjects according to their arousability, and I have argued that introverts are characterised by high arousal, extraverts by poor arousal (Eysenck, 1963, 1967). If this theory is along the right lines, we would expect extraverts to behave in the manner of the low arousal words in Fig. 5, and introverts in the manner of the high arousal words. In other words, for short recall times, extraverts should be superior, while for long recall times introverts should be superior. There are about half-a-dozen experiments in the literature demonstrating the superiority of extraverts over short-term intervals, including the work of Jensen already mentioned ; these have been summarized elsewhere (Eysenck, 1967), and all that need be said here is that results are in good agreement with prediction. Some unpublished work on pursuit rotor reminiscence also supports the prediction of better learning for introverts after long rest intervals.

A specially designed experiment by McLaughlin and Eysenck was undertaken to test, in addition to the hypothesis stated above, a further one relating

Intelligence Assessment

to the personality dimension of neuroticism, which we may regard as associated with drive (Spence, 1964). Subjects were tested on either an easy list of seven pairs of nonsense syllables, or on a difficult list, difficulty being manipulated through degree of response similarity. It was predicted that in accordance with the Yerkes-Dodson law the optimum drive level for the easy list would be higher than that for the difficult list, and it was further assumed that N subjects (high scorers on the N scale of the E.P.I.) would be characterized by higher drive than S subjects (stable, low scorers on the N scale of the E.P.I.). Extraverts, as already explained, were regarded as low in arousal, introverts as high. There are thus four groups of subjects, which, in order of drive, would be (from low to high) : stable extraverts ; neurotic extraverts and stable introverts ; neurotic introverts. (No prediction could be made about the position of the two intermediate groups relative to each other.) The results of the experiment are shown in Fig. 6 ; extraverts, as predicted, are significantly superior to introverts, and the optimum performance level of drive is shifted towards the low end as we go from the easy to the difficult list, thus shifting the SE group up and the NE group down. (The figures in the diagram refer to number of errors to criterion.)

If introverts, as hypothesized, are characterized by a more efficient consolidation process, due to their greater cortical arousal, then we should be able to predict that they should be superior to extraverts with respect to acquired knowledge. As an example, we may take vocabulary scores, which are clearly the product of learning, and which usually correlate very highly with other I.Q. tests. Eysenck (1947) has reported personality differences between 250 neurotic male soldiers whose Matrices scores were much superior to their Mill Hill Vocabulary scores, and 290 male soldiers whose scores showed a similar difference in the opposite direction ; he also studied 200 and 140 neurotic women soldiers showing similar differences. In both sex groups those subjects whose vocabulary was relatively good showed dysthmic (introverted) symptoms, while those whose vocabulary was relatively poor showed hysteric (extraverted) symptoms. Farley (unpublished) has carried out a study of forty-seven normal subjects in which he found a substantial positive correlation ($r = +0.48$) between introversion and vocabulary. This is of course in line with the alleged ' bookish ' character of the typical introvert. There was no such correlation between Introversion and Raven's Matrices.

It is possible to go further than this and argue that introverts should do rather better at school and university because of this superiority in consolidation of learned material ; there is much evidence to indicate that such a prediction may be along the right lines (Furneaux, 1962 ; Lynn and Gordon, 1961 ; Savage, 1962 ; Bendig, 1958, 1960 ; Otto, 1965 ; Otto and Fredricks, 1963 ; Child, 1964 ; Ranking, 1963a, 1963b). Not all the results are favourable, but the overall impression is certainly in accordance with expectation. It might be suggested that some form of zone analysis (Eysenck, 1966) which included the N variable as well as the E variable would throw much needed light on these relationships. It should be added that the results do not so much support the hypothesis, as rather fail to disprove it. There are so many alternative hypotheses to account for the finding that not too much should be read into the data.

VII.—INTELLIGENCE AND PERSONALITY.

It will be clear from this discussion that personality features such as neuroticism and extraversion-introversion interact with learning in complex though meaningful ways, and that great care has to be taken in the design of

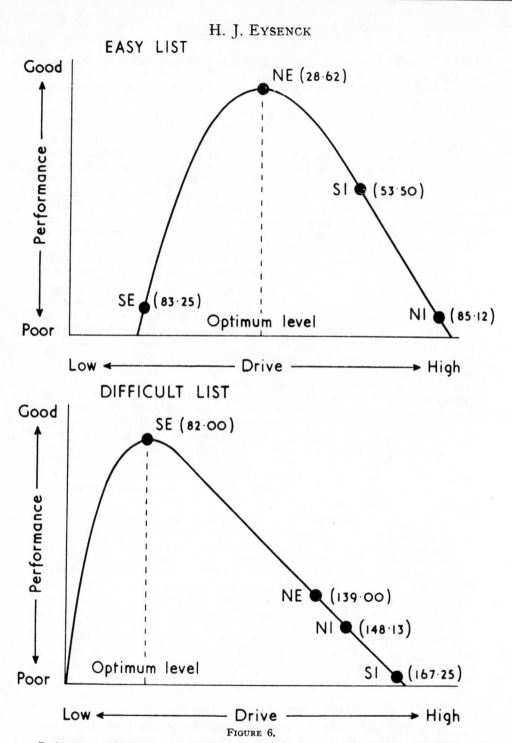

H. J. EYSENCK

FIGURE 6.

Performance of stable extraverts, neurotic extraverts, stable introverts and neurotic introverts on easy and difficult paired associate learning tasks (R. J. McLaughlin and H. J. Eysenck, unpublished data).

Intelligence Assessment

experiment not to fall foul of the complex laws relating performance to personality.* It might be objected that such relations only obtain when laboratory learning tasks are used, but that they fail to appear when orthodox intelligence tests are employed. This is not so. One of the earliest findings relating to extraversion/introversion was that extraverts opt for speed, introverts for accuracy, when there is the possibility of a choice in the carrying out of an experimental task (Eysenck, 1947), and we would expect this difference to appear in relation to intelligence tests also. Jensen (1964) correlated extraversion scores on the E.P.I. with time spent on the Progressive Matrices test and found a significant correlation of $-0 \cdot 46$; in other words, extraverts carried out the task more quickly. They also made more errors, but this trend was not significant. Farley (1966) applied the Nufferno test individually to thirty Ss, divided on the basis of their E.P.I. scores into ten extraverts, ten ambiverts and ten introverts. The mean log speed scores on all problems correctly solved for the groups were respectively: $\cdot 78$, $\cdot 88$ and $\cdot 93$. This monotonic increase in solution time with introversion was fully significant by analysis of variance. Other examples of this relation between speed and extraversion are given elsewhere (Eysenck, 1967); there seems little doubt about its reality.

Farley (1966) also discovered a significant relation with neuroticism, but as might have been expected (Payne, 1960) this showed a non-linear trend, subjects with average scores being superior to those with high or low N scores. Lynn and Gordon (1961) have also published a study showing a similar trend; they used the Progressive Matrices test. The rationale underlying the prediction of a curvilinear relationship in this context derives, of course, from the Yerkes-Dodson law; it is believed that the optimum drive level for complex and difficult tasks like those involved in an intelligence test lies below the high level reached by high N subjects, and above that reached by low N subjects. The general drive level of the group tested is, of course, quite critical in this connection, and it must be emphasized that unless this can be specified or measured, predictions will not always be fulfilled. Changes in difficulty level of the items, changes in the importance the result of the test assumes in the eyes of the subjects, and changes in the motivational value of the instructions may all lead to a general shift in the drive level of the subjects which may displace the optimum level in either direction. It would seem useful in tests of this prediction to have separate measures of drive, or of arousal, against which performance could be plotted (Eysenck, 1967): without such direct measures the subjects' N score may often be difficult to interpret, giving us essentially merely a measure of their *probability* of responding with antonomic activation to an anxiety-producing situation. If the situation is not perceived as anxiety-producing by the subjects, then differences in N cease to matter. This line of argument has led to a better understanding of the conditions under which N correlates with eyeblink conditioning (Eysenck, 1967), and it may be used to design experiments explicitly aimed at increasing the correlation posited.

This dependence of results on precise control of parameter values can also be illustrated by some recent unpublished experiments undertaken by M. Berger. We have noted that extraverts are faster and make more errors when

* The common belief that incentives and higher or depressed motivation generally do not affect intelligence test performance (Eysenck, 1944) may be mistaken; it is conceivable that here too we find the curvilinear Yerkes-Dodson relation, so that *overall* failure to find significant motivation and incentives may be due to compensating positive and negative effects of increased motivation on different types of subject. Some form of interaction terms should be included in analyses of this type, and by preference this should take the form of zone analysis. (Eysenck, 1966.)

H. J. EYSENCK

conditions are such that the test is administered without stress on speed ; in other words, when no explicit instructions are given emphasizing speed, extraverts opt for speed and neglect accuracy, whille introverts opt for accuracy and go slow. These are response styles well familiar from other types of activity (Eysenck, 1960). What would we expect to happen when stress was placed, explicitly and implicitly, on speed of problem solving activity ? Let us return to Fig. 6, in which we postulated that stable extraverts would have low drive level. neurotic introverts high drive level, with the other two groups (stable introverts and neurotic extraverts) intermediate. Given the specific stress on *speed* as the proper index of performance, we would expect the low-drive stable extraverts to have the slowest speed, and the neurotic introverts the highest, with the other two groups intermediate ; we might also expect that the neurotic introverts would produce more errors in order to make up for the excessive speed shown.

Berger tested twenty-one 13-year-old school children in each of the four personality groups ; the groups were equated for age, sex and intelligence, using their 11+ records for this purpose. Fifty problems were presented for solution individually, followed by a rest, and finally by another set of thirty problems. Each problem was shown to the child on a screen, with numbered alternative solution ; having selected the correct solution, the child pressed a numbered button, which activated a time switch, thus recording solution latency, and also caused the projector to project the next problem on to the screen. Instructions emphasized speed of working, and the whole experimental set-up added to this impression ; furthermore, the disappearance of the problem after the button had been pressed eliminated the possibility of checking the correctness of the answer. Figure 7 shows the results of the first fifty items ; the next thirty showed similar results. The Figure is arranged in the form of a cumulative time record, with time arranged along the ordinate and the problems, 1 to 50, along the abscissa. It will be clear that the stable extraverts are much the slowest, the neurotic introverts much the fastest, with the other two groups intermediate ; these differences are highly significant. It was also found, at a high level of significance, that neurotic introverts compensated for their speed by making more errors than the other groups. Thus, the Yerkes-Dodson law appears to be working here very much as it did in the case of the McLaughlin-Eysenck experiment : the low drive SE group does poorly because it is so slow, the high drive NI group does poorly because it makes too many errors, and the intermediate NE and SI groups do best because they work at an optimum level of motivation.

VIII.—FLUENCY AND INHIBITION.

This study illustrates the value of applying theories and laws from general and experimental psychology to intelligence testing.   Another example may serve the same function. From the point of view of the experimental psychologist, a typical intelligence test is a good example of a task undertaken in the condition of massed practice ; we would, therefore, expect it to generate reactive inhibition. Extraverts generate such inhibition more strongly and more quickly than do introverts (Eysenck, 1957, 1967), and consequently we would expect that when groups of extraverts and introverts are matched for performance during the earlier part of an intelligence test, then they will diverge towards the latter part, with the introverts superior in performance. Another way of saying the same thing would be to regard an intelligence test as a vigilance test, and use the well-known fact that introverts preserve vigilance better than extraverts

Intelligence Assessment

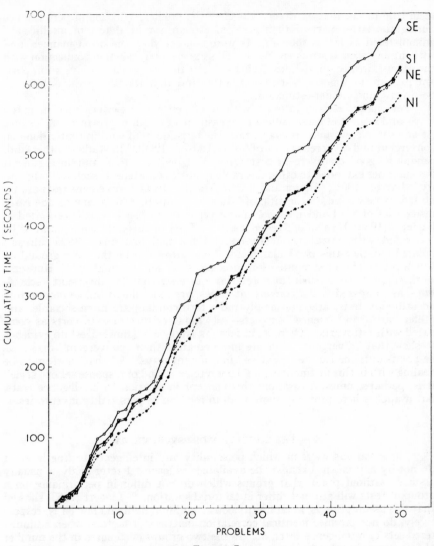

FIGURE 7.

Solution times of stable extraverts, neurotic extraverts, stable introverts and neurotic introverts on fifty intelligence problems, timed separately and cumulated. (M. Berger, unpublished data.)

to predict their better performance towards the end. Eysenck (1959) has reported such an experiment, in which he used sixty items from the Morrisby Compound Series test, individually but unobtrusively timed. Using speed of correct solutions, it was found that on the first forty-five problems introverts were slower than extraverts, but on the last fifteen items, the two groups reversed position and the extraverts were now the slower. On the last fifteen items, it was also found that the extraverts gave up more easily. It would thus

H. J. Eysenck

seem true to say that extraverts do show the predicted decline in performance during the latter part of their performance on a typical test of intelligence, administered as far as the subjects were concerned in the usual manner, and without any special stress on speed. This experiment, taken in connection with the others already quoted, leaves little doubt that personality plays an important part in intelligence test performance, and that its influence has hitherto been very much under-estimated.

Personality factors interact with intelligence test performance in many ways, and neglect of these factors may easily lead to quite incorrect conclusions. As an example, we may, perhaps, take the large body of work recently done on convergent and divergent types of tests (Hudson, 1966). In studies of this kind, candidates good on divergent tests are often called ' creative,' and the argument is sometimes extended to other desirable qualities of intellect, such as ' originality ' (Barron, 1963 ; Taylor and Barron, 1963). In fact, divergent tests are by no means new ; under the title of ' fluency ' tests they were among the early discoveries of the London school, and a typical set of such tests is reprinted in Cattell's (1936) *Manual of Mental Tests.* Tests of this kind were found to be correlated with extraversion (Eysenck, 1960) and Spearman (1926) already pointed out that this particular factor " has proved to be the main ground on which persons become reputed for ' quickness ' or for ' originality '." Hudson's work supports some such interpretation quite strongly ; ' divergent ' school-boys, as compared with ' convergent ' ones, are more fluent, make more errors on orthodox tests, are emotionally more forthcoming, are more sociable, and prefer ' arts ' to ' science ' subjects—all characteristics of extraverts as compared with introverts. There is, in fact (as Hudson acknowledges) no evidence to show that ' divergent ' boys are more creative than ' convergent ' ones ; as he points out, one can be ' creative ' in different ways. All that we seem to be dealing with in this distinction would seem to be a kind of response set or ' style'; it is, perhaps, unusual to apply this concept in relation to intelligence tests, but it applies here probably more than in relation to personality inventories.

IX.—The limitation of psychometry.

These various ways in which personality and intelligence testing interact do not by any means exhaust the available evidence. Factor analysts usually assume, without proof, that groups which do not differ in performance on a group of tests will also not differ in factorial solution. Lienert (1963) showed that.this assumption is, in fact, erroneous ; children high and low on N, respectively, do not produce identical correlation matrices or factors, when administered sets of intelligence tests, nor do the two groups even agree in the number of factors produced. As Eysenck and White (1964) have shown in a re-analysis of the data, " the stable group has a more clearly marked structure in the cognitive test field than has the labile group." (It has also been found that students differing in intelligence do not have identical factor patterns on personality questionnaires ; the evidence is presented by Shure and Rogers, 1963). It is not unlikely that some of the observed differences in factor structure are connected with the intellectual response styles which we have found to be characteristic of different personality groups, but at present there is no evidence to indicate precisely how this may have come about. Much further work is clearly required before we can be sure of our facts in this complex field.

All that has been said in this paper is only suggestive, and I do not in any way believe that the hypotheses stated, and sometimes supported by experimental data, are at the moment anything but guideposts pointing in the direction

Intelligence Assessment

of interesting and important factors which will almost certainly have a bearing on the proper measurement of intelligence. We have noted four stages in the development of intelligence tests ; it is the main purpose of this paper to suggest the importance of starting out on a fifth stage of intelligence assessment, a new stage based on theoretical and experimental work, and not divorced from the main body of academic psychology. Psychometrics and factor analysis have important contributions to make, but they can do so only in conjunction with other disciplines, not by ' going it alone.' What is required is clearly an integration of intelligence testing with the main stream of academic psychology, and a more determined experimental and laboratory approach to the problems raised by the various theories of intellectual functioning. Some obvious suggestions emerge from the inevitably somewhat rambling and unco-ordinated discussion of this paper. (1) Analysis of performance should always take into account individual items, rather than tests, i.e., averages taken over what may be, and usually are, non-homogeneous sets of items. Such analysis should be made in terms of latencies, i.e., speed of individual item solution, as well as of errors, persistence before abandoning items, and other similar differential indicators of response style. (2) Investigators should pay more attention to laboratory studies of learning and memory functions, of speed of information processing, and other experimental measures in the testing of specific hypotheses regarding the nature of intellectual functioning. Analysis of intelligence tests of the orthodox kind raises problems, but cannot in the nature of things go very far towards answering them. (3) Investigators should experiment with variations in experimental parameters, such as rest pauses, time from end of learning to recall, rate of presentation, degree of motivation, etc., in an effort to support or disprove specific theoretical predictions regarding the process of learning and problem solving. (4) Personality variables, such as stability-neuroticism and extraversion-introversion, should always be included in experimental studies of intellectual functioning, because of their proven value in mediating predictions and their interaction potential in all types of learning and performance tasks. Vigorous research along these lines carries with it the promise that notions such as intelligence, I.Q., ability and factor will cease to be regarded as poor relations, and will return to the eminent and successful status they held before the war; it also furnishes the only means of making these concepts scientifically meaningful, academically respectable, and practically more useful.

X.—REFERENCES.

BARRON, F. (1963). *Creativity and Psychological Health.* Princeton : Nostrand.

BENDIG, A. W. (1958). Extraversion, neuroticism and verbal ability measures. *J. Consult. Psychol.*, 22, 464.

BENDIG, A. W. (1960). Extraversion, neuroticism and student achievement in introductory psychology. *J. Educ. Res.* 53 263-267.

BINET, A., and SIMON, R. (1905). Méthodes nouvelles pour le diagnostic du nivean intellectuel des anormaux. *Annee Psychol.*, 11, 191-244.

CATTELL, J. McK. (1890). Mental tests and measurements. *Mind,* 15, 373-380.

CATTELL, R. B. (1936). *A Guide to Mental Testing.* London : University of London Press.

CATTELL, R. B. (1964). Fluid and crystallized abilities. In R. B. Cattell, *Personality and Social Psychology.* San Diego : R. R. Knapp.

CHILD, D. (1964). The relationships between introversion extraversion, neuroticism and performance in school examinations. *Brit. J. Educ. Psychol.,* 34, 187-196.

DUNCANSON, J. P. (1964). *Intelligence and the Ability to Learn.* Princeton, N.J. : Educational Testing Service.

EYSENCK, H. J. (1939). Primary mental abilities. *Brit. J. Educ. Psychol.,* 9, 270-275.

EYSENCK, H. J. (1944). The effect of incentives on neurotics, and the variability of neurotics as compared with normals. *Brit. J. Med. Psychol.,* 20, 100-103.

H. J. Eysenck

EYSENCK, H. J. (1947). *Dimensions of Personality*. London : Routledge and Kegan Paul.

EYSENCK, H. J. (1953). *Uses and Abuses of Psychology*. London : Pelican.

EYSENCK, H. J. (1957). *The Dynamics of Anxiety and Hysteria*. London : Routledge and Kegan Paul.

EYSENCK, H. J. (1959). Personality and problem solving. *Psychol. Rep.*, 5, 592.

EYSENCK, H. J. (1960). *The Structure of Human Personality*. London : Methuen.

EYSENCK, H. J. (1963). The biological basis of personality. *Nature*, 199, 1031-1034.

EYSENCK, H. J. (1966). Personality and experimental psychology. *Bull. Brit. Psychol. Soc.*, 62, 1-28.

EYSENCK, H. J. (1967). *The Biological Basis of Personality*. New York : C. C. Thomas.

EYSENCK, H. J., and HALSTEAD, H. (1945). The memory function. *Amer. J. Psychiatry*, 102, 174-180.

EYSENCK, H. J., and WHITE, P. O. (1964). Personality and the measurement of intelligence. *Brit. J. Educ. Psychol.*, 34, 197-202.

FARLEY, F. H. (1966). Individual differences in solution time in error-free problem solving *Brit. J. Soc. Clin. Psychol.*, 5. To appear.

FRANK, H. (1963). Informations psychologie and nachrichtentechnik. In Weiner, N., and Schade, J. P. *Progress in Brain Research, Vol. 2, Nerve, Brain and Memory Models*. Elsevier Publishing Co., Amsterdam, 79-96.

FURNEAUX, W. D. (1960). Intellectual abilities and problem solving behaviour. In H. J. Eysenck (Ed.) *Handbook of Abnormal Psychology*. London : Pitman.

FURNEAUX, W. D. (1962). The psychologist and the university. *Univ. Quart.*, 17, 33-47.

GALTON, F. (1883). *Inquiries Into Human Faculty and its Development*. London : Macmillan.

GUILFORD, J. P. (1966). Intelligence : 1965 model. *Amer. Psychol.*, 21, 20-26.

HICK, W. (1952). On the rate of gain of information. *Quart. J. Exp. Psychol.*, 4, 11-26.

HUDSON, L. (1966). *Contrary Imaginations*. London : Methuen.

HYMAN, R. (1953). Stimulus information as a determinant of recation time. *J. Exp. Psychol.*, 45, 188-196.

JENSEN, A. R. (1964). *Individual Differences in Learning : Interference Factors*. U.S. Depot. of Health, Educatisn and Welfare. Co-op. Project No. 1867.

KLEINSMITH, L. J., and KAPLAN, S. (1963). Paired-associate learning as a function and interpolated interval. *J. Exp. Psychol.*, 65, 190-193.

LIENERT, A. A. (1963). Die Faktorenstrukter der intelligenz als Funktion des Neurotizismus. *Zhstr. F. Exp. Angew. Psychol.*, 10, 140-159.

LYNN, R., and GORDON, I. E. (1961). The relation of neuroticism and extraversion to intelligence and educational attainment. *Brit. J. Educ. Psychol.*, 31, 194-203.

McNEMAR, R. (1964). Lost : our intelligence ?: Why ? *Amer. Psychol.*, 19, 871-882.

MERKEL, J. (1885). Die zeitlichen Verhältnisse der Willenstätigkeit. *Philos, Studien*, 2, 73-127.

OTTO, W. (1965). Inhibition potential in good and poor achievers. *J. Educ. Psychol.*, 56, 200-207.

OTTO, W., and FREDRICKS, R. C. (1963). Relationship of reactive inhibition to reading skill achievement. *Educ. Psychol.*, 54, 227, 230.

PAYNE, R. W. (1960). Cognitive abnormalities. In H. J. Eysenck (Ed.) *Handbook of Abnormal Psychology*. London : Pitman.

RANKIN, G. F. (1963a). *Reading Test Performance of Introverts and Extraverts*. Milwaukee 12th Yearbook of Nat. Reading. Conf.

RANKIN, G. F. (1963). Reading test reliability and validity as function of introversion: extraversion. *J. Devel. Reading*, 6, 106-117.

EYSENCK, H. J. (1967). *The Biological Basis of Personality*.

ROTH, E. Die Geschwindigkeit der Verarbeitung von Information und ihr Zusammmenharg mit intelligenz. *Atschr F. Exp. Angew. Psychol.*, 11, 616-622.

SAVAGE, R. D. (1962). Personality factors and academic performance. *Brit. J. Educ Pschol.*, 32, 251-252.

SCHMIDTKE, H. (1961). Zur Frage der informationstheoretischen Analyse von Wahlreaktionsexperimenten. *Psychol., Forschung*, 26, 157-178.

SCHONFIELD, D. (1965). Memory changes with age. *Nature*, 208, 918.

SHURE, G. H., and ROGERS, M. S. (1963). Personality factor stability for three ability levels. *J. Psychol.*, 55, 445-456.

SPEARMAN, C. (1904). " General intelligence " objectivity determined and measured. *Amer. J. Psychol.*, 15, 201-293.

SPEARMAN, C. (1923). *The Nature of " Intelligence " and the Principles of Cognition*. London : Macmillan.

SPEARMAN, C. (1927). *The Abilities of Man*. London : Methuen.

Intelligence Assessment

SPENCE, K. W. (1964).   Anxiety (drive) level and performance in eyelid conditioning.   PSYCHOL., BULL., 61, 129-139.

STAKE, R. E. (1961).   Learning parameters, aptitudes and achievements.   *Psychometric Mon.*, No. 9.

TAYLOR, C. W., and BARROW, F. (Eds.) (1963).   *Scientific Creativity.*   London : Wiley.

THORNDIKE, E. L. (1926).   *The Measurement of Intelligence.*   New York : Teachers' College Columbia University.

THURSTONE, L. L. (1926).   *The Nature of Intelligence.*   New York : Harcourt, Brace and World.

VERNON, P. E. (1965).   Ability factors and environmental influences.   *Amer. Psychol.*, 20, 273-733.

WOODROW, H. (1946).   The ability to learn.   *Psychol. Rev.*, 53, 147-158.

(*Manuscript received 21st July,* 1966)

From W. D. Furneaux (1960). Handbook of Abnormal Psychology, *Chapter 5, by kind permission of the author and Pitman Medical*

CHAPTER 5

Intellectual Abilities and Problem-solving Behaviour

W. D. FURNEAUX

THE INVESTIGATION OF "INTELLECT"

THE writer has for some years been concerned with the study of intellectual functions in humans, in particular with the examination of concepts such as those of *speed, power,* and *difficulty,* which in spite of the important role they must inevitably play in any theory of "intelligence," have been developed in a fashion so haphazard that even their definition is a matter for controversy. The results of these inquiries have circulated freely within the Institute of Psychiatry, but have not been widely reported elsewhere. The writers of some of the other sections of this HANDBOOK have thus found themselves in the difficult position of wishing to incorporate in their contributions a background of results and ideas with which their readers will not be familiar. The function of the present chapter is to sketch in this background, rather than to discuss in detail any aspect of abnormal function. It could well be regarded primarily as an introduction to the following chapter.

The study of the abnormal could proceed, in theory, in the absence of any clear understanding of normal mechanisms, but since these disparate fields must in the end be related in terms of concepts which are applicable to both, any change of outlook in the one will inevitably be reflected in the other. The point of view now to be described has been judged, by some, to be of value in connexion with the investigation of intellectual functions in patients demonstrating behaviour disorders, but it developed as a result of an attempt to investigate the normal determinants of score in so-called intelligence tests. The repeated demonstration that performance in "real-life" situations (e.g. success in examinations) can be predicted with reasonable accuracy from a knowledge of such scores provides ample justification for their use. The score given to a subject by such a test, however, describes his behaviour while taking it only very incompletely. This incompleteness does not arise because the score relates only to some *selected* aspect of the total behaviour, as do most scientific measurements. It arises because it attempts to summarize the results of the interaction of several apparently complex processes. The possibility must therefore be considered that the empirically demonstrated relationship between test score and real-life performance really reflects an even closer relationship between such performance and some restricted part of the total test-solving activity, with the other determinants of test score serving only to introduce an unnecessary error variance. In order to minimize error variance an attempt must thus be made to maximize the number of categories into which the subject's total test-taking behaviour can be subdivided, and in terms of which it is to be scored. Obviously, types of response which are logically distinguishable might involve separate determinants, so that ideally, the process of dissection should continue until further subdivision within any category becomes impossible.

It thus appears that the only really satisfactory approach to the study of test-taking behaviour is that of the thorough-going logical-atomist. This approach does not involve the rejection of the important theoretical and experimental contributions to the study of cognition which have been made by proponents of the various kinds of field theory (among whom, for the purposes of this discussion, must be included Piaget), but rather a refusal to recognize that there is any essential antithesis involved in the two kinds of formulation, except in so far as field theorists tend also to stress the importance of the concept of emergence. Any field can be specified in terms of the interaction of a set of discrete determinants, to just the same extent as can the output of a binary computer, and field theories *per se* do no more than direct attention to a particular type of possible interaction among determinants.

If the determinant A is associated with behaviours $a_1, a_2, \ldots a_r$, etc., and determinant B with $b_1, b_2, \ldots b_r$, etc., then according to the doctrine of emergence the interaction of A and B may lead to behaviours of the order (a, b, Δ) and not (a, b), where Δ is some component which cannot be predicted from a knowledge of A and B. This being the case, behaviours (a, b, Δ) can be predicted by tests involving A and B in interaction, but not by the manipulation of scores derived from separate tests of A and B.

In a situation where one has the determinants and is examining the results of their interactions the concept of emergence may have its uses. Where the behaviour is known and its determinants are sought, however, the concept seems to border on the metaphysical. If tests A and B, between them, predict only a part of the variance associated with a behaviour, it is difficult to imagine any experiment which would show that the remaining part depended on interaction effects between determinants A and B rather than on the effects of, say, C. The relevance of any particular C could always be subjected to scrutiny, but not that of all possible Cs. It is quite certain, however, that any attempt to pursue the problem at all would require the existence of measures for the individual determinants A, B, C, D, . . ., etc., rather than mixtures of several of them in unknown proportions.

The concept of emergence, in so far as it is not simply an acknowledgement of ignorance, does no more than re-state the fact that the relationships with which science is concerned are descriptive, and not explanatory. If the interaction of A and B leads to events of an order (A, B, Δ) rather than (A, B) all that matters is to discover whether a specific interaction leads repeatedly to a particular event (E_i) or not. If it does not, even to a useful degree of approximation, then the phenomena concerned cannot be made the subject of any kind of scientific study. If it does, then the successful prediction that E_i will occur would seem to depend entirely on our ability to distinguish A, B, E_i and the interaction concerned, from the general background of other irrelevant phenomena, i.e. successful prediction presupposes adequate atomization.

The development of cognitive tests does not seem to have been guided, to any great extent, by considerations of the type which have now been advanced. Thorndike (1926) was clearly aware of, and critical of, this defect. He asserted that tests of intellect displayed "ambiguity of content, arbitrariness of units, and ambiguity of significance," and suggested that at least three scores, rather than one, were needed to describe intellectual ability. The first of these was to be a measure of the range of operations a particular intelligence could perform, the second was concerned with the rate at which these operations could proceed, and the third with the maximum level of difficulty at which satisfactory operation could be achieved. The present writer's whole approach to the measurement of human intellectual function has developed out of

ideas which found their earliest systematic presentation in this volume. Thorndike's development of them seems to have been hampered, however, by an approach that was at times over semantic, and by a failure to define his fundamental concepts with sufficient rigour. He was particularly concerned with an attempt to define an entity called "the intellect" (Thorndike, *The Measurement of Intelligence*, 1926; cf. the long discussion on p. 25 *et seq.*), rather than to develop the atomistic framework of description which would seem to have been the logical result of his own insights.

Spearman himself attempted to define three different components of intellect, but there seems to have grown up, among British psychologists at least, a very strong tendency to use "g" as an explanatory concept not itself amenable to further subdivision. The preconceptions of the majority of workers are well demonstrated by the titles under which they have reported their results, the archetype involving some such formulation as: "An attempt to find a factor of 'speed' as opposed to 'g.' " The danger of such preconceptions is well illustrated in a paper by Sutherland (1934), who examined the intercorrelations between three measures of the time taken to solve simple problems correctly, and one measure of g. He argued that, since score in the g test was not a speed measure, the existence of a factor of "speed" within the three time tests could only be assumed if their intercorrelations remained significant when the contribution of g was partialled out. As their average residual correlation with g eliminated was only about $0 \cdot 12$ he concluded that no speed factor existed. He does not appear to have noticed that the average correlation between time scores and g scores was about $0 \cdot 57$, while the average of the reliabilities of the time scores was about $0 \cdot 57$ also. The greater part of the non-chance variance of each of the time scores must thus have been determined by g. If, therefore, g is assumed to be independent of speed the ludicrous conclusion must be accepted that the time taken to solve problems is not a measure of speed.

It is, of course, possible, although rather unlikely, that the perfect g test is concerned only with the effects of some single determinant. It seems much more probable, however, that cognitive tests display positive intercorrelations because rather similar interactions of the same set of determinants play an important part in determining score in all of them, and the foundations of an adequate knowledge of the nature of test-taking behaviour must be based on the study of these individual determinants and of their modes of interaction.

It seems to the writer that the application of the statistical technique of factor analysis to large batteries of psychological tests (e.g. Holzinger,

1934–5 and Thurstone, 1939) with the object of defining group-factors in terms of which intellectual function can be described, has done less to advance our knowledge of intellectual mechanisms than is commonly assumed. It is difficult to resist the conclusion that all this work has been rather too empirical, and that most of it will eventually have to be repeated. It is often very useful to know how particular test-scores relate together, but if, as seems probable, most test-scores reflect the interaction of a set of attributes whose composition and relative importance are a function both of the exact details of construction of the test (e.g. the range of difficulty covered by the items it embodies) and also of the characteristics of the group within which it is used, then generalization from the findings of a particular investigation becomes almost impossible. It is not without significance that, after three decades during which test-scores of the conventional kind have been the basic data upon which factorial studies have been erected, nothing even remotely resembling an acceptable theory of cognition has been evolved. This is not the fault of the technique of factor analysis, which has in fact the unusual power of serving at the same time as a means of analysis and also of synthesis. It could perhaps be claimed that the factor-analysts have, on the whole, given very adequate answers to questions which have not always been very carefully formulated.

Within even the most carefully designed of existing "single-factor" tests analysis will reveal the existence of logically distinguishable categories ·of response whose possible effects on score demand separate consideration. Thorndike's subdivisions of "speed" and "altitude," for example, together with related concepts such as "accuracy," seem to be applicable to most of them. It follows that it is impossible to know just what significance can legitimately be assigned to these "factors." Vernon (1950), for example, has suggested that the "w" and "f" (fluency) factors of the Primary Mental Abilities studies are differentiated from the verbal factor "v" only in terms of the level of difficulty at which the two kinds of score were obtained. The following brief analysis will perhaps serve to direct attention to a further ambiguity of a similar kind.

Suppose that there are two relatively independent attributes, say "speed" and "accuracy," each of which affects test performance separately in a way which varies with the difficulty of the test and with the time allowed for completion, but not with test content. In any heterogeneous set, tests will vary in difficulty and in the time allowed for completion, and the correlations between tests could therefore reflect these differences as well as, or even rather than, those associated with content. In view of this possibility each of the fifty-seven tests used in the original P.M.A.

experiment was considered in turn, and a decision made as to whether it was likely to have served as a measure for speed or for accuracy in the experimental population used. In making this decision consideration was given to any experience the writer might have had in using the same, or a similar test within a British population of university students, to the method of scoring adopted, to the shape of the distribution of scores, to the time allowed, and to the apparent difficulty of the test items as gauged from a brief scrutiny. In respect of thirteen tests no decision could be made with even moderate confidence. Sixteen seemed to be concerned mainly with speed, ten with accuracy, and eighteen with both. In order to simplify the analysis the factors isolated from Thurstone's matrix by Eysenck (1939), using Burt's group-factor method, were used instead of the oblique solution favoured by Thurstone himself. In Eysenck's study only four factors were of any great importance, the remaining five each accounting for less than 2 per cent of the total variance. One of the four factors concerned was a general factor accounting for some 31 per cent of the total variance, the others being Verbal-Literary (5 per cent), Arithmetical (4·6 per cent), and Visuo-Spatial (6·6 per cent).

After the speed/accuracy dependence of all fifty-seven tests had been estimated the nine tests having loadings greater than 0·3 on the Arithmetical axis were examined. Six of them had been designated measures of speed, one of accuracy, one mixed, and one unclassified. Of the fifteen tests defining the Visuo-Spatial factor, five had been designated measures of accuracy, seven mixed, two speed and one unclassified. Both speed and accuracy are represented to an approximately equal degree within the Verbal-Literary tests, four being measures of speed, three mixed, and two accuracy. Of the seventeen tests having loadings above 0·65 on the General-Factor only one represents speed, while no less than six had been designated accuracy. At g saturations below 0·4, on the other hand, four of the nine classifiable tests measured speed, and only one accuracy.

It would be absurd to make too much of so cursory an examination. The evidence could, however, be interpreted as supporting the hypothesis that at least part of the apparent differentiation between Visuo-Spatial and Arithmetical tests is not due to differences of content at all, but to differences in the extent to which they measure speed as opposed to accuracy. The association of tests measuring accuracy with·high loadings on the General-Factor is of interest in that it helps with the interpretation of the Factor. It is not however really relevant to the point under discussion, and in the present context the analysis will have served its purpose if it illustrates the difficulties which attend the use of the kind of complex test that still represents the psychologist's chief measuring instrument. It is rather as if the electrician had no means of measuring current and voltage independently, but could only use a wattmeter, to measure their product; or as if a tailor had to fit his customers from a knowledge of their weights.

In spite of its greater sophistication and range the monumental work of Guilford and his school, which is still proceeding, is of the same general kind as were the earlier studies (*see* Guilford, 1956, for a good summary of this work). The scores upon which the analyses are erected must all be based upon such complex interactions of material, operation, and context, that the disentangling of the true basic determinants, even with the aid of the most refined of correlational techniques, must be virtually impossible.

There has been an uneasy awareness of the unsatisfactory nature of psychological-test scores for several decades. It has been reflected in the work of Thorndike, and of the Factorists, but the approach of those who have participated in the speed-power controversy, although often extremely confused and unsatisfactory, seems to the writer to have displayed the most accurate assessment of the real nature of the problem. The search for a speed factor within intelligent behaviour began even before the first intelligence tests came into existence (e.g. J. Cattell's experiments at Columbia in 1894). Many workers, on the other hand, have denied the need for the separate measurement of speed, pointing to the high correlations between scores in timed and untimed tests in support of their contention. A paper by Sutherland was mentioned rather critically on a previous page (Sutherland, 1934), but its defects lay only in the initial acceptance of an unjustified assumption, in every other respect it displayed a standard of competence which could well have been taken as a model by the majority of participants in the controversy. Most studies have suffered from an astonishing degree of technical inadequacy. Speed was usually assessed by giving what was in part an accuracy score, such as the number of items solved correctly within a time-limit test. Alternatively, it was defined in terms of the total time required by the subject to complete a test, with complete disregard of the fact that correct and incorrect responses, as well as abandonments and omissions were thus assumed to be equivalent. Terms such as *power* and *level* seem sometimes to have been regarded as interchangeable, but at other times to involve important distinctions, while either might imply the total score under time-limit conditions, or alternatively under untimed conditions, at the whim of the author. Scores of these unsatisfactory types were then intercorrelated and the resulting coefficients interpreted with complete disregard of the part/whole

effects which they almost invariably incorporated. It is hardly surprising that the question as to whether speed of response demands separate consideration as a determinant of intelligent behaviour is still regarded by some as being an open one. The relevant literature cannot be reviewed here—it is far too voluminous—but two important studies are worthy of note. Slater (1938) has shown that within groups having a very small variance for score on a standardized intelligence test a very wide range of mental speeds (as measured by response-time per item correctly solved) can be demonstrated, and that these between-person differences in speed are associated with differences in school attainment. Tate (1950) has provided an able discussion of the problem of speed measurement, and has shown experimentally that such measurement can be accomplished with a very high degree of reliability and validity. Furneaux (1948) has also reported work which both supports and supplements that of Tate. Taken together these contributions suggest most strongly that the simple, unambiguous scores which result from properly considered measurements of response-rate are theoretically sound and also useful in practice. It occurred to the writer that they also have the merit of being scores of a kind which cannot easily be redefined in terms of sets of simpler determinants, and that they therefore satisfy the requirements elaborated in the opening paragraphs of this chapter. The question seemed to arise, therefore, as to whether it might not be possible and profitable to consider the human problem-solver (and thus the cognitive-test-taker) simply as a "black-box" whose input-output characteristics require to be specified in terms of unambiguously defined observations. This involves the setting on one side of the whole of the approach to cognitive function which originated with Binet and has come to be taken for granted ever since. Instead, we must approach problem-solving as if it were some kind of multiple-choice reaction, to be dealt with as far as possible by an extension of the classical stimulus-response approach which characterized the earliest days of systematized psychological research, and which was shown to be of value by such workers as Kirkpatrick (1900) and Kelly (1903). It is perhaps arguable that, if the orderly progress exemplified by such experiments had not been virtually halted following the publication of Binet's work in 1905, the whole field of psychometrics might by now have been far more soundly based than it is. This is not of course to argue that one should attempt to ignore the immensely valuable results which have been obtained by Binet and the mental-test movement which he founded. Binet's accomplishment in this field, however, was to devise a brilliant solution for an urgent practical problem, the solution involving the design of a novel form of school examination.

Psychologists have been feeling their cautious way back from this toward a genuinely scientific system of measurement ever since.

The relevance of the discussion, so far, to the study of abnormal (or normal) intellectual function can perhaps be illustrated by an example. At the present time one question frequently asked about the effects of psychoticism on intellectual function is something like: "Is the intelligence of psychotics reduced as compared with that of normals?" A very large number of studies has been made in an attempt to answer this question, with conflicting results. A typical experiment involves the administration of a standardized intelligence test to a sample of schizophrenics and to a sample of normals, followed by a comparison of the scores achieved by the two groups. The score a person achieves in a conventional intelligence test is a simple function of the number of problems which he can solve correctly, from a set which are given to him, in a particular specified time. His final score thus depends in part on how long he has to spend in obtaining those answers which prove to be right, in part on the amount of time he wastes in evolving answers which prove to be wrong, and in part on his ratio of right to wrong answers.[1] Unless these three determinants of score are highly correlated within both normal and schizophrenic groups it is impossible either to interpret the results of the experiment satisfactorily, or to generalize from them. If normals and schizophrenics achieve much the same scores, this may indicate that the problem-solving characteristics of both groups are virtually the same. The same result could arise, however, if schizophrenics were less accurate than normals but obtained both right and wrong answers more quickly. Alternatively they might be equally accurate, but might be quicker at arriving at incorrect solutions and slower at reaching correct ones. If this latter explanation were correct, then it would follow that if the experiment were repeated using an intelligence test in which the average difficulty of the problems was increased, then a different result would be obtained in that the schizophrenics would obtain higher scores than the normals. Even where the equality of scores arises from an identity of problem-solving performance between the two groups, it could not be assumed that a similar identity would arise in connexion with an easier or more difficult test, since this would be to assume that comparisons of performance made at one level of difficulty would be valid for problems at other levels. The methods of item analysis used in the construction of intelligence tests ensure that comparisons of accuracy made at one level of difficulty within normal groups bear some relation to those which

would be made at another,[1] but they take no account of rate at all, and the item analyses made within normal groups are never repeated within the abnormal groups for which the tests are nevertheless assumed to be valid.

This list of shortcomings is far from exhaustive, but it will probably suffice to show that little useful information about intellectual functions can be obtained from the use of conventional intelligence tests in the absence of an adequate theoretical and experimental analysis of the ways in which a person's responses, first to single problems and then to carefully defined sets of problems, can legitimately be scored. An attempt will now be made to sketch in the bare skeleton of such an analysis and to report briefly on the results of some experimental work to which it has led, and to discuss some of the implications of both theory and experiment.

The Analysis of a Formalized Problem-solver

Scientific investigation has always to start with the brutal oversimplification of the phenomena with which it is concerned. In order to lay the foundations of the study of problem-solving behaviour it is necessary to ignore many attributes which undoubtedly influence problem-solving responses, and to concentrate at first on a few limited fields of study. It facilitates such an approach if we formalize the human problem-solver, regarding him simply as a problem-solving-box (PB) having only such characteristics as we may explicitly assign to it.

Let PB be a problem-box containing an unspecified mechanism, of such a nature that when it is supplied with an input I in the form of a problem, an output is produced which represents an attempt to solve the problem. Suppose that each such output is designated an *essay*,[2] and is represented by the symbol O_e.

This input/output relationship can conveniently be set out in symbolic form, i.e.—

$$I[PB] \rightarrow O_e$$

Suppose that a time, t_e elapses between the feeding in of the input and the production of the output. We can incorporate this additional information thus—

$$I[PB] \rightarrow O_e, t_e$$

After it has been produced any O_e can be inspected and a decision made as to whether it is right or wrong. Let any O_e which represents a right answer be reclassified as O_r, while O_w stands for a wrong answer, and let t_r and t_w be the values of t_e relevant

---

[1] This analysis is not really adequate, as will appear, but will serve for the present illustration.

[1] As will appear, even this statement is not strictly true.
[2] The term *essay* has been used, because, although archaic, it leads to the use of e in suffix positions rather than other letters of a more ambiguous connotation. Thus the use of *trial* would involve the suffix *t*, which is already widely used in connexion with measurements of time.

to O_r and O_w respectively. Thus all O_r and all O_w are also O_e, and all t_r and all t_w are also t_e.

Suppose now that it is observed that the repeated application of a particular input $_pI$ to a particular Problem-box $_\alpha PB$ is followed by O_r on the proportion of occasions q_r, but by O_w on the remaining proportion, q_w, the sequence of responses being unpredictable save in cases where q_r has the value zero or unity. We can designate this symbolically thus—

$$\{_pI\}[_\alpha PB] \rightarrow \{O_r\}^p + \{O_w\}^q$$

where the curly bracket has in each case the usual connotation of "a set of." Suppose further that even if attention is confined to $\{O_r\}$ the associated values of t_r are not all equal but vary in unpredictable sequence between the limits R_t and $(R_t + H_{tr})$, defining a distribution having a mean of $\bar{t}_r$ and variance V_{tr}. Similarly let the $\{t_w\}$ associated with $\{O_w\}$ define a distribution having the limits W_t and $(W_t + H_{tw})$, variance V_{tw}, and mean $\bar{t}_w$. Then we can write—

$$\{_pI\}[_\alpha PB] \rightarrow \{O_r\}^p, \{t_r\} + \{O_w\}^q, \{t_w\}$$

In order that the terms on the right-hand side of this relationship can unambiguously be associated with the results of applying a particular $_pI$ to a particular $_\alpha PB$, even when set down in the absence of the left-hand side, it is convenient to add appropriate suffixes, thus—

$$\{_pI\}[_\alpha PB] \rightarrow \{_{p\alpha}O_r\}^p, \{_{p\alpha}t_r\} + \{_{p\alpha}O_w\}^q, \{_{p\alpha}t_w\}$$

while the addition of similar suffixes to the distribution statistics, e.g. $_{p\alpha}V_{tr}$, shows to which problem and to which PB they relate. It will be convenient to use the symbol M to stand for the whole set of parameters of a particular kind, or for a particular distribution. Thus we have—

$_{p\alpha}M_{tr}$ comprises $_{p\alpha}\bar{t}_r$, $_{p\alpha}V_{tr}$, $_{p\alpha}R_t$, and $_{p\alpha}(R_t + H_{tr})$
$_{p\alpha}M_{tw}$ comprises $_{p\alpha}\bar{t}_w$, etc., etc.,

while

$_{p\alpha}M_{qr}$ comprises only q_r.

Since both O_r and O_w are special cases of O_e it follows that we also have $_{p\alpha}M_{te}$, where

$$_{p\alpha}M_{te} = {}_{p\alpha}M_{tr} + {}_{p\alpha}M_{tw}.$$

It is not necessary to give separate consideration to $_{p\alpha}M_{qw}$ since $q_w = 1{\cdot}0 - q_r$.

Our assessment of the problem-solving characteristics of $_\alpha PB$ must start with the collecting of sets of observations from which the values of these various "M-statistics" can be computed, all with reference to the inputs provided by a particular problem p. We can then collect similar data using the same input $_pI$

to other problem-boxes, $_\beta PB$, $_\gamma OB$, etc., and in this way compare their characteristics in respect of this one problem. Although, for a particular purpose, interest may centre on a particular statistic, say $\bar{t}_r$, we must not make the mistake of assuming that one statistic is of greater intrinsic importance than another, or of attempting to define the behaviour of a PB in terms of one statistic only in the absence of clear evidence that all are highly correlated. Nor must we compare, say, the value of $\bar{t}_r$ derived from one PB with the value of $\bar{t}_w$ or q_r derived from another, and imagine that the comparison has a meaning. It would be equally unwise to set up a score which was a more or less undefined function of a lumping together of several of the statistics and then to imagine that it could have more than an accidental significance. All these strange operations are involved in current mental-testing procedures, although often to a rather mild degree.

The value of any measurement of behaviour can be assessed only in terms of the extent to which it relates to other measurements of different kinds (for the purpose of theory construction) and to various kinds of "real-life performance." There is no *a priori* reason why the sets of M-statistics associated with each of a properly selected set of single problems should not turn out to represent a set of scores which have a greater value, thus assessed, than scores derived from tests made up of assemblages of problems.[1] In order to pick out the most useful set of single problems from among all possible problems it is necessary to find ways in which problems can be classified, and it is at this stage that concepts need to be introduced similar to those of "difficulty" and "type" which are in current use.

The concept of difficulty arose originally because, on introspection, the sense of effort associated with attempts to solve some problems is stronger than that associated with others. By analogy with the fact that, for example, differences in experienced brightness intensities can be related to a measurable property of the relevant stimuli, an attempt was made to relate differences in experienced effort to a measurable property of problems—their "difficulty." Unfortunately, on inspecting problems, no such property can be observed, nor can it unambiguously be associated with any of those properties of problems which can be observed such as the number of symbols which are required for their presentation. In spite of this the idea that a problem "has" a difficulty, the value of which can be discovered by suitable measurement, has persisted, and the procedure commonly employed

---

[1] Once the discussion moves from the consideration of *PBs* to that of actual human subjects it becomes necessary to reconsider the validity of this statement, because of complications arising from the effects of practice, etc., when a single problem is solved repeatedly.

in order to discover the difficulties of problems is to scale them in terms of the number of individuals in some defined group who fail in their attempts to achieve an acceptable solution. Recognizing that the "difficulty-values" thus allotted are a function of the group within which the calibration has been made, the more sophisticated approaches involve attempts to transform the values thus obtained into the values which would have been observed in some such group as "an unselected normal population," or even to define a scale having an absolute zero (Thorndike, 1926). Controversies have arisen from time to time as to whether the measurement of difficulty is most accurately carried out in terms of observations of the number of people who fail a problem, or of the time taken for satisfactory solutions to be achieved.

The notions underlying this approach may be well founded, and the development of information-theory concepts may eventually make it possible to scale problems for difficulty in terms of the right kind of analysis of their structure. So far, however, they seem to have led only to confusion. It seems better to accept the fact that problems can only be classified in terms of the differences in response characteristics which they evoke. We can justifiably scale them in terms of the values of i_r, V_{tr}, q_r, etc., which are associated with them, but no useful purpose seems to be served by the choice of one particular statistic as being a measure of "difficulty," or by discussion as to which statistic affords the best measure of "difficulty." It is necessary to bear in mind, moreover, that any scale is intended to fulfil a particular limited classificatory function, and scales evolved in connexion with the responses evoked by problems must be constructed with this function in mind. Since all the components of response which have so far been discussed would seem to have much the same a priori importance, and since, in the absence of experimentation, their interrelationships are not known, it is necessary, in the first instance, to define a separate scale in connexion with each component, i.e. for our present purposes, in connexion with each of the M-statistics. It is convenient to call such scales "D-scales." That scale which is concerned with the ordering of problems in terms of the values of i_r which they evoke can usefully be designated the D_{tr} scale, and in terms of the same convention the D_{Vr} scale will relate to values of V_{tr}, D_{qr} to values of q_r, and so on.

To consider the D_{tr} scale as an example, the problem of scale construction is to assign to every problem a D_{tr} scale position such that if any $_{p\alpha}i_r$ is measured then for any other input set $\{_{q\alpha}I\}$ the relevant value of $_{q\alpha}i_r$ can accurately be forecast from a knowledge of $_{p\alpha}i_r$, the scale position of p, and the scale position of q. If the scale position allotted to q is denoted by

$_qD_{tr}$, then the requirement can be stated symbolically, and in a slightly modified form, thus—

$$_qi_r = f(_qD_{tr}, _\alpha K_{tr}) \tag{1}$$
$$= f(D, K)_{tr}$$

where $_\alpha K_{tr}$ is an individual constant assigned to $_\alpha PB$ in terms of the value of $_{p\alpha}i_r$ which is observed for it. The crucial requirement, of course, is that the form of $f(D, K)_{tr}$ must be the same for all individuals, only the value of K_{tr} differing from one person to another. Once the double task is completed of finding a form for $f(D, K)_{tr}$ and scale positions for p, q, etc., such that equation (1) is satisfied, all comparisons between individual PB's in terms of i_r can be made in terms of one measure per PB (i.e. K_{tr}) instead of in terms of all the values of i_r relevant to all possible problems.

Correlational studies using conventional test-scores have shown that performance in one kind of test cannot necessarily be forecast from a knowledge of performance in another kind. Such results suggest rather strongly that it may not be possible to arrange all possible problems along a single D_{tr} scale for use in conjunction with a particular form for $f(D, K)_{tr}$. We must be prepared to find that problems fall into sets (which may or may not involve differences of content analogous to the v, s, f, r, and other factors which result from the factor analysis of conventional test scores) for each of which a different D_{tr} scale and a different form for $f(D, K)_{tr}$ may be required. The members of any one set of problems may be said to define a particular *type* of problem. In the absence of experimentation it is impossible to say whether attempts at scale formation will lead to the discovery of a relatively small number of clearly discrete types, or to that of an infinite number which shade imperceptibly one into the other. In face of the latter eventuality it would be possible to define discrete types, for practical purposes, by assigning to the same type all those problems whose i_r values could be specified in terms of the same D_{tr} scale and the same form for $f(D, K)_{tr}$, within the limits of some specified degree of error. It is also possible that all attempts to construct D_{tr} scales, applicable without alteration to all PBs, might fail, but that subgroups of PBs could be defined within each of which all the members could be covered by a common scale. Although the construction of D scales can be carried out empirically and has a purely classificatory function it will be clear on reflection that the form of the function $f(D, K)$ which is relevant to a particular scale is contingent on the nature of the mechanism within PB whose functioning intervenes between the feeding in of an input and the appearance of an output. At this point the analysis thus has important implications in connexion with the study of abnormal behaviour. If it is found that the form of $f(D, K)$ relevant to a particular D scale is different in an abnormal group from that found for normal groups then it can be inferred that the actual nature of the problem-solving mechanism differs between normals and abnormals. If the $f(D, K)$ is common to both groups, however, then the nature of the mechanism is probably the same, although normals and abnormals might still be differentiated in terms of some of the Ks relevant to the M-statistics. So far as the writer knows there have as yet been no investigations of this kind.

The argument which has been conducted in terms of the D_{tr} scale is equally applicable to all the other scales implied by the statistics comprised within M_{tr}, M_{tw}, and M_{qr}. The primary concern of the psychometrician should thus be the construction of D scales, and in the absence of such scales there is no really satisfactory basis for the economical comparison of the problem-solving characteristics of different PB's or classes of PB. Given such scales, with each of which will be associated a particular $f(D, K)$, all comparisons will be made in terms of the K values relevant to the M-statistics associated with the types of problem which are being subject to study. Values of K can either be measured by the application of a particular $\{_{p\alpha}I\}$ or by computations based on the form of $f(D, K)$, following the single application of each of a number of problems which are members of the same D scale, and whose D positions are known.[1] Every kind of K value has an unambiguous meaning, however derived, in that it specifies the numerical value which would be observed for a particular M-statistic if a particular standard problem were applied to a particular PB. Questions of standardization, etc., do not therefore arise, although they are replaced, of course, by the problems involved in setting up D scales. As will appear, these latter are much more susceptible of solution than are those of defining, and collecting, a stratified sample from which can be deduced the characteristics of "an unselected normal population."

It is now necessary to modify the definition of a PB in order to take account of a property of the human problem-solver which has an important effect on his characteristics, although it seems never to be taken into account. When attempting a set of problems, as in a test, the subject is not willing to spend unlimited time on any one item. Faced with a difficulty which cannot be resolved within what, under all the circumstances seems to be a reasonable time, the reaction is to abandon the problem concerned, and to pass on to the next one. The length of time for which the subject continues to work at a particular problem has as one of its determinants his persistence, but this is

[1] Because of the effects of memory, this latter is the only feasible procedure with human subjects.

not the only factor involved, since the decision to abandon an item may sometimes be made on grounds which involve an intelligent assessment of the effects on score of attempting a lot of items rather than persisting with a few. It will be convenient, therefore, to designate the attribute as "Continuance," or C, a term free from any aetiological presuppositions. PB may be given characteristics analogous with those resulting from C by adding to it a device ST having the functions of a time-switch.

Let any input to PB be represented simultaneously at the input to ST. Let the normal state of ST be "off," but let it change to "on" immediately an input is received, and let it then remain in that state for a time t_s before reverting automatically to "off," at which time we can say that "Continuance has been exhausted." In the present context it is possible to consider only the simplest characteristics for ST, i.e. that it has no means of distinguishing between different problems as inputs, and that t_s varies between the limits S_t and $(S_t + H_{ts})$, defining a distribution M_{ts} of variance V_{ts} and mean $\bar{t}_s$, within which the sequence of t_s values cannot be predicted.

Let ST be coupled to PB, defining the composite device $(PB + ST)$, or PS. Let the ST relevant to $_\alpha PB$ be denoted $_\alpha ST$ and let the PS which results when they are coupled be $_\alpha PS$. Let the coupling be of such a nature that PB cannot start its problem-solving activity until ST is "on," and that the problem-solving process within PB is terminated as soon as it reverts to "off." Let such termination be signified by the appearance of an output O_s from PB, different in nature from the O_e which marks the production of an essay, and analogous to the entering of a dash or a question mark in the answer space on the part of a subject. If PB produces an O_e before C is exhausted, then ST moves to "off" immediately, and without the occurrence of O_s. A value of t_s which would have been observed if ST had not been coupled to PB is thus deleted from the M_{ts} distribution, whose characteristics are thus altered. In order that we can refer unambiguously and economically to the distributions which would have arisen in the absence of coupling and to those that are actually observed from the coupled device it will be useful to denote the former by M_{ts} as previously and the latter by M_{ts}. In a similar way, if C is exhausted before the value of t_e relevant to a particular input has elapsed, then an O_s will arise instead of the O_e which would have been observed in the absence of coupling, and a value of t_e will be lost from M_{te}. Let the resulting modified distribution be denoted by M_{te}. Any statistic relevant to any M can be distinguished from that relevant to the corresponding M in a similar way, e.g. by V_{te} instead of V_{te}. It will also be convenient to use the term "search" to denote the activity which is initiated within PB by an input I, and which terminates with the production of an O_e, or when ST moves to "off."

It is now possible to show that the evolution of D scales and the practical measurement of the various M statistics is considerably complicated by the effects of C. Unless these complications are taken into account, any attempt to compare normal and abnormal individuals, whether by using conventional tests or otherwise, may give rise to very misleading

never be switched off by the intervention of $_\alpha ST$, but always following the appearance of an O_e. In this region of D all M_{te} statistics are therefore unaffected. At D values greater than Z the $_\alpha PB$ will always be switched off by $_\alpha ST$ before an O_e can appear. In the region X to Y the number of O_e appearing after the lapse of times having values lying near to line B will be reduced, because on a proportion of occasions the $_\alpha PB$ will be shut off by $_\alpha ST$ before they have time to

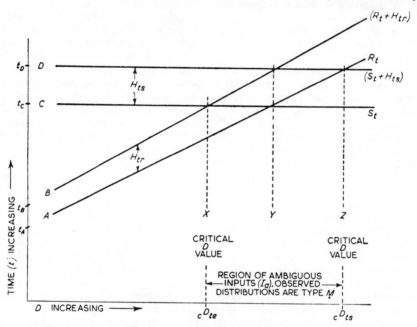

FIG. 5.1. THE INTERACTION OF SPEED AND CONTINUANCE, THEORETICAL

results. Terminological and other complications of considerable complexity result unless, in analysing the effects of C, the simplifying assumption is made that all types of D scale are identical. In the discussion which follows, therefore, the general term D scale will be used to cover all the scales D_{tr}, D_{tw}, D_{qr}, etc., unless the contrary is stated. Once the analysis has been completed in these terms the validity of the assumption can be tested experimentally.

Consider the relationships shown in Fig. 5.1 where the lines A and B, originating at t_a and t_b are supposed to define, for $_\alpha PB$, the longest and shortest times required for the production of an O_e at any value of D, there being no coupling between $_\alpha PB$ and $_\alpha ST$. The lines D and C define the longest and shortest values of t_s which relate to the uncoupled $_\alpha ST$, these values, $(S_t + H_{ts})$ and S_t, being the same at all values of D. If $_\alpha ST$ and $_\alpha PB$ are now coupled, the characteristics of the coupled device, PS, can be deduced from the diagram. At values of D less than X the $_\alpha PB$ will

appear. All those O_e appearing after times lying near to line A will however still arise. Between Y and Z the $_\alpha PB$ will always have been switched off before any O_e having $t_e > (S_t + H_{ts})$ can arise, so that for that small number of O_e that can emerge at all, values of t_e in the region of line A will predominate strongly. For D values greater than X, therefore, M_{te} will differ from M_{te} at all values of D, the difference becoming extreme at D values which approach Z.

It is important to realize that the actual values of D which correspond to the points X and Z will differ from one PS to another, depending in part on K_{te} and in part on i_s. It will be useful to refer to problems having D values in the range $D = X$ to $D = Z$, for a particular PS, as problems which, for it, constitute *ambiguous-inputs*, or I_a. (Strictly speaking, of course it is not the inputs which are ambiguous, but the statistics based on their outputs.) The term I_u (unambiguous-input) will have the obvious complementary meaning. It will also be useful to use the term *critical-D-value* for values of D, such as those which have so far been denoted by X and Z, at which there is a transition from I_a to I_u, or vice versa. The critical value for the M_e statistics can be denoted by $_cD_{te}$, and that for M_s by $_cD_{ts}$.

If the characteristics of $_aST$ be considered, then for $D > _cD_{ts}$ all the M_{ts} statistics are identical with those of M_{ts}, for no O_e arise. For $D < _cD_{ts}$, on those occasions when the uncoupled t_s approaches the value $(S_t + H_{ts})$ an O_e is more likely to intervene before switch-off occurs than is the case when it approaches the value S_t. In this region, therefore, M_{ts} will differ from M_{ts} at all values of D.

Given only the M statistics (relevant to the region where D has a value greater than $_cD_{te}$ but less than $_cD_{ts}$) there is no way of deducing from them the M statistics, and thus no way in which data can be obtained relevant to the problem of defining a form for, say, $f(D, K)_{tr}$, which is applicable to all PS. Any comparison between PSs which is made by using problems for which $D > _cD_{te}$ can apply only to the particular D value, or values, concerned. The statistics being compared, moreover, are not the carefully defined quantities $\bar{t}_e$, V_{te}, etc., but composite measures depending in unknown proportions on both the statistics of M_{te} and also of M_{ts}.

A human subject is always observed in his role as a PS, and can never be split up into the components PB and ST. There may well, therefore, be very considerable ranges of D values within which attempts to compare sets of subjects will be unsatisfactory in that the problems concerned will represent I_a for at least some members of at least some sets. For such a subject the statistics observed when problems are administered will be M rather than M, and will thus be useless. It follows that tests designed to measure M_{te} statistics within heterogeneous groups will probably have to consist of rather "easy" problems. The only alternative is to try to raise $\bar{t}_s$ to such a high value that interaction of M_{te} and M_{ts} does not occur even at high D values. This would mean ensuring very high motivation for all individuals tested, and administering problems one at a time in a face to face situation so that problems were not abandoned as a result of a desire to attempt all those appearing on a test-sheet.

Fig. 5.1 has been used to illustrate the general case of O_e responses, but it could be applied equally well in connexion with the temporal characteristics of either O_r or O_w responses separately. Since the $f(D, K)$ relevant to D_{tr} and D_{tw} scales may differ, and since the M_{tr} statistics may have numerical values different from those for M_{tw}, it follows that an input which is I_u when it results in an O_r response might be I_a if it gave rise to an O_w. It is thus necessary to refer to inputs which are $I_{a(tr)}$ or $I_{a(tw)}$ to prevent ambiguity.

In the same way there will be one *critical-D-value*, $_cD_{tr}$, which is relevant to O_r responses, and another, $_cD_{tw}$, for O_w responses.

If O_r responses are now considered, then by analogy with the argument which has just been considered for O_e responses in general, a proportion of potential O_r responses will be lost when $I_{a(tr)}$ inputs are employed, being replaced by an equal number of O_s responses. Given a knowledge of the form of $f(D, K)_{tr}$ and of the statistics of M_{tr} and M_{ts}, it is possible to compute exactly what proportion of potential O_r responses can actually arise at any specified value of D_{tr} for a particular PS. This proportion will be unity at $D_{tr} < _cD_{tr}$, and zero at $D_{tr} > _cD_{ts}$, so that the complete curve relating the proportion of potential O_r responses arising (P_{sr}) to the D_{tr} value of the input will have a form bearing some relationship to that shown by the curve B in Fig. 5.2. It will be convenient to call this curve the *completion-characteristic*. It should be noted that this characteristic cannot be computed, as might at first be thought, by making a direct count of the ratio of O_r to O_s responses at each value of D, since any particular O_s may represent an unrealized O_w rather than O_r.

To problems at any value of D there will be a relevant value of q_r. Let the relationship between q_r and D be something like that shown by the *accuracy-characteristic* represented by the curve A of Fig. 5.2.

The probability (P_{srq}) that an O_r will actually be observed at any value of D is clearly the product of P_{sr} and q_r. If K_{qr} has only a moderate correlation with K_{tr} and $\bar{t}_s$ then for different PS's the two curves A and B can differ in their relative and actual positions to a very considerable degree. Suppose that one untimed test of a conventional type involves items in the range P of D values (Fig. 5.2), while another covers the range Q. The curves A and B in Fig. 5.2 relate to a PS of low accuracy but high completion, and for it the only determinant of success in both tests is accuracy, since at D values such that completion is less than 1·0 all the responses would in any case be O_w. Suppose, however, that accuracy had been greater. Then the accuracy curve A would move to the right, towards the completion-curve. Accuracy would still be the only determinant of success in test P, but both accuracy and completion would be active in Q. If curve B moved to the left, indicating poorer completion, then test P would become a composite measure for both attributes, while if accuracy were a little greater and completion a little less then both tests would involve both determinants, but in different proportions.

Since completion is a function of the interaction of "speed" (as measured by K_{tr}) and "continuance" (as measured by $\bar{t}_s$) curve B will move to the left if either speed or continuance is reduced. The same mental test, if designed and scored in the conventional manner, will thus measure different combinations of speed, accuracy and continuance when applied to different *PS*s. Again, if a *PS* is fed with different tests, all of the same type, but all covering different ranges of *D*, then the score derived from each such test can relate to a different attribute or combination of attributes. It is an interesting corollary of this analysis that a test set without time-limit is not

these items are sufficiently "difficult" to lead to the production of some incorrect solutions by most members of the group, none are so difficult in relation to the range of mental speed existing within the group as to be given up as insoluble. If such a two-part test is set with time limit, the slowest members of the group will still be working on the N_e easy items when the time limit expires, and for them the determinants of success will be speed only. The moderately fast

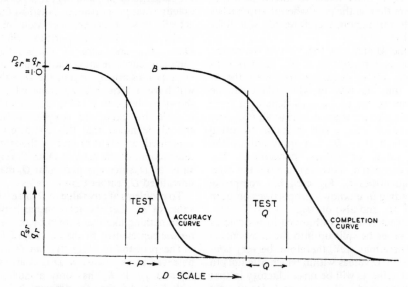

FIG. 5.2. THE INTERACTION OF COMPLETION AND ACCURACY, THEORETICAL

necessarily, or usually, a "speed-free" test. In any test which includes problems having *D* values which, for a particular subject, are greater than $_cD_{tr}$, score is determined in part by the completion characteristic, which is itself, in part, a function of speed (K_{tr}).

Some Implications

It seems that these conclusions, based on the analysis of a *PS*, must be applied equally to the human subject. Consider, as a further illustration, a test made up of items having such low *D* values that no individual in the population being examined returns any incorrect solutions. As the items are "easy" they will all be solved quite quickly, so continuance will not be a determinant of success. Under these circumstances the only factor influencing score if the test is timed will be K_{tr} for each subject, i.e. problem-solving speed. (If the test is untimed the group will of course exhibit zero variance.) Suppose now that following a set of N_e such easy items subjects have to proceed immediately to a set of N_m at higher values of *D*. To simplify the argument let us specify that although

individuals will all complete the N_e items, but at varying rates, so when the test finishes they will have been working for different times on the N_m items of moderate difficulty. During the time any individual is working on section N_m the rate at which his score will increase will be a function in part of his speed, but also in part, of his tendency to produce incorrect solutions. For this group of moderately fast individuals the final score attained will thus be determined in a fairly complex fashion both by speed and also by the frequency with which errors are produced. The very fast members of the group will all finish the test, but will be distributed in terms of their error tendencies. If, finally, a further set of N_d items, all at very high values of *D*, are added to the test, then the final score of the fast members of the group, who reach these N_d items within the time allotted will now depend in part on continuance, for those who are less continuant will lose possible increments of score through abandoning their efforts to obtain a solution before a sufficient time had elapsed for a solution to have a reasonable chance of emerging.

Any test can be regarded as consisting of $N_e + N_m + N_d$ items. If such a test is administered with time limit to a fairly homogeneous group it could measure mainly speed, mainly accuracy, or mainly continuance, depending on the interaction of the range of ability represented in the group, the time allowed for the test, and the numerical values of N_e, N_m, and N_d. In a fairly heterogeneous group the attributes measured, under certain conditions, could vary all the way from pure speed, for some individuals, and through various combinations of speed, accuracy and continuance. If unlimited time is allowed the manner in which these combine to determine the final score will be modified, but the same types of complication will arise as when a limit is imposed. It would thus appear that such a test cannot be said to measure any single, clearly defined trait, and that under some circumstances the same test will be comparing different subjects in terms of quite unrelated attributes. Conventional tests are therefore not very suitable for use in connexion with the comparison of normal and abnormal individuals, since if differences are demonstrated they will be as much a function of the range of D covered by the test items as of the attributes of the subjects.

If the same test measures different qualities in different individuals, it also seems to follow that each separate application of the same test to the same individual will tap different qualities if the intellectual powers are still developing during the period throughout which the test is repeated. Thus the determinants of score will be speed, accuracy and continuance in the case of (say) a ten-year-old child confronted with what is for him a rather difficult test. During the ensuing four or five years it is not unreasonable to assume that the child becomes more persistent, more accurate, and develops greater speed; although it does not appear that any measurements have as yet been made of the mode of development of these separate qualities. Should such changes in fact take place, the result would be to reduce the contribution made by the effects of continuance and accuracy to the test score, so that eventually the most important determinant becomes speed alone. The selection of tests for longitudinal studies, relating to the constancy, or otherwise, of "intelligence" and of cognitive structure in general, must inevitably be greatly complicated by the need to take such possibilities into account. Whether successive measurements are made in terms of the same test material or not there would seem to be a high probability that the various determinations are in fact concerned with different interactions of the three basic traits. If this should in fact be the case it would go a long way toward explaining the results obtained by Anderson (1939) who found that the intercorrelations of successive "intelligence"

scores reported for children were actually somewhat lower than those that would be expected on the basis of part/whole effects alone even if each successive yearly increment of score was completely uncorrelated with the score obtained at the beginning of that year. There certainly seems to be every reason to believe that developmental studies have little meaning unless they are carried out in terms of properly selected M-statistics, and that this demands a careful choice of D values for the problems that are to be utilized.

Since persistence will usually be one of the determinants of continuance, and may under some circumstances become its major determinant, it would seem to follow that persistence must be one of the factors influencing scores in so-called cognitive tests which embody problems for which $D > {_c}D_{tr}$ for those attempting them. That such a correlation would be observed was predicted by the writer (Furneaux, 1952, 1953) and subsequently confirmed by G. L. Mangan (Mangan, 1954) on the basis of a factor analysis of a battery which included both cognitive tests and measures of persistence.[1] Factor-analysing data reported by Bayley (Nelson, 1951), Hofstaetter (1954) too have suggested that persistence may affect cognitive test scores. In the writer's view no great weight can be given to Hofstaetter's findings, however, since as he himself is at pains to emphasize, the identification of the relevant factor as being one of persistence is based on a very tenuous argument. One would expect that in some forms of mental illness (such, perhaps, as the depressive psychoses) persistence might be greatly affected. The reduced cognitive-test scores sometimes reported as characterizing such illness might thus in reality be reflecting a change in an orectic attribute, as well as, or rather than, in a truly cognitive one.

The analysis also has other implications which are not directly relevant to the study of mental abnormality. For example, it would seem to follow that as the effective determinants of score are a function of the difficulty of the problems making up a test, then a factor analysis of inter-item correlations within a cognitive test should reveal one or more factors differentiating between items of different levels of difficulty. The emergence of such factors has in fact been reported from time to time (e.g. Guilford, 1941; Burt, 1942 and Vernon, 1950) and is clearly explicable in terms of the analysis here presented. It is only fair to add, however, that the cases so far reported might provide evidence for nothing of more significance than

---

[1] Readers of this chapter who also read Mangan's thesis may be puzzled to find that one or two of the arguments here presented also appear, word for word, in the thesis. Mangan was in fact quoting verbatim from material supplied to him by the present writer (Furneaux, 1953). The relevant acknowledgement was, unfortunately, accidentally omitted from his typescript.

a statistical artefact (Ferguson, 1941; Wherry, 1944 and Gourlay, 1951), so that too much significance should not be attached to them. The analysis is also obviously relevant to the theory and practice of item analysis, but as these are rather specialized topics they will not be discussed in the present context.

The discussion centred on Fig. 5.1 stressed the fact that for any particular $_\alpha PS$ numerical values for the M_{tr} statistics can only be obtained from the use of problems having D_{tr} values of less than $_cD_{tr}$ while the continuance statistics $\bar{\imath}_s$, V_{ts}, etc., have to be studied by using problems having D_{tr} values greater than $_cD_{ts}$. It may not be obvious that attempts to investigate the M_{qr} statistics too can only be useful if they are confined to observations of the outputs resulting from inputs having a restricted range of D. In the region $D_{tr} > {_cD_{tr}}$ a proportion of both potential O_r and potential O_w outputs will be lost because of the intervention of $_\alpha ST$, but the losses may be unequal if the numerical values of the M_{tr} statistics are different from those of M_{tw}. The ratio $N_r/(N_r + N_w)$ in this region does not necessarily define the statistic q_r, therefore, but only the interaction of the M_{qr} and M_{ts} statistics (where N_r and N_w are the number of O_r and O_w responses observed at a particular D_{tr} value). Data relevant to M_{qr} and $f(D, K)_{qr}$ can thus be collected only at D_{tr} values of less than $_cD_{tr}$ for each *PS*.

An Experimental Investigation

The discussion so far has rested on the logical development of a set of premises. It would lose most of its force if experiments should show, for example, that in the human problem-solver K_{tr}, K_{qr}, and $\bar{\imath}_s$, etc., were all very highly correlated; or that it was impossible to find forms for the various functions $f(D, K)$ which could be applied equally to all individuals (or at least to useful sets of individuals). At this stage it is therefore necessary to consider the results of some experimental work. Although a number of interim reports have been made, covering the gradual development of these experiments (Furneaux, 1948, 1950, 1952, 1955) no readily available account has previously been published. The exposition to be given here will therefore embody rather more detail than would usually be expected in a publication of this type. There appear to be no previous accounts of work directed to the kind of scaling problem which arises when the complications due to the effects of continuance are taken into account. The results of the analysis, moreover, are felt by some psychologists to be rather unexpected. Both these considerations reinforce the argument in favour of a reasonably detailed description.

The particular experiment which is to be discussed was performed with the help of two hundred and thirty-five soldiers, covering an age range of from 18 to 30 years, with a mean of 19·4. All had previously taken Anstey's Dominoes-Test, and the group had been selected to provide a roughly rectangular distribution between the limits of score defined by the points $+ 2 \cdot 0\sigma$ and $- 1 \cdot 5\sigma$, derived from the standardization distribution of this test. The upper limit was imposed by the failure to collect together a sufficient number of individuals having very high scores. The lower limit was deliberately chosen because of the need to use only subjects who were reasonably literate, and who could follow fairly complex instructions without too much difficulty. Each subject attempted letter-series problems of the kind used by Thurstone in his P.M.A. battery. Items had previously been scaled for "difficulty" in a rough-and-ready fashion, and were presented in cycles such that within any set of about five consecutive problems a very wide range of difficulty would be encountered. Instructions were designed to encourage high motivation, and the evidence suggests that this was achieved. Stress was laid on the need to persevere with items found to be difficult, rather than to attempt to reach the end of the test. All problems had to be worked through strictly in sequence, and once an item had been abandoned it could not be attempted again. An answer or a dash, signifying abandonment, was required in respect of each problem, and the time required for each response was measured to an accuracy of about two seconds, by using a device similar to that employed by Slater (1938). Testing was carried out in groups of about twenty, over a total time of three hours for each group. This was split up into two morning sessions of forty-five minutes each, separated by a fifteen minute rest period, followed by two similar periods after a break of one and a half hours for lunch.

Various corrections had to be made to the measured response times in order to eliminate the time spent recording answers and reading the timing device from the actual problem-solving time. These were made in terms of data derived from subsidiary experiments made on the same subjects. Corrected response times will be denoted by the symbols t_r, t_w, and t_s as heretofore. Of the two hundred and thirty-five problems available for presentation one hundred and twenty were attempted by every subject, and provided the basis for the analysis. A conventional item-analysis of these one hundred and twenty problems resulted in the rejection of forty. For the total experimental group the correlation between number right within the set of eighty surviving items, and Dominoes score, was 0·84.

If the investigation of the D_{tr} scale and its associated function $f(D, K)_{tr}$ are considered first, the object of the analysis must be to arrange as many as possible of the usable problems along a scale, and to find a function $f(D, K)_{tr}$, relating $\bar{\imath}_r$ and D_{tr}, which is equally valid for all subjects once each has been allocated his appropriate value for K_{tr}. In conducting this analysis we must take account only of responses at values of D_{tr} such that the observed M_{tr} statistics have not been affected by the interaction of continuance, i.e. all inputs considered must be $I_{u(tr)}$. We can only define such inputs rigorously, however, after a D_{tr} scale and a suitable form for $f(D, K)_{tr}$ have been evolved, and the associated M_{tr} statistics investigated. The escape from this circle of frustration lies via a series of iterations based on successive approximations. In order to simplify the description of the analysis the present tense will be used throughout.

Design of a D_{tr} Scale. Stage 1

For each of the eighty problems compute the proportion of the total experimental group who responded with O_r. Pick out, say, ten problems for which this proportion is highest, i.e. in conventional terms, the ten easiest problems, and assume that they will also have very low scale values for D_{tr}. These are thus problems which are unlikely to constitute $I_{a(tr)}$ inputs except in the case of subjects who have exceptionally poor continuance, or who are exceptionally slow. It will be convenient to refer to them as the *reference-problems*.

For each subject who has returned an O_r to at least five of the reference problems compute the mean of the values of t_r relevant to these problems. This is not a $\bar{\imath}_r$ measure, since it is unlikely that all the reference problems will turn out to occupy the same D scale position. It provides, in fact, a very rough-and-ready type of K_{tr} measure, say k_{tr}. A subject who has returned only a few O_r responses within the set of reference problems might well owe a high proportion of these successes to guessing, and would in any case receive only a very unreliable k_{tr} score from such a small number of responses—hence the rather arbitrary restriction with which this paragraph opens.

Let us now assume that for every subject, every type O_s response has equal status as a measure of t_s, contributing to an assessment of $\bar{\imath}_s$. Suppose that $\bar{\imath}_s$ is not a function of D_{tr}, and compute $\bar{\imath}_s$ for every subject. Pick out those whose continuance, thus computed, is above the mean. Other things being equal these subjects will have their values of critical-difficulty ($_cD_{tr}$) fairly high. There is thus a reasonable chance that the "easy" reference problems will all constitute type $I_{u(tr)}$ inputs for each of them.

From these continuant subjects pick out the forty with the lowest k_{tr} scores (i.e. the fastest) and designate these "Group F." Pick out the forty next in order, i.e. those of moderate speed, and designate these "Group M."

The most convenient function to use in defining a D scale calibrated in terms of t_r values is obviously of the form—

$$_\alpha \bar{\imath}_r = mD_{tr} + {}_\alpha K_{tr} \qquad (2)$$

where m has any convenient value. Assume that this function applies to each member of Group M, then it will follow that—

$$t_r(Av)_{\mathrm{M}} = mD_{tr} + {}_{\mathrm{M}}C_{tr} \qquad (3)$$

where $_{\mathrm{M}}C_{tr}$ is the mean of all the values of K_{tr} relevant to the group members, and $t_r(Av)_{\mathrm{M}}$ is the average value of t_r, within Group M, relevant to any problem which constitutes an input $I_{u(tr)}$ for all the members of the group. Since it is only the relative scale positions of items that are important, and not their absolute positions, we can decide to try the effects of adopting a scale such that in (3) above—

$$_{\mathrm{M}}C_{tr} = 0$$
$$m = 1$$

i.e. we take the $t_r(Av)_{\mathrm{M}}$ values as being also the D_{tr} values of the ten reference problems concerned.

Still on the assumption that the form of $f(D, K)_{tr}$ is identical for all subjects of Group M we can now compute the value of $_\alpha K_{tr}$ for each subject, in terms of the nucleus of the D_{tr} scale provided by the ten reference problems. For each $_\alpha S$ (subject) we have—

$$_\alpha K_{tr} = \Sigma(_{p\alpha}t_r - {}_pD_{tr})/_\alpha n \qquad (4)$$

where one value of $(_{p\alpha}t_r - {}_pD_{tr})$ is derived from each correctly solved item, p, from among the reference problems, and $_\alpha n$ is the number of such correctly solved items. If we assume for the moment that the value of the range H_{tr} (Fig. 5.1) is not a function of D_{tr}, then the value relevant to each subject is estimated by subtracting his smallest value of $(_{p\alpha}t_r - {}_pD_{tr})$ from his largest value, while the value of $(R_t +, H_{tr})$ is approximated, for each subject at $D_{tr} = 0$, by the largest of the values of $(_{p\alpha}t_r - {}_pD_{tr})$. It is easy to pick out the smallest observed value of t_s for each subject, and to assume that this gives an estimate of S_t (Fig. 5.1). The value of $_cD_{tr}$ for any subject is then that value of D_{tr} at which—

$$_{D=0}(R_t + H_{tr}) + {}_cD_{tr} = S_t \qquad (5)$$

i.e. $$_cD_{tr} = S_t - {}_{D=0}(R_t + H_{tr}) \qquad (6)$$

If, on computing this statistic, it were to turn out that for several subjects it had a value appreciably lower than the highest of the D values assigned to the reference problems, then it would follow that an appreciable proportion of the t_r data, derived from these problems, were relevant to $I_{a(tr)}$ inputs and not $I_{u(tr)}$. As has been explained, values of D_{tr} assigned to problems in terms of such data are quite useless for purposes of scale construction, and the observed

M_{tr} statistics are specific to the subject concerned, having no general validity.

In "Group M," however, the lowest value of $_cD_{tr}$ comes out to be 123, whereas the highest D value associated with a reference problem is 58. All inputs can therefore be assumed, with reasonable confidence, to have been of type $I_{u(tr)}$. If the form for $f(D, K)_{tr}$ assumed for equation (2) is universally applicable, it then follows that in any other group for which all the reference problems constitute $I_{u(tr)}$ inputs, the values of $t_r(Av)$ relevant to each of these problems, if plotted against their appropriate D_{tr} values, must define a straight line of slope 1·0 within the limits of sampling error. Group F, which has already been defined, constitutes such a group, for the average value of $\bar{i}_s$ for its members turns out to be a little higher than that for group M, and, by definition, they are also appreciably faster. On plotting the relevant data the best-fitting straight line has a slope of 0·74. A substantial part of the error variance of the array about this line is, of course, produced by the variance of K_{tr} between individuals. On subtracting this component and testing the significance of the difference between the two slopes we emerge with $p = 0·03$ (Snedecor, 1948). The plot strongly suggests, in fact, a curve having a negative acceleration. The form for $f(D, K)_{tr}$ assumed in equation (2) does not therefore provide an acceptable basis for the construction of the D_{tr} scale required.

Faced with such a result the next step must involve the formulation of a possible alternative form for $f(D, K)_{tr}$. The search is not, of course, a blind one, but can be guided by suitable graphical trials, and, in the present case, by hints obtained from other investigations. In 1948 (Furneaux, 1948) and 1950 (Tate, 1950) results were reported which showed that a logarithmic transformation of the response-time data relevant to problem-solving attempts resulted in improved homogeneity of variance between subjects. It seems reasonable therefore to try the effect of such a transformation in the case of the experiment now being reported, particularly as graphical inspection of the data suggests that it might be efficacious.

Design of D_{tr} Scale. Stage 2

Let $\log_{10} t_r = T_r$, then the revised form for equation (2) becomes—

$$_\alpha T_r = mD_{tr} + _\alpha K_{Tr} \tag{7}$$

The analysis now proceeds as from equation (2) in Stage 1, all statistics being concerned with values of T_r instead of t_r. The most suitable value for m, equations (2) and (3), is again 1·0, and the crucial stage is again the final check as to whether this statistic comes out to have the same value in group F as was specified for it in group M.

In the experiment being discussed this test produces a numerical value of 1·08. The analysis can therefore proceed on the assumption that equation (7) provides at least a reasonable approximation to the $f(D, K)_{tr}$ form required, over the range of K_{Tr} defined by groups F and M.

Design of D_{tr} Scale. Stage 3

For every subject in the experimental group a value of $_\alpha K_{Tr}$ can now be computed, using his O_r responses to reference problems according to the method described in Stage 1. His value of $_cD_{tr}$ is then calculated, again using the assumptions and methods of Stage 1. Those subjects for whom $_cD_{tr}$ is smaller than the largest D_{tr} value allotted to a reference problem are discarded, and analysis is continued with the remainder. For every subject retained there is an array of $_\alpha T_r$ values, relating to all the O_r responses made to the eighty problems being investigated. From each such value of $_\alpha T_r$ subtract the value of $_\alpha K_{Tr}$ relevant to the subject concerned. All arrays are thus superimposed at the point $D_{tr} = 0$, $\dot{T}_r = 0$, and if equation (7) is in fact of universal application the D value of any problem will be given by—

$$D = \dot{T}_r(Av) \tag{8}$$

Where $\dot{T}_r$ is the value of $(T_r - K_{Tr})$ obtained from any one subject in respect of the problem concerned, and $\dot{T}_r(Av)$ is the mean value of $\dot{T}_r$ for the whole experimental group. The transformation from T_r to $\dot{T}_r$ is necessary to correct for the fact that the sample of subjects obtaining O_r responses differs from problem to problem in a way which is a function of the D_{tr} value of the problem.

By comparing the D_{tr} values thus allocated with the $_cD_{tr}$ values of each subject it will now be observed that for nearly all subjects some of the $\dot{T}_r$ values contributed to these determinations of D_{tr} were relevant to $I_{a(tr)}$ inputs. A series of iterations are thus necessary to remove such data, and their effects, from the analysis. At the conclusion of this process a D value of probably moderate accuracy will have been assigned to the majority of the eighty problems. Some, however, will have D values greater than the value of $_cD_{tr}$ relevant to even the fastest and most continuant of subjects, and thus can only be calibrated as having D_{tr} values greater than such and such. For a similar reason others will have to be calibrated in terms of only a very few data, and thus inaccurately.

Design of D_{tr} Scale. Stage 4

It is now possible to examine the statistics of M_{ts} in greater detail, with a view to improving the estimates of S_t, and thus of $_cD_{tr}$. Since some sort of D_{tr} scale position has been allocated to most items, and a value of K_{Tr} assigned to each subject, the value of

D_{tr} at which the time R_t becomes equal to the time $(S_t + H_{ts})$ can be computed. This gives the numerical value of $_cD_{ts}$ for each individual, and by taking account only of those t_s values relevant to O_s responses evoked by problems for which $D > {_cD_{ts}}$ it becomes possible to investigate M_{ts}.

Assume again that $\hat{\imath}_s$ is not a function of D_{tr}, and compute V_{ts} for each subject, using only $I_{u(ts)}$ inputs as defined above. The application of Bartlett's test now shows these variances to differ significantly from one individual to another ($\chi^2 = 310$, $p \simeq 0.01$ with 228 d.f.). On introducing the transformation $\log_{10} t_s = T_s$, however, homogeneity is achieved ($\chi^2 = 242$, $p \simeq 0.30$). Compute $\bar{T}_s$ for each subject, and then the values of $\dot{T}_s$ obtained by subtracting $\bar{T}_s$ from each available value of T_s. All M_{T_s} distributions are thus superimposed with $\dot{T}_s = O$. Collect together all the values of $\dot{T}_s$ relevant to each particular problem, and compute their mean, $\dot{T}_s(Av)$, for the whole experimental group. On correlating $\dot{T}_s(Av)$ with D_{tr} over the whole set of problems we find a coefficient of 0.11 which with 31 d.f. is not significant. The assumption that T_s, and thus t_s, is not a function of D_{tr} seems therefore to be justified.

The method of timing used for the measurement of response times was such (Slater, 1938) that it is easy to find out how long a subject had already been working for when he attempted each problem. It is thus possible to plot each value of $\dot{T}_s$ contributed by each subject against this time already worked, and to see whether continuance varied appreciably during the time that testing was in progress. On plotting a single array including all $\dot{T}_s$ values derived from the whole group it becomes clear that no important variations occurred save during the concluding twenty minutes of both morning and afternoon testing periods. During each of these periods there is a steady fall in the values of $\dot{T}_s$, and an increase in the variance of the array. On further investigation this increase in variance is found to reflect the fact that subjects with high scores in the Dominoes test maintained their continuance virtually unchanged throughout the whole of each testing period, while those with low Dominoes scores were responsible for the general downward trend. The need to take account of variations in continuance would add formidable complications to the analysis, and to avoid these all data relating to the last twenty minutes of testing, in both morning and afternoon, are deleted from the analysis, for all subjects. After this has been done and revised values of V_{T_s} calculated, Bartlett's test gives $\chi^2 = 231$, $p \simeq 0.40$ with 220 d.f.[1], the best estimate of V_{T_s} being 0.0144 log sec.

The pooled distribution of $\dot{T}_s$, covering all subjects,

[1] At each stage of the analysis a few subjects fall out because of the nature of their test responses, scores, etc.

can now be taken as analogous to the M_{T_s} distribution that would result from a single subject of constant continuance who attempted a very large number of problems. There will be a small additional component of variance resulting from the sampling error associated with each individual determination of $\bar{T}_s$, but this will not be sufficiently large to produce any great distortion of the shape of the pooled distribution. On inspection this is clearly of normal type, so that it is reasonable to conclude that values of T_s which approach the extremes S_t and $(S_t + H_{ts})$ arise rather infrequently for any subject. The effective minimum value of T_s will in fact have a value of about $\bar{T}_s - 2\sqrt{V_{T_s}}$ for everyone, at all values of D_{tr}. Values of $_cD_{tr}$ computed in terms of this revised estimate of the minimum value of $\bar{T}_s$, for each subject, are of course higher than those resulting from the values of S_t, previously used, so that a larger number of $I_{u(tr)}$ become available for every subject. Iterations from this point result in revised values of D_{tr} for some problems, and in revised values of K_{T_r} for all subjects —all based on an increased number of data.

Design of D_{tr} Scale. Stage 5

If we take any two problems, p and q, and for each subject for whom they both constitute inputs $I_{u(tr)}$ compute $_{p\alpha}T_r - {_{q\alpha}T_r} = {_{(p-q)}}\dot{T}_r$, then if the value of V_{T_r} associated with each problem is equal, and is the same for all subjects, the variance of $_{(p-q)}\dot{T}_r$ within the whole group of subjects should equal $2V_{T_r}$. Starting with the problem having the lowest D value specify pairs of items of successive D_{tr} scale positions. For each pair compute the $_{(p-q)}\dot{T}_r$ variance within the total group, but taking account only of values derived entirely from inputs $I_{u(tr)}$.

Testing the resulting values for homogeneity the experimental data being considered give $\chi^2 = 45.7$, $p \simeq 0.04$ with 31 d.f. (Bartlett). The hypothesis that V_{T_r} has the same numerical value for all $I_{u(tr)}$ is thus untenable. On further investigation, however, it appears that the lack of homogeneity results from exceptionally large values of $2V_{T_r}$ associated with two particular problem pairs. On deleting these and repeating Bartlett's test on the remainder, we obtain a χ^2 of 36.1, i.e. $p \simeq 0.18$ with 29 d.f.

Now, compute separately within each subject, the variance of all the $_{(p-q)}\dot{T}_r$ values which arise from all those problem-pairs which constitute $I_{u(tr)}$ inputs, but ignore the two pairs deleted from the analysis above. On testing for homogeneity between subjects we find $\chi^2 = 227$, $p \simeq 0.4$ with 216 d.f. The variance estimate derived from the between-pairs-analysis was 0.1320, while the between-subjects-analysis gives a value of 0.1292. These clearly do not differ significantly, and their mean, 0.1306 log sec, provides an estimate of $2V_{T_r}$.

The analysis has provided no evidence inconsistent with the hypothesis of a numerical value for V_{Tr} which is constant over both subjects and problems, save in the case of one or both of the members of the two deleted problem-pairs. One can, however, imagine rather complicated (and unlikely) relationships between V_{Tr} and D_{tr} on the one hand and K_{Tr} on the other, which might also explain the results. No attempt will be made to dispose of them, in the present context, but the hypothesis of constancy will be accepted as being the simplest explanation of the data.

Up to the time of writing no rigorous analysis has been made of the exact form of the M_{Tr} distribution, but graphical inspections suggest that it is of normal type at all values of D_{tr} and for all subjects. Response times as long as $(R_t + H_{tr})$, at any value of D_{tr}, will therefore be rare, and the value of D at which any appreciable proportion of inputs turn out to be $I_{a(tr)}$ will therefore be rather higher than $_cD_{tr}$ as so far estimated. If the effective upper limit is taken to be $K_{Tr} + 2\sqrt{V_{Tr}} + D$, at any value of D, then a revised value of $_cD_{tr}$ can be computed for each subject. This revision will produce an increase in the

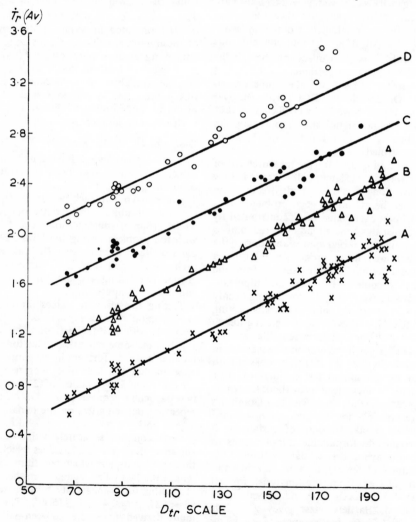

FIG. 5.3. $\dot{T}_r(Av)$ PLOTTED AGAINST $100 D_{tr}$ FOR GROUPS OF VARYING SPEED

(*See* text.)

Note. The curves *A, B, C, D* show the relationships to which the data should conform: they are *not* the best-fitting straight lines. To facilitate the examination of this graph 1·5 log units have been added to each value of $\dot{T}_r(Av)$ in Group *D*, and values of 1·0 and 0·5 log units in Groups *C* and *B* respectively.

number of $I_{u(tr)}$ available for each person, and thus provides the starting point for further iterations. When these have been completed final values of K_{T_r} and $\bar{T}_s$ are available for all subjects, and final estimates of D_{tr} for each problem.

A crucial test is now possible to see whether equation (7) is acceptable as the form of a relationship between D and t_r which is equally applicable to all subjects. Divide all subjects into four approximately

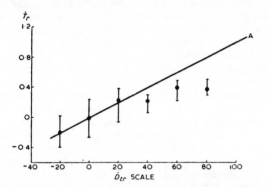

Fig. 5.4. Discrepancy between Relationship of T_r to D when I_a Inputs Are Used, and that Applying to I_u

The straight line A gives the relationship applying in the case of I_u inputs. Each point plotted shows the median observed value of $\dot{T}_r$ which relates to the set of inputs I_a having values of D_{tr} within the range ± 10 of the central value shown. The vertical lines terminate at the values of the upper and lower quartiles.

Values of $\dot{D}_{tr}$ have been multiplied by 100.

equal subgroups in terms of their K_{tr} scores, the fastest being allocated to Group A, the slowest to D, and the remainder, in order, to the intermediate groups. For each subgroup compute the value of $\dot{T}_r(Av)$ relevant to each problem, and plot these values against the D values of these problems. For each subgroup separately the slope of the relevant best-fitting straight line should have a value of $1·0$.

It will be clear from Fig. 5.3 that such a result was actually observed in the case of the experimental group concerned, so that the hypothesis that the relationship between D and $\bar{T}_r$ has the form set out in equation (7) for every subject is supported. The evidence presented in Stage 4 of the analysis also supported the hypothesis that the value of V_{Tr} is independent of D, and identical for all subjects. It must be remembered, however, that this latter result was only demonstrated after two item-pairs had been deleted from the analysis. Subsequent examination showed that one item from one of these pairs should have been rejected at the stage of item analysis; a correlation of $0·04$ with the criterion score had been wrongly computed as one of $0·40$. It was hoped that this initial item analysis might define a set of items all more or less of the same type, using this last term in

the rather unorthodox manner suggested earlier in the discussion. The results of the analysis, and the accidental finding with the wrongly calibrated item, suggest that this was in fact accomplished. Since it will be shown, in the further analysis, that separately designed D_{tr} and D_{qr} scales correlate very highly, this is more or less what one would expect to find, since a conventional item-analysis is clearly an approximate method of classifying in terms of M_{qr} characteristics. It achieves this classification only approximately, however, since it makes no distinction between O_w and O_s responses.

In the second discrepant item-pair the non-homogeneous value of $2V_{Tr}$ was found, on investigation, to be associated with one of the two items, rather than both, but no explanation for the discrepancy has as yet been found.

It must now be shown that the deletion of $I_{a(tr)}$ responses was necessary, and that their retention would have produced the kind of complication predicted by the theoretical analysis of a *PS*. If $I_{a(tr)}$ inputs give rise to the same relationships between T_r and D_{tr} as have been demonstrated for $I_{u(tr)}$ inputs, then the effort to distinguish between the two kinds of input is clearly unnecessary, and the theory which calls for the distinction is unsound.

For every subject compute the values of $\dot{T}_r$ which relate to $I_{a(tr)}$ inputs in the same way as was used for type $I_{u(tr)}$. For each subject separately, compute the values of $\dot{D}_{tr}$ which apply to all these inputs, where $\dot{D}_{tr} = D_{tr} - {}_cD_{tr}$. All such inputs are thus re-scaled in terms of a D scale which has its zero at that point on the D_{tr} scale above which continuance should, in terms of the theory being examined, begin to distort relationships. On plotting $\dot{T}_r$ v. $\dot{D}_{tr}$ as a single array covering all subjects, the relationship graphed in Fig. 5.4 is obtained. If $I_{a(tr)}$ inputs behaved in the same way as do type $I_{u(tr)}$ this array would have defined a straight line of slope $1·0$. As it clearly does not, the distinction between the two kinds of input appears to be justified. The nature of the array is in fact exactly of the kind that would have been predicted in terms of the discussion on pp. 175–176, both slope and dispersion decreasing as $\dot{D}_{tr}$ increases. When interpreting Fig. 5.4 it is important to bear in mind the fact that the problems which, as $I_{a(tr)}$ inputs, gave rise to this array are the same problems which, as $I_{u(tr)}$ inputs, led to the relationships shown in Fig. 5.3.

The results of the analyses justify the retention of the hypothesis that m, equation (7), and V_{Tr} are population constants. It is convenient to replace equation (7) by—

$$T_r = mD_{tr} + K_{Tr} + \varepsilon_i \qquad (9)$$

where ε_i is a positive or negative component arising on a particular occasion i, such that at every value of D the values of ε relevant to a large number of occasions are distributed with variance V_{Tr} about zero as mean.

Some psychologists, when discussing this hypothesis with the writer, have expressed surprise that such invariances should be found in a field where the discovery of substantial individual difference is the normal expectation. In the present study, however, such differences do not disappear, but are taken up in the individual-constants K_{Tr} and T_s which vary very considerably from one person to another. Equation (9) provides a form of relationship analogous to that embodied in, say, Fechner's law, which latter has served to clarify, rather than obscure, the study of individual differences in sensory thresholds. Equation (9) does, however, assert that there may be some cerebral mechanism involved in problem-solving activity, which is of the kind used in connexion with letter-series problems at least, and which has much the same form for at least a very wide range of individuals.

A Possible Problem-solving Mechanism

While the writer was speculating on the possible implications of these findings a report was published of a paper read by Hick (1950). In this paper Hick showed that the relationship between the time taken to react within a multiple-choice situation and the complexity of the choice situation could be expressed as—

$$RT = K \log M$$

where RT = choice reaction-time

K = an individual constant

M = a function of the complexity of the choice situation.

He developed the argument that this is the relationship one would expect to observe if multiple-choice activity involved successive binary classifications. As the brain seems to consist of a vast number of nearly identical units he argued that it might be permissible to posit that all its activities involve sequences of elementary operations of like kind and duration. Such a device might well function by carrying out successive binary switchings, with each "switch" taking the same time and involving the same sort of simple basic activity. This hypothesis of Hick's seems to imply that multiple-choice reaction-time is a measure of the time required for a search to be completed in the brain for the set of "connexions" which would initiate a required behaviour. It then occurred to the writer that problem-solving should perhaps be regarded as a special case of a multiple-choice reaction, and that it

would be interesting to see if the rather striking characteristics of equation (9) could be explained by postulating, within problem-solving processes, the repeated occurrence of some elementary activity which requires a substantially constant time for completion. The following hypothesis was eventually developed.

The brain structure of any individual, P, includes a set of $_pN$ neural elements which participate in problem-solving activities. It is not necessary at this stage to adopt any particular view as to the nature of these elements, which might be either single neurones or much more complex structures. The solution of a particular problem, h, of difficulty D, involves bringing into association a particular set, $_DN_h$, of these elements, interconnected in some precise order. (The terms "bringing into association" and "interconnected" should not necessarily be interpreted literally after the manner of, say, an electrical circuit. For example, the almost simultaneous firing of two otherwise independent units could constitute one method of bringing them into association, provided some device existed which could detect the simultaneity, while the exact order of firing might represent the mode of interconnexion.) When problem h is first presented single elements are first selected, at random, from the total pool $_pN$ and examined to see whether any one of them, alone, constitutes the required solution. A device must be postulated which carries out this examination—it must bring together the neural representations of the perceptual material embodying the problem, the rules according to which the problem has to be solved, and the particular organization of elements whose validity as a solution has to be examined. It must give rise to some sort of signal, which in the case of an acceptable organization will terminate the search process and will initiate the translation of the accepted neural organization into the activity which specifies the solution in behaviour terms. Alternatively, if the organization under examination proves to be unacceptable a signal must result which will lead to the continuation of the search process. It will be found useful to refer to this hypothetical device under the name of "the comparator."

If $D \neq 1$, the comparator will reject each of the $_pN$ trial solutions involving only a single element, and the search will then start for a pair of elements, which, when correctly interconnected, might constitute a valid solution. Suppose $D \neq 2$, then all possible organizations of the $_pN$ elements taken two at a time will also be examined and rejected, after which we can imagine that the search will continue among sets of three, four, five, etc. If $D = r$, then the comparator will reject in turn all the organizations involving from 1 to $(r - 1)$ elements, so that there will be a time

$\tau \sum\limits_{r-1}^{1} E$ sec within which a solution cannot occur, where—

τ (Tosouton) = the time required for completing a single elementary operation within the search process.[1]

$\sum\limits_{r-1}^{1} E$ = the number of elementary operations involved in the search process up to the level of complexity $(r - 1)$.

Similarly, after a time $\tau \sum\limits_{r}^{1} E$ sec all possible organizations embodying r elements will have been examined, so that correct solutions to problems of difficulty r will always arise within the period defined by the two limiting times $\tau \sum\limits_{r-1}^{1} E$ and $\tau \sum\limits_{r}^{1} E$. In terms of such a hypothesis, therefore, V_{Tr} is in no sense a function of error of measurement but results mainly from the range of times required to set up all possible modes of neural organization at a particular level of complexity. It is perhaps worth noting, in passing, that within the framework of such a hypothesis error would be accounted for by positing that during the search process organizations arise at levels of complexity $r - \delta_1, r - \delta_2, \ldots$, etc.,[2] which satisfy most, but not all, of the requirements of a true solution to a problem of difficulty r. If the comparator has characteristics analogous to those of "band-width" in electrical and mechanical discriminators, i.e. if its discriminating powers are such that neural organizations which closely resemble the organization representing a correct solution may be accepted as the required organization, then the possibility of error arises. The frequency of error, thus conceived, will be a function of the band-width of the comparator, and since the number of "nearly-correct" organizations will increase as D is increased, the likelihood of error will increase with D.

This probability is clearly dependent on the exact nature of the search process. Finally, continuance is easily defined in terms of such a "search" hypothesis; it is a measure of the length of time during which, following the initiation of search, the comparator remains "set" for a particular problem.

As has been explained, the hypothesis thus summarized seemed to grow naturally upon the foundations laid down by Hick, working with reaction-time data. It has the merit that it can be checked experimentally in virtually all its aspects, relationships of

---

[1] The Greek τοσοῦτον (Tosouton), meaning "so long," seems to be an appropriate name for this elementary period, particularly since τ is very appropriate as a symbol for a short period of time.

[2] If the possibility be accepted that the comparator might sometimes fail to respond to the "correct" organization, then response might also occur at levels of complexity $r + \delta$.

time against complexity which would characterize such a process can readily be computed, and compared with those actually observed. It can only be stated here that if it be considered that the search mechanism operates by setting up the orderly sequence of events outlined above, but takes account only of combinations rather than of possible permutations of neural organization, then time-complexity relationships approximating to those defined by equation (9) do in fact emerge. In the simplest, completely orderly case the observed distribution of log-times at a particular value of D should, of course, be rectangular rather than normal. This disparity between the requirements of the theory and observation can be removed by postulating that as time elapses after the initiation of the search for a particular solution the number of neural elements involved in successive interconnexions tends to increase steadily, but that interspersed with successive combinations involving a particular value of $_D N_h$ there also occur organizations involving either a larger or a smaller number of elements. In other words, an element of randomness must be imposed upon the type of order defined by the theory. It is interesting to note that if this is done then the theory predicts that with very low values of D, V_{Tr} should tend to increase as D decreases. This prediction from the theory has been confirmed by observations subsequently made. It is also of some interest that, if the theory is approximately true, then the solution of letter-series problems of such difficulty that they are correctly solved by only about 5 per cent of the unselected adult population involves the activity of less than one hundred neural elements.

A theory of this kind should not, of course, be taken too seriously. It might, for example, be objected that introspection during problem-solving reveals nothing comparable to the postulated search process, but then neither does visual experience in any way suggest the underlying complicated retinal and central processes. A more telling argument would be that it simply replaces the problem-solver by a little mannikin, the comparator. It could perhaps be claimed that it does serve the functions that a theory should, i.e. it accounts for such data as have been collected, suggests new experiments which could profitably be attempted, and predicts results for some of them.

One obvious prediction is that a change in the value of τ, such as one might expect to result from, say, an increase in drive, should leave unchanged the values of m and V_{Tr}, equation (9). A set of fifteen problems (set A) was therefore assembled, all having approximately the same low D_{tr} scale position, and a further set, B, all clustering around a slightly higher position. According to the theory, any group of subjects, no matter what their drive-state, should give rise to exactly the same value for $\bar{T}_r(Av)_B - \bar{T}_r(Av)_A$, where the two terms subtracted are the mean values of $\bar{T}$ relevant to the two sets of items, within the group concerned. This prediction has now been confirmed (within the limits of sampling error) for six different groups of university students, all comprising between thirty and seventy subjects, and covering a range of Faculties and ages. It has also been confirmed for one group of three hundred boys having a mean age of 14·4 years, in English grammar schools. For some of these groups the instructions given have stressed the fact that problems should be tackled at a comfortable, easy pace, while for others the fastest possible rate of work has been demanded. In every case adequate practice has preceded the actual testing.

V_{Tr} has behaved according to expectation in all those groups which have attempted the problems under what have come to be known as *unstressed* conditions, i.e. working at their own preferred pace. An appreciably discrepant value has been observed, however, in one of the groups of university students who were working under *stressed* conditions, i.e. at maximum rate. For this group the mean value of V_{Tr} among its members was significantly higher than expected. At the time of writing several lines of evidence appear to be converging to support the hypothesis that individuals who are working under a degree of drive in excess of that required for optimum performance in the task, display such exaggerated values of V_{Tr}. This single discrepancy may indicate an instability in the value of τ under such conditions.

The Investigation of M_{tw} and M_{qr}

Another prediction from the theory is clearly that the dispersion of the response-times arising in connexion with O_w outputs should be greater, at any value of D_{tr}, than that characterizing O_r outputs, since the former can arise at several levels of complexity, the latter only at one. Nothing has so far been said about the experimental investigation of the M_{tw} statistics, or of those of M_{qr}, nor of the problems which arise in connexion with the investigation of the associated functions $f(D, K)_{tw}$ and $f(D, K)_{qr}$. Space does not permit any detailed discussion of these topics. The general strategy used, a succession of iterations having the object of eliminating I_a inputs and of finding acceptable forms for the relevant functions $f(D, K)$, has been identical with that already described, but some of the detailed tactics have had to be modified. It must suffice to report of the M_{tw} statistics that values of $\bar{T}_w$ are smaller than values of $\bar{T}_r$ at the same D_{tr} value, the discrepancy increasing as D increases. Similarly, V_{Tw} is larger at all values of D_{tr} than is V_{Tr}, and again, the difference is greatest at high values of D. It is encouraging that these are just the characteristics which would be expected to arise from a device such as has been postulated. The

numerical values of these statistics, however, seem to be subject to a degree of individual variation which it has not yet proved possible to describe in terms of a few simple $f(D, K)$ relationships. In view of this failure the M_{tw} statistics cannot as yet be summarized in terms of scores which have the same significance for all subjects. In the particular groups of soldiers studied the correlations between $\bar{T}_r$ and $\bar{T}_w$, at various low values of D_{tr}, ranged around 0·58. At high values they fell below 0·50. These values, and the differences between them, reflect in part the low reliability of the $\bar{T}_w$ scores; resulting partly from the high value of V_{Tw} and partly from the fact that, at low values of D_{tr}, a comparatively small number of O_w responses are available for the making of $\bar{T}_w$ assessments. They do serve to make it clear, however, that the temporal characteristics of incorrect responses do not provide a very good estimate of those for correct ones, and this underlines the unsatisfactory nature of some frequently used rate measures.

In connexion with M_{qr} the analysis has been more successful. Using the D_{tr} scale as a starting point it has been possible to specify a normal ogive which, given an appropriate value of K_{qr}, gives an acceptable fit to the data relating q_r and D_{tr} for each member of the experimental group which has been described. In evolving the relevant function only type $I_{u(tr)}$ inputs were of course taken into account. An attempt to reduce the SE_{est} of individual arrays about the best-fitting ogive, by altering the D scale values allotted to the various problems, met with very little success, the correlation between the D_{tr} scale which served as a starting point, and the D_{qr} scale finally evolved, being 0·92. There are thus strong grounds for believing that, with letter-series type problems at least, the ultimate determinants within problems of both response-time and response-quality, are much the same. The use of the term "difficulty" embracing both kinds of D scale, seems thus to be justified. What must not be done, however, is to attempt to calibrate for D by lumping O_w and O_s outputs together as "wrong" and using a simple index such as percentage of wrong answers in a defined group. It will be clear that this procedure will result in the formation of an unstable scale of a multi-dimensional kind, because of the intervention of the effects of continuance. In the group which has been described, a D scale thus derived exhibited a correlation of only 0·68 with the D_{tr} scale when computed within the Group D relevant to Fig. 5.3, whereas for Group A, pertaining to the same figure, the coefficient rose to 0·79.

Interrelationships among Scores

The demonstration that D_{tr} and D_{qr} scales are very closely related does not imply a similar high correlation between values of K_{Tr} and K_{qr} for individuals.

Data relating to this latter relationship, and to those involving $\bar{T}_s$ as well, are given for the experiment which has been described, in Table V.1. From this it will be clear that these are all relatively independent

TABLE V.1

INTERCORRELATIONS OF K_{Tr}, K_{qr}, AND $\bar{T}_s$

	K_{Tr}	$\bar{T}_s$
K_{qr}	− 38	31
$\bar{T}_s$	− 27	

Notes: (a) A high value of K_{Tr} implies low speed.
(b) A high value of K_{qr} implies high accuracy.
(c) A high value of $\bar{T}_s$ implies high continuance.
(d) Of the total experimental group, only two hundred and nine could be scored for all three attributes.

scores which demand separate consideration. In more highly selected groups, such as university students, the coefficients concerned, as would be expected, are found to be considerably smaller. One cannot therefore justifiably talk of "letter-series test ability," but only of a person's standing in terms of each of the scores K_{Tr}, K_{qr} and $\bar{T}_s$. It seems difficult to resist the conclusion that results of a similar kind would be obtained if other types of problem material were investigated. Instead of intercorrelating conventional test scores, therefore, and describing cognitive structure in terms of such correlations, it seems that the foundation data for such analyses should be properly constituted measures of speed, accuracy and continuance, derived from each of the kinds of test material which it is desired to investigate.

It is very difficult to know whether K_{Tr} type scores derived from different kinds of problem material would display high intercorrelations, and thus define a useful speed-factor within all cognitive-test behaviour, since the speed scores used by nearly all those who have investigated this problem have been of the kind criticized in the earlier sections of this discussion. Rimoldi (1951), in a study remarkable for the range of activities it covered, showed that several fairly distinct speed factors were needed to describe his data, motor, perceptual, and cognitive rate measures each defining their own factor. His speed-of-cognition factor was a strong one, and included tests as disparate as "reasoning" and "space," together with measures of free-association rate, recognition rate, and speed of making judgements. On the other hand this cognition factor was only very slightly correlated with a perceptual-speed factor which included rate measures for reading, a verbal-meaning test, and a test of number. Nelson (1953), using reasonably well designed scores, found only very small intercorrelations

within a set of intellectual and motor speed-tests in a normal group, but as this group had a very restricted variance on the intellectual side, at least, this finding is of little significance. (With the "Nufferno" speed measures, for example, her group had a S.D. of about one quarter, of that characterizing an unselected normal population.) Nelson's abnormal groups, neurotics and psychotics, both of which displayed much larger variances than her normals, provided data which defined strong factors of mental and motor speed. In Thurstone's perceptual study (1949) a factor clearly analogous to Rimoldi's speed-of-cognition factor also emerged. There are in addition more than a score of correlational studies which have demonstrated intellectual-speed factors, but using unsatisfactory scoring methods.

The accuracy score (K_{qr}) derived from letter-series tests usually displays correlations with cognitive-test scores of the conventional kind which are higher than those associated with either speed (K_{Tr}) or continuance (C). This is not invariably the case, as everything depends on the relationship between the D values of the test items and the values of $_cD$ displayed by those taking them. In practice, however, accuracy does frequently emerge as the score which displays the closest relationships with those of the conventional kind. Since such conventional scores usually display quite high intercorrelations among themselves, this suggests that there may be quite a strong factor of accuracy underlying a wide variety of cognitive performances.

There would thus appear to be quite a strong justification for talking of a subject's *speed* and *accuracy* without making specific reference to the kind of problem-material in terms of which these attributes were measured. So far as continuance is concerned the position is less clear. In so far as test instructions can be designed in such a way that continuance becomes synonymous with persistence the results obtained from factorial studies of persistence tests are clearly applicable (e.g. Ryans, 1938). These investigators have shown that persistence tests do display intercorrelations which are sufficiently high to define a trait, or more probably two related traits. Unless instructions *are* so devised, however, continuance in a particular test will be affected by so many factors specific to that test that it would not be surprising if the continuance scores evoked by different instruments were only slightly related.

Until recently most psychologists have accepted the view that cognitive and orectic test-scores are relatively independent. A certain amount of evidence to the contrary has been available for some time, such as the work of Mandler (1952) who has shown that anxiety may reduce scores in certain kinds of test. Such demonstrations have usually been regarded as providing interesting exceptions, under rather unusual conditions, to well-established general rules. The analysis here presented, supported as it is by the results obtained by Mangan (1954) makes it difficult to accept such a viewpoint, since continuance will always involve orectic determinants. It is moreover quite obvious that speed in any problem-solving task will be a function of drive, and even if an increase in a subject's speed were always to be attended by just such a decrease in accuracy[1] as would serve to keep constant the overall score achieved in a conventional test, this would only serve to demonstrate rather clearly the inadequacy of such conventional tests for the purpose of making fundamental measurements.

The interdependence of cognitive and orectic traits seems to be demonstrated by the results of some experiments carried out by the writer in connexion with the relationship between stressed and unstressed speed. By subtracting K_{Tr} (stressed) from K_{Tr} (unstressed) for a particular individual one obtains a score which has been designated stress-gain, and which provides a measure of the extent to which he can improve his rate of production of O_r responses under the stressed instructions. This score was obtained for each of a group of seventy-five university students, who also completed the Guilford S.T.D.C.R. inventory. Taking the (D + C) score as providing a measure of neuroticism (Hildebrand, 1953) and the R score as a measure of extraversion, the whole group was divided up into four subgroups of approximately equal size—stable extraverts (SE), stable introverts (SI), neurotic introverts (NI), and neurotic extraverts (NE). The term neurotic is used here, of course, in a purely relative sense, and so far as is known no individual was actually neurotic in the overt, clinical sense. The mean values of stress-gain within each of these groups are displayed in Table V.2. The largest value is that associated with NE, whereas for NI a

negative value was obtained, indicating a slower rate of work under stressed than under unstressed conditions. The simplest explanation of these results is probably that which assumes that introverted students, because of their greater intrinsic susceptibility to conditioning (Franks, 1957) have come to respond to any formal test or examination situation by generating a high drive. If neuroticism is in any case associated with a state of high drive, then the convergence of the two determinants, within the NI subgroup, will result in such a state of high drive, even under the unstressed conditions, that the further increase produced by the stressed instructions takes it to a value greater than the optimum postulated by the Yerkes-Dodson law, and actually results in a performance decrement. The NE group, on the other hand, will exhibit much less drive under unstressed conditions, increasing to a value nearer to the optimum during the stressed test.

Whatever explanation may be accepted, the results demonstrate clearly that performance in a cognitive-test situation is influenced in very important ways by orectic determinants. A rough distinction between the cognitive and orectic manifestations of a disorder may often be useful, but to use cognitive tests as if they gave information about some independent, encapsulated part of the personality would seem to be a quite unjustifiable procedure. One could in fact go so far as to suggest that the study of the way in which cognitive performance changes under the influence of testing régimes designed to vary such factors as stress, motivation, and the like, should form an essential part of psychometric practice.

The Measurement of "Level"

The detailed design of tests which can be used for making accurate measurements of such individual constants as K_{Tr} and K_{qr} will not be discussed here, since the question is considered elsewhere (Furneaux, 1953, 1956). It need only be stated that a set of tests of such kinds have been developed (Furneaux, 1953, 1956) and that the use of these instruments has led to results of the kind which are discussed by Payne in his contribution to this HANDBOOK. Little mention has as yet been made in the present contribution, however, of such attributes as *power* and *level*, nor of the techniques which have been used for their measurement.

There are no generally accepted definitions for either of these terms, and both are frequently used without any attempt at definition being made at all. They are normally treated as if they referred to scores in untimed tests. It will be clear from the discussion so far that if an untimed test is made up of items constituting $I_{u(tr)}$ inputs for the individual being assessed, then it will constitute a measure of accuracy alone, whereas if a

TABLE V.2

RELATIONSHIP BETWEEN STRESS-GAIN
AND S.T.D.C.R. SCORES

		(D + C) score	
		$\leqslant 51$	> 51
R score	> 38	− 0·03	0·07
	< 38	0·00	0·05

Stress/gain scores in log sec units

Variance estimates: Between = 0·147 log sec units
Within = 0·036 log sec units
$F = 4.1$ with 3 and 71 d.f.
Sig. $\simeq 0.01$

[1] The writer knows of no evidence which indicates that this kind of compensation does in fact occur.

proportion of the items are $I_{a(tr)}$, being difficult for the subject concerned, then the test will measure an interaction of speed, accuracy, and continuance specific to the combination of test and subject. The normal use of the terms power and level thus imputes to the subject nothing more fundamental than the ability to achieve a particular score in a particular test, which may or may not exhibit a high correlation with the score he would achieve in a different untimed test using the same kind of material.

The writer has found it useful to reserve the term *Level-Test* for use in connexion with tests which have deliberately been designed in such a way as to provide the subject with the maximum possible reward for persistent effort (Furneaux, 1953). The basic unit in such a test is a set of items comprising a cycle. The first problem in each cycle is very easy, each succeeding item is of greater difficulty than its predecessor, and the last is so difficult that few can solve it correctly even when given unlimited time. The number of items in a cycle is quite small, so that difficulty increases fairly rapidly from item to item. On the initial easy items, score will be a function of accuracy only, but speed and continuance in interaction play an increasingly important part as the later problems are attempted, even for highly able subjects. The total number of items correctly solved within one cycle will thus provide a score for effectiveness within a situation designed to reward high continuance, as well as speed and accuracy, and the test instructions are so designed that continuance depends almost entirely on persistence. The score provided by one cycle will be rather unreliable, being based on a small number of items. If, however, several such cycles are arranged in series, the mean score-per-cycle, computed over all items attempted, provides a measure of adequate reliability. The maximum score possible is the same no matter how few cycles have been completed, so that a time limit can be imposed without penalty to the slow worker. Such a subject, if he is also persistent and accurate, can in fact obtain a higher score than one who is fast but lacks persistence. The reliability of the measurement is the only thing that varies with the number of problems attempted. Level-scores, thus defined, are not altogether free from the kind of ambiguity which has been criticized in connexion with conventional-type intelligence tests, since different level-tests, incorporating different numbers of items per cycle, and covering different ranges of difficulty,[1] will still give rise to scores which are not altogether comparable. It will be clear, however, that this kind of assessment approximates, rather roughly, to a measurement of the maximum

level of difficulty at which the subject can function successfully when motivated to persevere with items experienced as difficult. In so far as this is the case such level-tests measure a reasonably invariant property of the individual. The design and use of such tests is dealt with in greater detail elsewhere (Furneaux, 1953 and 1956). They serve the function of indicating the subject's intellectual ceiling, without however providing any clue as to the relative size of the contributions to his effectiveness which are provided by the more fundamental attributes of speed, accuracy, and continuance. In the less disabling forms of schizophrenia, for example, there appears to be a phase during which patients achieve level scores of the same magnitude as those characterizing normal individuals. Their illness has thus not impaired their effectiveness in certain kinds of situation. Tests of speed, however, reveal a marked slowness in the same patients, which is compensated for by an increase in persistence. The latter kind of test thus reveals an important aetiological characteristic, while the former shows that the organism as a whole is able, at least for a time, to compensate for its effects. Both kinds of measuring device would therefore appear to have their part to play in the investigation of abnormal function.

SUMMARY

The thesis has been argued that a subject's score in a cognitive test of the familiar kind is determined by the interaction of a number of determinants which should really all receive separate consideration. A logical analysis of the nature of the problem-solving act suggests that three attributes, speed, accuracy, and continuance, are concerned in any kind of "intelligent" behaviour, and that the valid and unambiguous measurement of these traits can only be accomplished after the problem of classifying problems in terms of both "type" and "difficulty" has been solved. The problem of scaling for difficulty has been shown to be a more complex one than has in general been assumed, and an example has been presented showing the kind of experimental analysis which can be undertaken in an effort to achieve a valid difficulty scale. Once such a scale had been achieved, in the experiment described, it showed up the existence of characteristics of problem-solving behaviour which seem to be invariant as between all subjects, and this suggests that the "mechanisms" involved in problem-solving may have a particular form, which has been described.

Once valid methods of defining the basic attributes of speed, accuracy, and persistence have been evolved, it becomes possible to see how they must interact in different kinds of conventional test, and how these interactions must complicate attempts to understand the nature of cognitive abnormalities. The whole

---

[1] It should be stressed that, by definition, a level-test *must* include items in each cycle which are experienced as being very difficult by those for whom the test was designed.

chapter should be regarded as providing an introduction to the more detailed discussions presented by Payne, in that it serves to describe concepts and results used by him, but which have not previously been widely reported.

In defining the device *PS* the human problem-solver or subject has of course been grossly over-simplified. Continuance, for example, has been accounted for in terms of a switch *ST* which is either "on" or "off." During the course of a particular attempt to solve a particular problem, however, the subject will presumably manifest a drive state of systematically varying intensity, so that the appropriate analogy is more likely to be a continuously variable impedance interposed between *PB* and its power supply. Again, although the question of between-persons correlations among scores for such attributes as speed, accuracy, and continuance has been touched upon, nothing has been said of the consequences which would arise as a result of within-person correlations between the several kinds of event which participate in determining the nature and characteristics of a particular output. The complications which arise when attributes such as memory, fatigue, conditioned inhibition, and the like, are introduced into the analyses, have not been considered at all.

The early introduction of too great a degree of complication, however, is likely to defeat its own objects, useful trends being obscured by a mass of detail so complex as to defy analysis. At the present time only a few very tentative steps have been taken towards the evolution of a theory of human problem-solving activity, and the present paper represents no more than an attempt to provide the beginnings of a vocabulary, of a conceptual framework, and of a technique of analysis.

The writer believes that the human problem-solver is rather like a self-programming calculator. The effectiveness of such a device depends in part on the characteristics of the computing mechanisms, but also on the adequacy of the programming. If a subject is attempting a highly structured test, such as may be made up of letter or number series, nearly all the programming is, in effect, imposed from outside, by the instructions. Under these circumstances the subject is functioning almost exclusively as a computer, and the characteristics he displays in a "pure" test of this kind are likely to give information about some relatively simple cognitive mechanism. In a more complex situation, however, part of the subject's task is to decide how best to tackle his problem, i.e. how to programme himself. The outcome of his attempts to solve the problem will therefore probably depend on the interaction of several more or less independent computing mechanisms and on the effectiveness of the programming. It is thus very unlikely that common descriptive functions $f(D, K)$ can be evolved which will describe the overall input/output characteristics of all subjects when they are attempting complex tasks, since the programming, and thus the computing mechanisms called into play and the order in which they are utilized, will vary from one subject to another. The analysis which has been attempted in the foregoing pages is thus applicable only to the computing aspects of human problem solving, and experimental work pertinent to the analysis can only be carried out by using highly structured tasks within which opportunities for differences of individual approach are as completely eliminated as may be possible. It may not be altogether fanciful to regard these computing mechanisms as making up an important part of "Intelligence A," as defined by Hebb (1949), while his "Intelligence B" would seem to result from the subject's gradual acquisition of sets of programmes suitable for bringing them into effective combination.

However this may be, it does seem probable that the investigation of both normal and abnormal cognitive function should take some account of the discussion here attempted, if it is to lead to fruitful results.

REFERENCES

ANDERSON, J. E., The limitations of infants and pre-school tests in the measurement of intelligence, *J. Psychol.*, **8**, 351–379 (1939).

BURT, C. and JOHN, E., A factor-analysis of Terman-Binet tests, *Brit. J. Educ. Psychol.*, **12**, 117–127, 156–161 (1942).

EYSENCK, H. J., Primary Mental Abilities, *Brit. J. Educ. Psychol.*, **9**, 3, 270–275 (1939).

FURNEAUX, W. D., The structure of "g" with particular reference to *speed* and *power*. *Proceedings of the 12th International Congress of Psychology*, Edinburgh (1948).

FURNEAUX, W. D., Speed and power in mental functioning, *Paper read before British Psychological Society*, London (1950).

FURNEAUX, W. D., Some speed, error, and difficulty relationships within a problem-solving situation, *Nature*, **170**, 37 (1952).

FURNEAUX, W. D., A note on the "Nufferno" tests of inductive reasoning abilities. Nuffield Research Unit (Inst. of Psychiatry) Internal Report F.1 (April, 1953).

FURNEAUX, W. D., The determinants of success in intelligence tests, *Proceedings of the British Association for the Advancement of Science*, Bristol (1955).

FURNEAUX, W. D., *The Nufferno Manual of Speed Tests*, and *The Nufferno Manual of Level Tests* (Publ. by the Inst. of Psychiatry, and distributed by the National Foundation for Educational Research, 1956).

FERGUSON, G. A., The factorial interpretation of test-difficulty, *Psychometrika*, **6**, 323–329 (1941).

FRANKS, C., Personality factors and the rate of conditioning, *Brit. J. Psychol.*, **48**, 119–126 (1957).

GOURLAY, N., Difficulty factors arising from the use of

tetrachoric correlations, *Brit. J. Statis. Psychol.*, **4**, 2, 65 (1951).

GUILFORD, J. P., The difficulty of a test and its factor composition, *Psychometrika*, **6**, 67–77 (1941).

GUILFORD, J. P., The structure of intellect, *Psychol. Bull.*, **53**, 267–293 (1956).

HEBB, D. O., *The Organization of Behavior* (New York, John Wiley & Sons, Inc., 1949).

HICK, W. E., Information theory in psychology, *Report of Proceedings of Symposium on Information Theory* (London, Ministry of Supply, 1950).

HILDEBRAND, P., A factorial study of introversion-extraversion by means of objective tests, *Unpub. Ph.D. Thesis, Univ. of London Lib.* (1953).

HOFSTAETTER, P. R., The changing composition of intelligence, a study in T-technique, *J. Genet. Psychol*, **85**, 159–164 (1954).

HOLZINGER, K. J., *Preliminary Reports on Spearman-Holzinger Unitary Trait Study.* (Chicago, 1935).

KELLEY, R. L., Psychophysical tests of normal and abnormal children, *Psychol. Rev.*, **10**, 345–352 (1903).

KIRKPATRICK, E. A., Individual tests of schoolchildren, *Psychol. Rev.*, **7**, 274–280 (1900).

MANDLER, G. and SARASON, S. B., A study of anxiety and learning, *J. Abnorm. (Soc.) Psychol.*, **47**, 2, 166 (1952).

MANGAN, G. L., A factorial study of speed, power, and related variables, *Unpubl. Ph.D. Thesis, Univ. of London Lib.* (1954).

NELSON, B., An experimental investigation of intellectual speed and power in mental disorders, *Unpubl. Ph.D. Thesis, Univ. of London Lib.* (1953).

NELSON, H., *Theoretical Foundations of Psychology* (New York, Van Nostrand, 1951).

RIMOLDI, H. J., Personal tempo, *J. Abnorm. (Soc.) Psychol.*, **46**, 283–303 (1951).

RYANS, D. G., An experimental attempt to analyse persistent behaviour, *J. Gen. Psychol.*, **19**, 333–353 (1938).

SLATER, P., Speed of work in intelligence tests, *Brit. J. Psychol.*, **29**, 1, 55 (1938).

SNEDECOR, G. W., *Statistical Methods* (327) (Iowa State College Press, 1948).

SUTHERLAND, J. D., The speed factor in intelligent reactions, *Brit. J. Psychol.*, **24**, 276 (1934).

TATE, M. W., Notes on the measurement of mental speed, *J. Educ. Psychol.*, **41**, 219 (1950).

THORNDIKE, E. L., *The Measurement of Intelligence* (Bureau of Publications, Teachers' College, Columbia University, 1926).

THURSTONE, L. L., *Primary Mental Abilities (Psychometric Monographs No.* 1) (Chicago, Univ. of Chicago Press, 1939).

THURSTONE, L. L., *A Factorial Study of Perception* (Chicago, Univ. of Chicago Press, 1949).

VERNON, P., An application of factorial analysis to the study of test items, *Brit. J. Statistic. Psychol.*, **3**, 1–15 (1950).

WHERRY, R. J. and GAYLORD, R. H., Factor pattern of test items and tests as a function of the correlation coefficient; content, difficulty, and constant-error factors, *Psychometrika*, **9**, 237–244 (1944).

The work described in Chapter 5 was carried out during the course of an investigation into the value of psychological tests as predictors of academic performance, and was financed under a Grant from the Nuffield Foundation.

From H. Brierley (1961). Brit. J. Psychol., *52*, 273–280, *by kind permission of the author and the British Psychological Association*

THE SPEED AND ACCURACY CHARACTERISTICS OF NEUROTICS

By HARRY BRIERLEY

Senior Psychologist, St George's Hospital, Morpeth

This experiment tests the psychiatric observation that the different groups of neurotics can be distinguished by their speed and accuracy. It is shown that introverted neurotics are characterized by low speed and extroverted neurotics by low accuracy. If regarded as measuring an aspect of personality, speed-accuracy patterns may be specially valuable because of their sensitivity to variations in time.

I. INTRODUCTION

Factorial investigations over the last 25 years have recognized individual differences in speed. Thurstone (1938) found three speed factors, involving fitting words into categories, arithmetical computation, and perceptual tasks. The Spearman–Holzinger Unitary Traits Study, Holzinger (1934), found a general speed factor over and above '*g*'. Woodrow (1938), Davidson & Carroll (1945), and Tate (1948) have also demonstrated an ability or preference for speed, using a variety of different methods of investigation. The problem now becomes one of deciding whether or not these speed differences have any importance. That is to say, it is necessary to find out whether measures of speed have any special value in predicting any aspect of human behaviour distinct from the arbitrarily mixed speed and accuracy scores of common intelligence tests and the like.

Baxter (1941) defined 'speed', operationally, as the time taken by a subject to finish the Otis Intelligence Test, and 'level' as the number of items correct in unlimited time, these being crude estimates of speed and accuracy. He found that the multiple correlation of academic rating with these scores was higher than the correlation with the normal Otis time-limit score. Myers (1952) also showed that there seemed to be an optimum value for the speeding of tests when they were used to predict naval academy results. In this limited field, therefore, there seems evidence of the utility of distinct speed and accuracy measurements.

Some investigations have found that the speed of mental functioning differs according to group and individual testing conditions (Hunsicker, 1925; Chapman, 1924). This may well be a result of the imposition of group speed standards by such slight cues as the sound of scratching pencils or of pages being turned. In some investigations the group speed standards would be clearly observable, as in the well known Ruch & Koerth (1923) experiment when subjects were allowed to leave once they had finished the tests. It also appears that the transient factors, such as change of tester and the rewards offered for success (Courtis, 1924; Sturt, 1921), or the minor cultural differences which might arise between one school and another (Chapman, 1924) might influence the balance of speed and accuracy of mental performance. It seems, therefore, that research into mental speed and accuracy requires specially carefully controlled conditions of testing which have not often obtained in past researches.

Speed and accuracy characteristics of neurotics

Three relevant variables—difficulty, accuracy and persistence—have also been ignored at various times. There is little purpose in deriving a speed score without specifying the difficulty of the tasks involved. On the whole harder tasks take longer; but the relationship is not a perfect one as Cane & Horn (1951) showed. It may be that the relationship between speed and difficulty is not the same for all individuals, and this could be one of the reasons why speed differences have always been more easily observed when the tasks are limited to those of low difficulty (see, for example, Sutherland, 1934).

There is some evidence that speed and accuracy are interchangeable (Sturt, 1921; Welford, 1958, p. 32), but again accuracy has often been left uncontrolled in studies of speed. Peak & Boring (1926), McFarland (1930), and others have controlled accuracy to some extent by rejecting all incorrect responses, and rejecting items which have been answered with less than a standard level of success by the group as a whole. This sort of method probably provides as near a measure of control as is practicable at the moment; but it should be noted that a correct response might follow inaccurate, but aborted, attempts at solution.

Many researches on mental speed have employed tests such as dotting and letter cancellation. There is a strong suggestion in the work of Studman (1935) that such tests are better regarded as measuring 'perseverance-industry-tenacity' or Webb's 'w' factor (Webb, 1918) than speed. Studman found that hysterics scored lower on these tests than did patients with anxiety states, whilst Himmelweit (1946) found that hysterics showed lower persistence than dysthymics. This is in contrast with the fact that in such researches as have been carried out into the speed characteristics of neurotics, hysterics seem to be the faster. Thus, if left uncontrolled, persistence differences can counteract speed differences.

Psychiatric literature abounds in references to speed of thinking in mental illness. For example, Curran & Partridge (1957) describe the slowness of thinking in depression (p. 53), the quick thinking of manic patients (p. 54), and the thoughts 'rushing' through the mind of the schizophrenic. The obsessional personality is usually described as slow and ponderous in his attempts to maintain high accuracy, whilst the hysteric is impulsive and erratic. Few of these clinical observations have been accurately examined by experiment, although Ogilvie (1954), Eysenck (1953), and Broadhurst (1958) report loss of intellectual speed in schizophrenia. Hetherington's (1956) work on the effects of E.C.T. leads him to suggest that depression is associated more with motor retardation than with psychic retardation.

Slater (1944) compared the test responses of different neurotic groups and concluded that, given time, the obsessional would score more highly than the hysteric on common intelligence tests. Himmelweit (1947) investigated the speed differences between hysterics and dysthymics as diagnosed by psychiatrists. Subjects were instructed to work as quickly and accurately as possible on tests of hidden words, cancellation, adding 7's, measurement, and the track tracer. The dysthymics were slower and more accurate than the hysterics; but the only speed difference for the groups to prove statistically significant was that derived from the track tracer. Nevertheless, Himmelweit concluded 'it has been possible to show that hysterics belong to the speed preference and dysthymics to the accuracy preference type'. Nelson (1953) applied the Nufferno Speed Test to groups of mentally ill patients including one group of twenty neurotics. Speed as measured by this test did not differentiate either between the abnormal groups themselves or between the abnormal and control groups. This seems rather contrary to general expectation as well as to the findings of such workers as Studman, Ogilvie, and others mentioned above. Nelson's groups were, however, selected to include only those patients who were fully co-operative and, in the writer's experience, only a fraction of psychotic patients, and not all neurotics, are able to respond adequately to this test. Whatever standards of full co-operation were accepted, it is quite possible that this selection vitiated the results of the experiment.

A series of studies by Foulds (1952) and Foulds & Caine (1958 *a*, *b*) have considered the speed of response of neurotic patients on the Porteus Maze Test in particular. In the earliest of these Foulds showed that the speed of starting and tracing the mazes decreased in the order: psychopaths, hysterics, anxiety states, obsessionals, and reactive depressions. In the later studies, Foulds & Caine found that timed test responses were more closely related to personality type than to diagnostic category. They showed that obsessive personalities take longer on the Mazes and Matrices than hysteroids. This finding is somewhat complicated by the fact that they employed a Hysteroid-Obsessive Rating Scale of their own design, based on psychiatric texts. (In this experiment psychiatrists' ratings on this scale correlated 0·40 with neuroticism but only 0·21 with introversion-extraversion, both as measured by the Heron Questionnaire (Heron, 1956).) These findings led them to the prediction that obsessives would show lower speed and higher accuracy than hysteroids in performance on the Nufferno Tests.

Intellectual speed or speed of thinking are used in this paper to refer to observable problem-solving behaviour. It may well be that this does not reliably indicate the actual mental processes taking place. For example, Hetherington (1956) found that electro-convulsive therapy reduced the output of depressives on tests of adding and letter substitution. He concluded from this that loss of thinking speed was a therapeutic effect of E.C.T. in depression and that this was consistent with the hypothesis that depressive psychic retardation was not a simple slowing of thoughts, but was due to the interference of a 'constant surge' of painful thoughts. The loss of output was not statistically significant on either test used, however, in contrast with the significant increases of speed in the later stages of treatment and the period following. Further, if output on tests of this type did measure an aspect of thinking speed, it was only a very limited one.

The evidence of speed differences between hysterics and dysthymics, presented above, is fairly strong when tasks which demand largely motor responses are concerned, i.e. the track tracer and maze tracing. There is no strong evidence that speed of thinking or problem solving, as distinct from motor performance, differentiates the groups. Moreover, persistence, accuracy, and difficulty of task are not controlled variables in any of the investigations which have studied the time of response to tests of the intelligence test type. There are features of the Nufferno Speed Tests which make them specially suitable for an investigation of the intellectual speed of neurotics, whilst controlling these three variables.

Speed and accuracy characteristics of neurotics

II. INVESTIGATION

The Nufferno Speed Tests consist of eighteen scored items, all of similar difficulty level and all of the Thurstone letter-series type. The speed score is derived from the mean of the log times for each item correctly solved. The reason for this scoring is discussed by Furneaux (1955). The subject is timed by a concealed stop watch and performs the test under the instruction to work at his own rate with 'no need at all to hurry'. All incorrectly solved or abandoned items are rejected for the speed scoring but the number correct is taken as an accuracy score. Thus accuracy is controlled in the manner used by previous workers. The tests are available at two levels of difficulty; test B 1 consists of items which are harder than those in test A 2, but as all the items in a test are of similar difficulty, difficulty is a controlled variable when comparing the groups on that test. Furneaux (1955) considers the problem of persistence and concludes that it is possible to measure speed at the level of difficulty involved in these tests, as distinct from the effects of persistence limits. Therefore, the three important variables appear to be satisfactorily controlled when speed is measured by this method.

The testing was carried out individually by the same examiner for all subjects. The testing situation was maintained as uniform as possible and all the subjects were instructed that the tests were purely for research purposes and would not help them in any way. In view of a work decrement effect reported by Eysenck (1957) on a similar test, rest pauses of 1 min. were introduced before each speed test. The subjects were instructed to sit quietly with their eyes closed and to try not to think about the testing.

Forty neurotic subjects of average or above average intelligence were referred by the consultants of the hospital for the purposes of the research. Patients undergoing treatment with E.C.T. were avoided and those being treated with appreciable doses of drugs such as 'Largactil' which might have a serious effect on mental functioning were not considered. The neurotic group

Table 1. *Association between psychiatric diagnosis and questionnaire classification*

	Questionnaire classification	
	Extravert	Introvert
Hysteria	6	3
Hypochondriasis	4	1
Phobic states	2	1
Psychopathic personality	3	2
Total	15	7
Anxiety states	4	9
Obsessive compulsive	1	4
Total	5	13

χ^2 for 2×2 table is 4·5. $0·05 > P > 0·02$.

was divided equally into introvert and extravert personality types according to their scores on the Heron Sociability Test (Heron, 1956) the median score being 6·5. This division significantly differentiated the anxiety and obsessive-compulsive diagnostic groups from the remaining neuroses (Table 1). On this evidence the two groups will be described as Dysthymics and Hysterics in accordance with Eysenck (e.g. 1957, p. 26).

The age range for the neurotic subjects was 16–53 years with a mean age of 32 years.

A control group of twenty normal subjects was drawn from hospital medical, clerical, and

HARRY BRIERLEY

artisan staff, and each was matched for age with one hysteric and one dysthymic subject. The maximum age range in each trio was 4 years. To effect this matching it was necessary to select patients, according to age only, to fill the last five places. The groups did not differ significantly in their scores on the Mill Hill Vocabulary Scale. This was accepted as indicating that they were of similar pre-morbid intelligence. The control group and the hysteric group included eleven males and nine females, the dysthymic group nine males and eleven females. Himmelweit (1947) suggested that females are quicker than males, therefore the bias in these groups would be contrary to the experimental hypothesis. Actually there were differences in intelligence between Himmelweit's male and female groups and it is not clear whether she had taken this into consideration in arriving at her conclusion.

III. RESULTS

The distribution of scores in this investigation sometimes becomes seriously non-normal and for this reason, especially, non-parametric statistics have been applied.

Table 2 summarizes the results and shows that the speed and accuracy differences are entirely as expected. At both levels of difficulty the dysthymic group is significantly slower than the control group in solving problems. The hysteric group also

Table 2. *Speed and accuracy scores*

Group	Mean speed score*	Wilcoxon T Dysthymics	Wilcoxon T Hysterics	Mean accuracy score	Wilcoxon T Dysthymics	Wilcoxon T Hysterics
		Test A 2 (low difficulty)				
Controls	193·2	42 $N = 19$ $0·025 > P > 0·01$ (one-tailed test)	97·5 (not sig.)	16·3	33 $N = 17$ $0·025 > P > 0·01$ (one-tailed test)	31 $N = 19$ $P = 0·005$ (one-tailed test)
Dysthymics	181·3 ·	—	64·0 (not sig.)	13·8	—	93 (not sig.)
Hysterics	189·7	—	—	13·3	—	—
		Test B 1 (higher difficulty)				
Controls	197·3	39 $N = 20$ $0·01 > P > 0·005$ (one-tailed test)	83·5 (not sig.)	15·1	44·5 $N = 17$ $P = 0·072$ (not sig.)	13·5 $N = 18$ $P = 0·005$ (one-tailed test)
Dysthymics	181·1	—	66·0 (not sig.)	13·3	—	55·5 $N = 20$ $P = 0·032$ (one-tailed test)
Hysterics	190·8	—	—	11·3	—	—

* The speed scores are stated as Nufferno Corrected Speed Scores.

appears somewhat slower although not to a statistically significant degree, but is also apparently faster than dysthymics. In accuracy the result is that the hysteric group shows the lowest score at both levels of difficulty and is significantly lower than the controls. Dysthymics also appear to be rather less accurate than controls, in fact significantly so at the lower level of difficulty. Moreover, it is only at the higher level of difficulty that the hysteric-dysthymic accuracy difference becomes statistically significant.

Speed and accuracy characteristics of neurotics

The pattern of speed and accuracy in problem solving is thus shown to be that hysterics are characterized by low accuracy and dysthymics by low speed. Each of the groups tends to be both slower and less accurate than the control group however.

IV. Discussion

The primary aim of this investigation was that of testing out a hypothesis derived from clinical observation. It is one of the important functions of clinical psychologists to attempt to find objective validity for such observations. In this case the psychiatric observations and the psychological experiment are in agreement. The outcome of this can be greater subjective confidence in psychiatric recommendations, as for example where the solution of employment problems in rehabilitation is based on clinical diagnosis. This sort of consideration is probably less important than the broader implications. The researches into skilled performance, e.g. those of Welford (1958), have emphasized the fundamental importance of speed. It is curious, therefore, that untimed, leisurely tests often seem intuitively preferred to time-limited tests. It may be that the attempt to remove time limits in psychological tests is to turn a blind eye to a crucial factor. In this investigation neurotic subjects were shown to be effectively inferior to normal persons either in speed or accuracy. The immediate question which arises is what the nature of this inferiority is. It may be that this is a real limitation in ability, or alternatively it could be more akin to a preference for a different pace of work or accuracy of response. The solution might be found in in attempts to pace performance so as to find out if neurotics are capable of adopting the normal pattern of performance and of becoming as quick and accurate as normals when the conditions demand it.

If these deficiencies are true limitations of ability, then either they may be of the nature of an impairment resulting from neurotic illness, or factors in the patient's personality which predispose him to neurosis. In the former case speed and accuracy may be associated with progress of treatment rather as Hetherington (1956) inferred, but in the latter case the predisposing factors may remain unrelated to the course of treatment. Framed in other terms, one is led to ask how far these speed and accuracy defects are the cause of neurotic breakdown, and how far the result of it. If they are the result, do they form part of a neurotic defence against more radical breakdown?

In this investigation, as in some of those referred to earlier, there is a clear relationship between patterns of speed and accuracy and questionnaire measures of introversion-extraversion, for neurotic patients. As they are consistent in many different types of material, they are likely to have some degree of stability in time. That is, a person showing high accuracy and low speed at one period will tend to show the same pattern at a later period when re-tested. There is, however, an important difference between these speed and accuracy testing methods and questionnaire methods. Investigations such as that of Bartholomew & Marley (1959) emphasize the temporal stability of questionnaire introversion-extraversion scores and that 'treatment in hospital has little effect on questionnaire response'. Demonstrations of this kind of reliability also indicate insensitivity to variations which might occur and this is what one would expect from the content of many questionnaires. One of the major difficulties patients raise in completing questionnaires of this type is that they seem to be able to answer in different ways according to whether they take them as referring to one period or another. In few, if any, questionnaires can the responses be made applicable to the here and now situation, although it is true that they will to some extent reflect present perception of a state of affairs which existed in the past. This sort of insensitivity is not a defect of the speed and accuracy test which can be used to assess the state of the patient at a well-defined and short period in time. Moreover, it seems that speed and accuracy testing is likely to be repeatable without serious re-test effects. There are many fields of research in which such methods of personality measurement may be useful to describe a situation existing at a particular instant in time and where methods with high temporal stability would be unsuitable.

This paper is an extract from an M.A. thesis presented by the author to Liverpool University. The help of the staff of the Department of Psychology is very gratefully acknowledged, as is the assistance of the hospital staff and patients.

REFERENCES

BARTHOLOMEW, A. A. & MARLEY, E. (1959). The temporal reliability of the Maudsley Personality Inventory. *J. Ment. Sci.* **105**, 238–40.

BAXTER, B. (1941). An experimental analysis of the contributions of speed and level in an intelligence test. *J. Educ. Psychol.* **32**, 285–96.

BROADHURST, A. (1958). Experimental studies of the mental speed of schizophrenics. II. *J. Ment. Sci.* **104**, 1130–6.

CANE, V. R. & HORN, V. (1951). The timing of responses to spatial perception questions. *Quart. J. Exp. Psychol.* **3**, 133–145.

CHAPMAN, J. C. (1924). Persistence, success, and speed in a mental test. *Ped. Sem.* **31**, 276–84.

COURTIS, S. A. (1924). The relation between speed and quality in educational measurement. *J. Educ. Res.* **10**, 110–31.

CURRAN, D. & PARTRIDGE, M. (1957). *Psychological Medicine*, 4th edn. London: Livingstone.

DAVIDSON, W. M. & CARROLL, J. B. (1945). Speed and level in time-limit scores—a factor analysis. *Educ. Psychol. Meas.* **5**, 411–27.

EYSENCK, H. J. (1953). Differential cognitive tests. Office of Naval Research Report, Contract no. N 625585, Bur. Med. Surg., U.S. Navy, London Branch.

EYSENCK, H. J. (1957). *The Dynamics of Anxiety and Hysteria.* London: Routledge and Kegan Paul.

FOULDS, G. A. (1952). Temperamental differences in maze performance. II. *Brit. J. Psychol.* **43**, 33–42.

FOULDS, G. A. & CAINE, T. M. (1958a). Personality factors and performance on timed tests of ability. *Occup. Psychol.* **32**, 102–5.

FOULDS, G. A. & CAINE, T. M. (1958b). Psychoneurotic symptom clusters, trait clusters, and psychological tests. *J. Ment. Sci.* **104**, 722–32.

FURNEAUX, W. D. (1955). The determinants of success in intelligence tests. Paper read at the Bristol meeting, British Association for the Advancement of Science.

HERON, A. (1956). A two-part personality measure for use as a research criterion. *Brit. J. Psychol.* **47**, 243–51.

HETHERINGTON, R. (1956). Efficiency and retentivity of depressed patients. *Brit. J. Med. Psychol.* **29**, 258–69.

HIMMELWEIT, H. T. (1946). Speed and accuracy of work as related to temperament. *Brit. J. Psychol.* **36**, 132–44.

HIMMELWEIT, H. T. (1947). The level of aspiration of normal and neurotic persons. *Brit. J. Psychol.* **37**, 41–59.

HOLZINGER, K. J. (1934). *Preliminary Report on the Spearman–Holzinger Unitary Traits Study.* Chicago: Statist. Lab. Dep. Educ. Univ. Chicago.

HARRY BRIERLEY

HUNSICKER, L. M. (1925). *A Study of the Relationship between Rate and Ability.* New York: Teachers' College, Columbia University.

McFARLAND, R. A. (1930). An experimental study of the relationship between speed and mental ability. *J. Gen. Psychol.* **3**, 67–97.

MYERS, C. T. (1952). The factorial composition and validity of differentially speeded tests. *Psychometrika,* **17**, 347–52.

NELSON, E. H. (1953). An experimental investigation of intellectual speed and power in mental disorders. Ph.D. thesis, University of London.

OGILVIE, B. C. (1954). A study of intellectual slowness in schizophrenia. Ph.D. thesis, University of London.

PEAK, H. & BORING, E. G. (1926). The factor of speed in intelligence. *J. Exp. Psychol.* **9**, 71–94.

RUCH, C. M. & KOERTH, W. (1923). 'Power' vs 'Speed' in Army Alpha. *J. Educ. Psychol.* **14**, 193–208.

SLATER, P. (1944). Scores of different types of neurotics on tests of intelligence. *Brit. J. Psychol.* **35**, 40–2.

STUDMAN, G. (1935). The measurement of speed and flow of mental activity. *J. Ment. Sci.* **81**, 107–37.

STURT, M. (1921). A comparison of speed with accuracy in the learning process. *Brit. J. Psychol.* **12**, 289–309.

SUTHERLAND, J. D. (1934). The speed factor in intelligent reactions. *Brit. J. Psychol.* **24**, 276–94.

TATE, M. W. (1948). Individual differences in speed of response in mental test materials of varying degrees of difficulty. *Educ. Psychol. Meas.* **8**, 353–74.

THURSTONE, L. L. (1938). *Primary Mental Abilities.* Chicago: University Press.

WEBB, E. (1918). Character and intelligence. *Brit. J. Psychol. Monogr. Suppl.,* no. 3.

WELFORD, A. T. (1958). *Ageing and Human Skill.* London: Oxford University Press.

WOODROW, H. (1938). The relation between abilities and improvement with practice. *J. Educ. Psychol.* **29**, 215–30.

(*Manuscript received* 1 *September* 1960)

Individual Differences in Speed, Accuracy and Persistence:
a Mathematical Model for Problem Solving[1,2]

by P.O. WHITE, *Institute of Psychiatry, University of London*

I Introduction

Traditional tests of cognitive abilities are of two main types. Some, exemplified by the Thurstone tests of primary mental abilities, include problems which span a broad range of specific types of ability. Tests of this type typically yield single scores for each of the ability types (such as verbal, numerical, spatial, or perceptual, for example), and a single, global score for what has usually been called "general ability". Other tests, exemplified by the Raven Progressive Matrices tests, include problems which, though differing in difficulty, are essentially of a single type. Tests of this sort also tend to yield but a single global score for general ability. More often than not the cognitive test of conventional design is administered in such a manner that the individual's score is the number of problems correctly solved within a time limit. Such scores depend in part on the choice of problems attempted, in part on the rate at which the subject works, in part on the accuracy of the subject's responses to the problems and in part on the extent to which he abandons problems which, given greater persistence, he might well solve. Furthermore, the extent to which these different aspects of the subject's performance influence his total score is quite unknown. Clearly, such a single score can be only an incomplete and quite inadequate summary of a very complicated problem-solving performance. In this paper we present a mathematical model which provides for the determination of separate speed, persistence, and accuracy scores for each of these logically distinct components; we show that it is feasible, though not at all easy, to fit the model to a set of empirical data; and we present and discuss some results from such an endeavour.

The model stems more or less directly from a conceptual model for problem solving reported by Furneaux (1960) and from a logistic latent trait model for test scores reported by Birnbaum (1968). It reformulates Furneaux's conceptual model in statistical terms and extends Birnbaum's statistical model to include speed, persistence, and response time variables.

II Mathematical Statement of the Model

A very condensed statement of the model has already appeared (1973). In this statement we go into considerably more detail, although some extremely simple steps in the derivation are left to the reader.

An attempt has been made to present the model in such a way that the reader with a limited mathematical background should be able to understand the basic features of the model if not its inner workings. Indeed, the

Individual Differences in Speed, Accuracy and Persistence

mathematical level of the paper is quite modest.

We assume that each of a set of n problems has been administered to each of a group of N subjects. We use the subscript j to index problems and the subscript i to index subjects. Thus there are $j = 1, 2, \ldots, n$ problems and $i = 1, 2, \ldots, N$ subjects. We note that when a particular problem is administered to a particular subject that one of three events must occur. The subject may abandon the problem and thus forfeit any chance of getting a correct response; or he may try to answer it, in which case he will either give a correct response or an incorrect response. We formalize this as follows.

Subject i is presented• with problem j. After some time $T_{ji} = t_{ji}$ he responds to the problem. His response is either to abandon the problem or to put forth an attempt at its solution. If he abandons the problem, the random variable Y_{ji} assumes the value $y_{ji} = 1$; otherwise it assumes the value $y_{ji} = 0$. If he makes an attempt to solve the problem, then his attempt is either correct or it is incorrect. If the attempt at solution is correct then the random variable X_{ji} assumes the value $x_{ji} = 1$; otherwise it assumes the value $x_{ji} = 0$. Thus, we have two observable discrete random variables X_{ji} and Y_{ji} with realizations x_{ji} and y_{ji}, and an observable mathematical variable T_{ji} with observed value t_{ji}. These relationships are summarized in equations (1) to (3).

$$X_{ji} = x_{ji} = \begin{cases} 1, \text{ correct response} \\ 0, \text{ otherwise} \end{cases} \tag{1}$$

$$Y_{ji} = y_{ji} = \begin{cases} 1, \text{ abandoned} \\ 0, \text{ otherwise} \end{cases} \tag{2}$$

$$T_{ji} = t_{ji} = \text{response time} \tag{3}$$

Equations (1) to (3) define the observed data to which we fit the model. We turn now to the unobserved quantities in the model. At this point we simply list these quantities in order to set up some required notation and we formally state some constraints which we impose on them.

For each subject we assume three unobservable random variables s_i (speed), p_i (persistence), and a_i (accuracy); and, for each problem, we assume two unknown parameters d_j (difficulty level) and D_j (discriminating power). We assume that speed, accuracy, persistence, and discriminating power are all positive quantities, and we assume that speed has an upper limit of unity. For the moment we defer any consideration of the interpretation of the subject variables and of the problem or item parameters. The constraints outlined above are stated in equations (4) to (7).

Thus far we have outlined both the observables $\{x_{ji}, y_{ji}, t_{ji}\}$ and the unobservables $\{s_i, p_i, a_i; d_j, D_j\}$ in the model. The reader may well have

Individual Differences in Speed, Accuracy and Persistence

$$a_i, p_i > 0 \left.\rule{0pt}{14pt}\right\} i = 1, 2, \ldots, N \tag{4}$$

$$0 < s_i < 1 \tag{5}$$

$$D_j > 0 \left.\rule{0pt}{14pt}\right\} j = 1, 2, \ldots, n \tag{6}$$

$$-\infty < d_j < +\infty \tag{7}$$

noticed that we seem to have five unobservables but only three observations. Note, however, that while there are $3N$ subject variables and $2n$ problem parameters, there are $3nN$ observations. For example with $n = 20$ problems and $N = 93$ subjects there are $3 \times 93 + 2 \times 20 = 319$ unobservables (quite a considerable number) but there are $3 \times 20 \times 93 = 5580$ observations (which is considerably more). Things are not as bad as they seem.

It may well assist the reader in following the development of the model itself if, at this point, we take a peek ahead and give him a glimpse at our ultimate goal. Note, first, that if $Y_{ji} = 1$ the subject has abandoned the problem and that $X_{ji} = 0$: it is not possible for both X_{ji} and Y_{ji} to be 1. Thus only three of the four logical X_{ji}, Y_{ji} combinations are empirically possible. These are $\{X_{ji} = 0, \quad Y_{ji} = 0\}$, $\{X_{ji} = 0, \quad Y_{ji} = 1\}$, and $\{X_{ji} = 1, \quad Y_{ji} = 0\}$. Associated with each of these observed combinations is an observed response time $T_{ji} = t_{ji}$. We plan to develop a mathematical function which will express the conditional probability of the observed X_{ji}, Y_{ji} combination (given the observed response time) as a function of the speed, persistence and accuracy of the subject, and of the difficulty level and discriminating power of the problem. Once this goal has been achieved we will be able to formulate the estimation problem in statistical terms and will be able to solve the estimation problem numerically using established computing procedures.

We now return to the development of the model and introduce the concept of effective ability, θ_{ji}. Effective ability is a function of the speed and accuracy of the subject, and of the time since presentation of the problem. It has a value of zero upon presentation of the problem and follows the well-known negatively accelerated exponential growth function. Effective ability grows asymptotically towards a_i at rate s_i as a function of increasing time. Its value when the response is elicited is given by equation (8). In this equation, θ_{ji} is effective ability, a_i and s_i are the subject's accuracy and speed scores, and t_{ji} is his response time to problem j.

$$\theta_{ji} = a_i \left[1 - \exp(-s_i t_{ji})\right] \tag{8}$$

We may see more clearly the role played by the speed parameter in

Individual Differences in Speed, Accuracy and Persistence

equation (8) if we look at the rate of change of θ_{ji} with respect to t_{ji}. To do this we take the derivative with respect to t_{ji} of equation (8). A simple algebraic manipulation leads directly to equation (9).

$$s_i = \frac{d\theta_{ji}/dt_{ji}}{(a_i - \theta_{ji})} \tag{9}$$

In this differential equation the numerator is the rate of change with respect to time and the denominator is the amount of change still possible.

Thus, as stated above, θ_{ji} grows towards a_i at "rate" s_i but the "rate" is a relative growth rate. The speed parameter in equation (8) is the growth rate relative to the amount of growth still possible.

We have now paved the way towards the statement of the two basic equations of the model. We have defined the observations $\{x_{ji}, y_{ji}, t_{ji}\}$, the subject variables $\{s_i, p_i, a_i\}$; and the problem parameters $\{d_j, D_j\}$; and we have defined effective ability θ_{ji} as a function of speed (s_i), of accuracy (a_i), and of response time (t_{ji}).

First, however, we must introduce the cumulative logistic function defined in equation (10).

$$\Phi[z] = \frac{1}{1+e^{-z}} = \frac{e^z}{1+e^z} \tag{10}$$

Even non-mathematical readers are probably on familiar terms with the S-shaped normal ogive or cumulative normal curve which is usually expressed in terms of a z-score. The cumulative logistic function defined in equation (8) is conceptually equivalent to the cumulative normal curve. As z approaches $-\infty$ both curves approach zero. As z increases towards zero both curves approach 0.5. As z passes through zero both curves pass through an inflexion point and change from upward concave to downward concave. Finally, as z approaches $+\infty$, both curves approach unity. We use the cumulative logistic function rather than the cumulative normal because the former is computationally more convenient and because its use tends in general to lead to more simple mathematical relationships.

We are now in a position to state the two main equations of the model.[3] These two equations, in conjunction with the well-known "law of compound probabilities" from elementary probability theory and the assumption of "local independence" determine all that follows.

$$\Pr[X_{ji} = 1 \mid Y_{ji} = 0, T_{ji} = t_{ji}; \omega_i] \tag{11}$$
$$= \Phi[D_j(\theta_{ji} - d_j)] = \alpha_{ji}$$
$$\Pr[Y_{ji} = 1 \mid T_{ji} = t_{ji}; \omega_i] \tag{12}$$
$$= \Phi[c(t_{ji} - p_i)] = \beta_{ji}$$

Individual Differences in Speed, Accuracy and Persistence

Equation (11) states that if subject i does not abandon problem j and thus puts forth an attempted solution at time t_{ji} the probability of a correct response is a cumulative logistic function of his effective ability θ_{ji}. The problem parameters d_j and D_j determine the precise shape of the curve.

The difficulty level (d_j) of the problem determines the amount of effective ability θ_{ji} required for this problem in order for the subject to have a 50-50 chance of a correct response (given of course that he does not abandon the problem). As θ_{ji} falls below this level the probability of a correct response falls towards zero. On the other hand, as θ_{ji} exceeds d_j the probability of a correct response approaches unity.

The discriminating power (D_j) of the problem is proportional to the slope of the curve at this point. Its name derives from the fact that, as the slope increases, small changes in effective ability about this point (d_j) cause greater changes in probability of correct response. Thus the problem is more sensitive to changes in effective ability or discriminates better among ability levels. Another way of putting it is that the steeper the slope the more likely it is that a subject who responds correctly has θ_{ji} greater than d_j. Conversely, the steeper the slope the more likely it is that a subject who attempts the problem but fails it has θ_{ji} less than d_j. In this sense, the discriminating power of the problem relates directly to its usefulness in classifying individuals according to their ability levels.

Equation (12) states that if subject i, with persistence score p_i, is presented with problem j and responds at time t_{ji}, the probability that his response will be an abandonment is a cumulative logistic function of his response time t_{ji}. His persistence parameter p_i determines the amount of time required to give him a 50-50 chance of abandoning the problem. A subject with the same response time but lower persistence would have a greater probability of abandonment while one with the same response time but greater persistence would have a lower probability of abandonment. In this equation c is a model parameter to be estimated from the data.

Equation (13) defines the well-known "law of compound probabilities" from elementary probability theory.

$$\Pr[E_1, E_2] = \Pr[E_1 \mid E_2]\Pr[E_2] \qquad (13)$$

Equation (13) expresses the joint probability of the two events E_1 and E_2 as the product of two factors: the conditional probability of E_1, given E_2; and the unconditional probability of E_2.

We may now write expressions for the probabilities of each of the X_{ji}, Y_{ji} combinations $\{X_{ji} = 0, \ Y_{ji} = 0\}$, $\{X_{ji} = 0, \ Y_{ji} = 1\}$, and

Individual Differences in Speed, Accuracy and Persistence

$\{X_{ji} = 1, \ Y_{ji} = 0\}$. Equations (14-16) follow directly from equations (11) to (13). The derivation is trivial and is left for the reader to verify.

$$\Pr[X_{ji} = 0, \ Y_{ji} = 0 \mid T_{ji} = t_{ji}; \ \omega_i] \tag{14}$$
$$= (1 - a_{ji})(1 - \beta_{ji})$$

$$\Pr[X_{ji} = 0, \ Y_{ji} = 1 \mid T_{ji} = t_{ji}; \ \omega_i] \tag{15}$$
$$= \beta_{ji}$$

$$\Pr[X_{ji} = 1, \ Y_{ji} = 0 \mid T_{ji} = t_{ji}; \ \omega_i]$$
$$= a_{ji}(1 - \beta_{ji}) \tag{16}$$

As indicated above, if the subject abandons the problem then he cannot give a correct response. Thus the event $\{X_{ji} = 1, \ Y_{ji} = 1\}$ cannot occur. Mathematically we say that the event occurs with probability zero. Equation (17) states this obvious fact.

$$\Pr[X_{ji} = 1, \ Y_{ji} = 1 \mid T_{ji} = t_{ji}; \ \omega_i]$$
$$= 0 \tag{17}$$

It is convenient at this point to combine equations (14) to (17) into the single equation (18).

$$\Pr[X_{ji} = x_{ji}, \ Y_{ji} = y_{ji} \mid T_{ji} = t_{ji}; \ \omega_i]$$
$$= a_{ji}^{x_{ji}} (1 - a_{ji})^{1 - x_{ji} - y_{ji}} \ \beta_{ji}^{y_{ji}} (1 - \beta_{ji})^{1 - y_{ji}} (1 - x_{ji} y_{ji})$$
$$= L_{ji} \tag{18}$$

This equation serves a dual purpose. On the one hand, by combining equations (14) to (17) into a single equation, it greatly simplifies the remainder of the derivation. On the other hand, in combination with equations (11) and (12), it highlights the relationships between this model and the two-parameter logistic model (Birnbaum, 1968). The form of equations (11) and (12) is instantly recognizable as that of a two-parameter logistic model. The form of equation (18) is virtually the product of two probability distribution functions of two-parameter logistic form.

For each subject we have observed x_{ji}, y_{ji}, t_{ji} for each of the n problems. In equation (18) we give the probability for the event $\{X_{ji} = x_{ji}, \ Y_{ji} = y_{ji}\}$ given that $T_{ji} = t_{ji}$. We now wish to give the probability for the simultaneous occurrence of the n events $(\{X_{ji} = x_{ji}, \ Y_{ji} = y_{ji}\}, j = 1, n)$ given that $\{T_{ji} = t_{ji}, j = 1, 2, \ldots, n\}$.

$$\Pr[X_{1i} = x_{1i}, \ Y_{1i} = y_{1i}, \ X_{2i} = x_{2i}, \ Y_{2i} = y_{2i}, \ldots,$$
$$\ldots, X_{ni} = x_{ni}, \ Y_{ni} = y_{ni} \mid T_{1i} = t_{1i}, \ T_{2i} = t_{2i}, \ldots, T_{ni} = t_{ni}; \ \omega_i]$$
$$= \prod_{j=1}^{n} L_{ji} = L_i \tag{19}$$

Individual Differences in Speed, Accuracy and Persistence

We may interpret equation (19) in either of two ways. We may say "making the usual assumption of local independence, equation (19) follows directly." Alternatively, we may just state equation (19) and regard it as a definition of local independence. In either event, equation (19) stands as the joint probability of the n response-pairs $\{x_{ji}, y_{ji}\}$ for subject i.

Finally, if we assume independent sampling across subjects we may write equation (20).

$$L = \prod_{j=1}^{n} \prod_{i=1}^{N} L_{ji} = \prod_{i=1}^{N} L_i \tag{20}$$

L is the likelihood of the set of response patterns of N different subjects to the same set of n items, expressed as a function of the $3nN$ observed quantities $\{x_{ji}, y_{ji}, t_{ji}\}; j = 1, 2, \ldots, n; i = 1, 2, \ldots, N$; of the $3N$ unobservable subject variables $\{s_i, p_i, a_i\}, i = 1, 2, \ldots, N$; and of the $2n$ unobservable problem parameters $\{d_j, D_j\}, j = 1, 2, \ldots, n$.

The likelihood function defined in equation (20) provides a basis for the computation of joint maximum likelihood estimates of the unobservable subject variables and of the unobservable problem parameters.

III Estimation

As indicated above, the estimation problem is that of obtaining joint maximum likelihood estimates of the speed, persistence, and accuracy variables for each subject and of the difficulty level and discriminating power parameters for each problem.

Three computer programs have been prepared for operation on the University of London CDC 6400-6600 computer system and a fourth, for operation on the CDC 7600 is in preparation. These we now describe briefly.

(1) The first program occupies minimal core store and thus gets good turnaround in the computer system. The price it pays for this convenience is that it requires multiple computer runs to yield a solution. This, however, occurs automatically, since the entire job environment is dumped to magnetic tape at the end of a run; computation then proceeds from that point on a subsequent run.

The program utilizes a well-known conjugate gradient method due to Fletcher and Reeves (1964) and gains its size advantage from the fact that this method does not have to store a large matrix of approximations to second derivatives of the function. Though effective, this program uses too

Individual Differences in Speed, Accuracy and Persistence

much computer time to be considered a satisfactory production program.

(2) A second program uses the well-known variable-metric algorithm of Fletcher and Powell (1963). Though more efficient than the first it requires some 50,000 words of core store for a matrix of approximations to second-order derivatives and gets very poor turnaround in our currently saturated system.

(3) A revision of the Fletcher-Powell program stores the large matrix on disk and brings it into core row-by-row as needed in the calculations. The increased computational efficiency of the variable metric algorithm is to some extent offset by a loss of speed due to the very large number of disk transfers involved. Nevertheless, it is about five times as fast as the Fletcher-Reeves program and, because of its decreased turnaround time, has made the in-core version of the Fletcher-Powell program obsolete.

(4) A new version of the Fletcher-Powell program is in preparation. In this version for the CDC 7600, the large matrix resides in "large core memory" rather than on disk. We anticipate that this strategy, coupled with the five-fold speed increase of the 7600 central processor, will yield a satisfactory production program.

IV Some Empirical Findings

The data which we present to illustrate an application of the model were provided by Michael Berger, Institute of Psychiatry. His subjects were all male volunteers and were paid to participate in a series of psychological investigations. They were quite heterogeneous both with respect to age (17-65 years) and with respect to occupation.

The results which we report are based on the responses of 93 subjects to 20 problems from the Advanced Progressive Matrices test of Raven (1962). Problems were arranged in cycles of ascending "difficulty" according to the proportions of subjects in the normative sample who failed them and were administered to all subjects in this order.

Subjects were tested individually in on-line sessions controlled by Berger's computer program operating on the augmented LINC-8 system in the Department of Psychology, Institute of Psychiatry. Problems were presented on a back-projection screen by a 35mm slide projector. Subjects responded by pressing keys on a small keyboard which the computer program monitored to determine which response alternative was chosen and to determine response times individually for each problem. A special key was reserved to indicate problem abandonment and subjects were instructed to indicate response alternatives only when quite sure of the correct response and otherwise to abandon the problem. In this way they were encouraged not to guess.

We turn now to some results from our analyses of these data.

In Table 1 we list difficulty levels and discriminating powers for each of the problems.

TABLE 1

Problem	Difficulty Level	Discriminating Power
1	−0·47	1·59
2	−1·28	1·19
3	−0·58	2·41
4	−1·08	0·40
5	1·47	0·92
6	−2·09	1·34
7	0·83	2·17
8	−0·18	1·55
9	4·23	0·25
10	−0·80	4·49
11	0·43	1180·50
12	−2·02	1·72
13	−0·85	0·23
14	6·02	0·18
15	−0·59	1·88
16	0·02	24·31
17	0·50	2·62
18	6·60	28·02
19	−2·93	1·25
20	−4·41	24·10

Parameters for 20 Problems

We note first that there are marked differences among problems on both sets of parameters. Problem 20 is extremely easy; problems 6, 12 and 19 are quite easy. Problems 14 and 18 are extremely difficult while problem 9 is quite difficult. The remaining problems are of intermediate difficulty. The model constrains the discriminating powers to be strictly positive but this constraint is not active for any problem. The low discriminating powers for problems 14, 13 and 9 indicate that, for these problems, the curve described by equation (11) is quite flat. The high discriminating powers for problems 11, 16 and 18 indicate that for these problems this curve is virtually a step function. A correct response to problem 11, for example, tells us that $\theta_{11,\,i}$ is almost certainly greater than .43 (the difficulty level); an incorrect response that $\theta_{11,\,i}$ is almost certainly less than .43. On the other hand, if we know that a subject attempts problem 14 and gets

Individual Differences in Speed, Accuracy and Persistence

it correct we know only that θ_{ji} is probably (i.e. $\Pr[\theta_{ji} > 6.02] > \frac{1}{2}$) greater than 6.02. We hope that these examples help to clarify the comments made following equations (11) and (12).

In Table 2 we present speed, accuracy and persistence scores and number of abandonments for 4 subjects each of whom have the same total score. Each of these subjects correctly solved 10 of the 20 problems.

TABLE 2

Subject	Abandonments	Speed	Accuracy	Persistence
1	3	·99	·40	·84
2	2	·99	·39	1·07
37	1	·99	·08	1·35
43	1	·97	·79	1·47

Results for 4 Selected Subjects

A test of conventional design would not differentiate among these four individuals: they all have the same total score. However, the model described in this paper responds vigorously and apparently with good sense to individual differences.

The four subjects selected for illustration not only had the same total score: they also were very similar in mean time to correct response. The model responds to this by giving them very similar speed scores (in the sample speed scores range from .01 to .99).

Subjects 1 and 2 have virtually identical scores on speed and accuracy. Subject 2 has 1 less abandonment and this is reflected in a higher persistence score.

Subjects 37 and 43 not only have identical total scores and similar mean times to correct response: they also have the same number of abandonments. The model wisely gives them very similar persistence scores.

Perhaps the most striking feature in Table 2, though, is the difference in accuracy scores for these same two subjects. Note again that they have identical total scores and the same number of abandonments as well as quite similar mean times to correct response and quite similar mean times to abandonment. Why then do they show such a striking difference in accuracy scores? Things seem even more striking when we note that of the 10 problems correctly solved 7 were the same problems for both subjects. The reason for this apparent discrepancy becomes quite clear when we note that the mean difficulty level of the remaining 3 correctly solved problems was considerably higher for subject 43 than for subject 37. It is indeed

Individual Differences in Speed, Accuracy and Persistence

gratifying that the model is sensitive to such small but quite important differences among response patterns.

We now turn from this consideration of results for individual subjects to some results from two correlational analyses.

The first analysis includes the following measures for each problem: (1) mean number of abandonments, (2) proportion of correct responses, (3) mean time to abandonment, (4) mean time to correct response, (5) mean time to incorrect response, (6) difficulty level, and (7) discriminating power. The correlations among these measures appear in Table 3.

TABLE 3

2	− ·85					
3	·63	− ·79				
4	·88	− ·91	·80			
5	·81	− ·90	·83	·94		
6	·83	− ·91	·74	·79	·80	
7	·13	− ·14	·09	·32	·16	·02
	1	2	3	4	5	6

Intercorrelations Among 7 Measures for 20 Problems

We comment now on some salient features of this matrix. Correlations appear in parentheses to aid the reader in identifying the measure on which the relationship is based.

Difficult problems are abandoned more frequently than are easy ones ($r = 0.83$) and they are failed by a higher proportion of subjects who attempt them ($r = -0.91$). They also show longer times to abandonment ($r = ·74$), to incorrect response ($r = 0.80$), and to correct response ($r = 0.79$). Problem difficulty level is uncorrelated with problem discriminating power though there is nothing in the model to constrain this to be so. These relationships make considerable psychological sense and this is as it should be. Indeed, if it were otherwise we would be in trouble. They are presented here not as striking facts but as confirmation that things seem to be working as they should.

In the second correlational analysis the following measures appear for each subject: (1) mean number of abandonments, (2) proportion of correct responses, (3) mean time to abandonment, (4) mean time to correct response, (5) mean time to incorrect response, (6) speed, (7) accuracy, (8) persistence, (9) psychoticism, (10) extraversion, (11) neuroticism, and (12) lie score. The final four measures were obtained from the Eysenck P.E.N. inventory which Berger also administered to his subjects. The correlations among these measures appear in Table 4.

Individual Differences in Speed, Accuracy and Persistence:

TABLE 4

	1	2	3	4	5	6	7	8	9	10	11
2	·02										
3	−·22	·49									
4	−·14	·40	·67								
5	−·28	·39	·67	·55							
6	−·02	−·09	−·30	−·75	−·26						
7	−·08	·74	·36	·32	·12	−·01					
8	−·76	·26	·68	·64	·69	−·35	·19				
9	−·03	−·29	−·24	−·13	−·08	−·03	−·24	−·06			
10	−·01	−·04	−·11	−·12	−·04	·16	−·13	−·05	·13		
11	·05	−·06	−·10	−·09	·04	·09	−·18	−·05	·43	−·06	
12	·23	−·05	·12	·12	·20	−·15	−·06	−·03	−·04	−·13	−·18

Intercorrelations Among 12 Measures for 93 Subjects

We now comment on some salient features of this matrix. As before, and for the same reason, we include correlations in parentheses. We include where relevant correlations with Advanced Progressive Matrices I.Q. score derived from a separate analysis.

Subjects with high persistence scores tend to abandon fewer problems ($r = -0·76$) and spend more time on those problems which they do abandon ($r = 0·68$). They also take more time to arrive at correct responses ($r = 0·64$) and to arrive at incorrect responses ($r = 0·69$).

Subjects with high accuracy scores correctly solve a higher proportion of the problems which they attempt than do those with low accuracy scores ($r = 0·74$).

Subjects with high speed scores take considerably less time to arrive at correct responses than do subjects with low speed scores ($r = 0·75$) but only slightly less time in abandoning problems ($r = 0·30$) and in arriving at incorrect responses ($r = -0·26$).

Speed is uncorrelated with accuracy ($r = -0·01$) and with I.Q. ($r = -0·06$), but is negatively correlated with persistence ($r = -0·35$).

Persistence is uncorrelated with accuracy ($r = 0·19$) but is moderately correlated with I.Q. ($r = 0·38$).

Accuracy is uncorrelated with speed ($r = -0·01$), and is strongly correlated ($r = 0·65$) with I.Q.

These relationships, too, indicate that the model seems to be functioning as it was designed to function. They tell us much more about the model than about the subjects.

We now summarize the relationships between the subjects' scores on the personality inventory and their speed, accuracy and persistence scores.

Extraversion, neuroticism and lie scale scores are all uncorrelated with speed, with accuracy, and with persistence. Psychoticism, however, correlates negatively both with accuracy ($r = -0.24$) and with I.Q. ($r = -0.36$).

Since speed, accuracy, and persistence scores were highly skewed, logarithmic transformations were carried out on these measures before computation of the correlations.

By now the reader may be wondering how well, or how badly, perhaps, the model actually fits the data. To this point we now turn.

The speed, accuracy, and persistence scores and the difficulty level and discriminating power parameters were chosen to minimize minus log likelihood. The value of this statistic by itself is of little use to us. If we had an alternative model which made use of precisely the same data we could fit the parameters of that model to the same data to minimize minus log likelihood under the alternative model. We could then compute the ratio of the likelihood functions under the two models and conclude, perhaps, that the data were more likely under our model than under the alternative model.

The only model which we can propose as an alternative to be fitted to precisely these data is a version of the present model which uses the same speed, accuracy, and persistence scores for all subjects. It is, if you like, an individual differences model without individual differences. Such a model seems psychologically sterile and its use would be merely a device to enable us to compute a likelihood-ratio statistic. This we have not done.

Instead, we have computed the contingency table which we display in Table 5.

There are 93×20 observed response pairs $\{x_{ji}, y_{ji}\}$ each with its observed t_{ji}, and its associated $\{a_i, s_i, p_i\}$ and $\{d_j, D_j\}$. For each j, i combination we can compute the following three probabilities $\Pr[X_{ji} = 0, Y_{ji} = 0]$, $\Pr[X_{ji} = 0, Y_{ji} = 1]$, and $\Pr[X_{ji} = 1, Y_{ji} = 0]$. The event corresponding to the largest of these probabilities is the event expected under the model. This assigns the "expected" event to one of the columns of the contingency table. The observed event $\{X_{ji} = x_{ji}, Y_{ji} = y_{ji}\}$ is assigned to the corresponding row of the contingency table. Thus, the observations are assigned to columns of the contingency table by the model; to rows by the behaviour of the subject. Thus, the entry n_{pq} in the p, q'th cell of the table is the number of observations of type p that the model says should be of type q. For example, there were 1140 observations of type $\{X_{ji} = 1, Y_{ji} = 0\}$. Of these 1053 are correctly classified by the model, 23 are incorrectly classified as type $\{X_{ji} = 0, Y_{ji} = 0\}$.

We wish to test whether the model is doing significantly better than

Individual Differences in Speed, Accuracy and Persistence:

TABLE 5

Observed \ Expected	$X_{ji}=0$, $Y_{ji}=0$	$X_{ji}=0$, $Y_{ji}=1$	$X_{ji}=1$, $Y_{ji}=0$	
$X_{ji}=0$, $Y_{ji}=0$	255	29	184	468
$X_{ji}=0$, $Y_{ji}=1$	128	58	66	252
$X_{ji}=1$, $Y_{ji}=0$	64	23	1053	1140
	447	110	1303	1860

Contingency Table for Observation Classification

chance in assigning the observations to the response categories. If the number of correct classifications, or "hits" is less than or equal to the number expected by chance then the model is clearly not doing significantly better than chance. Thus our test is a one-sided test. We compute the expected number of "hits" (926), the expected number of "misses" (934), the observed number of "hits" (1366 = 255+58+1053), and the observed number of "misses" (494). The number of "hits" is greater than the expected number so we compute $\chi^2 = (1366-926)^2/926+(494-934)^2/934 = 416{\cdot}35$ which, on 1 degree of freedom, is clearly significant.

But what does this mean? Surely, having fitted 320 parameters we would expect to do better than chance. We see no clear way to take this factor into account and suggest that χ^2 should perhaps be regarded merely as a descriptive statistic. At any rate, it is clear at a glance where the discrepancies are occurring and we hope that further study of the table may suggest modifications to the model. For example, 252 abandonments occur but the model only "expects" 110. We have already noted that difficult

Individual Differences in Speed, Accuracy and Persistence:

problems tend to be abandoned more frequently than easy ones. This suggests that we might improve things by modifying equation (12) in some way to take account of problem difficulty d_j as well as the subject's persistence p_i. This matter is under consideration.

We have now presented the model. We have shown that, though not easily done, it is feasible to fit the model to a non-trivial set of data. We conclude that the fitted subject scores and item parameters make very good psychological sense both in terms of their mutual inter-relationships and of their inter-relationships with other measures and with I.Q.

[1] This piece by Owen White was specially written for this book, as nothing suitable was available (Ed.).

[2] The research reported here has been supported, in part, by a grant from the Social Science Research Council.

[3] We use the symbol ω_i for a vector of subject variables for subject i. Thus, $\omega_i = \{a_i, s_i, p_i\}$.

REFERENCES

BIRNBAUM, A. Some latent trait models and their use in inferring an examinee's ability. Chapters 17–20 in Lord, F. M. and Novick, M. R. *Statistical theories of mental test scores*. Reading, Mass.: Addison-Wesley, 1968.

FLETCHER, R. and M. J. D. POWELL. A rapidly convergent descent method for minimization. *Computer Journal*, 1963, *6*, 163–168.

FLETCHER, R. and C. M. REEVES. Function minimization by conjugate gradients. *Computer Journal*, 1964, *7*, 149–154.

FURNEAUX, W. D. Intellectual abilities and problem-solving behaviour. Chapter 5 in Eysenck, H. J. (ed.) *Handbook of abnormal psychology*. London: Pitman, 1960.

RAVEN, J. C. Advanced progressive matrices (Set II, 1962 Revision). London: Lewis, 1962.

WHITE, P. O. A mathematical model for individual differences in problem solving. Chapter 20 in Elithorn, A. and D. Jones. *Artificial and human thinking*. Amsterdam: Elsevier, 1973.

PART VI

HEREDITY AND ENVIRONMENT: I, TWIN AND FAMILIAL STUDIES

The question of the degree to which differences in intelligence test performance are determined by heredity and environment respectively is a thorny one; clearly both are needed to produce any effect, and accordingly some form of interactionism, giving proper weight to both aspects, is the only proper scientific answer to the question. However, this still leaves us with the further, quantitative question of how much? Some critics have claimed that such a question cannot meaningfully be posed, but modern methods of genetic analysis, taking their root in Fisher's famous 1918 paper and adopting the methods developed by Mather and Jinks (1972), make such a stand impossible. Certain restrictions must of course be acknowledged for any generalizations, and it is important to bear these in mind in reading the papers here reprinted. Any estimate of heritability is inevitably tied to a given population, at a given point of time; it cannot and should not be extrapolated to populations at a different point of time. Nor should it be applied to a given individual; because the heritability of intelligence in the population is 80%, it does not follow that for every individual person in that population heredity plays a part twice as important (not 8:2 but $\sqrt{8:2}$) as the environment. But given these limitations, and also granting that the ratio might be drastically altered by some new and as yet unthought of invention, it is clear that modern work has thrown much light on these ancient disputes, and any student of intelligence should be *au fait* with these developments. (As an example of such an invention which might make a great deal of difference to our ideas, consider the recent work on "decompression" in South Africa; it was claimed that by putting the pregnant mother in a kind of decompression chamber, the child's IQ could be raised by 15 points. (Heyms, 1963). These claims have been shown to be false, (Liddicoat, 1968; Nelson 1969), but this example illustrates what sort of experimental procedure might fulfill this function. Administration of such drugs as glutamic acid is another method tried, as yet without very much success; there is no reason why eventually success should not attend a better understanding of the way in which the cortex works).

Most discussions of the nature-nurture problem consider genetic evidence, i.e. empirical studies deriving from predictions made on the basis of some sort of genetic model. Some of these studies are reprinted in this section. But equally important are studies which consider environmental evidence, i.e. empirical work deriving from predictions made on the basis of some sort of environmental model. Some of the most famous of these studies are reprinted in the next section. What is so impressive is the fact that these two series of studies converge on very similar estimates for the contribution of heredity (80%) and environment (20%) to the total variance; when we bear in mind that within each group of studies there are several different methods which have been used, and that these different methods also converge on the self-same values, we will appreciate that we are beginning to have solid ground under our feet.

As Jinks and Fulker (1970) point out, "there are currently three alternative approaches to the genetical analysis of human twin and familial data. There is what might be termed the classical approach through correlations between relatives, culminating in the estimation of various ratios describing the relative importance of genetic and environmental influences on trait variation. . . . There is the more systematic and comprehensive approach of the Multiple Abstract Variance Analysis (MAVA) developed by Cattell (1960, 1965) leading to both the estimation of nature:nurture ratios, and an assessment of the importance of the correlation between genetic and environmental influences within the family as well as within the culture. This approach is open-ended and based on the comparison of within- and between-family variances of full- and half-sib families, as well as monozygotic and dizygotic twins. Finally, there is the biometrical genetical approach initiated by Fischer (1918), and extended and applied by Mather (1949), which includes the first two approaches as special cases, and attempts to go beyond them to an assessment of the kind of gene action and mating system operating in the population." (P. 311). The Jinks and Fulker paper is too long to be reproduced here, but it is the corner-stone on which any future argument about heritability must be based. The authors split the total trait variation into four components, G_1 (within-family genetic component), G_2 (between-family genetic component), E_1 (within-family environmental component), and E_2 (between-family environmental component). They then elaborate models which exclude G/E interaction, and others which make provision for it, and lay down methods for estimating the values appropriate to a testing of the existence and degree of interaction. When the appropriate model has been chosen, it becomes possible to calculate the narrow and broad heritabilities, to assess dominance and assortative mating, and to deal with the problem of interaction and correlated environments. "The biometrical genetical approach . . . poses the question whether or not the correlation of interaction items in the model are essential or redundant by means of a number of statistical tests (scaling tests) that specifically detect their presence. . . . As may be seen later from the reanalysis of the data, these scaling tests allow us to suggest with some confidence that very simple genetical models are quite adequate to account for most of the data." (P. 313).

This is a very important conclusion. The early attempts to arrive at estimates of heritability, including the H coefficient of Holzinger (1929), the E coefficient of Neel and Schull (1954), and the HR of Nichols (1965), could all be criticized justifiably because of assumptions made in their derivation which could not be proved, such as the relative lack of importance of between-family environmental effects (E_2), lack of interaction effects, absence of correlated environments, etc. Critics could rightly point to these assumptions and say that in the absence of proof justifying them, no reasonable estimate of heritability could be made. Now that we know, thanks to Jinks and Fulker, that a relatively simple model accounts for most of the facts, we can assert with much more confidence that the estimates made on the basis of the older formulae are not very far out, and that the assumptions then made are sufficiently near the truth to render the estimates reasonable, if not quite accurate. Critics will have to come to terms with this new approach, and re-learn their genetics; the old and time-worn objections will not do any longer.

The first paper here reprinted is a famous review of some 50 empirical studies of genetic relationship categories and their bearing on performance on intelligence tests. Agreement, as the authors point out, is impressive in view of the heterogeneity of sources; the results strongly suggest that "the composite data are compatible with the polygenic hypothesis which is generally favoured in accounting for inherited differences in mental ability." The authors also conclude that "sex linkage is not supported by the data." (P. 1478). The second paper deals with early mental develop-

ment in twins, and links up with our discussion of the "overlap" hypothesis and the testing of early intelligence in infants. The hypothesis tested here is that spurts and lags in development of intellectual ability would be found much more highly related in monozygotic twins than in dizygotic ones; these spurts and lags are of course much more relevant at an early stage of development than is level, if we assume that level and gains are poorly or not at all correlated. The conclusion arrived at was that "infant mental development was primarily determined by the twins' genetic blueprint and that, except in unusual cases, other factors served mainly as a supportive function." (P. 914). These results are valuable in relation to suggestions that at an early stage of development environmental factors may be particularly important and relevant; these data do not suggest that this point of view has much empirical support.

The third paper deals with the IQ's of identical twins reared apart; it reviews what is perhaps the most cogent evidence in favour of the genetic determination of intelligence, and should therefore be read with particular care. It represents an impressive combination of scholarship and empirical evidence difficult to refute; if the genetic case rested on just one kind of support, this would be the one chosen by most experts. Fortunately, we are not in that position; the calculations carried out in relation to these twins give results which can be checked in other ways, and the results, as noted already, agree to a satisfactory extent.

There is one criticism which must be made of most calculations which are based on twin material, viz. a disregard of certain biological factors which seriously lead one to doubt the assumption that monozygotic twins share 100% heredity. As Darlington (1970) has pointed out, "it has long been clear that environment has a special meaning for one-egg twins since what is external to each is internal to the two. For one-egg twins there are therefore sources of discordance which are neither genetic nor environmental in the ordinary sense. And they can now be individually distinguished. These may be provisionally classified as follows:

1. Nuclear differences: arising by gene mutation or chromosone loss or gain in one of the two products of splitting (Bruins, 1963; Dekaban, 1966; Edwards et al., 1966).
2. Cytoplasmic differences: arising by the actions of deleterious genes in an assymmetrical cytoplasm (Darlington, 1954).
3. Embryological differences: arising from errors fo late splitting (Lieberman, 1938).
4. Nutritional differences: arising from errors of joint placentation (Price, 1950; Uchida et al., 1957).

A number of lines of enquiry arise from this classification. For example in the Edwards' twins the plane of splitting between the twins does not follow the cell-lineage divisions as shown either by the chromosomes or by the sexual character which they determine. Each twin is therefore a mosaic, a sexual mosaic, just as he is when cells migrate through the placenta between two-egg twins. Again in the remarkable case described by Walker (1950) when two one-egg twins have two different abnormalities, the one retinoblastoma, the other cleft palate, we have the opposite possibility that a reciprocal chromosome difference due to bridge-breakage at mitosis is directly responsible; the difference between the twins is then precisely a cell-lineage difference."

Bulmer (1970) discusses another problem, namely that of mirror imaging. As Darlington points out, "if we agree that left-handedness and situs inversus of the viscera occur no more frequently than by chance in one-egg twins there remains the question of whether we assign the difference to heredity or to environment." He concluded: "Surely to neither. It is the effect of an uncertainty in development. It resembles that primary uncertainty in the position of partner chromosomes at meiosis which underlies the almost universal uncertainty in frequency of crossing-over. But it differs inasmuch as it seems to lie close to the limit of selectable variation." Darlington concludes: "When all these questions have been considered we may return to ask ourselves where we stand with the classical assumption that one-egg twins are genetically identical and their discordances assignable to the 'environment'. It seems we have to withdraw this assumption and replace it with the principle that their discordance gives us a maximum estimate, and statistically always an over-estimate of environmental influence." This is an important conclusion, and one which few behavioural geneticists have borne in mind in assessing heritability of intelligence.

The evidence here presented is not all that could be adduced, and attention is drawn to the discussion of additional sources of information in Burt's paper which constitutes the first reprint in this book, and the data on "regression to the mean" contained in the same author's paper reprinted in a later section (Burt, 1961, Table 1). This argument from regression is too important to leave with just a mention; in the absence of any single paper which could be reprinted to emphasize its importance a brief discussion here may not be out of place. In this discussion I have followed the treatment adopted by Jensen (1972), who reanalyzed some data from the famous Terman "gifted children" study. In this monumental study, Terman (1926) selected over 1,000 children with Stanford-Binet IQ's of 140 or above from Californian schools; this selection took place in 1922. Since then, the educational and occupational careers of these children have been followed into adulthood (Terman and Oden, 1959), and the Stanford-Binet IQ's of more than 1,500 of the children of these gifted parents have been obtained. These data, therefore, permit an interesting genetic prediction. Jensen uses a formula given by Crow (1970), based on a simple additive genetic model which is not too dissimilar to that found adequate by Jinks and Fulker (1970); this

formula is used to predict the mean value of some attribute in the offspring of a specially selected parent population:

$$\bar{O} = M + h_N{}^2(P - M)$$

where $\bar{O}$ =predicted mean of the offspring, M =general population mean, $h_N{}^2$ =narrow heritability, and P = parental mean. (Note that this formula implies a randomized allocation of individuals to environments; if this is not true, then a correction must of course be made in the formula).

The following figures may be taken from Terman. The mean IQ of the gifted group (as children) was 152. The estimated mean Stanford-Binet IQ of their spouses (derived from his Concept mastery test) was 125, showing considerable assortative mating. Thus the parental mean IQ would be P=(152+125)/2=138·5. The population mean, M=100, by definition and by demonstration. The best available estimate of narrow heritability ($h_N{}^2$) for intelligence is that given by Jinks and Fulker (1970, P. 343, 346) as 0·71 ± ·01. Substituting these values in the Crow formula, we have as the predicted mean IQ of the offspring:

$$\bar{O} = 100 + 0·71\,(138·5 - 100) = 127·33$$

The actual observed IQ is 132·7, with a S.D. of 16·5, a discrepancy of 5·4 IQ points. But, as Jensen points out, "the prediction was based on the assumption of no difference between the average environment provided by the gifted parents and the average environment in the general population. Therefore, the discrepancy of 5·4 IQ points over the predicted IQ may be viewed as due to the environmental advantages of the offspring of the gifted. This would be a 'between-families' environmental effect, one S.D. of which, according to our MZ twin analysis, is equivalent to 3·35 IQ points. So the offspring of the Terman gifted group could be regarded as having enjoyed environmental advantages 5·4/3·35 = 1·6 S.D.s above the average environment in the general population. It is interesting, therefore, that the average family income of the gifted is 1·45 S.D.s above the national average. Using only income as an index of environmental advantage, we would estimate the IQ of the offspring of the gifted as the genetic prediction (IQ = 127·3) plus the environmental advantage (1·45 × 3·35 = 4·9 IQ points) as 132·2, which does not differ significantly from the obtained mean IQ of 132·7. Thus, our model fits the Terman gifted data very well."

I have quoted these simple calculations because they illustrate to perfection a feature of the paradigm or model we are dealing with which is of the utmost importance for any proper critical assessment. We can take quantitative assessments, such as that of narrow heritability, from one study, and apply these assessments to another, in the full expectations that when these data are inserted in the equation, the appropriate result will follow.* In other words, we have a model of mental ability which can be considered truly quantitative, demonstrating proper invariance; this at once does away with much facile and arid argumentation. If the figure derived for heritability from twin studies were indeed as arbitrary and subject to criticism as many writers have suggested, then it would not be possible to use it in connection with a heritability study using, not twins, but regression effects; the results should fail completely to agree with the facts as observed. Yet as we have seen, this is not so; agreement is almost too complete! It is this kind of quantitative agreement which is so impressive, and which seems to render nugatory the purely verbal criticisms often made of intelligence testing, and the derivation of heritability estimates. The only way in which the paradigm could be dethroned would be the elaboration of another, better paradigm, which does all that the existing model does, and which in addition caters for anomalies which at present remain unexplained. Such a paradigm is no-where in sight.

Yet there is a curious tendency among most psychologists to disregard the paradigm in their eagerness to offer environmentalistic explanations of inconvenient findings, however far-fetched these might be, rather than acknowledge the close agreement between fact and genetic hypothesis. This failure to even consider genetic

* An alternative method of dealing with the data would of course be to treat $h_N{}^2$ as the inknown, insert the known values of P and M, and the actual value for O instead of treating this as the value to be predicted. We can now solve this question and derive the narrow heritability directly; this is in fact identical with that derived from the twin data by Jinks and Fulker, provided we make the correction for environmental effects discussed in the text. This is probably a more useful way of using Crow's equation than that adopted by Jensen.

The degree to which different estimates of heritability of intelligence agree, even though they are derived from quite different sources, and employ different assumptions and methods of calculation, is perhaps the firmest ground for believing in the essential accuracy of the final figure reached. The agreement is probably closer than that achieved in determining Avogadro's number from an array of diverse phenomena in the early years of this century (Perrin, 1914). Thus determination through gas viscosity by van der Wals equation gave a value of 62, Brownian movement values ranging from 65 (rotations) to 69 (diffusion), black body radiation a value of 64, radioactivity values ranging from 60 to 71, and so on, for $N/10^{22}$. Thus the range of estimates was about 25% of the lowest estimate, (Nye, 1972); the range of estimates for the heritability of intelligence is less than this, and could in turn be much reduced if all workers in the field agreed to use identical tests, increased the reliability of these tests by making them longer, and made certain that the populations used were not restricted in range. Even as they stand, however, the figures show considerable agreement; only a non-scientist would expect greater agreement at such an early stage.

causes, in spite of the overwhelming evidence in support of their importance, may be worth illustrating. Gross (1967) compared two Brooklyn Jewish groups on a variety of cognitive tests. The children were around 6 years of age, all their mothers were native-born, and English was the household language; all were middle-class and lived in the same community. It was found that the Ashkenazic boys (whose parents had immigrated from Europe) had IQ's very much higher than the Sephardic boys (whose parents had immigrated from Arabic or Oriental countries). In spite of a thorough search for relevant environmental variables to explain this difference, no divergencies could be found in a host of family training and background experiences—except for one item in the questionnaire of parental attitudes (which might of course have given a statistically "significant" difference, on a chance basis, being one item out of hundreds). Twice as many Ashkenazic mothers said that earnings were "unimportant" in their desires for their children, and three times as many Sephardic mothers said they wanted their children to be "wealthy". Havighurst (1970, P. 321) cites this study as an example of how subtle environmental differences can influence cognitive development, and this curious notion that the mother's desire for her son to be wealthy can decrease his IQ by 17 points has been echoed by other writers. Yet no known method of teaching or environmental manipulation has ever produced differences anything like as large as this within non-disadvantaged groups! One would have thought that the genetic explanation would be more likely to explain the observed facts. This failure to apply the known and demonstrated truths embodied in the paradigm in explanations of experimental findings is a sad comment on the present state of psychology.

The genetic hypothesis has of course also been applied to racial differences, although here difficulties are very great, and indeed almost overwhelming; it would be impossible to go into the many and varied arguments which have been advanced in this field since Jensen published his well-known monograph in the Harvard Educational Review (reprinted in Jensen, 1972a). A thorough review of the evidence has been given elsewhere (Eysenck, 1971). However, it may be interesting to illustrate possible applications of the model with which we are here concerned to this problem, and note how it can facilitate the use of the hypothetico-deductive method. The study chosen for discussion is outlined by Jensen (1973), in connection with his introduction to the concept of sibling regression; the argument is complex, but convincing. He first points out that if we match black (American) children with white (American) children for IQ, their performance on scholastic achievement tests is for all practical purposes identical; in other words, IQ tests give the same prediction of scholastic performance for Negro as for white children. Now let us match a number of Negro and white children for IQ, and then look at the IQ's of their full siblings with whom they were reared. "Technically speaking, of course, the white and black children were matched on 'regressed true scores', i.e. the IQ scores they would be expected to obtain if errors of measurement were eliminated; this is a standard statistical procedure used in studies calling for matching of two or more groups. Under these conditions it is found that the Negro siblings average some 7 to 10 points lower than the white siblings. Further, the higher the IQ of the matched black-white pair, the greater is the absolute amount of regression shown by the IQ's of the siblings; if the IQ's of the matched children is 120, the white siblings will have IQ's around 110, the black siblings IQ's around 100. In other words, the siblings of both groups have regressed halfway to their respective population means and *not* to the mean of the combined population. (The same is of course true when children from the low end of the IQ scale are matched; Negro and white children matched for IQ 70 will have siblings whose average IQ's are about 78 for the Negroes and 85 for the whites). The regression line shows no significant departure from linearity through the range from IQ 60 to 150.

"This very lawful phenomenon would seem difficult to explain in terms of a strictly environmental theory of the causation of individual differences in IQ. If Negro and white children are matched for IQ's of, say, 120, it must be presumed that both sets of children had environments that were good enough to stimulate or permit IQ's this high to develop. Since there is no reason to believe that the environments of these children's siblings differ on the average markedly from their own, why should one group of siblings come out much lower in IQ than the other? Genetically identical twins who have been reared from infancy in *different* families do not differ in IQ by nearly so much as our siblings reared together in the same family. It can be claimed that though the white and Negro children are matched for IQ 120, they actually have different environments, with the Negro child, on the average, having the less intellectually stimulating environment. Therefore, it could be argued he actually has a higher genetic potential for intelligence than the environmentally more favoured white child with the same IQ. But if this were the case, why should not the Negro child's siblings also have somewhat superior genetic potential? They have the same parents, and their degree of genetic resemblance, indicated by the theoretical genetic correlation among siblings, is presumably the same for Negroes and whites."

It will be seen that this application of the paradigm neatly sidesteps the obvious difficulties inherent in any comparison between two groups differing in social status and other environmental determinants of IQ. Matching black and white children on IQ ensures that the genetic potential of the black child is *at least* as great as that of the white child (and probably superior if his IQ is depressed by environmental deficits); why then does his sibling regress to the black population mean, leaving the white sibling, who has regressed to the white mean, superior to the extent predictable from the simple regression equation? The sibling's environment, in each case, is sufficiently like that of the proband to make an environmentalistic explanation difficult, if not impossible; this leaves us with a purely genetic hypothesis for at least the major part of the observed difference. The argument is of course not conclusive; no scientific argument is ever conclusive in an absolute sense. In any case, it is not quoted here to decide on the issue of racial differences; it is quoted to illustrate ways and means of applying the general paradigm, and the regression formula which forms such an important part of it, to an applied problem. Such applications could with advantage be made in many cases where experimenters, instead of considering both genetic and environmentalistic causes for their findings with some degree of impartiality, plump for the latter, without consideration of the former; simple quantitative considerations of the data, or a better-informed design, could often make possible a suitable partition of the variance between causal influences without reliance on preconceived notions.

REFERENCES

Bruins, J. W. Discordant mongolism in monozygotic twins. *Proc. 11th Int. Congr. Genet.*, 1963, *1*, 307.

Bulmer, M. G. The biology of twinning in man. Oxford: Clarendon Press, 1970.

Burt, C. Intelligence and social mobility. *Brit. J. stat. Psychol.*, 1901, *14*, 3–24.

Cattell, R. B. The multiple abstract variance analysis equations and solutions for nature-nurture research on continuancy variables. *Psychol. Rev.*, 1960, *67*, 353–372.

Cattell, R. B. Methodological and conceptual advances in evaluating hereditary and environmental influences and their interaction. In: S. G. Vandenberg (Ed.) Methods and goals in human behaviour genetics. New York: Academic Press, 1965.

Crow, J. F. Do genetic factors contribute to poverty? In: V. L. Allen (Ed.), Psychological factors in poverty. Chicago: Markham, 1970. Pp. 147–160.

Darlington, C. D. Heredity and environment. Caryologia, 1954. Suppl. to Vol. VI, Pp. 370–381.

Darlington, C. D. Twin biology. Heredity, 1970, Pp. 25. Notes and Comments section.

Dekaban, A. Twins probably monozygotic: one mongoloid with 48 chromosomes, the other normal. *Cytogenetics*, 1966, *4*, 227–239.

Edwards, J. H. et al. Monozygotic twins of different sex. *J. med. Genet.*, 1966, *3*, 77–158.

Eysenck, H. J. The IQ argument. New York: The Library Press, 1971. (Race, Intelligence and Education. London: Maurice Temple Smith, 1971).

Fisher, R. A. The correlation between relations on the supposition of Mendelian inheritance. *Transaction Roy. Soc.*, (Edinburgh), 1918, *52*, 399–433.

Gross, M. Learning readiness in two Jewish groups. New York: Center for Urban Education, 1967.

HEYNS, O. S. Abdominal decompression. A monograph. Johannesburg: *Univ. Press.* 1963.

HAVIGHURST, R. J. Minority subculture and the law of effect. *American Psychologist,* 1970, *25,* 313–322.

HOLZINGER, K. J. The relative effect of nature and nurture influences in twin differences. *J. educ. Psychol.,* 1929, *20,* 245–248.

JENSEN, A. R. Genetics and Education. London: Methuen, 1972.

JENSEN, A. R. Genetics, educability, and subpopulation differences. London: Methuen, 1973.

JINKS, J. L., FULKER, D. W. Comparison of the biometrical genetical, MAVA, and classical approaches to the analysis of human behaviour. *Psychol. Bull.,* 1970, *73,* 311–349.

LEIBERMAN, L. Zwillingspathologische Untersuchungen. *Ztsch. mensche. Vererb. u. Kaustl.,* 1938, *22,* 373–417.

LIDDICOAT, R. The effects of maternal antenatal decompression treatment on infant mental development. *Psychologia Africana,* 1968, *12,* 103–121.

MATHER, K., JINKS, J. L. Biometrical Genetics (2nd Edition). London: Methuen, 1972. (First edition, 1949, by Mather, K.).

NEEL, J. V., SCHULL, W. J. Human Heredity. Chicago: Univ. of Chicago Press, 1954.

NELSON, G. K. Effects of maternal antenatal decompression treatment on infant development. Johannesburg: *Nat. Inst. Personnel Res.* 1969.

NICHOLS, R. C. The National Merit twin study. In: S. G. Vandenberg (Ed.) Methods and goals in human behaviour genetics. New York: Academic Press, 1965.

NYE, M. J. Molecular reality. London: *Macdonald,* 1972.

PERRIN, J. Les atomes. Paris: *F. Alcan,* 1914, p. 293.

PRICE, B. Primary biases in twin studies: a view of prenatal and antenatal differences in producing factors in monozygotic twins. *Amer. J. Human Genetics,* 1950, *2,* 293–352.

TERMAN, L. M. Genetic studies of genius. Vol. I. Mental and physical traits of a thousand gifted children. Stanford: University Press, 1926.

TERMAN, L. M., ODEN, M. The gifted groups at mid-life. Stanford: University Press, 1959.

UCHIDA, I. A., ROWE, R. D. Discordant heart anomalies in (one-egg) twins. *Amer. J. Human Genetics,* 1957, *9,* 133–140.

WALKER, N. F. Discordant monozygotic twins (a) with retino-blastoma, and (b) cleft palate. *Amer. J. Human Genetics,* 1950, *2,* 375–384.

From L. Erlenmeyer-Kimling and L. F. Jarvek (1963). Science, 142, 1477–1479. Copyright (1963), by kind permission of the authors and The American Association for the Advancement of Science

Genetics and Intelligence: A Review

Abstract. *A survey of the literature of the past 50 years reveals remarkable consistency in the accumulated data relating mental functioning to genetic potentials. Intragroup resemblance in intellectual abilities increases in proportion to the degree of genetic relationship.*

Nomothetic psychological theories have been distinguished by the tendency to disregard the individual variability which is characteristic of all behavior. A parallel between genetic individuality and psychologic individuality has rarely been drawn because the usual assumption has been, as recently noted in these pages (*1*), that the organisms intervening between stimulus and response are equivalent "black boxes," which react in uniform ways to given stimuli.

While behavior theory and its analytic methods as yet make few provisions for modern genetic concepts, the literature contains more information than is generally realized about the relationship between genotypic similarity and similarity of performance on mental tests. In a search for order among the published data on intellectual ability, we have recently summarized the work of the past half century (*2*). By using the most commonly reported statistical measure, namely, the correlation coefficient, it has been possible to assemble comparative figures from the majority of the investigations.

Certain studies giving correlations had to be excluded from this compilation for one of the following reasons: (i) type of test used (for example, achievement tests, scholastic performance, or subjective rating of intelligence); (ii) type of subject used (for example, mental defectives); (iii) inadequate information about zygosity diagnosis in twin studies (*3*); (iv) reports on too few special twin pairs.

The 52 studies (*2*) remaining after these exclusions yield over 30,000 correlational pairings (*4*) for the genetic relationship categories shown in Fig. 1. The data, in aggregate, provide a broad basis for the comparison of genotypic and phenotypic correlations. Considering only *ranges* of the observed measures, a marked trend is seen toward an increasing degree of intellectual resemblance in direct proportion to an increasing degree of genetic relationship, regardless of environmental communality.

Furthermore, for most relationship categories, the *median* of the empirical correlations closely approaches the theoretical value predicted on the basis of genetic relationship alone. The average genetic correlation between parent and child, as well as that between siblings (including dizygotic twins) is 0.50. The median correlations actually observed on tests of intellectual functioning are: 0.50 for parent-child, 0.49 for siblings reared together, and 0.53 for dizygotic twins, both the opposite-sex and like-sex pairs. Although twins are presumably exposed to more similar environmental conditions than are siblings spaced apart in age, the correlations for mental ability do not indicate a sizable difference between the groups. Since only two studies dealt with siblings reared *apart*, it is possible to state only that the reported correlations for that group fall within the range of values obtained for siblings reared together and exceed those for unrelated children living *together*.

For unrelated persons in a large random-mating population, the theoretical genetic correlation is usually considered to be zero; for smaller populations, or those that deviate substantially from panmixia, however, the genetic correlation between presumably unrelated individuals in fact may be considerably higher. The observed median for unrelated persons reared apart is −0.01. Medians for unrelated individuals reared together (children reared in the same orphanage or foster home from an early age) and for the fosterparent-child group are 0.23 and 0.20, respec-

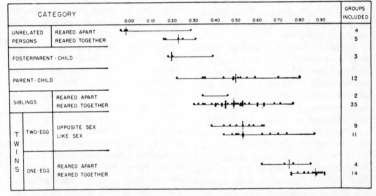

Fig. 1. Correlation coefficients for "intelligence" test scores from 52 studies. Some studies reported data for more than one relationship category; some included more than one sample per category, giving a total of 99 groups. Over two-thirds of the correlation coefficients were derived from I.Q.'s, the remainder from special tests (for example, Primary Mental Abilities). Midparent-child correlation was used when available, otherwise mother-child correlation. Correlation coefficients obtained in each study are indicated by dark circles; medians are shown by vertical lines intersecting the horizontal lines which represent the ranges.

tively. The relative contributions made by environmental similarity and sample selection to these deviations from zero are still to be analyzed.

At the other end of the relationship scale, where monozygotic twins theoretically have 100 percent genetic correlation, medians of the observed correlations in intellectual functioning are 0.87 for the twins brought up together, and 0.75 for those brought up apart (5). The correlations obtained for monozygotic twins reared together are generally in line with the intra-individual reliabilities of the tests. The median for the separated twins is somewhat lower, but clearly exceeds those for all other relationship groups.

In further reference to twin studies, our survey (2) shows that mean intrapair differences on tests of mental abilities for dizygotic twins generally are between 1½ to 2 times as great as those between monozygotic twins reared together. Such a relationship appears to hold also for the upper age groups, as suggested by a longitudinal study of senescent twins (6).

Taken individually, many of the 52 studies reviewed here are subject to various types of criticism (for example, methodological). Nevertheless, the overall orderliness of the results is particularly impressive if one considers that the investigators had different backgrounds and contrasting views regarding the importance of heredity. Not all of them used the same measures of intelligence (see caption, Fig. 1), and they derived their data from samples which were unequal in size, age structure, ethnic composition, and socioeconomic stratification; the data were collected in eight countries on four continents during a time span covering more than two generations of individuals. Against this pronounced heterogeneity, which should have clouded the picture, and is reflected by the wide range of correlations, a clearly definitive consistency emerges from the data.

The composite data are compatible with the polygenic hypothesis which is generally favored in accounting for inherited differences in mental ability. Sex-linkage is not supported by these data (for example, under a hypothesis of sex-linkage the correlations for likesex dizygotic twins should be higher than those for opposite-sex twins), although the possible effects of sex-linked genes are not precluded for some specific factors of ability.

We do not imply that environment is without effect upon intellectual functioning; the intellectual level is *not* unalterably fixed by the genetic constitution. Rather, its expression in the phenotype results from the patterns laid down by the genotype under given environmental conditions. Two illustrations of the "norm of reaction" concept in relation to intellectual variability are seen in early total deafness and in phenylketonuria. Early deafness makes its stamp upon intellectual development, in that it lowers I.Q. by an estimated 20 score points (7). Phenylketonuria is ordinarily associated with an even greater degree of intellectual impairment. However, early alteration of the nutritional environment of the affected child changes the phenotypic expression of this genetic defect (8). Individual differences in behavioral *potential* reflect genotypic differences; individual differences in behavioral *performance* result from the nonuniform recording of environmental stimuli by intrinsically nonuniform organisms.

L. ERLENMEYER-KIMLING
LISSY F. JARVIK
Department of Medical Genetics,
New York State Psychiatric Institute,
Columbia University, New York 32

References and Notes

1. J. Hirsch. *Science.* this issue.
2. This material was included in a report presented at the XVII International Congress of Psychology. Washington, D.C., 1963 (L. Erlenmeyer-Kimling, L. F. Jarvik, and F. J. Kallmann). Detailed information about the data presented here is available upon request and is in preparation for publication.
3. This survey does include reports on opposite-sex (hence dizygotic) twin pairs from these studies.
4. Correlational pairings refer to the number of individual pairs used in deriving the correlation coefficients. Some investigators constructed a large number of pairings on the basis of a relatively small number of individuals. Altogether, we have been able to identify the following minimum numbers: twins, 3134 pairs (1082 monozygotic and 2052 dizygotic); sibs apart, 125 pairs plus 131 individuals; sibs together, 8288 pairs plus 7225 individuals; parent-child, 371 pairs plus 6812 individuals; fosterparent-child, 537 individuals; unrelated apart, 15,086 pairings; unrelated together, 195 pairings plus 287 individuals.
5. Correlational data are now available on 107 separated pairs of monozygotic twins from four series: H. H. Newman, F. N. Freeman, K. J. Holzinger, *Twins: A Study of Heredity and Environment* (Univ. of Chicago Press, Chicago, 1937); J. Conway, *Brit. J. Stat. Psychol.* 11, 171 (1958); N. Juel-Nielsen and A. Mogensen, cited by E. Strömgren. in *Expanding Goals of Genetics in Psychiatry,* F. J. Kallmann, Ed. (Grune and Stratton, New York, 1962), p. 231; J. Shields, *Monozygotic Twins Brought Up Apart and Brought Up Together* (Oxford Univ. Press, London, 1962).
6. L. F. Jarvik and A. Falek, *J. Gerontol.* 18, 173 (1963).
7. R. M. Salzberger and L. F. Jarvik, in *Family and Mental Health Problems in a Deaf Population,* J. D. Rainer et al., Eds. (N.Y. State Psychiatric Institute, New York, 1963).
8. F. A. Homer. C. W. Streamer, L. L. Alejandrino, L. H. Reed, F. Ibbott, *New Engl. J. Med.* 266, 79 (1962).

From R. S. Wilson (1972). Science, 175, 914–917. Copyright (1972), by kind permission of the author and the American Association for the Advancement of Science

Twins: Early Mental Development

Abstract. *Mental development was appraised periodically for infant twins, and the twins displayed high within-pair concordance for level of mental development during the first and second years. Twins were also concordant for the spurts and lags in development in this period (monozygotic twins more so than dizygotic). From these results it was inferred that infant mental development was primarily determined by the twins' genetic blueprint and that, except in unusual cases, other factors served mainly a supportive function.*

For several years the Louisville Twin Study has recruited newborn twins for participation in a longitudinal study of growth and development. The twins are seen at 3, 6, 9, 12, 18, and 24 months of age, and at each age they are tested with the research version of the Bayley scales of mental and motor development. This report gives the results for the mental scale for 261 pairs of twins (*1*).

Infant mental development is a matter of particular interest in its own right. Infant test scores are essentially unrelated to adult intelligence except in cases of marked retardation, and in fact the correlations are relatively low between tests given at 6-month intervals during early childhood (*2*).

The interpretation of these results is that the functions measured during infancy undergo rapid changes as new capabilities emerge and become fully developed. But the rate of gain is not uniform for all children, and consequently for any particular infant there may be significant changes in relative maturity from one age to the next.

At this point, the test data for twins take on added significance. If the emergence of mental functions depends upon genetically determined growth processes, then the level of mental development attained at each age should be comparable for twins. Further, if these processes alternate between phases of accelerated growth and of drift, then the rate of gain between ages for both twins should be subject to the same spurts and lags. Finally, if gene segregation is a significant factor, then the exact duplication of genotypes for identical twins should make them more concordant than fraternal twins.

The Bayley scale was administered within 1 week of the twins' birthday for ages 3, 6, 9, and 12 months, and within 2 weeks for ages 18 and 24 months. The total sample included 225 white same-sex pairs and 36 white opposite-sex pairs. The number of valid tests actually obtained at each age was affected by missed visits due to illness, occasional substitution of other tests, and so forth, so the sample size is reported separately for each analysis. The mean scores and standard deviations for twins are given in Table 1, along with the comparable singleton means at each age as reported by Bayley (*3*).

The results show that the average score for twins was somewhat lower at each age (significantly so at 6, 12, and 18 months), but the size of the difference was comparatively small. With a modest allowance made for prematurity, it appears that the developmental processes tapped by the Bayley mental scale unfold at essentially the same rate for twins as for singletons.

A separate analysis for sex differences revealed a slight but inconsequential advantage for females at all ages; the difference was significant only at 18 months. In line with Bayley's results, the present data support the view of sex equivalence in performance on the mental scale.

All twin scores were then transformed into standardized developmental quotients for each age, with a mean of 100 and standard deviation of 16. Subsequent analyses were performed with these standardized scores.

To verify the previous reports of low order correlations during infancy, I computed intercorrelations between the individual test scores obtained at each age, and the resulting coefficients ranged from .53 to .08. They were highest for adjacent ages (typically $r > .40$), but even the largest between-age correlation accounted for less than 30 percent of the variance and was well below the estimated reliability of the scale at each age ($r = .88$ to .94).

Since the low order correlations cannot be attributed to poor test reliability, they may be reflecting the influence of some systematic factor or factors, perhaps genetic in origin, that modulated the rate of gain in mental development from one age to the next. For example, an infant that was precocious at 6 months of age may have made a relatively slow gain over the next 6 months, and consequently by his first birthday he may have fallen behind the average child. Other infants would be subject to their own idiosyncratic rates of gain; and as a result, changes in relative precocity would be the rule, not the exception, for mental development during infancy.

This interpretation would be considerably strengthened by data showing that two infants that shared the same genetic blueprint actually followed the same course of mental development. Accordingly, the sample was separated into monozygotic (MZ) and dizygotic (DZ) pairs, on the basis of blood-typing tests for 22 or more antigens (*4*). All same-sex pairs that were discordant for one or more antisera tests were classified as DZ and combined with the opposite-sex pairs to form the entire DZ sample. The remaining concordant pairs constituted the MZ sample. For technical and psychological reasons the blood-typing is deferred until the twins are 3 years old, so there are some pairs for whom zygosity has not yet been established. These pairs are omitted from the current analysis.

The expectation was that DZ pairs would show a moderate degree of concordance in mental development by

Table 1. Means and standard deviations (SD's) of Bayley mental scale scores for twins.

Age (months)	Twin Means*	Twin SD's	Bayley singleton means	Number of pairs MZ	Number of pairs DZ	Within-pair correlations (r) MZ	Within-pair correlations (r) DZ
3	33.0	6.08	33.6	71	79	.84‡	.67
6	65.0	7.77	69.6†	85	98	.82	.74
9	83.6	4.51	84.3	82	101	.81‡	.69
12	97.2	5.73	99.6†	86	104	.82‡	.61
18	121.8	6.05	125.0†	88	91	.76	.72
24	141.4	8.62	143.0	57	77	.87‡	.75

* $N \geqslant 400$ through 18 months; $N = 298$ at 24 months. † Singleton mean significantly higher than twin mean ($P < .05$). ‡ MZ correlation significantly higher than DZ correlation ($P < .05$).

virtue of originating from the same gene pool and growing up in the same family, whereas MZ pairs would be significantly more concordant because all genes were held in common. The analysis was made by computing intraclass (within-pair) correlations for the test scores at each age, and the results are presented separately for MZ and DZ twins in the final columns of Table 1.

The results show that the MZ correlations were significantly higher at most ages and in fact approached the limits set by the reliability of the scale. The duplication of genotypes for MZ twins appears to have had a profound influence on the course of mental development. Further, even the within-pair correlations for DZ twins were higher than the between-age correlations reported earlier, so it is evident that twin A was a better predictor of twin B's score at the same age than he was of his own score at an adjacent age. The short-term developmental changes during infancy produced greater age-to-age deviations for one child than the accumulated differences in biological makeup and experience produced within the average DZ pair.

If the members of a twin pair resembled one another at each age, the next question was whether they followed the same pattern of mental development across ages, with correlated spurts and lags. The score profiles for several sets of MZ twins are presented in Fig. 1; these profiles were selected to illustrate the high degree of congruence that may be found among twins who follow quite different trends in mental development during infancy.

As the curves show, the score profile for each twin may be distinguished both in terms of contour and overall elevation. The profile contour is a function of age-to-age changes in precocity —the spurt-lag factor—while the overall elevation reflects a more enduring degree of developmental maturity (or immaturity) which persists across several ages. From an analytic standpoint, it would be informative to compute the within-pair concordance for twins on both of these aspects of infant mental development.

The analysis of the test scores was performed separately for each zygosity group by a repeated-measures analysis of variance that was adapted for use with twin data (5). The test scores obtained within the first and second years were analyzed separately to determine whether the degree of concordance remained the same for both years, or whether there was some notable change linked to age and zygosity (6). The results are presented in Table 2.

When the correlations for overall developmental level are examined, it is evident that the MZ pairs displayed a very high level of concordance within each year; that is, if the cumulative score for one twin were known, the corresponding score for his co-twin could be predicted with a small margin of error. If these correlations for overall level are compared with the MZ correlations in Table 1, it is clear that combining scores across ages minimized the errors of measurement and yielded a within-pair correlation that equaled the estimated reliability of the scale. In fact, the MZ correlations might be said to represent the purest measure of reliability for the developmental scale, since they are based on scores from two genetically identical infants who were raised in the same home and tested at the same age.

There was also a substantial degree of concordance within DZ pairs for overall developmental level, the implications of which are discussed later; but nevertheless the MZ correlations significantly exceeded the DZ correlations in both years. And when the profile contour correlations were examined, it was evident that the MZ correlations were significantly larger than the DZ correlations for this aspect of mental development as well. Since profile contour represents the age-to-age changes in relative precocity, these correlations signify that MZ twins were more closely aligned for the spurts and lags in development.

This analysis suggests that MZ twins and DZ twins constitute two significantly different subpopulations as far as concordance in early mental devel-

Table 2. Analysis of Bayley mental scale scores for twins in first and second years. The within-pair correlation is given by $R = (MS_b - MS_w)/(MS_b + MS_w)$, where MS_b is the mean square between pairs and MS_w is the mean square within pairs.

Source of variance	Within-pair correlations (R)	Test for MZ > DZ (P)	Range of 98 percent level of confidence	Mean square Between pairs	Mean square Within pairs	Degrees of freedom
Ages 3, 6, 9, and 12 months						
Overall level						
MZ pairs	.90	< .01	.80 – .95	645.5	35.6	44/45
DZ pairs	.75		.57 – .86	871.8	122.4	50/51
Profile contour						
MZ pairs	.75	< .01	.65 – .83	280.0	39.1	132/135
DZ pairs	.50		.34 – .63	228.5	76.0	150/153
Ages 12, 18, and 24 months						
Overall level						
MZ pairs	.89	< .05	.79 – .94	677.8	40.7	50/51
DZ pairs	.79		.62 – .89	614.5	71.0	45/46
Profile contour						
MZ pairs	.67	< .05	.53 – .78	272.4	53.1	100/102
DZ pairs	.52		.33 – .68	200.7	62.4	90/92

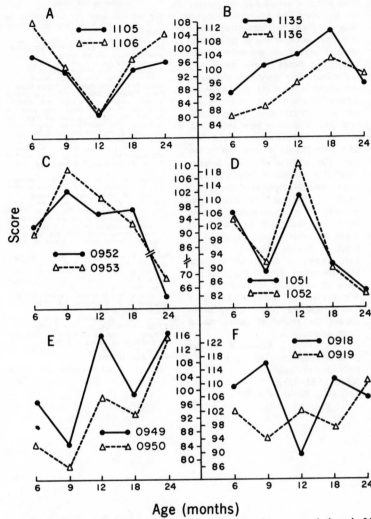

Fig. 1. Profiles of mental development scores for MZ twins at ages 6 through 24 months. The pairs in A to E exhibit moderate to high profile congruence; the pair in F is obviously noncongruent.

opment is concerned. If the difference is real and large enough to take seriously, the obtained within-pair correlations for MZ twins should fall outside the expected range for DZ twins, and the reverse should also be true. The ranges as set by the 98 percent confidence level are shown in Table 2 for all correlations, and the expectation is met—the MZ correlations are at least as large as the upper 1 percent limit for the DZ range, and conversely the DZ correlations fall below the lower 1 percent limit for the MZ range. So the difference in concordance level between MZ and DZ twins appears to

be a stable feature of early mental development which is evident in the first year and maintained throughout the second.

The results clearly reveal a significant genetic influence on both aspects of infant mental development. They confirm the interpretation offered earlier that the age-to-age changes in relative precocity are conditioned by genetic factors; and the manner in which these genetic factors exert their age-linked influence presumably follows the pattern that Thompson and Grusec described (7): "Thus the expression of certain genes may be so timed that certain types of behavior and certain capacities for discrimination and for articulated response will emerge at particular times." Further, while this conclusion is limited to the infancy period by the present data, we believe that the rate of gain throughout the preschool years will also be found to depend upon genetic factors.

Besides the significantly higher level of concordance for MZ twins, another equally important feature of the twin data is the relatively high degree of concordance for overall developmental level in DZ twins. It signifies that the differences within DZ pairs produced by gene segregation and different life experiences are comparatively small in relation to the sizable differences between pairs. What inference about the role of genetic and environmental factors might be drawn from these results?

The primary source of genetic variance in any nonrandom mating system is between families (technically, between parental mating combinations); and in a nuclear family society, the primary source of environmental variance is also between families. The reference behavior exhibited by offspring from each family is jointly affected by both sources of variance, but the proportion of influence from each source is not necessarily equal.

The influence of home environment will be considered first. The families in this study range from the welfare case to the wealthy professional family, and each family was assigned a socioeconomic status score (SES) by the classification system of Reiss (8). When the correlation was computed between SES scores and overall level of development for each year, the relation was very weak for the first year ($r = .11$) and improved only slightly for the second year ($r = .20$). Comparable results were reported by Bayley for her large norm sample (3); and taken on balance, both sources of data argue against a significant linkage between precocity of infant mental development and the socioeconomic quality of the home.

Stated more broadly, the conclusion is that the caretaking and stimulation needed to support infant mental development are sufficiently supplied by most home environments that fall above the level of impoverished. In all likelihood, however, there may be a cumulative latent influence absorbed from the home environment during infancy that combines with genetic predisposition and gradually becomes manifest as school age approaches; since the child's measured IQ becomes increasingly related to his parents' IQ, educational level, and socioeconomic status as he gets older (9).

Aside from these variables, there are other dimensions of the parent-child relationship that do have some immediate influence upon infant mental development, notably maternal love and acceptance as opposed to hostility and rejection (10). The effects of these maternal behaviors are inconsistent by age and sex, however; females develop more precociously during infancy under the shelter of a warm maternal attitude but lose their advantage by school age, whereas the opposite is true for males. A satisfactory explanation is still awaited for these sex differences in response to maternal care; and in any event, the demonstrable relation between maternal care and infant mental development is modest in size and falls below the concordance level for twins.

Therefore, the hypothesis is proposed that these socioeconomic and maternal care variables serve to modulate the primary determinant of developmental capability, namely, the ge-netic blueprint supplied by the parents. On this view, the differences between twin pairs and the similarities within twin pairs in the course of infant mental development are primarily a function of the shared genetic blueprint.

Further, while there is a continuing interaction between the genetically determined gradient of development and the life circumstances under which each pair of twins is born and raised, it requires unusual environmental conditions to impose a major deflection upon the gradient of infant development. For example, there will be some pairs where development of one or both twins is suppressed by serious prematurity or an impoverished environment; and there will be some pairs where the twins become discordant because of deviant prenatal conditions, birth trauma, or sharply differentiated life experiences. But for the great majority of pairs, life circumstances fall within the broad limits of sufficiency that permit the genetic blueprint to control the course of infant mental development.

RONALD S. WILSON

Child Development Unit,
University of Louisville
School of Medicine,
Louisville, Kentucky 40202

References and Notes

1. The complete report will be published by R. S. Wilson and E. B. Harpring, in preparation.
2. N. Bayley, *Genet. Psychol. Monogr.* **14**, 1 (1933); *J. Genet. Psychol.* **75**, 165 (1949); *Amer. Psychol.* **10**, 805 (1955).
3. ———, *Child Develop.* **36**, 379 (1965).
4. R. S. Wilson, *Human Hered.* **20**, 30 (1970).
5. ———, in *Progress in Human Behavior Genetics*, S. G. Vandenberg, Ed. (Johns Hopkins Press, Baltimore, 1968), p. 287. As a prelude to this analysis, the means and standard deviations of the test scores were compared for MZ and DZ twins, and no significant differences were found at any age. In addition, the between-subject variability (from which the between-pair and within-pair variances are derived), was found to be comparable among MZ and DZ twins for all analyses of overall developmental level and profile contour.
6. Another reason for performing a separate analysis for each year is that the analysis requires test scores from both members of the pair at all ages, so if any score is missing, the pair is excluded. The sample shrinkage in each zygosity group due to exclusions is within tolerable limits for the set of scores obtained within each year, but it becomes prohibitive when the entire age range is covered.
7. W. R. Thompson and J. Grusec, in *Carmichael's Manual of Child Psychology*, P. H. Mussen, Ed. (Wiley, New York, 1970), p. 633.
8. A. J. Reiss, *Occupations and Social Status* (Free Press, New York, 1961).
9. N. Bayley, in *Carmichael's Manual of Child Psychology*, P. H. Mussen, Ed. (Wiley, New York, 1970), p. 1163.
10. ——— and E. S. Schaefer, *Monogr. Soc. Res. Child Develop.* **29**, (No. 97), 6 (1964).
11. I thank J. Buren, J. Gresham, E. Harpring, P. McGinty, M. Moseson, J. Parker, and B. Slaven for testing the twins. Supported by NIH grant HD 03217.

14 April 1971; revised 12 October 1971 ∎

From A. R. Jensen (1970). Behaviour Genetics, *Vol 1, No. 2, 133–146, by kind permission of the author and Plenum Publishing Corporation*

IQ's OF IDENTICAL TWINS REARED APART

Arthur R. Jensen

Institute of Human Learning

University of California, Berkeley

ABSTRACT—A new analysis of the original data from the four largest studies (Newman, Freeman and Holzinger, 1937; Shields, 1962; Juel-Nielsen, 1965; Burt, 1955) of the intelligence of monozygotic twins reared apart, totaling 122 twin pairs, leads to conclusions not found in the original studies or in previous reviews of them. Statistical analysis of the twin differences reveals no significant differences among the twin samples in the four studies; all of them can thus be viewed statistically as samples from the same population. They can therefore be pooled for more detailed and powerful statistical treatment.

The 244 individual twins' IQ's are normally distributed, with the mean $= 96.82$, $SD = 14.16$. The mean absolute difference between twins is 6.60 ($SD = 5.20$), the largest difference being 24 IQ points. The frequency of large twin differences is no more than would be expected from the normal probability curve. The overall intraclass correlation between twins is .824, which may be interpreted as an upper-bound estimate of the heritability (h^2) of IQ in the English, Danish, and North American Caucasian populations sampled in these studies. The absolute differences between twins (attributable to nongenetic effects and measurement error) closely approximate the chi distribution; this fact indicates that environmental effects are normally distributed. That is, if $P = G + E$ (where P is phenotypic value, G is genotypic value, and E is environmental effect), it can be concluded that for this population P, G, and E, are each normally distributed. There is no evidence of asymmetry or of threshold conditions for the effects of environment on IQ. The lack of a significant correlation ($r = -0.15$) between twin-pair means and twin-pair differences indicates that magnitude of differential environmental effects is not systematically related to intelligence level of twin pairs.

COMPARISON of monozygotic (MZ) twins reared apart is conceptually the simplest method of estimating the broad heritability of a characteristic. Theoretically, the characteristic's total phenotypic variance (V_P) in the population is analyzable into a genetic component (V_G), a nongenetic (or "environmental") component (V_E), a component attributable to the covariance of genotypes and environments (V_{GE}), a component due to the interaction (i.e., the non-additive effects) of genetic and environmental factors (V_I), and a variance component due to measurement error (V_e). Thus:

$$V_P = V_G + V_E + V_{GE} + V_I + V_e.$$

Heritability in the broad sense is defined as $h^2 = V_G/V_P$, or, if corrected for attenuation (errors of measurement), as $h_c^2 = V_G/(V_P - V_E)$.

The correlation between pairs of individuals can be expressed as the proportion of the variance components that the members of each pair have in common:

$$r = \frac{\text{Sum of Variance Components in Common}}{\text{Total Variance}}$$

Behavior Genetics

In an idealized experiment to estimate h^2, therefore, we would assign each member of a pair of genetically identical individuals to different environments entirely at random at the moment of conception, and then determine the correlation between the pairs at some later stage of their development. Since the environmental conditions are randomized there would be no correlation between pairs due to environmental effects and there would be no correlation between genotypes and environments, at least at the outset. (Different genotypes can influence the environment differently, thereby producing some genotype X environment covariance. This component is usually regarded as part of the genetic variance in heritability studies of socially conditioned characteristics.) V_G, therefore, is the only component our idealized pair would share in common, and so the correlation between them would be equal to $V_G/V_P = h^2$.

The closest approximation to this idealized experiment in reality is the study of MZ twins separated soon after birth, or in infancy and early childhood, and reared separately. Unfortunately, in such studies there is always some uncertainty about the degree to which the nongenetic variance components are common to the separated twins. There is little, if any, real doubt in the major studies about the genetic component. Errors in the determination of zygosity in these studies are highly improbable. Any such errors, of course, would subtract from V_G and thus would result in a lower value of h^2. The nongenetic components are much more questionable. There is never truly random assignment of separated twins to their foster homes. Some separated twins are reared, for example, in different branches of the same family. And twins put out for adoption rarely go into the poorest homes. Furthermore, separated twins have the same mother prenatally, and to whatever extent there are favorable or unfavorable maternal conditions that might affect the twins' intrauterine development, these conditions are presumably more alike for twins than for singletons born to different mothers. On the other hand, twin correlation due to common nongenetic factors is counteracted to some unknown extent by effects occurring immediately after fertilization which create inequalities in the development of the twins. Darlington (1954) points to nuclear, nucleocytoplasmic, and cytoplasmic differences occurring in the first stages of cell division that would cause MZ twins to be less alike than their genotype at the moment of fertilization. Some of these conditions of embryological asymmetry do not affect singletons or dizygotic (DZ) twins. Partly for this reason DZ twins are more alike in birth weight than MZ twins. Although the biologic discordances referred to by Darlington affect only a minority of MZ twins, he concludes that their total effect is sufficient to lead to a gross underestimate in all twin studies of the force of genetic determination.

The correlation between MZ twins reared apart, therefore, cannot be taken at its face value as the most valid estimate of h^2. It must be checked against estimates of h^2 obtained by other means which involve more complex formulas (and often additional assumptions) for estimating heritability from a variety of kinship correlations, including unrelated children reared together and the comparison of correlations for MZ and DZ twins. Estimates of h^2 from MZ twins reared apart are, so to speak, cross-validated when similar values of h^2 are found by other methods, assuming that similar biases do not operate in the same direction or that they are statistically controlled. There is, in fact, quite substantial agreement among the various methods and types of data for estimating heritability. Using practically all the appropriate data to be found in the literature, heritability estimates for intelligence are distributed about an average value of close to 0.8 (Jensen, 1969). MZ twins reared apart show a correlation of similar magnitude for intelligence.

The questions posed by the present study are: do the major researches on MZ twins reared apart show consistency with one another in estimates of the heritability of intelligence? Are the main parameters of these samples sufficiently alike to permit the data from the several studies to be analyzed as a total composite that would allow new and stronger inferences than would be possible for any one of the studies viewed by itself?

METHOD

The published literature contains only four major studies of the intelligence of MZ twins reared apart (Newman et al., 1937; Shields, 1962; Juel-Nielsen, 1965; Burt, 1966). There are a few single sets of separated MZ twins scattered in the literature, but they are either psychiatric cases or do not present adequate intelligence test data for the purpose of the present analysis. The four major studies, based on twins from the Caucasian populations of England, Denmark, and the United States, comprise a total of 122 sets of MZ twins separated early in life and reared apart. Details concerning the twins' sex, age of separation, environmental circumstances, case histories, and so on, are to be found in the original publications. The present analysis is based on the individual intelligence test scores of the 244 subjects.

The data

Burt (1966). The 53 pairs in Burt's sample were obtained largely from schools in London. All had been separated at birth or during their first six months of life. Their IQ's were obtained from an individual test, the English adaptation of the Stanford–Binet, with mean = 100, SD = 15.

Shields (1962). The 44 pairs in Shield's sample were adults obtained from all parts of the British Isles. (One twin was found as far away as South America.) All of Shields' twins were separated before 6 months of age and 21 of the pairs were separated at birth. Complete intelligence test scores were obtained on only 38 of the 44 sets of twins. Two tests were used: Raven's Mill Hill Vocabulary Scale (a synonyms multiple-choice test), and the Dominoes (D48) test (a timed twenty-minute nonverbal test of intelligence). The Dominoes test has a high g loading (.86) and correlates .74 with Raven's Progressive Matrices. Since Shields presented the results of these tests in the form of raw scores, it was necessary to convert them to the standard IQ scale. A raw score of 19 on the Vocabulary scale and of 28 on the Dominoes Test correspond to IQ 100 in the general population. The raw score means were transformed in accord with these population IQ values and the standard deviation was transformed to accord with the population value of SD = 15. The IQ's thus obtained on each test were then averaged to yield a single IQ measure for each subject.

Behavior Genetics

Newman, et al. (1937). These 19 twin pairs were obtained in the United States and were tested as adults. In 18 cases the age of separation was less than 25 months, and in 9 it was less than 6 months. About the one pair that was separated at 6 years (and tested at age 41) Newman *et al.,* states: ". . . the twins were separated at six years, somewhat late for our purposes; but we had information that the environments of the twins had been so markedly different since separation that we decided to add the case to our collection" (p. 142). (These twins differed by 9 IQ points.)

Stanford–Binet IQ's were obtained on all subjects.

Juel-Nielsen (1965). These 12 pairs were obtained in Denmark. The age of separation ranges from 1 day to 5¾ years; 9 were separated before 12 months. IQ's were obtained by an individual test, a Danish adaptation of the Wechsler-Bellevue Intelligence Scale (Form I), which in the general population has a mean $= 100$ and $SD = 15$.

TABLE 1

IQ's for MZ Twins Reared Apart

Burt (1966), $N = 53$ Pairs

A	B	A	B	A	B	A	B	A	B
68	63	94	86	93	99	115	101	104	114
71	76	87	93	94	94	102	104	125	114
77	73	97	87	96	95	106	103	108	115
72	75	89	102	96	93	105	109	116	116
78	71	90	80	96	109	107	106	116	118
75	79	91	82	97	92	106	108	121	118
86	81	91	88	95	97	108	107	128	125
82	82	91	92	112	97	101	107	117	129
82	93	96	92	97	113	108	95	132	131
86	83	87	93	105	99	98	111	......	......
83	85	99	93	88	100	116	112	......	......

Shields (1962), $N = 38$ Pairs*

A	B	A	B	A	B	A	B	A	B
95	87	109	102	102	108	76	79	84	68
96	100	98	110	113	111	91	84	121	121
95	79	101	87	89	93	103	116	107	111
71	75	99	108	88	110	98	94	74	69
86	84	99	97	96	99	94	76	79	84
105	105	69	71	85	84	95	101	107	106
93	76	86	85	89	84	96	97	......	......
83	89	107	105	90	107	63	73	......	......

Newman *et al.* (1937) $N = 19$ Pairs

A	B	A	B	A	B	A	B	A	B
85	97	89	93	102	96	94	95	105	115
78	66	94	102	122	127	84	85	96	77
99	101	105	106	116	92	90	91	79	88
106	89	77	92	109	116	88	90	......	......

Juel-Nielsen (1965) $N = 12$ Pairs

A	B	A	B	A	B	A	B	A	B
120	128	100	94	99	105	114	124	......	......
104	99	111	116	100	94	114	113	......	......
99	108	105	97	104	103	112	100	......	......

*IQ's transformed from raw scores on Mill Hill Vocabulary tests and the Domino D48 Test. (See text for explanation.)

IQ's of Identical Twins Reared Apart

The IQ's of all the twins in the four studies are given in Table 1.

RESULTS

The main statistical parameters of the separate studies and of the combined data are shown in Table 2. The few instances of slight discrepancies between these statistics and the corresponding figures of the original authors are all within the range of rounding error. All the present analyses were calculated by computer, with figures carried to five decimals and not rounded till the final product.

TABLE 2

Statistics on IQ's of MZ Twins

Study	N (Pairs)	Mean IQ	SD	$|d|$	SD_d	r_i	r_d
Burt	53	97.7	14.8	5.96	4.44	.88	.88
Shields	38	93.0	13.4	6.72	5.80	.78	.84
Newman *et al.*	19	95.7	13.0	8.21	6.65	.67	.76
Juel-Nielsen	12	106.8	9.0	6.46	3.22	.68	.86
Combined	122	96.8	14.2	6.60	5.20	.82	.85

Distribution of IQ's

The mean IQ of the MZ twins is slightly below the population mean. This is a general finding for twins reared together or apart and is probably related to the intrauterine disadvantages of twinning, including lowered birth weight. The small Juel-Nielsen sample is atypical in having a mean IQ above 100. The stand-

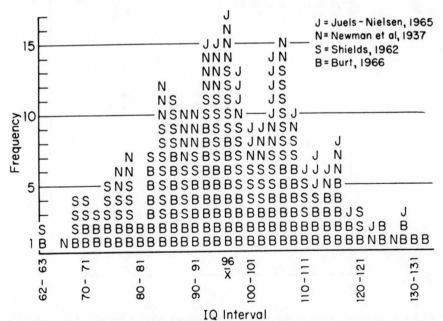

FIGURE 1. IQ distribution of 244 MZ twins reared apart, from four studies. The distribution does not deviate significantly from normality.

Behavior Genetics

ard deviation of the twin IQ's is only slightly less than the 15 points in the general population. Figure 1 shows the form of the IQ distribution. It extends over a range of 71 IQ points, or 4.7 sigmas, which would include approximately 98 percent of the general population. A chi square test of the goodness of fit shows that the IQ distribution of Figure 1 does not depart significantly from normality. The chi square based on eight subdivisions of the distribution is only 3.08, $p = 0.80$. (Chi square with 7 degrees of freedom must exceed 14.07 for significance at the .05 level.) It can be concluded that the IQ's of the total sample of 244 twins are quite typical and representative of the distribution of intelligence in the general population.

Correlation between twins

The intraclass correlations (r_i) between twins are given in Table 2. A correlation scatter diagram for all twins is shown in Figure 2. Twins were assigned to the A and B axes in such a way as to equalize the means of the two distributions. The intraclass correlation (r_i) represented by the scatter diagram is .82. Corrected for attenuation (i.e., test unreliability), assuming the upper-bound for Stanford–Binet test reliability of .95, the twin correlation would be .86.

It is interesting to compare the scatter diagram for IQ's shown in Figure 2 with a scatter diagram for the socioeconomic status (SES) of the homes in which

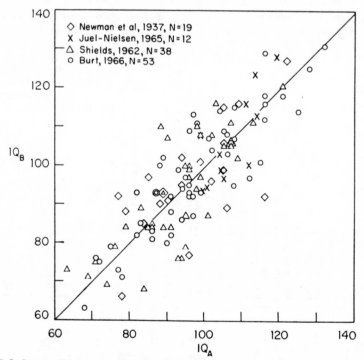

FIGURE 2. Scatter diagram showing correlation between IQ's of 122 sets of co-twins (A and B assigned at random). The obtained intraclass correlation (r_i) is 0.82. The diagonal line represents perfect correlation ($r_i = 1.00$).

IQ's of Identical Twins Reared Apart

the twins were reared. The one study which classified subjects in terms of *SES*, based on parents' or foster parents' occupation, is Burt's. The six categories were (1) higher professional, (2) lower professional, (3) clerical, (4) skilled, (5) semi-skilled, (6) unskilled. The seven cases reared in residential institutions are omitted from this analysis, since there is no basis for assignment to one of the six *SES* categories. The scatter diagram is shown in Figure 3. It represents a correlation of 0.03 between the SES of the homes of the separated twins in Burt's

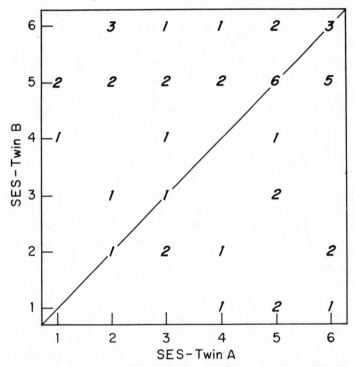

FIGURE 3. Scatter diagram of socioeconomic status (SES, based on six occupational categories of the parents, from "professional" (#1) to "unskilled" (#6)) for 46 co-twins in the Burt (1966) study. The numbers in the scatter diagram represent frequencies of twin-pairs. (Assignment to A and B is the same as in Figure 2.) The intraclass correlation (r_i) between co-twins' SES is 0.03.

sample. Obviously virtually none of the correlation between twins' IQ's is attributable to similarities in their home environments when these are classified by *SES* in terms of the parents' occupation.

The intraclass correlations for IQ in the four studies differ from one another mainly because of differences in the restriction of range of IQ's in the various samples. The magnitude of r_i is, of course, partly a function of the sample variance. The magnitude of r_i by itself, therefore, can be a somewhat deceptive indicator of the actual magnitude of twin differences (or similarities) relative to the population variance. For this reason the most crucial statistic in twin data is the absolute difference between twins.

Behavior Genetics

Twin differences in IQ

The mean absolute difference ($|\bar{d}|$) between twins and the standard deviation of the differences (SD_d) are shown in Table 2. Since the absolute difference between twins also contains measurement error due to imperfect reliability of the tests, the $|\bar{d}|$ of 6.60 should be compared to the value of 4.68, which is the mean difference between forms L and M of the Stanford–Binet administered to the same persons. The SD of these differences is 4.13 (Terman and Merrill, 1937, p. 46). Some of this difference, of course, reflects gains due to the practice effect of the first test upon the second. But the mean difference of 6.60 can be corrected for attenuation assuming the upper bound reliability for the Stanford–Binet of .95, which results in a "true" absolute difference of 5.36

It is proposed that the absolute differences between twin's IQ's can be used to compute a correlation coefficient which has the same scale as the Pearson and intraclass correlation but indicates the degree of similarity between twins relative to the similarity between persons paired at random from the general population. This can be called a "difference correlation," signified as r_d. This is a useful statistic in studying kinship resemblance because it preserves the actual magnitude of the difference between kinship pairs. For example, even if there were a perfect Pearson r (or intraclass correlation) between relatives, r_d would be less than 1.00 if there was any mean difference between the related persons (as would be the case if one member of each pair of MZ twins were reared in a very unfavorable environment and one member in a very favorable environment). Thus r_d should be reported in twin studies (and other kinship studies) to supplement the usual correlation coefficient (Pearson or intraclass). The value of r_d is not sensitive to the sample variance. Imagine that by some fluke we obtained a sample of twins with no differences between the means of the twin pairs; even if the average difference between members of each pair were small, the intraclass correlation (or Pearson r) between twins would be zero, suggesting that the heritability is zero. Especially when twin samples are small, it makes more sense to ask what is the magnitude of the twin differences relative to differences among unrelated persons in the general population. The answer is provided by r_d. The formula for r_d is

$$r_d = 1 - \left(\frac{|\bar{d}_k|}{|\bar{d}_P|} \right)^2 \quad ,$$

where

$|\bar{d}_k|$ = mean absolute difference between kinship members,
$|\bar{d}_P|$ = mean absolute difference between all possible paired comparisons in the general population, and

$$|\bar{d}_P| = \frac{2\sigma}{\sqrt{\pi}} = 1.13\sigma.$$

Unless one has an estimate of σ in the population from which the kinship groups are a sample or to which one wishes to generalize concerning r_d, this statistic cannot be used.

IQ's of Identical Twins Reared Apart

It can be seen in Table 2 that the values of r_d are much more consistent than r_i among the four studies. Corrected for attenuation (reliability $= .95$) the composite r_d of .85 becomes .88. This value should be interpreted as an estimate of h^2 only with caution, since it is uncertain just how much of the nongenetic variance is common to the separated twins. The studies do not differ significantly in r_d, because the values of $|\bar{d}|$ themselves do not show significant differences among the studies. An analysis of variance to test the significance of differences in $|\bar{d}|$ in the four studies yielded an $F = 0.87$, $df = 3$ and 118, $p < 0.46$. Thus the studies clearly do not differ significantly in the magnitude of twin differences. Bartlett's test was performed on the standard deviations of the absolute differences (SD_d) and revealed that on this parameter the differences among the studies are nonsignificant at the .01 level.

Figure 4 shows the frequency distribution of the absolute differences between twins. These are, of course, composed of environmental effects plus errors of

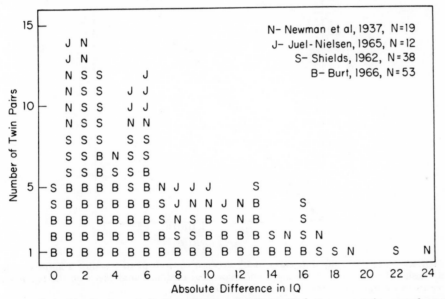

FIGURE 4. Distribution of absolute differences ($|d|$) in IQ between co-twins reared apart. This distribution closely approximates the chi distribution.

measurement. Extreme differences are rare; in only 3 cases does $|\bar{d}|$ exceed the average difference of 17 IQ points between all possible pairs of persons in the population; and in only 19 cases (16 percent) do the differences exceed the average difference of 12 IQ points between full siblings reared together, while 16 percent of the differences exceed the mean difference of about 11 IQ points generally found between DZ twins reared together. Since the differences shown in Figure 4 represent environmental effects (and random errors of measurement), these results should permit some inference about the distribution of environmental effects on IQ.

Behavior Genetics

Distribution of environmental effects

The distribution of absolute differences shown in Figure 4 closely resembles a chi distribution. If one draws pairs of values at random from a normal distribution, the absolute differences between the values in each pair yield the chi distribution, which, in effect, is one half of the normal distribution. One can think of the chi distribution as consisting of the normal distribution folded over on itself, with the fold at the median. (The corresponding deviations above and below the median, of course, are added together.) Therefore, one can graphically test a distribution for goodness of fit to the chi distribution by plotting the obtained distribution on a normal probability scale after the percentiles of the distribution have been "unfolded" at the median. This "unfolding" is simply achieved by the transformation 50 + %ile/2. If these values when plotted on the normal probability scale fall approximately along a straight line, it is evidence that the distribution does not differ significantly from chi. Figure 5 shows

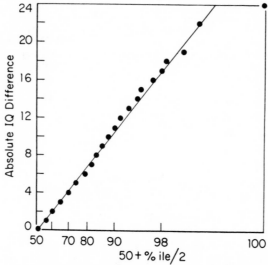

FIGURE 5. The absolute differences in IQ between co-twins plotted against a normal probability scale. The close fit to the straight line shows that environmental effects on the IQ, as represented by co-twin differences, are normally distributed.

this plot. The goodness of fit of the data to a straight line is practically perfect with the exception of the one most extreme case among the 122 twin pairs—an IQ difference of 24 points. This is the frequently cited case of Gladys (IQ 92) and Helen (IQ 116) in the study by Newman *et al.* (p. 245). They were separated at 18 months and tested at the age of 35 years. They had markedly different health histories as children; Gladys suffered a number of severe illnesses, one being nearly fatal, while Helen enjoyed unusually good health. Gladys did not go beyond the third grade in school, while Helen obtained a B.A. degree from a good college and became a high school teacher of English and history.

What Figure 5 means is that the nongenetic or environmental effects, which are wholly responsible for the twin differences, are normally distributed. (The absolute differences are due to environmental effects plus measurement error; it is assumed that errors of measurement are distributed normally.) Note that this says nothing about the distribution of environments *per se*. The conclusion refers to the *effects* of environment on IQ. There is no evidence in these data of asymmetry or of threshold conditions for the effects of environment on IQ.

Since the IQ's (i.e., phenotypes) are themselves normally distributed (Figure 1), and since the environmental effects on IQ have been shown to be normally distributed in this sample, it follows that the genotypes for IQ also are normally distributed. (The sums of two normal variates also have a normal distribution.) That is to say, if $P = G + E$ (where P is phenotypic value, G is genotypic value, and E is environmental effect), it can be concluded that for these IQ data, P, G, and E are each normally distributed.

Since P, G, and E are distributed normally, it is meaningful to estimate the standard deviations of their distributions. (We assume test reliability of .95 and normally distributed errors of measurement.) Given these conditions and a twin correlation (r_d) of .85, the estimates that would obtain in a population with $\sigma = 15$ are shown in Table 3. Since in a normal distribution six sigmas encompass

TABLE 3

Components of Variance in IQ's Estimated from
MZ Twins Reared Apart

Source	σ	σ^2	% Variance
Heredity	13.83	191.25	85
Environment	4.74	22.50	10
Test Error	3.35	11.25	5
Total (Phenotypes)	15.00	225.00	100

virtually 100 percent of the population (actually all but 2×10^{-7} percent), and since the standard deviation of environmental effects on IQ is 4.74, it can be said that the total range of environmental effects in a population typified by this twin sample is $6 \times 4.74 = 28.4$ I.Q. points.

Genotype X environment interaction

A corollary to the finding that environmental effects are normally distributed is the question of whether a favorable environment raises the IQ more or less than an unfavorable environment depresses the IQ. If favorable and unfavorable environmental effects were asymmetrical, we should expect to find that the higher and lower IQ's from each pair of twins would have different distributions about their respective means. This is in fact not the case. Probably the way to see this most clearly is to plot the IQ's of the higher and lower twins in each pair against the absolute difference between the twins. This plot is shown in Figure 6. The mean IQ's of the higher and lower twins are 100.12 and 93.52, respectively. The difference is significant beyond the .001 level. The corresponding *SD*'s are 13.68 and 13.86; the difference is nonsignificant. The straight lines through the data points are a least squares best fit. The slopes of these lines (in opposite directions) are not significantly different. The correlation (Pearson *r*) between IQ and

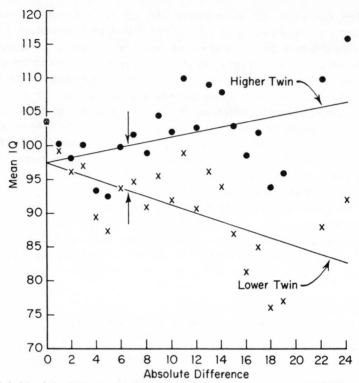

FIGURE 6. IQ of the higher twin (H) and the lower twin (L) plotted against their absolute difference in IQ. The straight lines are a least squares best fit to all the data (122 twins). The straight arrows indicate the bivariate means.

absolute difference is $+ 0.15$ for the lower twins and $- 0.22$ for the higher twins. The difference (disregarding the sign of r) is completely nonsignificant.

We can also ask: Is there an interaction between environment and genotype for intelligence? If there is, we should expect a correlation between the mean IQ of each twin pair (reflecting their genotypic value) and the absolute difference between the twins (reflecting environmental differences).[1] This correlation (Pearson r), based on the 122 pairs, turns out to be $- 0.15$, which is not significantly different from zero. These data, then, do not show evidence of a genotype X environment interaction for IQ.

Sources of environmental differences

The present data do not permit any strong inferences about the sources of environmental variance, but other twin research indicates that a substantial and perhaps even a major proportion of the nongenetic variance is attributable to prenatal and other biological influences rather than to differences in the social-psychological environment. The cytoplasmic discordances and the like pointed

---

[1] This method of assessing the GXE interaction was originally suggested and explicated by J. L. Jinks and D. W. Fuller in "Comparison of the biometrical genetical, MAVA, and classical approaches to the analysis of human behavior." *Psychological Bulletin*, 1970, 73, 311–49.

IQ's of Identical Twins Reared Apart

out by Darlington have already been mentioned. Differences in the favorableness of the intrauterine environment are reflected in differences in birth weight between twins (the differences being greater for MZ than for DZ twins), and the differences in birth weight are known to be related to IQ disparities in twins. In a review of this evidence, Scarr (1969) found that MZ twins who were both over 2500 grams in birth weight differed in later IQ by 4.9 points in favor of the heavier twin; when one twin was less than 2500 grams, the IQ difference was 13.3; and when both twins were less than 2500 grams, the IQ difference was 6.4. The mean difference of 6.9 IQ points between the heavier and lighter MZ twins (52 pairs) in the studies summarized by Scarr is not far from the mean IQ difference of 6.6 between all the twins in the present study.

It is sometimes argued that the IQ resemblance between MZ twins reared apart is largely attributable to similarities in their home environments. To the extent that this is true, it should lead to the prediction that characteristics with *lower* heritability (and consequently greater susceptibility to environmental influences), should show even less difference between MZ twins reared apart, as compared with MZ twins reared together, than characteristics of *higher* heritability. In this connection it is instructive to compare the IQ with tests of scholastic achievement for MZ twins reared together and reared apart. A review of studies of the heritability of scholastic achievement has shown much lower values of h^2 (the average being about 0.40) than for IQ (Jensen, 1967). The studies by Burt and Newman *et al.* provide the necessary scholastic achievement data for the relevant comparisons. These are shown in Table 4. Note that when twins are reared together (MZT), they differ much less in scholastic achievement than when

TABLE 4

Mean Absolute Difference ($|\overline{d}|$) Between MZ Twins Reared Together (MZT) and Reared Apart (MZA) for IQ and Scholastic Achievement
(Both scaled to $\sigma = 15$)

Study	IQ MZT	IQ MZA	Sch. Ach. MZT	Sch. Ach. MZA	Number MZT	Number MZA
Burt	4.79	5.96	2.40	10.29	95	53
Newman *et al.*	5.90	8.21	3.39	11.86	50	19
Combined	5.17	6.55	2.74	10.70	145	72

reared apart (MZA). No such large difference is found for IQ between MZT and MZA. If the MZA twin resemblance in IQ were due to environmental similarities, these similarities should be even more strongly reflected by scholastic achievement, and this is clearly not the case. Estimates of *within* and *between* family environmental effects may be obtained by subtracting (MZT)^2 from (MZA)^2 and obtaining the square root. For IQ the *within* environments effect is 5.17 and the *between* environments effect is $(6.55)^2 - (5.17)^2 = \sqrt{16.2} = 4.02$ IQ points. For scholastic achievement the *within* envirnments effect is 2.74 and the *between* environments effect is 10.34. The fact of much greater *within* than *between* environmental effects for IQ strongly suggests that the differences between identical

Behavior Genetics

twins in IQ arise largely from prenatal factors rather than from influences in the social-psychological environment. Just the opposite conclusion would pertain in the case of scholastic achievement.

CONCLUSION

Analysis of the data from the four major studies of the intelligence of MZ twins reared apart, totaling 122 twin pairs, leads to conclusions not found in the original studies or in previous reviews of them. A statistical test of the absolute difference between the separated twins' IQ's indicates that there are no significant differences among the twin samples in the four studies. All of them can be viewed as samples from the same population and can therefore be pooled for more detailed and powerful statistical treatment.

The 244 individual twins' IQ's are normally distributed, with the mean $= 96.82$, $SD = 14.16$. The mean absolute difference between twins is 6.60 ($SD = 5.20$), the largest difference being 24 IQ points. The frequency of large twin differences is no more than would be expected from the normal probability curve.

The overall intraclass correlation between twins is .824, which may be interpreted as an upper-bound estimate of the heritability of IQ in the English, Danish, and North American Caucasian populations sampled in these studies.

The absolute differences between members of twin pairs (attributable to non-genetic effects and measurement error) closely approximate the chi distribution; this fact indicates that environmental effects are normally distributed. If $P. = G + E$ (where P is phenotypic value, G is genotypic value, and E is environmental effect), it can be concluded that for this population P, G, and E are each normally distributed. There is no evidence of asymmetry or of threshold conditions for the effects of environment on IQ. The lack of a significant correlation between twin-pair means (reflecting genotype values) and twin-pair differences (reflecting environmental effects) indicates a lack of genotype X environment interaction; that is to say, the magnitude of differential environmental effects is not systematically related to the intelligence level of twin pairs. Additional evidence from comparison of the difference between MZ twins reared together with the difference betwen MZ twins reared apart suggests that most of the small twin difference in IQ may be attributable to prenatal intrauterine factors rather than to later effects of the individual's social-psychological environment.

REFERENCES

Burt, C. (1966). The genetic determination of differences in intelligence: A study of monozygotic twins reared together and apart. *British Journal of Psychology*, **57**, 137–53.

Darlington, D. C. (1954). Heredity and environment. Proc. IX International Congress of Genetics. *Caryologia*, **190**, 370–81.

Jensen, A. R. (1967). Estimation of the limits of heritability of traits by comparison of monozygotic and dizygotic twins. *Proceedings of the National Academy of Sciences*, **58**, 149–57.

Jensen, A. R. (1969). How much can we boost IQ and scholastic achievement? *Harvard Educational Review*, **39**, 1–123.

Juel-Nielsen, N. (1965). Individual and environment: a psychiatric-psychological investigation of monozygous twins reared apart. *Acta psychiatrica et neurologica Scandinavica*, (Monogr. Suppl. 183).

IQ's of Identical Twins Reared Apart

Newman, H. H., Freeman, F. N., and Holzinger, K. J. (1937). *Twins: A study of heredity and environment*, University of Chicago Press, Chicago.

Scarr, Sandra. (1969). Effects of birth weight on later intelligence. *Social Biology*, **16**, 249–56.

Shields, J. (1962). *Monozygotic twins brought up apart and brought up together*, Oxford University Press, London.

Terman, L. M., & Merrill, Maud A. (1937), *Measuring intelligence*, Houghton-Mifflin, Boston.

RÉSUMÉ—Une nouvelle analyse des données originelles tirées des quatre plus importantes études (Newman, Freeman and Holzinger, 1937; Shields, 1962; Juel-Nielsen, 1965; Burt, 1966) sur l'intelligence de jumeaux monozygotes élevés séparément et portant au total sur 122 paires de jumeaux, conduit à des conclusions qui n'apparaissent pas dans les études originelles ou leurs critiques faites jusquà présent. L'analyse statistique des différences entre les jumeaux montre qu'il n'y a pas de différence significative entre les échantillons de jumeaux des quatre études; ainsi, toutes les paires peuvent être considérées, d'un point de statistique, comme des échantillons d'une même population. Elles peuvent donc être regroupées afin de donner lieu à une analyse statistique plus poussée et plus détaillée.

Les quotients intellectuels des 244 jumeaux, pris individuellement, sont distribués suivant une loi normale, de moyenne = 96,82 et d'écart-type = 14,16. La différence moyenne, en valeur absolue, entre les jumeaux est 6,60 (écart-type = 5,20), la différence la plus grande étant égale à 24 points de quotient intellectuel. La fréquence d'occurrence de grandes différences entre jumeaux n'est pas plus grande que ce que l'on pouvait attendre en se basant sur la courbe normale de probabilité. Globalement, le coefficient de corrélation entre jumeaux à l'intérieur de chaque classe est égal à 0,824, évaluation qui peut être considérée comme au-dessus de la moyenne des estimations du degré de transmission héréditaire (h^2) du quotient intellectuel parmi les populations anglaises, danoises et causiennes de l'Amérique du Nord, d'où ont été tirés les échantillons pour effectuer ces études. Les valeurs absolues des différences entre jumeaux (attribuables à des effects non génétiques et à des erreurs de mesure) approche de très près la distribution du χ^2; ceci indique que les effects dûs à l'environnement sont distribués d'une façon normale. C'est-à-dire que si $P = G + E$ (où P est la valeur phénotype, G est la valeur génotype et E l'effet dû à l'environnement), on peut en conclure que, pour cette population, P, G, et E sont chacun normalement distribués. Rien ne laisse supposer qu'en ce qui concerne les effets de l'environnement sur le quotient intellectuel, il puisse y avoir une assymétrie ou un seuil. L'absence de corrélation significative (r = —0,15) entre les moyennes et les différences se rapportant à chaque paire de jumeaux indique que l'ampleur des effets différentiels dûs à l'environnement ne peut pas être systématiquement liée au niveau d'intelligence des paires de jumeaux.

ZUSAMMENFASSUNG—Eine erneute Auswertung der in den vier umfangreichsten Studien (Newman, Freeman and Holzinger, 1937; Shields, 1962; Juel-Nielsen, 1965; Burt, 1966) enthaltenen Daten über die Intelligenz von eineiigen Zwillingen, die getrennt erzogen worden sind (insgesamt 122 Zwillingspaare), führt zu Folgerungen, die in den ursprünglichen Studien bzw. in früheren Besprechungen derselben nicht enthalten sind. Die statistische Auswertung der Unterschiede zwischen den Zwillingen zeigt, dass zwischen den Zwillings-Auswahlgruppen. in den vier Studien keine bedeutsamen Unterschiede bestehen, sodass man sie statistisch alle als Auswahlgruppen der gleichen Gesamtmasse betrachten kann. Folglich können sie zum Zwecke einer detaillierteren und überzeugenderen statistischen Behandlung zusammengelegt werden.

Die Intelligenzquotienten der 244 eineiigen Zwillinge weisen eine Normalverteilung mit dem arithmetischen Mittel = 96,82 und der Standardabweichung $SD = 14,16$ auf. Der mittlere absolute Unterschied zwischen Zwillingen beträgt 6,60 (Standardabweichung $SD = 5,20$), der grösste Unterschied beträgt 24 IQ-Punkte. Die Häufigkeit der grossen Unterschiede zwischen Zwillingen ist nicht grösser als die normale Wahrscheinlichkeitskurve erwarten lässt. Die Gesamtkorrelation innerhalb der Gattung zwischen Zwillingen ist 0,824, was als Schätzung des oberen Grenzwertes der Erblichkeit (h^2) des Intelligenzquotienten für die kaukasische Gesamtmasse in Dänemark, England und Nordamerika, deren Auswahlgruppen in

Behavior Genetics

diesen Studien betrachtet wurden, gedeutet werden kann. Die absoluten Unterschiede zwischen Zwillingen (nichtgenetischen Einflüssen und dem Messfehler zuschreibbar) kommen der chi-Verteilung sehr nahe; dies bedeutet, dass die Umwelteinflüsse eine Normalverteilung aufweisen. Das heisst, wenn $P = G + E$ (P steht für den phänotypischen Wert, G für den genotypischen Wert und E für die Umwelteinflüsse), so kann geschlossen werden, dass im Falle dieser Gesamtmasse P, G und E jeweils eine Normalverteilung aufweisen. Es bestehen keine Anzeichen für das Vorliegen einer Asymmetrie oder von Schwellenwertbedingungen bezüglich der Umwelteinflüsse auf den Intelligenzquotienten. Die Abwesenheit einer bedeutsamen Korrelation ($r = -0,15$) zwischen den Zwillingspaar-Mittelwerten und den Zwillingspaar-Unterschieden deutet darauf hin, dass das Ausmass unterschiedlicher Umwelteinflüsse nicht systematisch mit dem Intelligenzniveau von Zwillingspaaren zusammenhängt.

Manuscript received April 27, 1970

PART VII

HEREDITY AND ENVIRONMENT: II, FOSTER AND ORPHANAGE CHILDREN

What twins are to the genetic analysis of inheritance of intelligence, as illustrated in the last section, foster children are to the genetic analysis of inheritance of intelligence through manipulation of the environment. In the first group we are dealing with experiments of nature in which we know, at least approximately, the degree of consanguinity and hereditary determination; in the second group we are dealing with experiments of society in which we know, at least approximately, the change of environmental circumstances that has taken place. And just as in the former case we have many different ways of using the outcome of the accidental experiment, so here too there are several ways of making use of the sad events which give rise to the fostering of children, or their arrival in an orphanage.

One of the most ingenious of these methods of analysis is due to Lawrence (1931), in a study which has been rather forgotten. He studied the Binet test scores of children in an elementary school, and those of same-age children in an orphanage, given the fictitious name of Dr. Smith's Home.

"Dr. Smith's Home is a large and important charitable institution, subsisting mainly on the funds of a 200-year-old foundation. Its purpose is to provide a healthy and moral home for illegitimate children who would otherwise be brought up under degrading conditions; and secondly, by relieving the mother of the trouble and humiliation involved in the possession of an illegitimate child, to enable her to start afresh and recover what she may have lost of social status.

For these reasons only the first illegitimate child of any mother is received. It is felt that to take others would be encouraging her in immorality. Where the father can by some coercion be compelled to provide for the child, the mother is assisted in applying that coercion, in preference to being relieved of the baby. As a result, all the cases are ones of desertion by the father. Careful enquiries into all the circumstances of the case are made, and it is insisted on that the mother should give the father's name and occupation as well as her own. No child more than a year old is taken. The numbers admitted at from 1 to 6 months are about equal to those from 6 months to a year. This means that the average age of admission is 6 months. British born children from any part of the British Isles are eligible. If a child is accepted into the institution, the mother resigns all claim to it, and in most cases does not see it again. A mother wishing to reclaim her child later is permitted to do so if she satisfies the authorities that she is able to maintain it and that it is in the interests of the child that she should do so. The children are given fictitious names, and are entirely ignorant of their parents' identity and circumstances.

The babies, on leaving their mothers, are boarded out in approved cottage homes in the country, at convenient distances from the town from which the organisation is controlled. The cottagers who receive the children are usually agricultural labourers of the better type. All homes are inspected at intervals. The children become very attached to their foster-mothers, whom they usually regard as their real mothers. When they give up the children, many of the foster-mothers keep in touch with them for years, visiting them at intervals, writing to them and sending them presents.

At between 5 and 6 years old all children are brought to headquarters, which is the original building of the foundation. This is their home until they are 15 or 16. It is near the centre of a big town, but is entirely secluded within its own walls. The building has sufficient space around it to form playgrounds for the children. The older boys and girls live almost entirely separately, though under the same wide roof. Each group has its own dormitories, dining hall, play-room, and its own side of the big playground. They see each other at Sunday Chapel, across the playground, and once or twice a week at singing practice, but the only occasion on which they meet socially is a yearly party, when they are allowed to play together freely.

The food of these children is very plain, but its nutritive value is carefully calculated, and to judge from the appearance of the children, is entirely adequate. As a group they look exceptionally strong, healthy, and well developed.

The Home has its own school within the grounds. There is an infant school where boys and girls between 5 and 7 years of age are educated together for about a year after admission to headquarters. They are then promoted to separate schools for boys and girls, where the instruction is about that of an ordinary good elementary school. The buildings are old-fashioned and the classes large.

All the children in Dr. Smoth's Home were given intelligence tests. This material, consisting as it does of children removed from their parents in earliest infancy, was felt to be sufficiently important for particular care in testing to be taken. Each child was therefore given an individual Stanford-Binet test. In addition all the children over 9 were given a Simplex group intelligence test. It was not possible, by the rules of the institution, for the investigator to see the case papers of these children, but the mother's occupation and that of the father were obtained."

After dealing with the average intelligence levels of the children, which are not of interest here, Lawrence goes on to say:

"Something might be learnt by a comparison of the range of intelligence within groups. If environment can affect intelligence scores we should expect the children reared in a uniform environment to be more alike than those brought up in dissimilar surroundings. The children within a single residential institution should show a smaller range of intelligence than for instance, those living in their own homes and attending a day school. The usual way of expressing the range of intelligence is by the coefficient of variation. Comparing Dr. Smith's Home and the London elementary school, as giving the extremes of uniformity and diversity within the limits of the present study, we find that the coefficients of variation are as follows:

	Boys	Girls
Dr. Smith's Home	13·93	12·94
Elementary School	15·39	14·04

These increases are very small, and are barely significant. They are in the direction one would expect, but are certainly smaller than might be assumed, considering the very great uniformity of environment inside Dr. Smith's Home."

The number of children involved (over 200 in Dr. Smith's Home, nearly 500 in elementary school) is large enough to make one have faith in the meaningfulness of the figures given. They show clearly that even the "very great uniformity of environment inside Dr. Smith's Home" does not reduce to any marked extent the variability of intelligence as manifested on Binet tests. The mean difference in variability is 1·46 for boys, 1·10 for girls, i.e., well under 10% of the variability of the

elementary school children. The difference in variability between elementary school boys and girls is 1·35, i.e. of about the same size, and probably quite accidental. The conclusion seems inescapable that reducing environmental variability during the childhood of a group of boys and girls hardly affects the variation in IQ resulting; this conclusion is in good accord with an hypothesis putting much more stress on heredity than on environment.

This conclusion has not always been the result of studies of foster children, and the work of the Iowa school, under the leadership of Dr. George D. Stoddard and Dr. Beth L. Wellman, on changes brought about by school and environmental factors is still often quoted as proving the great differences which good and poor environment can produce.

The first selection here reprinted, therefore, is a thorough examination of the rich material produced by these writers and their colleagues by a master of statistical evidence, Quinn McNemar. It points out all the many statistical pitfalls into which these investigators have stumbled, and may serve as a warning to later writers who have not always heeded the advice contained in this masterly survey. It may also serve as a warning to the reader not to take too seriously the frequent articles appearing in the popular press, or even in more serious journals, which advise him that this or that psychologist or educator has achieved remarkable successes in raising the IQ, or the school achievement quotient, of a group of dull or disadvantaged children. It is only after the most thorough reporting, and the most searching examination of the results, the design, and the statistical treatment of the data, that such reports should be considered seriously; most investigators have not unfortunately learned their lesson from McNemar's critical survey, and the selfsame errors and omissions are still too prevalent.

In complete contrast to the poorly designed and badly analyzed studies reviewed by McNemar is our second selection, a rightly famous study by Barbara Burks (1928), whose untimely death cut short a promising career. Unfortunately this monograph is much too long to be quoted in full, and accordingly only the main argument, and the data supporting it, have been extracted. The reader is advised to read the whole monograph as an example of the quality of work in those remote days preceding the great recession. There is very little work done nowadays that would begin to compare with this study in design, statistical treatment, care to consider alternative hypotheses, or the sheer quality of the thinking that has gone into the work. For better or worse, they don't write monographs like this any more!

The point of Burks' paper is a very simple one. Having located foster children assigned on what amounts to a random principle to their foster parents, she looked into the circumstances prevailing in the foster home, taking great care to include in her survey as many measurable features of the environment as possible; she then correlated these features with the IQ of the children involved, to determine the degree to which these features could be said to determine IQ. She also combined all the environmental aspects to determine the total amount which they might be said to contribute to IQ variance; the figure she arrived at was 17%. Thus the most thorough study of the influence of environmental variation on IQ variance gives a figure which neatly complements the figure of 80% for genetic influence.* It is interesting to note how close these figures are to an early estimate made by Thorndike (1940, P. 320–321) long before most of the results on which we now base our conclusions were available. He ascribed the following percentages to the components of variance in individual differences in intelligence:

Genes 80%
Training 17%
"Accident" 3%

The discussion of empirical results, such as those reported by the Iowa school, by B. Burks and others, is much facilitated and rendered more quantitative by reference to the "reaction range of IQ." Geneticists define the reaction range of a phenotypic characteristic as the range through which it varies in the population due to nongenetic influences; in the case of IQ it is best expressed in terms of probabilities under the normal curve. Assuming the heritability of the IQ to be ·80, then the phenotypic reaction range, i.e. the total distribution of environmental effects on IQ, is as shown in Figure 1; the shaded curve in this Figure is the normal distri-

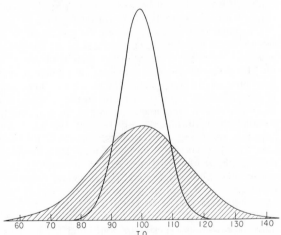

Figure 1. Shaded curve is distribution of IQs in population. Unshaded curve is hypothetical distribution if all genetic variance (when $h^2 = ·80$) is removed. From Jensen (1972).

* An interesting re-analysis of Burks data has been made by Wright (1931) using his method of "path coefficients to good advantage; this should be consulted by serious students.

bution of the IQ's in the population (Jensen, 1972). If we remove the 80% of the variance due to genetic factors and leave only the 20% of variance due to non-genetic factors, we see in the unshaded curve the resulting total distribution of IQ's for identical genotypes that express phenotypic IQ's in average environmental conditions (including intrauterine and pre-natal factors under the term "environmental"). In other words, the variance of the unshaded curve is only 20% of that of the shaded curve. Figure 2 shows what happens if we remove the effects of environmental influences on the total phenotypic variance; this removal shrinks the total variance by 20%, a change which is hardly noticeable.

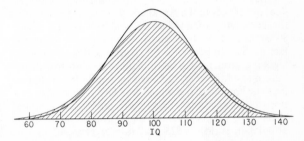

Figure 2. Shaded curve is distribution of IQs in the population. Unshaded curve is hypothetical distribution if all environmental variance were removed (when $h^2 = ·80$). From Jensen (1972).

When we talk about "environmental" influences in this context, we are using a term which is easily misunderstood; "non-genetic" might be a better term. As understood popularly "environmental" refers to causes which are reasonably well understood, and which can be manipulated, causes such as type of school, presence or absence of books in the home, poverty vs. affluence, and all the sundry causes so carefully studied by Burks in her paper. But environmental variance includes many more or less random effects with unknown, unpredictable, or as yet uncontrolled causes, many of them intrauterine. After all, even ·MZ twins brought up together are not phenotypically identical, and accordingly it cannot be suggested realistically that all members of the population would be subject to as little environmental variance as identical twins reared together? The manipulable or equalizable aspects of the environment probably affect much less of the IQ variance than would appear from the notion of the total reaction range, as shown in Figure 1. It may be useful to employ different terms in this connection, such as *innate*, *hereditary*, and *congenital*. Not everything that is innate is hereditary, since mutations can produce in a person innate tendencies not present in the parents; nor is everything that is congenital (i.e. something a person is born with), innate, since processes at birth, or influences in gestation, can produce marked effects.

Jensen (1972) has analyzed the Skodak and Skeels (1949) experiments in terms of the concept of the reaction range, and his discussion is quoted to illustrate the quantitative manner in which such findings should be treated in order to test properly the paradigmatic model we are discussing.

"The Skodak and Skeels study is usually held up as an example of evidence which supposedly contradicts the high heritability of intelligence. The fact that the adopted children in the Skodak and Skeels study turned out to have considerably higher IQs than their biological mothers is thought to constitute a disproof of the conclusion from many heritability studies that genetic factors are more important than environmental factors (in the ratio of about 2 to 1) in the causation of individual differences in IQ. Another way of saying this is that the heritability of intelligence is about ·80, i.e. about 80 per cent of the IQ variance is attributable to genetic factors. The 20 per cent of the variance due to environmental differences can be thought of as a normal distribution of all the effects of environment in IQ, including prenatal and postnatal influences. This normal distribution of environmental effects has a standard deviation of about 7 IQ points since the total variance of IQ in the population is $15^2 = 225$ and the 20 per cent of this which is attributable to environment is $·20(225) = 45$, the square root of which gives $SD = 6·71$. Is there anything in the Skodak and Skeels data that would contradict this conclusion? Skodak and Skeels based their study on 100 children born to mothers with rather low IQs (a range from 53 to 128, with a mean of 85·7, SD of 15·8. The children were adopted into what Skodak and Skeels described as exceptionally good, upper-middle class families selected by the adoption agency for their superior qualities. Of the 100 true mothers, 62 were given the 1916 form of the Stanford-Binet IQ test at the time of the adoption. Their children, who had been reared in adoptive homes, were given the same test as adolescents. The correlation between the mother's and the children's IQs was ·38. Now the *difference* between the mother's IQs and the children's IQs is not really the relevant question. Yet it is on this point that the interpretation of this study has so often gone wrong. What we really want to know is, how much do the children differ from the IQs we'd predict from a genetic model? Using the simplest model, which assumes that the children represent a random selection of the offspring of mothers having a mean IQ of 85·7 and are reared in a random sample of homes in the general population, the children's average predicted IQ would be 96. In fact, however, their average IQ turns out to be 107, or 11 points higher than the predicted IQ. If 20 per cent of the IQ variance is environmental, and if one standard deviation of environmental influence is equivalent to about 7 IQ points, then it might be said that the Skodak and Skeels children were reared in environments which averaged 11/7ths or about 1·6 standard deviations above the average environment of randomly

selected families in the population. This would be about what one should expect if the adoption agency placed children only in homes they judged to be about one standard deviation above the average of the general population in the desirability of the environment they could provide. From what Skodak and Skeels say in their description of the adoptive families, they were at least one standard deviation above the general average in socioeconomic status and were probably even higher in other qualities deemed desirable in adoptive parents. So an eleven-point IQ gain over the average environment falls well within what we should expect, even if environmental factors contribute only 20% of the variance. But this 11 IQ points of apparent gain is more likely to be an over-estimate to some extent, since these children, it should be remembered, were selected by the agency as suitable for adoption. They were not a random selection of children born to low IQ mothers. Many such children were never put out for adoption. (Most of the children were illegitimate, and as indicated in Leahy's (1935) study, illegitimate children who become adopted have a higher average IQ than illegitimate children in general or than legitimate children placed for adoption). Even so, it is interesting that Skodak and Skeels found that the 11 adopted children whose true mothers had IQs below 70 averaged 25 points higher than the 8 adopted children whose true mothers had IQs above 105. There are also certain technical, methodological deficiencies of the Skodak and Skeels study which make its results questionable; these deficiencies were trenchantly pointed out many years ago in critiques by Terman (1940, pp. 462–467) and McNemar (1940). In summary, the Skodak and Skeels study, such as it is, can be seen to be not at all inconsistent with a heritability of ·80 for intelligence."

The same type of analysis may be employed to a recent (as yet unpublished) experiment by R. Heber, in which two groups of genotypically similar children in the Milwaukee ghetto were compared, one group reared from birth in what may well be the lowest 1 or 2 per cent of environmental conditions found in the U.S.A., and the other reared experimentally in the most mentally stimulating environment well beyond the scale of naturally occurring environments. These children are now 5 to 6 years old, and Heber finds IQ differences between the group of between 20 and 30 points. This is not incompatible with the reaction range, as illustrated in Figure 1; yet popular accounts of this experiment have suggested that it in some way "disproves" the genetic model which we are considering. Even if the differences should persist into adulthood (as we have seen, gains are uncorrelated with status at such an early age, and it seems unlikely that the terminal difference will be anything as large as that obtaining now), the experiment gives results well within the range of our model to accommodate. We may conclude that before experimental results are considered to invalidate the model, accurate and informed quantitative calculations should be made to see whether in fact the results found are outside the genetic reaction range of the model. Verbal and literary interpretations and "common sense" conclusions have no place in science; what is required is a proper quantitative approach.

This discussion of the Heber study should not be taken as endorsement of the claims made therein, i.e. that gains of up to 30 IQ points were actually achieved; we are concerned entirely with the theoretical point of whether such gains, if actually produced, would invalidate the paradigm. There are good reasons for believing that the claims made for the Heber study are in fact grossly exaggeråted, and that in fact no proper conclusions can be drawn from it at all. Page (1973) has given a detailed criticism of the study, relying for his facts on Heber's 1971 Progress Report, which is the only available document relating to this experiment. He criticizes the experiment on three main grounds. (1) Assignment of subjects to experimental and control groups was not random. This point is absolutely crucial for experiments of this sort, and there is no doubt from Heber's own description that random allocation did not in fact take place. Instead Heber made use of a poorly described grouping procedure which could not be relied on to produce the desired effects. Furthermore, it is clear from some figures on morphology which Heber has published that gross differences in this respect existed between the E and C groups, differences which caused the E children to be two standard differences shorter than the C children by the age of two years! Such large differences rule out of court any attempt to treat the two groups as random samples from a given parent population, and invalidate any conclusions based on that assumption. (2) "Teaching the test". One of the perennial faults of educational experiments designed to improve performance is the failure to recognize the difference between *trait* and *score*. The aim is to produce generalizable improvement in the *trait* (intelligence, in this instance), but improvement in the *score* (on a specific IQ test) can be achieved by "teaching the test", i.e. by specific instruction on the problems contained in the final test, without any generalization. It seems clear from Heber's own description that at least some such "teaching the test" has taken place in his study, and this again would invalidate the conclusions. (3) Failure to specify treatments. There is practically no discussion of the details of the treatments given to the experimental group of children; what is said is so general as to be practically meaningless. Consequently it would be impossible to assess or replicate the study, and this failure, although unlike the other subject to remedial action in later reports, again makes it impossible to accept the recorded results as scientifically meaningful. Each of these three criticisms by itself would be serious; the three together seem fatal to any serious consideration of the claimed "30 IQ points improvement" through any environmental action.

It is to be hoped that a proper account of this experiment will soon be published, taking into consideration the criticisms mentioned; so far only uncritical and often enthusiastic press comments have been available, and it is on the basis of these that millions of people (including some psychologists) have come to the unwarranted conclusion that miraculous-sounding increases in IQ can be produced by environmental manipulation. Certainly the popular impression is that Heber's study has seriously impugned the paradigmatic position put forward in this book—even though he himself has stated that "Professor Jensen and I both agree that, regardless of the outcome in terms of data, the Milwaukee Project is in no sense a test of his position on heritability." This is a curious statement, because obviously any study of the effects of environment on IQ must also of necessity constitute a test of the paradigm's position on heritability, and indeed elsewhere Heber stated that "We are proceeding to test the social deprivation hypothesis." (Page, 1973). There is clearly some confusion here; were it not for the widespread if indirect knowledge that many people have of the existence of this project it would have been preferable to await clarification before commenting on it. However, such a course of action would to many people have looked like discussing Hamlet without mentioning the Prince of Denmark; hence these few comments on the Heber study seemed necessary in order to set the record straight. Perhaps social scientists will learn the lesson implicit in the history of this study, viz. that no news from an investigation should be issued to the press until a full and detailed scientific report has been made, and has been studied and if need be criticized by the scientific community. Unless this rule is followed, confusion will be made more confounded, and the popular view that "experts always disagree" will receive damaging support.

REFERENCES

BURKS, B. The relative influence of nature and nurture upon mental development: a comparative study of foster parents-foster child resemblance and true parent-true child resemblance. *Yearbook Nat. Soc. Studies in Education*, 1928, *27*(I), 219–316.

HEBER, R. Rehabilitation of families at risk for mental retardation: a progress report. Madison: University of Wisconsin, 1971.

JENSEN, A. On "Jensenism": a reply to critics. Invited address, American Educational Research Association, Chicago, 1972.

LAWRENCE, E. M. An investigation into the relation between intelligence and inheritance. *Brit. J. Psychology*, Monograph Supplement 1931, *16*, No. 5.

LEAHY, A. M. Nature-Nurture and intelligence. *Genetic Psychology Monographs*, 1935, *17*, 241–305.

MCNEMAR, Q. A critical examination of the University of Iowa studies of environmental influences upon the IQ. *Psychological Bulletin*, 1940, *37*, 63–92.

PAGE, E. B. The Miracle of Milwaukee. In press, 1973.

SKODAK, M., SKEELS, H. M. A final follow-up study of one hundred adopted children. *J. genetic Psychology*, 1949, *75*, 85–125.

TERMAN, L. M. Personal reactions of the Yearbook Committee. In: G. M. Whipple (Ed.) Intelligence: its nature and nurture. 39th Yearbook of the National Society for the Study of Education, 1940, Part I, 460–467.

THORNDIKE, E. L. Human nature and the social order. New York: Macmillan, 1940.

WRIGHT, S. Statistical methods in biology. *J. American Statistical Association*, 1931, *26*, 155–163.

From Q. McNemar, Psychological Bulletin, *37*, 63–92. *Copyright* (1940), *by kind permission of the author and the American Psychological Association*

Psychological Bulletin

A CRITICAL EXAMINATION OF THE UNIVERSITY OF IOWA STUDIES OF ENVIRONMENTAL INFLUENCES UPON THE IQ

BY QUINN McNEMAR
Stanford University

INTRODUCTION

During the last year or so the educational journals of the country have contained many articles from the pen of either Professor George D. Stoddard or Dr. Beth L. Wellman on changes in the IQ brought about by school and environmental factors. This popularization of research results has not been confined to learned journals, but has been spread abroad *via* more popular routes such as the newspapers and the radio. In an article in the *New York Times* under the signature of Dr. Wellman (28) will be found such statements as: " The extent of change under especially favorable circumstances may be sufficient to move a child from average intelligence to the so-called genius or extremely high levels. Or it may when conditions are especially unfavorable change children from average intelligence to feeble-mindedness." In *Childhood Education* (27) Dr. Wellman writes that the " group mental level of the children in a school is an important factor in the change in IQ of a particular child." In the *Journal of Consulting Psychology* Dr. Wellman says that " results from long-time consecutive studies of intelligence of children are demanding certain changes in our concept of intelligence in order that our concept conform with the facts. Data showing large changes in IQ have been steadily piling up, until they can no longer be summarily waved aside. There is no escape from the fact that the IQ's of children have possibilities of change over a large portion of the IQ range from genius to feeble-mindedness " (25, p. 97).

In an article under the co-authorship of Dr. Wellman and Professor Stoddard in *Social Frontier* (31) it is said that " some geniuses are made " and " some children are made feeble-minded " by their environments. Professor Stoddard, in *National Parent-Teacher* (17), after discussing marked changes in IQ says: " Such changes are not to be considered artificial or transitory." " They are durable." In a lecture on " The IQ: its ups and downs," by Professor Stoddard, one finds the statement: " The children of definitely moronic mothers and laboring class fathers, if placed early in good foster homes, will turn out to be above average in mental ability " (18, p. 49).

In *Progressive Education* Professor Stoddard (14) writes that " even scientific rigor and caution need not prevent us from saying flatly " that better nursery schools foster mental development. In the *Proceedings of the National Education Association* (15) Stoddard goes on record to the effect that " some of our recent well-documented work at Iowa . . . indicate[s] definitely that the intelligence quotients of young children can be raised by environmental stimulation." A recent issue of *School & Society* (16) contains an address of Professor Stoddard's in which he speaks of " the reaffirmation, in a most technical and substantial way, of the idea that the child is plastic," and states that " the scientific evidence against such a stand [that plasticity does not apply to the intelligence quotient] is mounting and cannot be denied."

That the new gospel is being carried beyond the educational journals is again evidenced by Dr. Wellman's article in the *Journal of Home Economics* (30), in which will be found the usual citation of changes for *selected* cases and the extraordinary statement that the orphanage children not enrolled in preschool " moved swiftly in the direction of feeblemindedness." We thus see from all of these quotations not only how positive are the generalizations from the Iowa studies, but also how widely the news is being spread.

The average reader will naturally assume that claims so extreme would surely not be made by well-known psychologists without the best of evidence. That the claims may sound exaggerated is anticipated in a statement of Wellman, Skeels, *et al.:* " These statements may seem unbelievably extreme " (10, p. 185). The writer does not believe that either the environmentalist or the hereditarian can be blamed for expressing a word of skepticism, but he believes that skepticism should lead to a minute examination of the research findings instead of resulting merely in sweeping condemnations thereof. In the critique to follow, we shall first examine in some detail the orphanage preschool project of Skeels, Updegraff, Wellman, and Williams, and then scrutinize the foster children study of Skodak

ENVIRONMENTAL INFLUENCES UPON THE IQ

and Skeels. Other studies will then be briefly considered, and finally we shall devote a section to a type of statistical treatment which is common to all the IQ studies of the Iowa Child Welfare Research Station.

The Orphanage Preschool Project

"A study of environmental stimulation" is the title of a monograph under the co-authorship of Skeels, Updegraff, Wellman, and Williams (**10**). On the grounds of an orphanage, which is described as a nonstimulating atmosphere intellectually, a model preschool was established. For every child, age 18 months to 5½ years, who attended this preschool there was a control child whose activities were only those of the restricted orphanage environment, and who had been paired with the preschool child on the basis of CA, MA, IQ, sex, nutritional status, and length of residence in the orphanage. There were 21 such pairs of children at the beginning of the project, but, due to the placement of children in foster homes, only a few of these continued for the full three years of the study. As children dropped out of either the preschool or control groups, new admissions were added with an attempt continually to equalize the two groups in relation to the factors considered in the original matching. Data are given to show that the original groups were equal with regard to CA, MA, and IQ, but the information given for the total groups, 46 preschool and 44 controls, indicates that the preschool group averaged 4.5 IQ points higher on the initial tests.

Initial IQ's were available for both the preschool and control individuals prior to school experience by the former. Over a period of three years retests were given at intervals of "approximately six months." Since, save for the five or six hours of daily school attendance of the one group, the two groups experienced the same living conditions in a nonstimulating orphanage environment, it would seem that any found differences in the mental development of the two groups could be attributed to school attendance. However, that the setup is not nearly so ideal as one might at first suppose is evidenced by the fact that, for any given comparison regarding the effect of preschool experience on IQ's, it was not possible to control more than two or three of the following variables at a time: (1) age, (2) initial intelligence, (3) orphanage residence, (4) actual number of days of school attendance, (5) days of residence between tests or retest intervals, (6) various examiners, (7) practice effects, (8) Kuhlmann-Binet or Stanford-Binet, (9) possible unintentional coaching in pre-

QUINN McNEMAR

school on material similar to many items in the tests used, and (10) differences in rapport in testing.

The first, and perhaps chief, finding regarding changes in intelligence is summarized herewith in Table I, which is a condensation of the authors' Table 2. The reader will readily see that no allowance has been made here for certain variables mentioned above (though the authors in their complete table do make some allowance for initial IQ by separate treatment for those initially above and below

TABLE I

IQ Changes According to Days Residence Between Tests

Residence	Preschool		Control		Difference in Change	D/σ_D
	N	Mean IQ	N	Mean IQ		
1 to 199 days	91	87.6	76	82.4		
	91	86.9	76	82.6		
		—.7		.2	.9	.7
200 to 399 days	90	82.3	96	77.7		
	90	86.0	96	76.5		
		3.7		—1.2	—4.9	3.3
400 or more days	40	80.1	65	77.2		
	40	84.7	65	72.6		
		4.6		—4.6	—9.2	4.2

80 IQ). The excess of the N's in this table over 46 and 44 is due to the fact that " a child was included as a separate case as many times as he met the requirement of residence interval " (days between tests). Thus, a child who had four tests was included in the appropriate residence group for first to second, second to third, third to fourth, first to third, first to fourth, and second to fourth tests. In other words, a child with n tests contributes $n(n-1)/2$ to the N's of Table I. This is the first of a series of jugglings in a monograph which is literally filled with highly questionable procedures. In the first place, one can raise a question as to the meaning that can be attached to an average change so determined, but, granting that it does have a definite meaning, one must ask about the proper formula for evaluating the changes in terms of sampling. If the authors care to dig deep enough into the statistics of sampling, they will find that the fundamental conditions for sampling are that each unit or individual in the universe being sampled must have an equal chance of being included in the sample, and that the drawing of one unit or individual must in no way affect the drawing of any other unit or individual. This latter condition can be stated differently: The drawing of each unit or individual must be independent of the drawing of any other unit or individual. These two conditions are the

ENVIRONMENTAL INFLUENCES UPON THE IQ

basic assumptions for all ordinary standard error formulas, and any departure from either of these two fundamental conditions invalidates the use of such formulas.

That the authors have violated the second condition of sampling is so obvious that we should not have to elaborate thereon. Once a child has been included, he is automatically included two more times if he has had three tests, or five more times if he has had four tests, or nine more times if five tests have been administered. Nevertheless, he is just one out of a defined universe of individuals who might be drawn for the sample. To say that this type of thing has operated similarly for the preschool and control groups, and therefore has not affected the results, is to miss the point.

In the absence of any adequate sampling error formulas for testing significance where we have this double type of sampling—a sample of individuals and a varying number of observations as we pass from individual to individual—we must either manufacture a formula for the situation or alter the situation in such a way as to permit the proper use of available formulas. Mathematical statisticians have found that formulas for similar situations are not easily derived unless certain simplifying assumptions are permissible which, when made, so restrict the obtained formulas as to make them inapplicable to the practical situation.[1] How, then, can we handle such data as these authors have collected? A reasonable way for surmounting the difficulty would be to state the problem as follows: Given two groups with known (measured) IQ's at the beginning of a project, one group being subject to stimulating nursery school conditions, the other group (control) remaining submerged in an intellectually stifling orphanage, then we can easily check the effect of preschool attendance on mental development providing we are willing to grant two assumptions: (1) that the initial IQ's can be taken as representing the intellectual status of the two groups at the beginning of the experiment, and (2) that the last, or final, IQ's can be taken as reflecting the later intellectual standing of the groups. A straightforward comparison of the mean changes from initial to final IQ's will permit conclusions as to the difference in gain or loss for the two groups. The sampling evaluation of found differences between the groups will involve nothing more complicated than the standard errors of two mean changes and avoids the indefensible procedure of using inflated N's.

[1] See Fisher, R. A. The statistical utilizations of multiple measurements. *Ann. Eugen., Camb.*, 1938, **8**, 376–386.

QUINN McNEMAR

For those who object that such a simplifying procedure does not take into account progressive changes, let it merely be noted that, after it has been demonstrated that a real difference in change between the groups has taken place, it will not be too late to examine the progress of the changes.

From the original data, which have been kindly supplied by Dr. Wellman, we have determined the mean changes from initial to final test for three residence intervals. In doing this we have not attempted to make any allowance for the aforementioned uncontrolled variables. The results of this treatment of changes, summarized in Table II,

TABLE II

IQ CHANGES BETWEEN INITIAL AND FINAL TESTS ACCORDING TO RESIDENCE
BETWEEN INITIAL AND FINAL TESTS

Residence	Preschool		Control		Difference in Change	D/σ_D
	N	Mean IQ	N	Mean IQ		
1 to 199 days	15	98.5	11	90.8		
	15	96.9	11	94.6		
		—1.6		3.8	5.4	1.2
200 to 399 days	10	79.4	11	80.4		
	10	84.5	11	82.8		
		5.1		2.4	—2.7	.9
400 or more days	21	82.9	22	81.4		
	21	85.7	22	75.7		
		2.8		—5.7	—8.5	2.2

should be compared with the authors' findings as given in our Table I. In view of the fact that a proper statistical treatment of the data has reduced their two significant critical ratios of 3.3 and 4.2 to .9 and 2.2, we are inclined to say that the authors' first, and main, finding has resulted from faulty statistics rather than from preschool attendance. Incidentally, the use of inflated N's not only exaggerates the statistical significance of the findings, but is also apt to mislead the layman into placing undue confidence in a result. For instance, in one of Dr. Wellman's popular articles we find the passage: " In two years' time a group of twenty-six children who averaged 90 in IQ dropped 16 points " (27). The correct N happens, in this case, to be only 11. It will be noted that such changes as have taken place, though of doubtful statistical significance, are in the direction of gains for the preschool and losses for the control group, but before we can attribute such changes to the stimulating effect of the preschool environment and the progressively degrading influence of the orphanage, we must ask about other factors which might account for the changes.

ENVIRONMENTAL INFLUENCES UPON THE IQ

One of the most important of the uncontrolled variables in the study has to do with the rapport between child and examiner. Nothing is said in the report about shyness, negativism, distractibility, or general coöperativeness of the children during the testing. The report does contain some information (pp. 23–25) which is highly pertinent. In their picturesque description of the children and their habits and attitudes which prevailed at the beginning of the project the authors make such assertions as the following: " The language of the children was in the great majority of cases either entirely or practically unintelligible "; " any constructive conversation seemed out of the question "; the children were " not accustomed to listening to the words of adults "; " the attitude toward adults was a strange mixture of defiance, wish for affection, and desire for attention "; there existed " a feeling of the individual against the world, expecting no quarter and giving none "; reaction to strangers was " the same [as] to wax figures "; there was " an almost invariable negative response to anything which the child could possibly interpret as potential coercion " and a " highly emotional response to unwelcome requests "; the children were " full of suspicion and mistrust " and " seldom in the frame of emotion or mind to face a situation "; they showed " lack of confidence in adults " and " generally violent and moblike reactions to new situations."

If this description is not highly journalistic, then the initial tests were invalid to begin with and unworthy of further consideration. It might be argued that this lack of rapport would be alike for the initial tests on the two groups, but what about later tests? The controls remain in the " bad " orphanage and would therefore be expected to become even less coöperative with the passing of time, whereas the preschool children would become more coöperative as a result of decent treatment by adults in the preschool. This factor alone might serve as an adequate explanation (if a statistically insignificant difference calls for explanation) for such divergences as exist. It is difficult to understand just how the authors could overlook this long-recognized and exceedingly important matter of rapport. At this point one is made to wonder why they forget a previous paper by one of them, Updegraff, in which it was reported, with substantial data, that " it has been found that an intelligence quotient obtained just previous to a young child's first experience in preschool is not reliable " (20, p. 164).

Let us now turn to the second main finding with regard to environmental effects on intelligence. The changes for both groups were analyzed according to initial IQ level: below and above 80, and by 10-point classifications. Inflated N's are again used in determining standard errors, with the result that all the critical ratios are spuriously high. Here we note a failure to appreciate the phenomenon of regression, which must be taken into account in this type of analysis. Without elaboration at this time on regression effects, which will be dealt with more fully later, we note a most amazing statement made by the authors with regard to the leveling effect of the orphanage environment on the control children: " Regardless of the original classification, all the groups headed for a final classification between 70 and 79 IQ. The effect of long residence for the control children was thus a leveling one, tending to bring all children to high grade feeble-mindedness or borderline classification " (p. 45).

This conclusion is based on a completely erroneous line of reasoning. The authors might have been expected to know that the only thing which kept their constructed curves from showing a greater leveling effect was the fact that the test-retest correlation was not zero. The interpretation of the authors can be exploded with a bang by asking for data on the variability of the group on the final tests as compared with that for the initial tests. This pertinent information is not included in the monograph. Direct computation (from the original data supplied by Dr. Wellman) shows a S.D. of 13.2 for the final test as opposed to 13.9 for the initial test. No doubt the authors will themselves be surprised to learn that the leveling effect was such as to reduce the S.D. by .7 of an IQ point, or to reduce the variance by less than 1%. Even for the long-residence group the S.D. is reduced only from 15.0 to 13.1—an unreliable drop. Evidently the leveling effect of the orphanage environment did not take place until the data had passed through the statistical laboratory.

In the subsequent analysis and discussion of the gains, the most important finding to emerge is a correlation of .28 between the actual number of days attendance by the preschool individuals and change in IQ's. The probable error of .04 attached to this r is evidently based on a combination N, partly individuals and partly observations; otherwise, the probable error for 46 individuals would be .09. How much of this obtained correlation reflects changes as due to " increased ability " and how much has resulted from increased rapport cannot be determined. Further analysis shows the changes in relation to percentage of attendance, and here (p. 50) we have the following remarkable finding: "Although between the 91 to 100 per cent group and the 61 to 70 per cent group there was only seven days' difference in actual attendance, the difference in IQ change was 7.0 points." This should be too much even for the most ardent nurturite.

We come next to a striking graph (Fig. 8, p. 54) which tells only a part of the story concerning IQ changes for the control group, in that it portrays individual curves only for *decreases* in IQ. The casual reader is likely to be much impressed by this visual demonstration of the effect of unfavorable circumstances on the IQ, but the critical reader's first reaction will be to raise a question concerning possible cases which might show an increase. The data for the seven curves in this figure may be briefly summarized in terms of loss from initial to final IQ: 103 to 60, 98 to 61, 86 to 62, 83 to 60, 85 to 71, 80 to 70, and 79 to 69. Elsewhere (25, p. 99), Wellman states that "these cases represent the trend for the larger group of which they were members." We are about to see that this is a gross misstatement of fact. Since no significance can be attached to the losses of 10 points by the last two cases, we have left four cases which show marked losses of 43, 37, 24, and 23 points, and one case which shows a loss of 14 points. But an examination of the original data reveals two control children who showed gains of 27 (70 to 97) and 22 (61 to 83) points, and one who gained 14 points. We find, moreover, that of 15 individuals in the control group who had received only two tests, one showed a loss of 18 points and four showed gains of 16 or more points. Evidently, residence in the orphanage did not tend " to bring *all* children to high grade feeble-mindedness or borderline classification" (p. 45; italics ours). Further examination of the original scores leads to the discovery of only three in the total preschool group, as compared to seven in the control group, who showed gains from initial to final of more than 14 points. These three children gained 25, 19, and 17 points. Thus, the greatest individual gains took place not in the preschool but in the control group. This fact is not mentioned, nor can it be discovered from their published data.

Further perusal of the data supplied by Dr. Wellman discloses additional facts which are highly pertinent. Despite the fact that the groups had comparable mean ages, 41.9 and 41.4 months, at the time of the initial tests (p. 17), there were seven in the control, as opposed to three in the preschool, group who were tested prior to 20 months of age. Now it happens that the three controls showing the largest losses (43, 37, and 24 points) were tested initially at less than 20 months of age. If we count the number tested prior to 24 months, we find seven for the preschool group and eleven for the control group, and five of these eleven are among the seven control children who provided the conclusion " that children of average ability may be made feebleminded " (p. 57). Surely some consideration should have been given to the question of the comparability of measures of " intelligence " at age 18 months with such measures at age 4 before even suggesting such a conclusion.

In summarizing a section on the later development, we learn that " of the children later adjudged feebleminded and transferred to the school for feebleminded, 75 per cent were from the control group " (p. 60). This percentage, coupled with the claim that the preschool and control groups were " originally equated " on the basis of intelligence, sounds quite impressive until it is recalled that the IQ's only of those in the groups at the beginning of the project were equated. For some unexplained reason the " attempt continually to equalize the two groups " when new admissions were added was not very successful. The 21 controls added five or more months after the beginning of the project averaged 83.3, as contrasted with 90.6 for the 23 new admissions to the preschool group. Another reason why the above percentage loses significance for all but casual summary-readers is the fact that it is based on only eight cases, six from the control and two from the preschool group.

The remaining part of the monograph deals principally with Merrill-Palmer tests, language development, general information, social maturity, and motor achievement. It is not our purpose to discuss these additional findings in detail, since a few major criticisms will illustrate the authors' general method of dealing with these topics.

The only result for the Merrill-Palmer test which approached statistical significance (critical ratio of 2.5) was a difference of nine IQ points in favor of the preschool group. How much of this is due to differences in rapport is unknown. In general, the analysis of the data on the Merrill-Palmer leads the authors to make strong claims for the effect of preschool, but when, for instance, one finds the statement that " the preschool subjects gained 21.5 points, while the control subjects lost 1.1 points " (p. 67), one wonders why the statement wasn't made to read: the *four* preschool subjects gained 21.5 points, *but one child contributed 11 points to this average,* while *seven* control subjects lost 1.1 points. This is just one of many unqualified statements in this monograph which are apt to mislead the hurried reader.

Despite the fact that the largest critical ratio for the language achievement data was only 1.5, the summary to the section is replete

ENVIRONMENTAL INFLUENCES UPON THE IQ

with positive statements regarding the superiority of the preschool group. Turning to the results for vocabulary, we find that " the preschool group clearly excelled the control group " (p. 97) in vocabulary quotient, but nowhere prior to this statement can one find a single critical ratio, either large or small. Furthermore, the vocabulary quotient used is a highly questionable concept in that it was obtained by dividing the median score made by the orphanage children by the median score made by normal or average Iowa City children of the same age. That the authors did not appreciate the artifacts which result from such a quotient is evident from the following quotation: " It is not clear why the quotients rose with age [from about 20 at age 2 to about 60 at age 5] in the control as well as in the preschool group " (p. 97). A few pages later one finds vocabulary and language achievement quotients being compared and the paradoxical conclusion that " the course of vocabulary development and of language achievement was in opposite directions " (p. 118). Apparently the authors were unaware of the fallacious nature of ratios based upon arbitrary score points. It may be that neither the numerator nor the denominator of such quotients represents anything remotely like a deviation from a real zero point. Make the vocabulary test either easier or more difficult and, presto, the quotients will bounce about.

The chapter on general information contains a statistical " believe it or not ": a critical ratio for the difference between means based on N's of 1 and 2; another for N's of 1 and 3; and still another for N's of 2 and 4 (p. 126).

In concluding this discussion of "A study of environmental stimulation " we quote from the authors' final chapter: " Taken all in all, the preschool exerted a profound influence upon the children during the period of preschool enrollment "; " the effect of long residence for the control group was that of tending to bring all children, regardless of initial intelligence classification, to high grade feeble-mindedness or borderline classification "; " the greatest decreases . . . arose for children originally of average intelligence who became feeble-minded." The authors say that these and other statements in the final chapter " may seem unbelievably extreme." We agree. In view of the questions and criticisms which we have raised, we are prepared to make a few statements which may seem unbelievably extreme to the authors and to psychologists and educators who may have uncritically accepted the claims made on the basis of this study. In the first place, there is not a single finding in regard to the influence of preschool upon mental development which could not be explained on the basis of rapport. In the second place, a critical study of the statistical jugglery reveals that differences in rapport need only be invoked to explain slight, statistically insignificant findings. And finally, the authors are guilty of continually playing up unreliable differences and ignoring not only alternative explanations, but also those parts of their data which do not fit with the environmental hypothesis.

CHILDREN IN FOSTER HOMES

The major part of Skodak's monograph (12) is devoted to a study of 154 foster children who had been placed prior to the age of six months. Of this group, 140 were illegitimates. After at least a year's residence in the foster homes all were tested on either the Kuhlmann or the Stanford Revision of the Binet, and some two years later retests were given. The Kuhlmann was used with children of ages 3½ or younger, while the Stanford was employed with the older children. The median age at first test was one year, seven months, and at the second test four years, one month. The average IQ of the true mothers was 87.7, their average education, 10 grades completed; the average education of the true fathers was also 10 grades completed, and their mean occupational status was 5.4, or .6 of a class below that for the general population. The foster fathers and mothers had, on the average, finished the twelfth grade, and the foster fathers rated 3.1, or 1.7 points better than the general population in regard to occupational status. Let us first consider the major finding of the study, namely, that 154 children, the offspring of parents assertedly much below average and who were placed in superior foster homes prior to the age of six months, were found after a year or more of residence to be above average in intelligence (mean IQ, 116 on first test; 111.5 on second test). This has been hailed by Skeels (8), who also reports on the same study, as " unexpected," and Stoddard speaks of this finding as a " shock to our expectations " (18, p. 47).

One might have anticipated that such shocking results would have led to a close scrutiny of the data rather than hasty acceptance. Just what are the facts?

Let us first examine the claim that " on the basis of information on the intelligence, occupation, and education of the mothers, and the general social status of the true families, it may be stated that on the whole the true family background of these children was inferior to that of the general population on these criteria, which are usually

ENVIRONMENTAL INFLUENCES UPON THE IQ

considered to be indications of ability and intelligence" (p. 102). The true parents are characterized by Stoddard (18, p. 48) as "poor stock." In contrast, the foster homes are described as superior to the average. Now to the evidence.

On the basis of Stanford-Binet tests of only 80 of the 154 true mothers, an average IQ of 87.7 was found. A chronological age divisor of 16 was used; had 15 been used, the average would have been 93.5. The mothers were tested by "various individuals" at three institutions, and "so far as could be determined" the Stanford-Binet was used "either in the completed or abbreviated form." Nothing is said about the expertness (or inexpertness) of the examiners, nor are we told when the tests were given. If, as presumably was the case, the tests were given just before or just after the birth of the illegitimate child, the results would be highly questionable. One would need to have a sublime faith in numerical test scores to take much stock in IQ's determined at a time of such profound emotional stress. The mean education of 144 of the true mothers was 9.9 grades completed, a value which is said to be below the average for the general population.

The intellectual level of the true fathers is inferred from the educational level attained by 88 of the 154 fathers and from the occupational status of 110 of the 154. The mean occupational status was 5.4, or 6 of a point (one-fourth of a sigma) below the general population mean of 4.8. It can thus be seen that the true fathers for whom information was available differed but little from the generality with regard to occupational status. When one considers that many of the fathers were doubtless young (nine were still students, hence unclassified) and therefore had not reached their ultimate occupational level, and when one further considers the likelihood that the 35 unknown fathers were above average, it seems doubtful that the occupational level of the true fathers was inferior. As to their educational achievement, it is reported that the mean grade finished by 88 known fathers was 10.2. This and the corresponding figure for the true mothers form part of the basis for the claim that the parents were subaverage.

At this point it might be well to do what Dr. Skodak did not do, *i.e.* find data on the average education of the generality of adults. In a bulletin of the U. S. Department of Education it is stated that "the median education in 1934 is only completion of elementary school" (32, p. 14), elementary school being defined as up to and including the eighth grade. This figure is for all U. S. adults and is likely lower than that for adults of ages corresponding to the true parents. No information is given, however, as to the ages of the parents, but it seems safe to guess that their ages ranged from about 16 up, with a majority under 30. The national school survival figures of Foster (4) indicate that those who were in the fifth grade in 1924 completed about nine grades. This figure agrees with that reported by Bell (1) for the median grade completed by 10,898 youths, 16 to 24 years of age in 1930. This sample was carefully chosen to be representative of the State of Maryland. Even allowing for the fact that the above findings may not hold for Iowa, we are compelled, on the basis of these three sources, to question the assertion of Skodak that the education of the known true parents was below the general adult population level. Perhaps they were actually superior.

Aside from the fact that the mean grade finished by the known fathers is above that for the generality, we have to inquire about the educational achievement of the 66 fathers for whom this was unknown. The best that one can do here is to make a conjecture, then check this with the opinion of others. Our guess is that the " unknown " fathers of illegitimate children are apt to be intellectually superior to known fathers, the intellectual superiority being a factor in their remaining unknown. The reader of this paper can judge for himself the reasonableness of this conjecture.

The above considerations lead the writer to believe that the true fathers were probably above average and that the true mothers were at least average. That the foster homes were above average cannot be doubted, but it has not been demonstrated that the true parents were so far below average as to provide a genuine set for a shock to one's expectations regarding the IQ's of the children. Furthermore, the shock might have been somewhat lessened by reference to norms for the Kuhlmann-Binet (85% of the first tests were Kuhlmann's). According to Kuhlmann (6, p. 13), children of 6, 12, and 18 months of age average 115, whereas, according to Skeels (8, p. 37), the foster children examined prior to 24 months averaged 119. For ages 2 and 3, Kuhlmann gives an average of 107, while Goodenough (5, p. 40) finds an average of 105. The average for the two-year-old foster children was 108. It is therefore possible that these foster children did not really score higher than the average.

Thus, when we consider the intellectual background of the known true parents, the possible level of the unknown parents, and the failure of the children to exceed appreciably the averages found for more nearly unselected children, we are forced to conclude that the

ENVIRONMENTAL INFLUENCES UPON THE IQ

intellectual level of the children is not above that to be expected from their parentage.

The above discussion has been concerned with the major finding based on a foster group placed prior to six months of age. Questions of more or less importance can be raised concerning several points in connection with the treatment of the data for this foster group. There is an indiscriminate mixing of Kuhlmann and Stanford-Binet test results with no thought to the generally admitted faults of the Stanford Revision at the preschool levels. Throughout the discussion, the characterization of the true parents is made to sound as if information were available on all. The difference between the means, 116 and 111.5, for the first and second tests on the children is said to be "slight" (p. 56), although the difference, when the complete formula for the standard error of the difference is used, happens to be 4.5 times its standard error instead of the reported value of 2.99, which Skodak obtained by ignoring the correlational term in the standard error of the difference formula. No concern is shown for the unreliability of testing at the tender age of one year, nor does the author ever seem to appreciate that what is called "intelligence" at these extremely young ages may be decidedly different from what is measured by the Stanford-Binet at ages 4 or 5. She contrasts her findings with researches on older children as though the measures of intelligence for the several ages had been proven comparable.

The correlation of mid-true-parent education with the first test IQ was .08 and with the second test IQ, .33. It is said (p. 78) that at the time of the second examination the correlation had increased "slightly," but was still "substantially" below correlations reported for own-parent-child comparisons. At this juncture she might have reproduced the correlations for own children, given earlier (p. 67), as reported by Goodenough, .35; by Burks, .27; and by Leahy, .48 and .50. Apparently the r of .33 is not "substantially" below that for own-parent-education child IQ relationships. Perhaps the hereditarian could here rescue something from Skodak's study which might tend to support his hypothesis.

On page 84 it is reported that the correlation between the IQ of the mothers and the IQ of the children on the first test was .06, and on the second test, .24. To show that these low figures are consistent with values previously reported in the literature, Snygg and Skeels are cited, but no hint is given that Skeels's data were based on 147 of Skodak's 154 cases. No mention is made of the fact that

QUINN McNEMAR

the *r* of .24 was attenuated (1) by unreliability of tests at young ages, (2) by the mixture of Kuhlmann and Stanford-Binet tests, and (3) by the circumstances under which the mothers were tested. Parenthetically, it might be noted here that Snygg (13) ignores a selective factor: the mothers who had passed the high school entrance tests were not included. This definitely restricted the range, and consequently reduced the parent-child correlation by an unknown amount.

It was also found that the older children in foster homes of superior occupational status had IQ's some 12 points higher than those in lower homes. This finding and the correlation of .18 between mid-foster-parent education and second test IQ are of reduced significance in view of the admitted selective placement as shown by the correlation of .30 for the education of true with foster parent, and as evidenced by Skodak's Table 9 (p. 74). From this table we note that there is a correspondence between foster-father's occupational classification and the following: true-father's occupation, true-mother's education, and IQ of true mother. It can be determined from the data given that the correlation ratio for true-mother's IQ on foster-father's occupational status is .35. This definitely indicates selective placement.

Thus, when the obvious selective placement is taken into account, it cannot be claimed that the child's IQ is causally related either to the foster-parental education or to occupational status. This factor of selective placement seems to have been entirely forgotten during most of the discussion and especially when points 2, 3, 5, 6, and 8 in the final summary (pp. 128–129) were written.

A highly questionable finding is the correlation of .49 between final IQ's of the children and an inventory which was devised to provide a measure of the intellectually stimulating value of the environment furnished by the foster homes. Obviously, a part of the obtained correlation can be accounted for on the basis of selective placement. Furthermore, examination of the items in the scale reveals that at least seven of 22 items pertaining to the nonphysical aspect of the home environment may actually be a reflection or function of the child's IQ rather than a producer thereof. For instance, does the child who spends a considerable amount of time reading thus raise his IQ, or does this activity merely reflect a high degree of intelligence? Does conversation of a child with adults lead to increased intelligence or result from native intelligence? That the factors measured by this inventory are not instrumental in changing intelligence is evidenced by the finding that those who gained 6 points or more from the first to second test were in homes with a mean inventory value of 85.2 as compared to 85.0 for the homes of those who lost 6 to 15 points and 81.7 for the homes of those who lost 16 or more points. (The S.D. for the scale was 14.3.)

From Skodak's study of the IQ's of 16 children of claimed feebleminded mothers flow the following momentous conclusions: " Thus mother's intelligence appears to have little if any relationship to or influence on the mental development of a child who is removed from her care in early infancy " (p. 91), and " The mental development of children of feebleminded mothers and the most inferior true-family backgrounds is indistinguishable from that of children whose mothers are not feebleminded " (p. 104). Wishful thinkers will accept such statements on faith, but others will insist on additional information concerning the intelligence and testing of the mothers and concerning the " other criteria " by which the mothers were judged feebleminded. Certainly, only the careless will accept the statement that the mean education of the true fathers was ninth grade, but not even the critical will glean from this monograph the fact that information on education was available for only seven of the 16 fathers of these children. This important bit of information was found in another report. More data on the tests and the testing of the children would also be needed for a proper evaluation, and the nongullible prospective foster parent might also ask for data on more than 16 cases before accepting Professor Stoddard's dictum, based on these 16 cases, that " the children of definitely moronic mothers and laboring class fathers, if placed early in good foster homes, will turn out to be above average in mental ability " (18, p. 49).

In closing these comments on the foster children study, we refrain from doing the obviously needed thing—recasting Dr. Skodak's many unsubstantiated conclusions regarding the potency of environment. It is clear that her findings not only fail to support the environmental hypothesis but that they are, in fact, entirely consistent with the hereditarian viewpoint.

Other Studies

The first two papers of Wellman (21, 22) set the pace for those to follow. Here we find the beginning of the indiscriminate mixing of Kuhlmann and Stanford-Binet IQ's; the first of many analyses in which changes are related to initial IQ level; the abundant use of graphical presentation and failure to give essential tabular material; and gross misuse of percentiles—IQ's are converted into percentiles, then the percentiles and percentile gains are averaged. How much distortion has been introduced *via* percentiles will never be known unless the original data are reworked.

In Wellman's third paper (23), data are presented to show that IQ changes are not only related to preschool attendance (as claimed in the first two papers) but also to the type of school. The evidence in the first two parts of this third study is in line with claims made in the two earlier studies to the effect that IQ's tend to increase during preschool attendance. Aside from the points raised in the last paragraph and the additional fact that the greatest gain takes place from the first to the second test, it is difficult to criticize this finding on the basis of the data given. Perhaps it may sound unfair to make the general statement that the presentation of the data in these early papers is such as to annoy the reader who is anxious to evaluate critically the results. This is particularly unfortunate in that those who would prefer to accept the claims, but who are cautious, may find the treatment of the data and the control of pertinent variables somewhat obscure.

In the third part of this third study, information is given, then ignored, to the effect that a group of non-preschool children " had had several infant examinations " prior to their first Binet. One wonders, in the absence of information, to what extent experience with infant examinations was an additional uncontrolled variable in these early studies. In so far as the results for this particular non-preschool group are concerned, we have here a possible explanation for their failure to gain from their first to second Binet test. The fact that their initial mean IQ was higher than that for the preschool group is interpreted as indicating that they were rather highly selected, but why stop at this when it might be possible to check on the selection? Surely, information was available on the education and economic levels of the parents. We suspect, however, that their initial test scores were high because of the rapport built up by frequent prior infant examinations. For this group, passing from the first to second test was comparable to going from, perhaps, the fourth to the fifth test for the preschool group, who, it will be recalled, made their greatest gains from first to second or third tests.

Wellman's fourth paper (24) cannot help being a nightmare to statisticians who have for so long held the position that averages and correlations involving percentiles are fallacious. If Dr. Wellman has analytic proof to the contrary, the statistical world has a right to examine that proof. There are a few other points in this paper that seem questionable. In Table 2 we learn that the correlation between initial IQ and years attendance is .04, but, when it is found in Table 4 that the long-attendance group had an initial mean IQ 6.8 points higher than the short-attendance group, a difference which yields a biserial *r* of about .27, error can be suspected. In Table 4 one also finds the omission of two disturbingly large critical ratios— the corresponding lower values *were* included in Table 3. These omissions have to do with differences in initial IQ's for the long- and short-attendance groups. These differences are large enough to make one question the reality of the later differences on American Council on Education test percentiles. In fact, when the groups are equated on the basis of initial IQ's (Table 5), the critical ratios drop to 1.9 or less. This mere fact does not lead the author to qualify the summary: " Long attendance children (six or more years in the University schools) consistently made significantly higher scores than short attendance children (one to five years) of equal initial ability " (**24**, p. 136).

It is in this paper that we note the beginning of the stunt of show- ing curves for *selected* individuals, and it is here that we find the first mention of the now much-publicized cases who gained from average to the genius level (because of the University school system?). Here one finds certain maximum, and startling, changes pointed out. The greatest change is an increase from 98 at age 3½ to 167 at age 5. This gain is stressed, but the reader is not reminded of the pertinent fact that this individual dropped to 143 at age 10 or to an average of 148 for four tests from ages 9 to 12. Another jump from 89 to 149 is pointed out, but the subsequent drop to 130 is not specifically mentioned. These large individual gains from initial Stanford-Binet tests at age 3 and 3½ may have some meaning, but when it is noted that big gains of 30, 69, and 28 points occur prior to age 6, one becomes somewhat skeptical. In view of the fact that individual cases were found among the data of the orphanage preschool project which showed changes opposite to the cases selected by the authors, and for other reasons, the present writer feels sure that cases among the University school group could be found which would show decrease. In a later paper we find Wellman saying, with regard to four children who showed marked gains, that " these children were not atypical but are representative of a fairly large group " (**25**, p. 98). Until supporting evidence is given—and it cannot be found in any of her papers—v are compelled to characterize this statement as a gross exaggeration.

We turn next to the recent monograph by Wellman on " The intelligence of preschool children as measured by the Merrill-Palmer scale of performance tests " (26), but our remarks will be confined to the chief conclusion of that part of the study which has to do with the effects of preschool attendance on Merrill-Palmer scores. The main conclusion is stated as follows: " From these various analyses a sufficient number of positive and significant differences was obtained to justify the conclusion that preschool attendance materially affected ability on the Merrill-Palmer test " (p. 77). It is said that the IQ method of scoring reflected these changes more clearly than sigma scores or percentiles, so let us examine the IQ evidence for the above conclusion. It should be noted that different methods of scoring the test results for the same children will not add to the sampling significance of the results. Accordingly, if we demolish the finding with respect to IQ scoring, the method which " reflected these changes more clearly," it should not be necessary to state here the detailed argument which could be produced to explain away the findings with regard to other scoring schemes.

Let us now evaluate the data upon which the above-quoted conclusion is based. It is reported (Table 11, p. 41) that 72 " cases " gained 9.1 IQ points from fall to spring tests, the gain yielding a critical ratio of 3.37 (one of two significant ratios for results dealing with effects of preschool upon Merrill-Palmer IQ), and that 46 " cases " gained 3.7 points from spring to fall tests, a gain which is 1.09 times its standard error. Now there are three important questions, or issues, to be raised here. First, in determining the significance of the gains, the correlation term in the standard error of the difference formula was ignored. This is a frequent error in these Iowa studies, and one which does not always lead to a conservative statement of significance, e.g. see Skodak's (12, p. 56) " slight " change which, properly evaluated, is 4.5 times its standard error. The gains of 9.1 and 3.7 IQ points given above are, on the basis of the given N's and r's, actually 5.32 and 2.10 times their standard errors, respectively, for fall to spring and spring to fall. Second, the 72 " cases " given are not 72 different children, nor can one be sure that the 46 " cases" are 46 different children (see the bouncing N's in Table 10, and subsequent discussion on page 40), and therefore we again have another instance in which one of the assumptions of sampling has been violated. Since the true N's are not given, we

ENVIRONMENTAL INFLUENCES UPON THE IQ

cannot make an adjustment for this incorrect use of error formulas; we can only state that such a correction would tend to increase the standard errors and hence lower the critical ratios. Third, Dr. Wellman has been content to stop with evidence for a significant gain for one group and an insignificant gain for the other, but in reality an adequate statistical treatment must evaluate the *difference* between the gains.

Using the error formula proper for correlated means, but with no adjustment for the real (and unstated) N's, we have the gain from fall to spring as 9.1 ± 1.71 and the gain from spring to fall as 3.7 ± 1.76; then the difference between the gains, 5.4, is readily found to be 2.2 times the standard error of the difference. This ratio is too high because of the use of inflated N's. In order to make a justifiable comparison so far as the N's are concerned, we note the results (Table 11) for 42 children having a first test in the fall and whose gain to spring of 10.7 IQ points is reported to be 3.35 times its standard error (the second of two significant ratios for results dealing with effects of preschool upon Merrill-Palmer IQ), while 20 children having a first test in the spring made a gain of 5.2 points (.97 times its sigma). In evaluating the significance of the *difference,* we first recompute the standard errors of the gains by the formula which includes the r term. The needed r's are not given; presumably, they will not differ much from those reported for the total groups, as given in Table 14 (p. 54). The difference between gains, 10.7 minus 5.2, is found to be only 1.56 times its standard error. The fact that this gain is consistent with that found for the larger groups adds nothing to the significance of the finding, since it is based on subsamplings of the larger groups. Thus, it is seen that the author's conclusion regarding the effect of preschool attendance on Merrill-Palmer IQ's resulted from faulty statistical treatment of the data.

In a paper by Skeels and Fillmore (9) it is concluded that the longer subaverage children remain in their underprivileged homes, the lower are their IQ's. This conclusion was based on a comparison of means for older as opposed to younger children, but the significant drop with age was not properly evaluated in that no allowance was made for the fact, reproduced in their paper, that the 1916 Stanford Revision yielded a negative correlation for IQ with age for unselected children. An adequate statistical analysis must determine the significance of the difference between the drop for their group and that for the unselected group. This can readily be accomplished by either of two methods. One can determine from their data that the mean for ages 12 to 14 combined is 11.8 points lower than the mean for ages 5 to 7 combined. The corresponding figure for unselected cases is 7.5. The difference, 4.3, between the differences happens to be only 1.6 times its standard error. The second method, which is preferable in that it utilizes all the cases from 5 to 14, inclusive, is to compare the slopes of the two regression lines for IQ on age. From the data given one cannot ascertain exactly the two regression coefficients, but an excellent approximation can be obtained by fitting lines to the age means, weighted according to their respective N's. The difference between the two regression coefficients, *i.e.* the slopes, so computed is 1.8 times its standard error. When we also consider the data in Wellman's (21) earlier study, which showed that above-average children in above-average homes drop about 10 or 11 IQ points with age (ages 5 to 7 combined compared to ages 12 to 14 combined), it appears that the conclusion of Skeels and Fillmore is entirely unwarranted.

IQ CHANGES AND REGRESSION

The analysis of changes in IQ according to initial IQ level has been persistently pursued in all the Iowa studies so far mentioned, and has been given such prominence in the monograph by Crissey (3) as to lead Professor Stoddard in his foreword thereto to point out the main finding as being the fact that " changes in brightness tend to be related to the general IQ level of the group: the relatively dull move upward and the relatively bright show losses." In Wellman's study of the Merrill-Palmer scale we find that IQ's on this scale are analyzed in terms of Binet IQ level, and vice versa, with the resultant finding " that children who receive low Merrill-Palmer scores can be expected to receive higher Binet scores than their Merrill-Palmers, and children who receive low Binet scores can be expected to receive higher Merrill-Palmer scores . . ." (26, pp. 99–100). This is just the result which any competent statistician would have confidently predicted, providing he had been told the fact that the standard deviations for Binet and Merrill-Palmer IQ distributions were approximately the same and that the correlation between the two sets of scores was low (say, less than .80).

Our main concern here, however, is with the test-retest changes according to initial IQ level. Except for a couple of instances, all of the Iowa analyses on this point have yielded results consistent with the finding, cited above, of Crissey. These findings can be summarized in correlational terms by saying that there is a negative correlation between changes expressed as gains and initial IQ level. So stated, one type of divergence from Crissey's result can be brought into line. We refer to the situation where gains are shown at all initial IQ classifications, but are still inversely related to initial level; or to the situation where losses occur at all levels, but those initially lower lose less than those initially above the group average. The other exception to the Crissey result is to be found in Wellman's analysis of retests at a week's interval on the Merrill-Palmer. It was found that "the amount of gain increased with successively higher initial IQ classifications" (**26**, p. 30). The explanation of this in terms of practice effects, with superior children profiting more, is acceptable to the writer.

That IQ changes from one test to a later retest are related to IQ level on the first test cannot be denied, but when an environmental explanation is advanced, we begin to feel that the environmental hypothesis is being overworked. It is suggested by Dr. Wellman (**26**, p. 53) that the superior do not find their environments sufficiently challenging and hence tend to lose on retest, and Crissey (**3**, p. 21) suggests that those initially below average tend to gain because they find their environments stimulating. Dr. Wellman has maintained that ordinary statistical regression has nothing whatever to do with the inverse relationship between gains and initial IQ level, but we are forced to readvance the concept of regression, which has been labeled by Dr. Wellman as an "hypothesis," despite the position of qualified statisticians that regression is a "fact."

Before turning to Dr. Wellman's arguments against regression, let us consider an unpublished finding of the present writer. Fifty-four children of initial IQ's between 140 and 149 lost an average of five points (CR of 3.00) on a retest. Shall we attribute this loss to lack of environmental stimulation? To do so would stretch the imagination of even the most hopeful environmentalist, since this loss occurred within a week. The loss represents nothing more than statistical regression as we pass from Form M to Form L of the New Stanford-Binet, and is due solely to errors of measurement. A similar loss occurs when we pass from Form L to Form M, and gains occur for those classified as inferior on either form and tested a week later on the other form.

It should be explicitly noted that we are not claiming that all the gains for the inferior and all losses for the superior reported by the Iowa investigators are explicable on the basis of errors of measurement. However, the reliabilities of the Kuhlmann and Stanford-

Binet and the Merrill-Palmer at ages 2 to 5 are not high enough to preclude the possibility that a large part of such gains and losses is due to errors of measurement. The remaining portion of the changes, differential with regard to IQ level, from test to retest six or more months later may be attributable to differences in maturation or, conceivably, to differences in environmental stimulation. But before we accept the hypothesis that losses for those initially above the group average are due to a lack of environmental stimulation, and that gains for those below the group average are due to the environment being stimulating for them, we must ask about a further result which should follow if this hypothesis is to be tenable. If the hypothesis were true, we would expect a reduction in variability from initial to later test, but this happens not to be the case, not even for the control group in the orphanage. Perhaps the Iowa people, who are quite adept at finding an environmental explanation for all changes, can produce one to account for the fact that the number of people in the several IQ classifications is approximately the same for later tests as for the initial test, despite the fact of differential changes.

If these investigators should insist on the correctness of their concept concerning the " stimulating value of the group," they must explain the fact that individuals classified above average on the basis of a final test will, in general, have had lower initial IQ's, while those below average on the final test will have been higher on the initial test. Perhaps the " stimulating value of the group " has acted retroactively! But we hasten to point out that this merely describes the fact that some (a large number) of the individuals initially above average do gain, while some below average do lose—gains and losses which occur in spite of the supposed stimulating value of the total group.

Let us look at the problem from the analytical viewpoint. Given an initial IQ, x_1, and a retest IQ, x_2, and let the gain be defined as $g = x_2 - x_1$, then it can be shown by easy algebra that the correlation between initial IQ and gain is

$$r_{1g} = \frac{r_{12}\sigma_2 - \sigma_1}{\sqrt{\sigma_1^2 + \sigma_2^2 - 2r_{12}\sigma_1\sigma_2}}$$

from which it can readily be seen that, unless the variability increases from first test to the second or later test, the correlation between gains and initial IQ *must* be negative, since in practice r_{12} will never be unity. This, of course, does not explain the negative correlation; it merely indicates that the Iowa investigators have gone to an enor-

ENVIRONMENTAL INFLUENCES UPON THE IQ

mous amount of work to demonstrate a fact which even a mediocre statistician could prove analytically in less than five minutes. Perhaps we should not object to empirical demonstrations, but when these lead to such fallacious conclusions as that concerning the "leveling effect" on intelligence of residence in an orphanage (discussed earlier in this paper), it is time for the artifactual nature of the finding to be reviewed.

It is difficult to understand how Dr. Wellman could discuss the relationship between Merrill-Palmer and Binet IQ's, or study her graphs (**26**, p. 98), without recognizing regression, but no mention is made of this fact when she speaks of those with high Binets having lower Merrill-Palmers, etc. Earlier in this same monograph, however, we do find Dr. Wellman discussing and rejecting regression as it affects test-retest changes. Her argument is so pertinent that we reproduce it here in full:

"Another hypothesis is that commonly referred to as regression towards the mean. According to this hypothesis very superior children are expected to lose and below average children to gain, both extremes approaching the mean. This phenomenon when observed has been interpreted at times as purely statistical, the chances of loss of high-scoring children and the chances of gain of low-scoring children being automatically greater. At times the phenomenon has received a biological interpretation of the tendency of the organism to veer toward the general level of the race. There are two difficulties in acceptance of the regression-towards-the-mean hypothesis here: (1) the facts of change on retest at one week do not fit the expected trend, and (2) the winter and summer groups are selected superior groups. Instead of gaining, the children at 0.0 sigma score should not have changed, and the children at 0.5 and 1.0 sigma score should have lost" (**26**. p. 53).

Following this rejection of the regression "hypothesis," Dr. Wellman proposes the earlier-mentioned explanation of the differential gains as being a matter of environmental stimulation. Let us examine her argument. In the first place, the regression phenomenon is, of course, in this case purely statistical as opposed to any notion of biological regression. As we understand the latter concept, it has to do with progeny as compared with parent, and, as such, the latter concept is absolutely not applicable to the test-retest situation. The first of the two difficulties has already been mentioned earlier by the present writer as an exception to Crissey's finding, and at that time we accepted Wellman's explanation in terms of practice effects—the superior are better able to profit therefrom, and consequently we have a factor of such potency as to overcome the ordinary statistical regression. This, in terms of the formula given above, really means that σ_2 had to be greater than σ_1 (about $1.2\,\sigma_1$).

In regard to the second difficulty, it should first be noted that the changes over a six-months period for the selected superior groups *do* exhibit regression, as is evidenced by Wellman's Table 13 (26, p. 52) and by the negative correlations of .38 and .43 between changes and initial IQ. This regression, however, is about the means of the groups concerned and not about the population mean. This should not be surprising, since their original classification as " selected superior groups " was not made on the basis of the first test. They earned this classification *via* whatever factors operate to fill pre-schools with superior children. This differs from, for example, Terman's selection of " gifted " children as those above 140 IQ and the consequent drop (regression) on later tests. Perhaps an analogy may help us understand why Wellman's selected superior children did not, and need not, as a group, regress toward the population mean from test to retest. Suppose we choose a group of eight-year-old boys of Swedish extraction and determine that their mean height was one-half a sigma above the mean for the generality of American boys of that age. After a period of eight years we remeasure them; the correlation between the two sets of measures will not be high— changes in the relative standing of the individuals will have occurred, but we would not expect the group as a whole to be nearer the mean of all 16-year-old American boys than one-half a sigma (this second sigma must, of course, be based on 16-year-olds). We would expect regression *within* the Swedish group, but this would not tend to reduce their superiority nor would it lead to a reduction in the abso-lute or relative variability of the group. In contrast, if, on the basis of *measurement*, we had chosen a group of boys as above average, we would find a general tendency for the group, so selected, to be nearer the universe mean upon subsequent measurement.

Perhaps the point can be better illustrated by a mental test situ-ation. Suppose it has been established (1) that the father-child IQ correlation is .50 for each of the child age levels 6 to 14, (2) that the average IQ for each age level and for fathers is 100, and (3) that the S.D.'s for each level and for the fathers is 16. Now let us select for study those six-year-old children whose fathers have IQ's of 80; the average IQ of these children will be 90, the S.D. will be 13.86. It should be obvious that if we retest these children at age 14 they will again average 90 (since the average IQ for all 14-year-old chil-dren of fathers with 80 IQ will be 90). That is, the test-retest

ENVIRONMENTAL INFLUENCES UPON THE IQ

regression will not have brought them nearer the population mean, but, within the group, regression about the mean of 90 will have taken place. In other words, an inferior or superior group will not move toward the general mean on a retest unless they have been selected as inferior or superior on the basis of an initial test.

Aside from the general, and easily anticipated, finding of Crissey that changes are inversely related to initial IQ level, it is of some interest to follow through a different type of analysis which purports to substantiate the hypothesis that " the rate of mental development of a child in an institution designed for normal and dull-normal children should vary from that of a child of similar mental ability in an institution designed for the feeble-minded " (3, p. 52). To check this hypothesis the method of matched groups was used, and one of the matching criteria was that the individuals had to be within three points in IQ on initial test. Since the average initial IQ for the individuals in the institution for dull-normals was about 85, as compared to an average of about 62 for those in the institution for feeble-minded, it follows that in order to equate on initial IQ it was necessary in general to match children from the lower end of one distribution with children from the upper end of the second (or feebleminded) distribution. This type of thing tends definitely to capitalize on errors of measurement, with the result that the individuals drawn from the first group will regress upward, while those drawn from the second group will regress downward on a later test. It is not surprising, therefore, when Crissey (3, p. 53) finds that, for four different sets of matched groups, the groups selected from among dull-normals gain and those selected from among feebleminded lose. A significant difference in changes does not, of course, preclude the possibility that the changes were due to errors of measurement *via* regression.

There are two methods for making allowance for the regressive effect of measurement errors on IQ changes of the sort being discussed in this section. We can make our classification on the basis of regressed ($x_{\infty} = r_{11}x$) initial IQ's and then determine the changes (gains or losses) from these regressed scores. By this method any mean gain on the part of the initially low or mean loss on the part of the initially high will not be due to errors of measurement. The second scheme for eliminating the effect of errors of measurement is to state the relationship between initial IQ and changes in terms of the correlation coefficient and then correct this for attenuation. It has long been known that this correction will *reduce* (bring nearer zero) the correlation, or, conversely, that the effect of measurement errors is to *produce* a negative correlation between initial sc ·es and gain (19).

In closing this rather lengthy discussion of regression we agree with Dr. Wellman that regression " is really more of a descriptive than an explanatory term " (26, p. 32), but it does not follow from this that pages of tedious analysis need to be devoted to pointing out that those initially high tend to lose and those initially low tend to gain. This can readily be inferred from the test-retest correlation and the sigmas and means for a given group. Neither does it follow that regression from test to retest exemplifies a leveling effect. Furthermore, no definite conclusions can be drawn from the many analyses showing losses for those above the group average and gains for those below until due allowance is made for the portion of these changes which is attributable to regression because of errors of measurement.

Summary and Conclusion

So far in this critical examination of the Iowa studies on IQ changes we have been content to raise specific questions concerning definite methodological and statistical inadequacies. In summarizing, we find it necessary to make a few general statements, the validity of which can be judged by the reader. In brief, we have found much of the supposed evidence for environmental influences on the IQ to be entirely nonexistent. We have cited instance after instance, and have left unmentioned many more examples of minor importance, in which the findings have resulted from either uncontrolled factors or erroneous statistical treatment or both. We have noted, but not stressed, the fact that these studies are replete with misleading, *i.e.* not properly qualified, statements regarding the influences of school and environment. We have said little about the fact that insignificant findings in favor of the environmental viewpoint have been constantly played up while contrary findings have been ignored. We have also noted a disturbing tendency to a dramatic use of selected cases, falsely claimed to be typical, and a simultaneous disregard for other cases which would just as dramatically disprove their contentions.

In conclusion, the writer would like to express two personal opinions. First, in view of the fact that we have discovered startling inadequacies in those studies reported in monographic detail and in

ENVIRONMENTAL INFLUENCES UPON THE IQ

view of the fact that it was not until the original data were secured that we were able properly to evaluate—in this case demolish—the evidence based on the orphanage preschool project, we are strongly skeptical as to the dependability of the results which have been reported all too briefly in the shorter papers, by which we mean specifically the earlier papers of Dr. Wellman. Second, if it is the responsibility of the scientist to establish, and the educator to disseminate, truths, then our scientists who have turned educators should take the responsibility for dispelling error, especially that which has been the result of their own hasty promulgation of unverified and largely invalid research results.

BIBLIOGRAPHY

1. BELL, H. M. Youth tell their story. Washington: American Council on Education, 1938.
2. COFFEY, H. S., & WELLMAN, B. L. The role of cultural status in intelligence changes of preschool children. *J. exp. Educ.*, 1936–1937, **5**, 191–202.
3. CRISSEY, O. L. Mental development as related to institutional residence and educational achievement. *Univ. Ia Stud. Child Welf.*, 1937, **11**, No. 1.
4. FOSTER, E. M. School survival rates. *Sch. Life,* 1936, **22**, 13–14; 1938, **23**, 265–267.
5. GOODENOUGH, F. L. The Kuhlmann-Binet tests. Minneapolis: Univ. Minnesota Press, 1928.
6. KUHLMANN, F. A handbook of mental tests. Baltimore: Warwick & York, 1922.
7. SKEELS, H. M. Mental development of children in foster homes. *J. genet. Psychol.,* 1936, **49**, 91–106.
8. SKEELS, H. M. Mental development of children in foster homes. *J. consult. Psychol.,* 1938, **2**, 33–43.
9. SKEELS, H. M., & FILLMORE, E. A. The mental development of children from underprivileged homes. *J. genet. Psychol.,* 1937, **50**, 427–439.
10. SKEELS, H. M., UPDEGRAFF, R., WELLMAN, B. L., & WILLIAMS, H. M. A study of environmental stimulation. *Univ. Ia Stud. Child Welf.,* 1938, **15**, No. 4.
11. SKODAK, M. The mental development of adopted children whose true mothers are feeble-minded. *Child Develpm.,* 1938, **9**, 303–308.
12. SKODAK, M. Children in foster homes: a study of mental development. *Univ. Ia Stud. Child Welf.,* 1939, **16**, No. 1.
13. SNYGG, D. The relation between the intelligence of mothers and of their children living in foster homes. *J. genet. Psychol.,* 1938, **52**, 401–406.
14. STODDARD, G. D. What of the nursery school? *Progr. Educ.,* 1937, **14**, 440–451.
15. STODDARD, G. D. Our children: their intelligence. (Abstract.) *Proc. nat. Educ. Ass.,* 1938, **76**, 61–62.
16. STODDARD, G. D. Child development—a new approach to education. *Sch. & Soc.,* 1939, **49**, 33–38.

17. STODDARD, G. D. Education for self-realization. *Nat. Parent-Teach.*, 1939, **33**, 5–8.

18. STODDARD, G. D. The IQ: its ups and downs. *Educ. Rec. Suppl.*, January, 1939, 44–57.

19. THOMSON, G. H. An alternate formula for true correlation of initial values with gains. *J. exp. Psychol.*, 1925, **8**, 323–324.

20. UPDEGRAFF, R. The determination of a reliable intelligence quotient for the young child. *J. genet. Psychol.*, 1932, **41**, 152–166.

21. WELLMAN, B. L. Some new bases for interpretation of the IQ. *J. genet. Psychol.*, 1932, **41**, 116–126.

22. WELLMAN, B. L. The effect of pre-school attendance upon the IQ. *J. exp. Educ.*, 1932–1933, **1**, 48–69.

23. WELLMAN, B. L. Growth in intelligence under differing school environments. *J. exp. Educ.*, 1934–1935, **3**, 59–83.

24. WELLMAN, B. L. Mental growth from preschool to college. *J. exp. Educ.*, 1937–1938, **6**, 127–138.

25. WELLMAN, B. L. Our changing concepts of intelligence. *J. consult. Psychol.*, 1938, **2**, 97–107.

26. WELLMAN, B. L. The intelligence of preschool children as measured by the Merrill-Palmer scale of performance tests. *Univ. Ia Stud. Child Welf.*, 1938, **15**, No. 3.

27. WELLMAN, B. L. Guiding mental development. *Childhood Educ.*, 1938, **15**, 108–112.

28. WELLMAN, B. L. New tests attack theory of fixed IQ. *New York Times*, July 17, 1938, Section II, 4.

29. WELLMAN, B. L. How the child's mind grows. *Nat. Parent-Teach.*, 1939, **33**, 17–18.

30. WELLMAN, B. L. The changing concept of the I. Q. *J. Home Econ.*, 1939, **31**, 77–80.

31. WELLMAN, B. L., & STODDARD, G. D. The IQ: a problem in social construction. *Social Front.*, 1939, **5**, 151–152.

32. ———. Biennial survey of education, 1933–1934. *U. S. Off. Educ. Bull.*, 1935, No. 2.

From Barbara Burks (1928). The 27th Year Book, 221–310, *published by the National Society for the Study of Education*

THE RELATIVE INFLUENCE OF NATURE AND NURTURE UPON MENTAL DEVELOPMENT; A COMPARATIVE STUDY OF FOSTER PARENT-FOSTER CHILD RESEMBLANCE AND TRUE PARENT-TRUE CHILD RESEMBLANCE [1]

BARBARA STODDARD BURKS
Stanford University, Palo Alto, California

The investigation in hand approaches the aspect of the problem which concerns heredity and *home environment* through a comparison of mental test resemblances obtaining between parents and their children on the one hand, with those obtaining between foster parents and their foster children on the other. Thus, it seeks to evaluate the effects of nature and of home nurture through a study of two kinds of familial resemblance, one of which is dependent upon nurture influence alone, and the other upon a combination of both nature and nurture influences. Through its use of foster parents and their foster children as subjects, it applies to its purpose the end results of the social experimentation which is going on in many homes all about us.

PUBLISHERS NOTE

Limitations in space have prevented us from printing in full this remarkable paper. Professor Eysenck has selected the key sections from the original 100-page article. The original figure and table numbers have been retained and consequently are not consecutive.

It should be emphasized at this point that whatever tendencies and conclusions can be found in this study are valid only for populations as homogeneous in racial extraction, social standards, and educational opportunities as that from which our subjects are drawn. The distribution of homes of the children studied in this investigation was probably nearly as variable in essential features[3] as homes of the general American white population (though somewhat skewed toward a superior level). It was not as variable, however, as if the homes of southern negroes, poor mountain whites, or Philippine Negritoes had been included; and consequently, home environment cannot be expected to have as large a proportional effect upon the mental differences of the children we studied as though they were being reared in families unselected as to race or geographical location throughout the world.

Reference should also be made to the educational opportunities of the children examined, which were good. (All children were living in California communities.) If the children had varied considerably in educational opportunity, so that a number of them had as limited amount of schooling as that, for example, of Gordon's English canal-boat children, and if, in addition, home environment and educational opportunity had been correlated, it would have been quite difficult to separate the effects of the two upon the mental variability of our children. In this study, not only is the possible complication of differences in educational opportunity averted, but the confusing issue of possible cumulative effects of schooling is averted as well, since the measuring instrument used—the Stanford-Binet test of intelligence—was standardized upon California school children covering the same age range as our children, who themselves had undergone a cumulative educational process.

Other factors causing real or apparent impairment in mental ability, such as language handicap, deafness, pathological trauma (as from spastic birth paralysis, lethargic encephalitis or other diseases leaving permanent mental deficiency) were also ruled out.

Thus, the study is based upon children homogeneous as to race and educational opportunity; sufficiently homogeneous in health

---

[3] This seems probable because the variability in intelligence of both the control and foster children coming from these homes is as large as that of unselected children.

and physique to avoid confusion; and about as variable in hereditary endowment and in home environment (including kindred social mores) as white children of ordinary communities.

The study does not purport to demonstrate what proportions of the *total* mental development of an individual are due to heredity and to environment. Biologists have frequently pointed out the futility of attempting such a demonstration, since *any development whatever would be impossible without the contributions of both nature and nurture.* But if we direct our attention to the contributions of ordinary differences in heredity and ordinary differences in environment to *mental differences* (*i. e.,* I. Q. variance), it is possible to draw some significant conclusions. The causes which affect human differences, rather than the causes which condition the absolute developmental level of the human species have, after all, the more vital bearing upon social and educational problems.

Given a group of school children such as our subjects (which surely are representative of the largest single element in the American juvenile population), it will later be seen that the data gathered in this investigation lead to the conclusion that *about 17 percent of the variability of intelligence is due to differences in home environment.* It will further appear that the best estimate the data afford of the extreme degree to which the most favorable home environment may enhance the I. Q., or the least favorable environment depress it, is about 20 I. Q. points. This amount is larger, no doubt, than some of the firmest believers in heredity would have anticipated, but smaller than the effects often attributed to nurture by holders of an extreme environmentalist's view. To the writer, these results constitute an important vindication of the potency of home environment. But even more significant appear to be the implications of these basic results, *e. g.,* that *not far from 70 percent of ordinary white school children have intelligence that deviates less than 6 I. Q. points up or down from what they would have if all children were raised in a standard (average) home environment;* that, while home environment in rare, extreme cases may account for as much as 20 points of increment above the expected, or congenital, level, heredity (in conjunction with environment) may account in some instances for increments above the level of the generality which are five times as large (100 points).

III. METHODS EMPLOYED

1. Approach

The program for family study required four to eight hours of a field worker's time per family. Much of the testing and interviewing had to be done at night to suit the hours when the fathers of the children could be at home.

It was our invariable rule to make no first approaches by telephone, as it seemed probable that our chances of gaining the interest and coöperation of families would be far better by personal interview. Consequently, much time was lost in attempted calls when the family were out, away from town, moved, etc. This condition, linked with the wide areas it was necessary to travel, and the difficulty of dove-tailing appointments at unusual hours with any degree of efficiency, resulted in slower progress than we had at first contemplated. From two to three completed cases weekly was the ordinary average per field worker.

2. Schedule

The items of our family case schedule were these:

1. Stanford Binet Test, administered to parents and children.

2. A home-information blank, containing an adaptation of the Whittier Scale for Home Grading and a culture scale of our own, filled out by field assistants.

3. Rating of the child on ten character and temperament traits made independently by the two parents.

4. Personal information blank filled out by each parent.

5. Woodworth-Cady questionnaire (to test emotional stability) filled out by children ten years old or over.

6. Information was also obtained from the files of the placement agenices, in the case of the foster group. This included heredity (if known), age at placement, age at adoption, national descent, etc.

The Stanford Binet Test and record booklet are so well known as to require no description here.

The nature of the Whittier Scale and the culture scale are made evident in the section later on wherein the scoring standards for these scales are described.

The ten traits upon which the parents rated their children were: (1) will power and perseverance; (2) cheerfulness and optimism; (3) musical appreciation; (4) sense of humor; (5) permanency of moods; (6) leadership; (7) sympathy and tenderness; (8) conscientiousness; (9) originality; (10) general intelligence. The traits were selected from a large number of traits used in connection with the Stanford study of gifted children; and ratings were made upon a seven-category graphic rating scale, as reproduced in *Genetic Studies of Genius,* I (15).

The personal information blank filled out by each parent called for data upon the following points: birthplace; occupation; highest school grade reached; special interests, hobbies or accomplishments; positions of honor, trust, or recognition which have been held; distribution of time during the day (at home or away from home); children's hobbies or interests; occupations which parents think may be suitable for child in future; where child spends his leisure time; discipline of child. In addition, the blank filled out by the mother asked for information upon the kind and amount of home reading done by the child at various ages; the home instruction or attention received by the child in such matters as reading or writing, story-telling to child, number work, or nature study; and the private tutoring received by the child (in music, dancing, or other subjects).

The Woodworth-Cady questionnaire—reproduced in full in *Genetic Studies of Genius,* I, pp. 500 ff. (15)—is a questionnaire of 85 questions designed to sift out psychotic tendencies. A number of questions are inserted as 'padding' to lull the suspicions of the subject as to the purpose of the test. Samples of the questions are:

"Do your teachers generally treat you right?"
"Did you ever have a nickname you didn't like very well?"
"Are you happy most of the time?"

IV. Selection, Location, and Coöperation of Cases

1. Foster Group

a. Criteria of selection. The following criteria were satisfied in selecting cases for the study from the files of the Native Sons and Native Daughters of the Golden West Central Committee on Homeless Children, and the Children's Home Society of California:

1. Children were placed in their foster homes before the age of

12 months. (The average age of placement of our group proved to be 3 months, 2 days.)

2. Children were legally adopted—not merely cared for in free or boarding homes.

3. Children were between 5 and 14 years, inclusive, at the time of the investigation.

4. Foster parents were white, non-Jewish, English-speaking, and American, British, or north-European-born.

5. True parents (so far as was definitely known) were white, non-Jewish, Americans, British, or north-Europeans.

6. Children were placed in the home of a married couple, both members of which were alive and living together at the time of the investigation.

7. Cases must be accessible to the three centers—San Francisco Bay region, Los Angeles, and San Diego.

These criteria require little discussion. The first one was laid down (1) to insure that each child had lived in the environment of a single home from early infancy, and (2) to avoid the type of selective placement that might easily have been exercised if the children had been old enough at the time of their adoption to give clear evidence of their mental potentiality.

The second criterion confined the study to children who were being reared as though they were the actual offspring of the foster parents.

The third confined it to children within a range for which the I. Q. is fairly comparable at all ages.

The fourth and fifth criteria enabled us to avoid the confusion in results that would ensue from a foreign language handicap in any of the subjects who were tested, and precluded the possibility of an adventitious resemblance between foster parents and children due to the practice by placement societies of matching foster parents and children for racial descent.

The sixth insured that all the children should be homogeneous in having both a paternal and a maternal influence; and the seventh merely made the study administratively feasible.

INFLUENCES UPON MENTAL DEVELOPMENT

TABLE II.—REASONS FOR UNAVAILABILITY

	Number of cases
One foster parent dead	15
Foster parents separated or divorced	10
"No time"	10
Foster child died	8
Sickness in family	4
Home in inaccessible region	3
Field workers told by organization secretaries not to visit case	3
Part of family away	2
Mother works	2
Deafness of foster parent	2
Child had been returned to organization because of feeble-mindedness	1
Possible secondary feeble-mindedness of foster child	1
Child was feeble-minded and in an institution	1
Test of child was invalidated by having foster parents come in and talk during test	
Case was known by field visitor to be too confidential to approach	1
Total	64

2. Control Group

a. Function of Control Group. The function of the array of families comprising parents and their true offspring which we have termed the 'Control Group' should be clearly defined at this point. The group serves two significant ends. It permits an estimate of the strength of mental *heredity*, after the strength of environment has been evaluated in the foster group; and it furnishes a most important check upon the validity of methods used.

Regarding the first end, more will be said in the final section. With regard to the second end, it is easy to see how indispensable the Control Group really is. If our test data and environmental data had been obtained only for the Foster Group alone, the low 'environmental' correlations reported in a subsequent section of this study could not have been said with any assurance to represent the actual limits of the type of influence we sought to measure. The unanswerable criticism could have been made that our methods might simply be unadapted to measuring the force of environment, and that better methods in the future might contravert our findings. But here we have a control group for which data were gathered by the same field workers and by the same procedure as that employed for the Foster Group. In marked contrast to the results for the Foster Group, we shall find in the Control Group that parent-child mental resemblances are of about the same magnitude as those ordinarily found in the case of hereditary *physical* traits. Such results will offer a solid basis upon which to interpret results.

The point was made in an earlier section that our conclusions are valid (at least in numerical terms) only for populations resembling in important respects the ones tested. It follows that if the results from the Foster Group and the Control Group are to furnish a valid comparison, the two groups must be 'matched' in a very rigid sense with respect to all the factors that could directly or even remotely influence the results. The effort which we made to secure such matching is manifest in the criteria that follow for selecting the Control Group. That the criteria were successful in attaining good matching will be seen in fifth section, headed "Composition of Groups."

b. Criteria of selection. Control cases were chosen by the following criteria:

1. Children of the Control Group were matched with those of the Foster Group for age, sex, and number of five-year-olds who had had no kindergarten attendance.

2. Control families were matched with foster families for locality, type of neighborhood, and occupational field of the father.

3. Non-Jewish, white American, British, or north-European families who spoke English were taken.

4. Both parents were alive and living together at the time of the investigation.

5. Only one child per family was tested (though families were not selected with respect to size).

Only 50 percent as many control cases as foster cases were selected, since our resources and time were becoming limited. As it turned out, the correlations in the Control Group, despite smaller numbers, had no greater probable errors for the most part than the corresponding correlations for the Foster Group, because the control correlations were in general so much larger.

As a possible source of cases, we considered the advisability of seeking the coöperation of parents who had an application for a foster child pending with one of the California child-placement agencies, and at the same time had a true child. Several such cases were looked up, who gave coöperation readily, but it soon became evident that to secure enough cases through this source would require the field visitors to travel prohibitive distances. Accordingly, it was arranged to select cases from the files of the public schools in the general localities represented by the Foster Group. The listing of subjects was as impartial as we were able to make it. At each school coöperating, the procedure was:

1. Select two or three names under each letter in the alphabet to avoid siblings.

2. Take about twelve cases for each age group.

3. Ask principal to check list for divorces, step children, race, etc.

4. Ascertain occupations of fathers from the children.

5. Locate a few children who have five-year-old siblings who have never attended kindergarten.

6. Check list with teachers.

7. Get letter of introduction from principal to parents.

This scheme gave us a working list far greater than the total number of cases we intended to gather, and allowed us sufficient leeway to insure good matching of controls with fosters in all the criteria laid down.

The Control Group, as finally completed, consisted of:

Cases selected through public schools...................... 93
Cases of 'true children' in our foster families who were
    tested while our foster records were being compiled.... 6
Cases of 'true children' of parents with applications pending
    for a foster child.................................... 3
Other cases of families interested in project.............. 3
                                                          ———
                                                          105

In the Foster Group all the tests were made by the three field workers mentioned, with the exception of one 'outside' case contributed by Miss Elizabeth Briggs, who was doing field work on another Stanford project, and a test of one foster child contributed by a Berkeley school. In the Control Group tests which were not made by one of the three field workers were administered as follows:

Tests of children in Palo Alto, by students trained by Dr.
    Merrill, of Stanford University...................... 4
Test of child contributed by a school..................... 1
                                                          ———
                                                          5

VI. Main Results of the Study

As this investigation was conceived, the chief emphasis was laid upon intelligence and the factors conditioning its development. It was decided to touch upon traits other than intelligence only to the extent that this was possible without undue expenditure of time. A consideration of the factors influencing vocabulary was possible, since a vocabulary test is one element of the Stanford-Binet Scale for mental levels beyond the seventh year. The Woodworth-Cady questionnaire was administered to children of ten or over in the hope that trends might appear that would suggest the factors underlying emotional instability. Unfortunately, the number of children eligible to answer this questionnaire was smaller than we had anticipated, and the results are consequently not very significant. Rough measures of several other mental and character traits of the children were secured through ratings and estimates by their parents (or foster parents), and a crude index of the children's school achievement was obtained by noting their grade placement. The results from our statistical treatment of all these aspects of the problem will be presented, but the data for other traits than intelligence can not be regarded as very reliable.

1. Factors Underlying Differences in Intelligence

Table XXXI presents corresponding correlation coefficients for the Foster and Control Groups between child's I.Q. and the environmental and hereditary factors for which we obtained measures.

INFLUENCES UPON MENTAL DEVELOPMENT

TABLE XXXI.—CHILD'S I. Q. CORRELATED WITH ENVIRONMENTAL AND HEREDITARY FACTORS*

Factor	Type of r	Foster			Control		
		r	P.E.	N	r	P.E.	N
Father's M. A.	P.M.	.07	.05	178	.45	.05	100
Mother's M. A.	P.M.	.19	.05	204	.46	.05	105
Mid-parent M. A.	P.M.	.20	.05	174	.52	.05	100
Father's vocabulary	P.M.	.13	.05	181	.47	.05	101
Mother's vocabulary	P.M.	.23	.04	202	.43	.05	104
Whittier index	P.M.	.21	.04	206	.42	.05	104
Whittier index (using 5-yr.-olds only)	P.M.	.29	.08	63	....	....	....
Culture index	P.M.	.25	.05	186	.44	.05	101
Culture index (using 5-yr.-olds only)	P.M.	.23	.08	60	....	....	....
Grade reached by father	P.M.	.01	.05	173	.27	.06	102
Grade reached by mother	P.M.	.17	.05	194	.27	.06	103
Parental supervision rating 3 or 4 vs. 5 or 6	B.	.12	.05	206	.40	.09	104
Income	P.M., K.	.23	.05	181	.24	.06	99
No. of books in home library	P.M., K.	.16	.05	194	.34	.06	100
Owning or renting home	B.	.25	.07	149	.32	.10	100
....	....	......	......	......	......	......	......
No. of books in child's library	P.M., K.	.32	.04	191	.32	.06	101
Private tutoring (in music, dancing, etc.)	B.						
Boys		.06	.10	77	.43	.11	46
Girls		.31	.08	108	.52	.09	56
Five-year-girls only		.50	.12	31	....	....	....
Home instruction by members of household (hrs. weekly)	P.M.						
Ages 2 and 3		.34	.04	181	−.05	.07	101
Ages 4 and 5 (children over 5)		.15	.06	129	−.03	.08	71
Ages 6 and 7 (children over 7)		.03	.07	88	.24	.09	46
Ages 2 and 3 (5-yr.-olds only)		.18	.09	51	....	....	....
Ages 4 and 5 (5-yr.-olds only)		.13	.09	52	....	....	....
Father's rating of child's intelligence	P.M.	.49	.04	164	.32	.06	98
Mother's rating of child's intelligence	P.M.	.39	.04	181	.52	.05	101

*The following abbreviations are used in this table: M.A. for mental age. P.M. for product-moment correlation. B. for biserial correlation. K. for Professor Kelley's auxiliary score method.

See also the tables of correlation arrays for child's I. Q. with Father's M. A. and Mother's M.A., from which the corresponding r's in this table were computed. (Appendix, II).

The significance of the division of the table by the dotted line is explained in the text, p. 338

In the field work it proved to be impossible to obtain full supplementary information upon all the cases tested, but correlations are given which utilize all the information we have with respect to each item. The number of cases entering into each correlation consequently varies somewhat.

Kelley's auxiliary score method, described in full in his text on *Statistical Method* (9), pp. 185 ff., is a device for straightening curvilinear regression lines empirically in such a way as not to capitalize chance. It was employed in the correlations with income and books in library.

Sheppard's correction was applied to all standard deviations used in the study—those published in tabular form as well as those entering correlation computations.

A word should be inserted at this point regarding the probable errors of the correlations reported. They have all been computed by standard formulae. Now, it can be shown that if, in two correlated series, some of the items in one variable enter the correlation array in more than one pair of measures, the effective N to use in computing the probable error of the coefficient is less than the total number of pairs. The effective N lies at some value intermediate between the total number of pairs and the total number minus the number of items entering the correlation more than once. We have such a situation in the Foster Group, for it contains 21 pairs of *double cases, i.e.,* foster siblings being reared in the same home. Correlations of various factors with measures of the children consequently have about 21 items which enter the correlations twice. We have ascertained, however, that within the limits that the effective N must lie in our Foster Group, no change occurs in the first or second decimal place of the P.E.'s in most of the correlations, nor greater than 1 point in the second decimal place in the remaining correlations. This difficulty can therefore be neglected, and was mentioned only to·avert possible criticism of the P.E.'s that are published. There is no such difficulty in the Control Group, of course, since only one child was considered from any one family.

In addition to the correlations of Table XXXI, a few coefficients were computed for the Foster Group only. These (Tables XXXII and XXXIII) were based upon specially selected groups of subjects.

As a matter of interest, a biserial correlation was computed between the child's I.Q. and his knowledge or lack of knowledge that he was an adopted child. With 189 cases for which we had data upon this point, the biserial correlation was .10 $\pm$ .06, to which we can attach no significance. Telling or not telling a child of his

INFLUENCES UPON MENTAL DEVELOPMENT

TABLE XXXII.—CORRELATIONS BETWEEN I. Q.'S OF CHILDREN AND FACTORS INFLUENCING THESE I. Q.'S IN THE CASE OF CHILDREN WHO WERE LESS THAN ONE MONTH OLD WHEN TAKEN BY FOSTER PARENTS

Factor	r	P.E.	N
Foster father's M.A.	.02	.09	60
Foster mother's M.A.	.15	.08	66
Mid-foster parent M.A.	.08	.09	58

TABLE XXXIII.—CORRELATIONS BETWEEN THE I.Q.'S OF FOUNDLINGS* AND FACTORS INFLUENCING THESE I.Q.'S

Factor	r	P. E.	N
Foster father's M.A.	.15	.21	10
Foster mother's M.A.	.14	.18	13
Mid-foster parent M.A.	.24	.20	10

*"Foundling" defined as a child picked up on a doorstep, in an automobile, etc., without any means of identification.

adoption is related much more to the age of the child and the intelligence of his foster parents than to his I.Q., as is evident in the following correlations:

	Biserial r	P.E.	N
Foster father's M.A. and whether or not child was told	.21	.07	156
Foster mother's M.A. and whether or not child was told	.43	.06	156
Age of child and whether or not he was told	.25	.07	156

When age of child is partialled out from the correlations with father's and mother's mental age, the first two correlations above are .21 and .42, respectively.

Correlations between the I.Q's of the pairs of unrelated foster siblings which are encountered are also of interest. Pairs were correlated against one another using chance arrangement.

	r	P.E.	N
Two unrelated foster children reared in same home	.23	.14	21
Same cases plus 7 in which a foster child and a true child were reared in same home	.11	.13	28

The first (which is also the higher) of these correlations is probably the more valid, since the seven true children in the second correlation introduce a sample from a non-comparable population of children having a higher central tendency than that of the foster group.

Another point of interest lies in the possible effect of schooling upon intelligence. The five-year-olds provide the only group in which this point can be considered, since practically all the older children had attended school. In the Foster Group our records show that 30 five-year-olds had attended kindergarten or first grade, and that 30 five-year-olds had not. The mean I.Q. of those who had attended kindergarten or school was 111, and of those who had not attended, 107. The difference of 4 points in favor of the first group is quite possibly due to schooling, but since the probable error of the difference is 2.8 points, it cannot be considered as reliably established. Moreover, even if the difference were a reliable one, nothing in our data could show that part of the difference was not due to a tendency on the part of parents to enter bright children in school at an earlier age than dull ones.

The following correlations were found between the mental ages of fathers and mothers in the two groups:

	r	P.E.	N
Foster	.42	.04	174
Control	.55	.05	100

Let us now return to the data of Table XXXI. A dotted line was there inserted to separate from the more important coefficients certain coefficients that are ambiguous because they represent relationships between variables that might conceivably have reciprocal effects upon one another. For example, do the books in a child's library stimulate the growth of his I.Q. or does the child of high intelligence tend to collect more books around him? Does reading the Burgess bedtime stories to a two-year-old enhance his mental potentiality or does the child with high mental potentiality clamor loudest for the bedtime stories? Such considerations relegate these correlations to the realm of speculation; they are presented only for what interest they possess.

However, the first correlations of the table offer a clearer picture. The variables listed there could scarcely be thought of as influenced to any appreciable degree by the intelligence of the children in a home (at least by the intelligence of children as young as ours). Consequently, these correlations, when significantly greater than their own probable errors, can be taken as actual measures of the effect of environment in the Foster Group, and as measures of the combined effects of heredity and environment in the Control Group. The point is emphasized in this section—where results are first presented which are to serve as a basis for subsequent statistical treatment and final conclusions—that *the differences between corresponding correlation coefficients in the Foster Group and Control Group are striking and consistent.*

2. Corrections for Attenuation

While the raw correlations of Table XXXI show the drift of the evidence, they do not tell the complete story. In Spearman's nomenclature they are ''attenuated,'' owing to the unreliability of the measures upon which they are based. Spearman's formula of correction for attenuation was applied to some of the most important correlations to yield the best available estimate of what the relationships would have been if perfectly reliable, *i. e.*, 'true' measures, could have been used. Coefficients so computed represent more accurately than raw coefficients the actual contributions of various factors to variability in a criterion.

In computing coefficients corrected for attenuation, the problem of ascertaining sound reliabilities to be used in the Spearman formula was a perplexing one.

To find the reliability of the Stanford Binet Test for children and for adults, the Spearman-Brown formula[11] was applied to 'split halves.' This formula, which is based upon an assumption that the 'split halves' are fully comparable with respect to the function that both halves purport to measure, does not provide an entirely satisfactory measure of reliability for a battery as variegated as the Stanford Binet. Unless we may make the additional (as yet unproved and possibly untrue) assumption that the function we call intelligence is due to a general factor plus no specific factors, the measures of Stanford Binet reliability which are reached by methods described below may probably be considered as too low. Possibly, the high correlations reported by Herring (6)

---

[11] The formula is:

$$r_n = \frac{2r_{\frac{1}{2}} \, I/II}{1 + r_{\frac{1}{2}} \, I/II}$$

between I.Q's measured on the Herring and on the Stanford revisions of the Binet Test (.97 to .99) provide a better estimate of the true reliability of the Binet Scale, although these reliabilities, too, seem open to question. The material in the two versions is so similar as possibly to capitalize chance skills, techniques or information that an individual has happened to acquire during the course of his life.[12]

Fortunately, the indeterminate error in the reliability coefficients for the Stanford Binet does not seriously affect the results based upon the reliabilities. This is because the total corrections (by the formula for correcting attenuation) amount to only a few points in the second decimal place when reliabilities are even approximately as high as those found and when the raw correlations to which the corrections are applied are not high themselves.

The specific procedure employed to determine the reliabilities was as follows:

a. Children. From the test files of the Stanford Psychology Department, a distribution of fifty complete tests was built up. The subjects represented by the tests matched the Foster Group in age and I.Q. The reliability of half the test was computed by correlating I.Q.'s based upon halves split by the alternate item method, and then the Spearman-Brown formula was applied to find the reliability of the test as a whole.

Next the correlation between the complete form and the 'lopped' form (see explanation of 'lopped' form p. 230) was computed for this group. The reliability of the lopped form was then inferred by a formula derived for this purpose by Professor Kelley,

$$r_{2\,II} = r^2_{12}\, r_{1\,I} \text{ where}$$

$r_{2\,II}$ is the reliability of the lopped form

$r_{1\,I}$ is the reliability or the complete form

r_{12} is the correlation between the composite and the lopped form.

The following coefficients were found in using the successive steps:

$r_{\frac{1}{2}I\,/\,II} = .79$
$r_{1\,I} \quad = .88$ (correction by Spearman-Brown formula)
$r_{12} \quad = .97$
$r_{2\,II} \quad = .83$, the value of reliability used in this study.

The same reliability coefficient was used for the tests of the control children as for the foster children, since the variabilities in I.Q. of the two groups were exactly the same.

---

[12] In this connection, see Professor Kelley's *Note on the Reliability of a Test* (8) in which the conditions tending to raise or lower reliabilities spuriously are set forth.

INFLUENCES UPON MENTAL DEVELOPMENT

By way of interest it may be noted that the above values for $r_{1\,I}$ and r_{12} agree quite well with similar values found by James DeVoss (2) and by Floyd Ruch (14), respectively. The former found I.Q. reliabilities clustering around .92 for single age groups; the latter found a correlation of .98 between the complete and lopped Binet forms, using an adult population.

b. Adults. One third (59) of the tests of foster fathers were selected in such a way that the numbers from each mental age level would be proportional to the corresponding numbers in the entire group. These were split by the alternate item method; the halves were correlated, and the correlation corrected by the Spearman-Brown formula, yielding .86. But this 'reliability,' based upon lopped tests, is spuriously high, since the lopped test assumes perfect performance on all tests below the lowest level given, and consistent failure on all tests above the highest level given. Now in the built-up distribution of tests of children, the complete tests had a Spearman-Brown corrected reliability of .88, and a similar procedure yielded .90 for the lopped version—a value only .02 points higher. The empirical assumption was made that the 'reliability' .86 found for the lopped adult tests was .02 higher than a real reliability based upon complete tests would have been. Letting

$$r_{1\,I} = .84$$
$$r_{12} = .97$$

then, by Kelley's formula, $r_{2\,II} = .79$, the value of reliability used in this study.

The reliabilities of adult and children's vocabularies were easily determined by correlating one list of the vocabulary test against the other list, and inferring the reliability for the complete test by the Spearman-Brown formula. This was done for fathers, mothers, and children in the Foster Group, and the reliabilities thus determined were used also in the Control Group.

Reliabilities for the Whittier Scale and the Culture Scale were taken to be the correlations between independent ratings by Mrs. Jensen and myself upon all the Whittier and Culture blanks in the Control Group. Strictly speaking, these correlations are not reliabilities, for they are almost certainly somewhat higher than two series of ratings based upon data gathered twice from the same homes with a month or a year intervening would have been. They represent rather the upper limit of reliability.

The reliability of family income was assumed to be unity, which, of course, is too high, although our impression was that the parents attempted to give us accurate information upon this point.

While fully realizing that the determination of reliabilities of these variables is not without flaws, I think it probable that the correlations forthwith presented represent a closer approximation to the truth than the raw correlations. It is possible for reliabilities to vary several points in the second decimal from their proper value without seriously distorting the correlations corrected for attenuation. Moreover, it is probable that some reliabilities estimated too high are compensated for by others estimated too low; so that in the multiple correlations which have been computed very reasonable values may be obtained.

Summarizing this discussion, the following reliabilities were used:

Stanford Binet, children's I.Q. 83
Stanford Binet, adult mental age 79
Vocabulary, fathers 96
Vocabulary, mothers 96
Vocabulary, children (age 8-14) 93
Whittier index 92
Culture index 95
Income 1.00

TABLE XXXIV.—CHILD'S I. Q. CORRELATED WITH ENVIRONMENTAL AND HEREDITARY FACTORS AND CORRECTED FOR ATTENUATION*

	Foster		Control	
	r	N	r	N
Father's M.A.	.09	178	.55	100
Mother's M.A.	.23	204	.57	105
Father's vocabulary	.14	181	.52	101
Mother's vocabulary	.25	202	.48	104
Whittier index	.24	206	.48	104
Culture index	.29	186	.49	101
Income	.26	181	.26	99

*The P.E.'s are all in the neighborhood of .06.

It is obvious that the fairly high correlations between I.Q. and environmental factors in the Control Group are due to a large extent to the high association between parental intelligence and environmental factors. Such association can be shown by the correlations of Table XXXV.

It is perhaps surprising that income correlates somewhat less with parents' mental level than do the other environmental measures. Nevertheless, the income correlations probably approximate their true values, in as much as the correlation of foster father's mental age and income, .31, agrees with the corresponding value in the Control Group fairly well.

In interpreting all the foregoing correlation comparisons between the Foster Group and the Control Group, it should be borne in mind that the *squares* of the correlations, rather than the corre-

TABLE XXXV.—PARENTAL CORRELATIONS IN CONTROL GROUP

Factor	Father's Mental Age		Mother's Mental Age	
	Raw	Corr. for atten.	Raw	Corr. for atten.
Whittier index................	.60	.70	.60	.70
Culture index.................	.67	.77	.71	.82
Income (by aux. score meth.)...	.38	.43	.40	.51
Father's education............	.46	....	....	....
Mother's education...........	....	....	.62	....

lations themselves, represent the portion of the variance of children's I.Q's that can be accounted for by reference to the respective variables [I.e $\sigma_{1.2} = \sigma_1^2 (1 - r_{12}^2)$]. This consideration emphasizes the differences in strength of relationship found in the two groups.

3. Multiple Correlations

It should also be pointed out that the foregoing correlations do not provide an absolute basis for evaluating the relative influence of various environmental factors. The intercorrelations between these factors are so complex, and the status of the factors as possible causes and effects of one another is so uncertain, that their unique contributions to the variance of the children's I.Q.'s are impossible to extricate. Because of the difficulties just mentioned, partial correlation technique is obviously unadapted to the problem (1). It is possible, however, to arrive at an estimate of the *total* effect of our measured environmental factors through multiple correlation technique.

Accordingly, we determined the multiple correlation of the following factors with child's I.Q. in the foster and control groups:

Father's mental age   Father's education
Mother's mental age   Mother's education
Father's vocabulary   Whittier index
Mother's vocabulary   Culture index
                      Family income

To have gone through the operation of computing multiple correlations that utilized all nine of the variables in question would have been enormously time-consuming. To save labor, certain variables were eliminated, after first demonstrating, through multiples using three of four variables, that they contributed practically nothing to an estimate of the child's I.Q. not already contributed by variables retained for the final multiple. For example, in the foster multiple, income was retained, but Whittier and Culture indices were dropped out, because the multiple of I.Q. with all three together (.34) was only .01 higher than the correlation (.33) between I.Q. and income alone; again, mother's vocabulary was retained, but mother's mental age and mother's education were dropped out because the multiple of I.Q. with all three together (.254) was only .005 higher than the correlation (.249) between I.Q. and mother's vocabulary alone. Similarly, in the Control Group, certain variables were not used. The variables finally employed no doubt yield values for the multiple correlations that attain, within one or two points in the second decimal, to what the values would have been had we used all nine variables.

The factors retained for the foster multiple were: father's mental age, father's vocabulary, mother's vocabulary, income. Those retained for the control multiple were: father's mental age, father's vocabulary, mother's mental age, Whittier index. The unexpected predictive prepotency of parental vocabulary over parental mental age is probably an adventitious fact, due to the higher reliability of the vocabulary test.

The multiple correlations of Table XXXVI summarize the chief statistical results of the study in two clear-cut comparisons. They

TABLE XXXVI.—MULTIPLE CORRELATIONS OF HEREDITARY AND ENVIRONMENTAL FACTORS WITH CHILD'S I. Q.

	Foster			Control		
	r	P.E.	N	r	P.E.	N
Raw multiple................	.35	.05	164	.53	.05	95
Multiple using r's corrected for attenuation*............	.42	...	164	.61	...	95

*The P.E.'s of the multiples using correlations corrected for attenuation are not subject to calculation by any methods at present available, but they are, of course, somewhat higher than the P.E.'s for the raw multiples.

show more distinctly than do any of the results from previous sections the significant differences between the outcomes for the Foster Group and those for the Control Group.

INFLUENCES UPON MENTAL DEVELOPMENT

VIII. Interpretation and Conclusions

The way has now been cleared to answer, if possible, the questions regarding the relative contributions to intelligence of nature and nurture which were raised in the beginning of the study. The interpretation of results to be presented will embrace the following aspects of the problem of factors conditioning children's intelligence:

1. Proportional contribution of total home environment to variance.

2. Unique contribution of parental intelligence to variance.

3. Estimate of total contribution of heredity to variance.

4. Numerical estimate of the potency of home environment to raise or depress the I.Q.

1. Proportional Contribution of Total Home Environment

Considering the correlations which have been reported, we have logical ground for believing that the multiple correlation corrected for attenuation (.42) is a measure in the Foster Group of the effect of home environment upon differences in children's intelligence. More precisely, the *square* of this multiple (.17) represents the portion of the variance of children in ordinary communities that is due to home environment.[16]

---

[16] In discussing the portion of the *variance* of the children due to this factor and that one, I follow Fisher (3). The justifications for dealing with contribution to variance (*i. e.*, squares of the S. D.) rather than with contributions to the first power of the standard deviation or to any other power are: (a) that such contributions to variance combine additively to give the total variance of the criterion, but contributions to any other power of the S. D. do not; and (b) contributions to variance, but not to other measures of variability, can readily be interpreted by a concept of the proportional number of *common factors* underlying the influences and the criterion. For example, a criterion composed of four equally variable factors, a, b, c, and d, correlates $1/\sqrt{4}$, or ½ with any of the 'influences'—a, b, c, or d. The square of the correlation ½, or ¼, gives the contribution of each factor to the variance of the criterion, and expresses the proportion of factors in the criterion contributed by each factor.

In this connection may be cited a paper by Pearson, "On Certain Errors with Regard to Multiple Correlation Occasionally Made by Those Who Have Not Adequately Studied this Subject" (11). In this article Pearson demonstrates that nearly the maximal predictivity, with respect to a criterion, of a large group of variables all showing considerable correlation among themselves is attained when only a few of such variables are used in a multiple correlation. It follows that the square of our multiple probably represents nearly the maximal effect of home environment, especially since various factors of home environment that were not used in the final multiple could be legitimately dropped out because they were found to contribute to I.Q. variance practically nothing in addition to the contribution of the variables retained.

2. Unique Contribution of Parental Intelligence

In the Control Group, the square (.37) of the multiple correlation corrected for attenuation (.61) represents the *combined* effect of home environment and parental mental level upon the variance of children's intelligence. Neglecting the variable 'father's vocabulary,' which contributes only an insignificant amount in addition to father's mental age, it is extremely interesting to apply the Wright path coefficient technique to the correlations for the Control Group, to find out how much of the children's I.Q. variance can be accounted for by reference to parental intelligence alone.[17]

This situation is a particularly favorable one for using the Wright technique, for the assumptions regarding casual relation-

---

[17] The path coefficient method, to quote Sewall Wright (20) "depends on the combination of knowledge of the degrees of correlation among variables in a system with such knowledge as may be possessed of the causal relations." The method is limited by the rarity with which we have actual knowledge of causal relations; but it provides a tool of the nicest precision in such situations as do offer an adequate basis for postulating causation. It cannot, itself, uncover what is cause and what is effect, though in the absence of definite knowledge regarding causal relationships between variables, the method "can be used to find out the logical consequences of any particular hypothesis in regard to them." Conservatively stated, in any situation in which we feel justified in drawing conclusions regarding the effects of certain phenomena upon others, the Wright method provides a numerical expression of such conclusions. For a detailed explanation of its application, the reader is referred to two articles by Wright (20) (21).

INFLUENCES UPON MENTAL DEVELOPMENT

ships are here at a minimum. It is only necessary to assume that parental intelligence and home environment affect the child's I.Q., but that the child's I.Q. does not contribute to these. It is not necessary to make any assumption at all regarding a possible casual or interacting relationship between parental intelligence and environment; merely the known correlation between the two is sufficient. The relation between the variables is represented in the 'set-up' shown herewith, in which

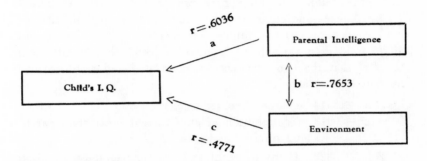

r (parental intelligence) (I.Q.) is the multiple, corrected for attenuation, between the I.Q. of the child and the mental ages of the two parents;

r (parental intelligence) (environment) is the multiple, corrected for attenuation, between the Whittier index and the mental ages of the two parents; and

r (I.Q.) (environment) is the correlation, corrected for attenuation, between the child's I.Q. and the Whittier index.

a represents the direct path of influence between parental intelligence and child's I.Q. and a^2 the percentage of I.Q. variance attributable to parental intelligence. The coefficients c and c^2 represent corresponding coefficients of environmental influence other than that reflected in a and a^2. The coefficient b represents the known correlation between parental intelligence and environment.

The directions of the arrows indicate the relationship of the variables with respect to cause, effect, and possible reciprocal action.

By Wright's formulas:

r (I.Q.) (parental intelligence) $= .6036 = a + bc$

r (I.Q.) (environment) $= .4771 = c + ab$

r (parental intelligence) (environment) $= .7653 = b$

Solving these three equations for the two unknowns,

$$a = .5757 \qquad\qquad a^2 = .3314$$
$$c = .0367 \qquad\qquad c^2 = .0013$$

In addition to a and b, there is an effect upon the child's I.Q. due to the *combined* working of the two correlated variables, parental intelligence and environment. This effect is equal to 2abc, or .0322, and expresses the minute increment of variance, over and above what each variable contributes by itself, that results from the fact that the two variables are correlated and reënforce one another to some extent.

$$a^2 = .3314 \quad \text{(parental contribution)}$$

$c^2 = .0013$ (contribution of environment *other* than parental intelligence)

$2abc = .0322$ (joint parental and environmental contribution over and above separate contribution of each)

$$\overline{.3649}$$

The sum of a^2, c^2, and 2abc is equal to the square of the multiple correlation of I.Q. with parental intelligence and environment.

A question of great interest concerns the difference between the contribution (.17) of total environment in the Foster Group and the contribution (.0013) of environmental influence (other than the direct influence of parental intelligence) in the Control Group. This difference is probably due to several facts, viz:

(1) The environmental as well as the hereditary contribution of parental intelligence is contained in a^2, and is consequently lacking in the value, .0013, of c^2. We should not expect this *environmental* contribution of parental intelligence to be over four or five percent, however, because the correlations (even when corrected for attenuation) between child's I.Q. and foster parents' M.A. are so very low (see Table XXXIV). The correlation squared is .0081 with foster father, and .0529 with foster mother; and both these values represent more than the unique foster parent contri-

butions, because they are increased by the relationship of parental M.A. to other influences of environment.

(2) Part of the joint parental and environmental contribution (.0322) should be properly attributed to environment when a comparison is made of environmental influences in our two groups.

(3) The probable errors of our determinations of degrees of influence could well account for the remaining discrepancy. It is not known exactly what the magnitude of these probable errors is; however, we do know that the P.E. of the multiple correlation (corrected) of child's I.Q. with environment in the Foster Group is greater than .05; and that the P.E. of path coefficients based upon corrected correlations of the size of the ones entering our calculations is fully as large as that.

3. Estimate of Total Contribution of Heredity

As has been noted above, a^2, or 33 percent, represents the proportion of I.Q. variance that is attributable to parental intelligence alone. Now, 37 percent is the proportion of I.Q. variance that we have already found attributable to parental intelligence and environment, alone and in combination. It follows that, if we could, without at the same time narrowing the range of parental intelligence, level all other aspects of home environment to a standard or average, the variance of children's intelligence would be reduced by 37 minus 33, or 4 percent. The contribution of parental intelligence to variance would then be equal to .33/.96, or 34 percent.

Such a contribution corresponds to a multiple correlation of $\sqrt{.34}$, or .58,—the multiple correlation (corrected for attenuation) which would be found between child's I.Q. and parental intelligence if the home environment of all families were made constant, but *parental intelligence continued to vary as much as before.* In this latter respect the coefficient differs radically in theory from the partial correlation coefficient, which in comparable situations has sometimes been interpreted erroneously (1). The partial correlation of I.Q. and parental intelligence with environment constant is here only .42, as contrasted with .58.

The value .58 probably represents fairly closely the actual degree of resemblance between children and their two parents based upon heredity alone. The undoubted fact that a small amount of parent-child resemblance due to environment, but not measured by the Whittier Scale, is still concealed in the coefficient probably enhances its value slightly. But the fact that parents were themselves molded in part by environment, and in consequence vary somewhat from their congenital mental level, and the further likelihood of slight random *environmental* effects (such as those from pre- and post-natal nutrition), suggest that the intrinsic genetic resemblance between parents and offspring is somewhat depressed thereby. The elevating and depressing effects undoubtedly cancel one another to some extent. The coefficient .58 can consequently be taken as a tentative approximation to the true genetic relation. Its probable error could in this case be computed similarly to the probable error of a regression coefficient if the coefficient .58 were not based upon correlations corrected for attenuation. It can only be observed that its probable error must be somewhat greater than the probable error (.06) of an ordinary regression coefficient based upon raw intercorrelations equivalent to the corrected ones used here.

We have now seen that the total contribution of systematic (or measurable) home environment is close to 17 percent, and that the contribution of home environment and parental intelligence together is represented by a multiple correlation coefficient (corrected) of .61, or by a percentage of .37. If not more than 35 or 40 percent of the variance of children's I.Q.'s is accounted for by reference to these factors, what contributes the other 60 or 65 percent?

Possibly a portion of this residual variance is due to the "random somatic effects of environment," to quote Fisher (3). But it seems reasonable to suppose that not a great deal is due to this effect, since numerous studies have shown a marked tendency for the I.Q. to remain constant over a period of years, while other studies have shown that identical twins correlate in intelligence about as closely as the reliability of the tests employed will permit (10). Probably the major share of the residual variance is due to congenital endowment, since in known modes of hereditary transmission the influence of heredity is *always* far stronger than parental correlations alone would indicate. This is necessarily the case because only half the chromosomes of each parent are passed on to the offspring. Hence, the parental deviation for any trait in question is determined by a number of factors other than the ones transmitted to the child. In hereditary traits such as stature, which are known to be influenced relatively little by ordinary differences in environment, the multiple correlation of child with parents is .64, but the contribution of heredity to variance approaches 100 percent. The closeness of our estimated value of the "genetic" multiple correlation for intelligence to this value of the multiple correlation for stature is striking. *Probably, then, close to 75 or 80 percent of I.Q. variance is due to innate and heritable causes.*

This estimate makes allowance for the 17 percent which the data of this study show is due to measurable home environment, plus an additional 5 or 10 percent due to the possible "random somatic effects of environment." In the opinion of the writer, the estimate is the most reasonable one that can be made from available data with available methods. But a determination of the total contribution of heredity can probably never be made beyond cavil until the genetic mechanics of mental heredity are first established by methods analogous to those used by Fisher in the study of physical traits (3).

4. A Numerical Estimate of the Potency of Home Environment to Raise or Depress the I.Q.

One further angle of interpretation will be especially pertinent to the general problem of the possibilities and limitations of training. From a practical outlook the point to be raised is undoubtedly of even greater significance than the more general problem of the proportional contributions of nature and nurture to mental variability. It is concerned with the question: "How far, in terms of measurable I.Q., is environment potent to increase or inhibit the development of innate intelligence?"

Let us turn to the data of Section V. It was there seen that empirical considerations, based upon facts given, strongly suggested that the 'congenital mental level' of the foster children was not more than two or three points above 100 I.Q. But the average I.Q. level actually found in this group was 107. Can this discrepancy be accounted for through superior environmental advantages?

Probably it can be. The average mental age level of the foster fathers is 16 years, 11 months, and of the foster mothers is 16 years,

3 months. The average *mid-parent* level, 16-7, is about one standard deviation above that of parents in general.

The army intelligence data (22) strongly imply that the average adult mental level of Americans is closer to 14 years than to the 16-year level which had been tentatively established previously. But the Army Alpha group test was different in many respects from individual tests, and psychologists have hesitated to assume without further evidence that the same outcome would necessarily hold for tests of the Binet type. However, our control data rather bear out the army conclusions when treated in the following manner: Summary cards for the cases were arranged from lowest to highest in order of father's mental age. Starting with the first case, the children's I.Q.'s were added and averaged as each additional case was inserted. When a point was reached at which the children's I.Q.'s averaged as close to 100 as our limited number of cases permitted (within three points of 100), the fathers' and mothers' mental ages for those cases were averaged separately and together with the following result:

		N
Fathers' mental age	12.9	21
Mothers' mental age	14.5	21
Average	13.7	

The same procedure was repeated with cases in which mothers' mental age was arranged from lowest to highest, with the result:

		N
Fathers' mental age	14.6	20
Mothers' mental age	12.4	20
Average	13.5	

Finally, first with the fathers and then with the mothers, and starting with 13.5 as a median, paired cases in which parent scores showed equal positive and negative deviations from 13.5 were selected until all possible pairs had been used. The average of fathers and mothers was 13.8 in the first instance and 14.1 in the second instance. The corresponding average I.Q.'s of children were 105 and 104, respectively, suggesting that 14 years may be a little high to represent the average adult level. But it seems justifiable on the basis of the foregoing to use 14 for an approximation to the truth. As the standard deviation of our mid-parent mental age is close to two years, the average level of the control parents (and similarly of the foster parents) is about one standard deviation superior.

It is difficult to say just how high above the mean of the generality are the other environmental measures (culture index, Whittier index, income, etc.) because no satisfactory norms for unselected populations are available upon them. Since most of the correlations between the measures of environment and the measures of parental intelligence are quite high, a safe estimate would be that the total complex of environment (including parental intelligence) is between one half and one standard deviation above average.

The multiple correlation (corrected for attenuation), .42, can now be used as a regression coefficient for predicting the average standard score of the Foster Group. A positive increment of .42 times one standard deviation (or 15 I.Q. points) would equal 6 I.Q. points; or times one half a standard deviation would equal 3 I.Q. points. An increment of 3 to 6 I.Q. points would bring the I.Q. level of our foster children very close to that actually found (107), provided my judgment is correct that their average innate intelligence is about 102 or 103.

We may now go through some of the variables which were correlated with the I.Q's of the foster children and ascertain, when various factors of environment are, say, one standard unit above or below the mean of American communities, how much the I.Q's of the children have been shifted from their "congenital" value in consequence. The column in the following table headed "Measured" is based upon raw correlations, and the column headed "Actual"is based upon correlations corrected for attenuation. Correlations used for the computations are those reported in Tables XXXI, XXXIV, and XXXVI. The values of Table XLV are

TABLE XLV.—AVERAGE SHIFT, DUE· TO ENVIRONMENT, IN POINTS OF I.Q., OF FOSTER CHILDREN, WHEN VARIOUS FACTORS ARE ONE S. D. ABOVE OR BELOW THE POPULATION MEAN

Factor	Measured	Actual
Foster father's mental age...........................	1.0	1.4
Foster mother's mental age...........................	2.9	3.5
Foster mid-parent mental age	3.0	....
Whittier rating of foster home.......................	3.1	3.6
Culture rating of foster home........................	3.7	4.4
Total environment...................................	5.3	6.3

found merely by multiplying the correlations of foster children's I.Q.'s with the factors in question by the S.D., 15, of the children's I.Q.'s

The implications of this table seem to the writer of more profound significance than those of any other part of the study. While the intercorrelations between these environmental factors are so complex that the relative influences of the separate factors are probably not represented linearly by the differences in the corresponding I.Q. "shifts," the *order* of their influence is probably so indicated. From this argument two outstanding conclusions emerge:

1. The total effect of environmental factors one standard deviation up or down the scale is only about 6 points, or, allowing for a maximal oscillation in the corrected multiple correlation (.42) of as much as .20, the maximal effect almost certainly lies between 3 and 9 points.

2. Assuming the best possible environment to be three standard deviations above the mean of the population (which, if "environments" are distributed approximately according to the normal law, would only occur about once in a thousand cases,) the excess in such a situation of a child's I.Q. over his inherited level would lie between 9 and 27 points—or less if the relation of culture to I.Q. is curvilinear on the upper levels, as it well may be.

An influence of this magnitude, although significant, is emphatically not sufficient to account for genius upon a theory of environment. Francis Galton, whose I.Q. in childhood Professor Terman has estimated to have been close to 200 (16), was reared in a home of exceptional cultural advantages. Yet even without the possible 9 to 27 points contributed by his environment, he would still have ranked as a genius such as occurs in unselected populations only once in many thousands of individuals. Whether or not he would have succeeded in using his gifts with such telling effect if he had not had the training, education, and inspiring associates that were his, is of course another question. While many men and women have surmounted unbelievable obstacles to achieve eminence, there is no telling how many others, of weaker stamina, have crumpled by the way.

It is of further interest to note that, while the environmental conditions of gifted men, women, and children indisputably show a somewhat superior tendency, they are not, as a rule, so exceptional as those to which the fortunate young Galton was born. The average Barr rating of fathers of the California gifted children studied by Professor Terman is 12.77—a value close to that of the foster fathers and of the control fathers. Thus, the superiority of the gifted group must be due preponderantly to endowment and, on an average, less than 10 points of I.Q. must be due to environment. *Home environment in the most favorable circumstances may suffice to bring a child just under the borderline of dullness up over the threshhold of normality, and to make a slightly superior child out of a normal one; but it cannot account for the enormous mental differences to be found among human beings.*

If environment cannot account for men, like Galton, who far and away outstrip the majority of their fellows coming even from such a favorable environment as theirs, still less can it account for an impressive number of eminent men whose early conditions of life have been of the kind that depress rather than enhance the I.Q.: men like Lincoln of the backwoods; Carlyle, whose simple peasant mother learned writing while he was at college so that she might correspond with him; Dickens, whose nursery was a London slum; or Canning, a neglected little boy who "longed for bread and butter" as he followed the ragged fortunes of a band of strolling players in eighteenth century England.

5. Summary of Conclusions

By methods which have permitted the effects of environment to be studied separately from those of heredity in conjunction with environment, this study has sought to evaluate the factors conditioning the intelligence of a group of white American school children living in ordinarily variable circumstances. The main conclusions thereby reached are as follows:

1. Home environment contributes about 17 percent of the variance in I.Q.: parental intelligence alone accounts for about 33 percent.

2. The total contribution of heredity (i. e., of innate and heritable factors) is probably not far from 75 or 80 percent.

3. Measurable environment one standard deviation above or below the mean of the population does not shift the I. Q. by more than 6 to 9 points above or below the value it would have had under normal environmental conditions. In other words, nearly 70 percent of school children have an actual I.Q. within 6 to 9 points of that represented by their innate intelligence.

4. The maximal contribution of the best home environment to intelligence is apparently about 20 I.Q. points, or less, and almost surely lies between 10 and 30 points. Conversely, the least cultured, least stimulating kind of American home environment may depress the I.Q. as much as 20 I.Q. points. But situations as extreme as either of these probably occur only once or twice in a thousand times in American communities.

5. With regard to character and personality traits, upon which the data presented are less reliable and less objective than those upon intelligence, the indications are that environment is at least as potent as in the case of intellectual traits—possibly much more potent.

A more comprehensive study of such traits, however, must await the future. Whatever clear contribution is made to the general nature-nurture problem by this investigation must rest only upon the data which deal with intelligence. On this point, it is believed that the study finds support for the conclusion reached by the first pioneer to study mental heredity by statistical methods—that heredity is a force in the determination of mental ability by the side of which all other forces are "dwarfed in comparison."

IX. References

(1) BURKS, BARBARA S. "On the inadequacy of the partial and multiple correlation technique." *Jour. Ed. Psych.*, 17: 1926, 522-540.

(2) DEVOSS, JAMES C. "*The Unevenness of the Abilities of Gifted Children in California.*" Ph.D. dissertation, Stanford University, 1924.

(3) FISHER, R. A. "Correlation between relatives on the supposition of Mendelian inheritance." *Trans. Royal. Soc. Edinburgh*, 52: 1918, 399-433.

(4) GORDON, KATE. "The influence of heredity in mental ability." Children's Dept., Calif. State Board of Control, 4th Bienn. Rept., 1918-1920.

(5) GORDON, HUGH. "Mental and scholastic tests among retarded children." Ed. Pamphlets, No. 44, Bd. of Ed., London, 1923.

(6) HERRING, JOHN P. "Reliability of the Stanford and the Herring revision of the Binet-Simon tests." *Jour. Ed. Psych.*, 15: 1924, 217-223.

(7) HILDRETH, GERTRUDE H. *Resemblance of Siblings in Intelligence and Achievement.* New York, 1925, (Teachers College, Columbia, Contributions to Education, No. 186).

(8) KELLEY, T. L. "Note on the reliability of a test." *Jour. Ed. Psych.*, 15: 1924, 193-204.

(9) KELLEY, T. L. *Statistical Method.* New York, 1924.

(10) MERRIMAN, CURTIS. "The intellectual resemblance of twins." *Psych. Monographs*, 33: 1924, pp. 58.

(11) PEARSON, KARL. "On certain errors with regard to multiple correlation occasionally made by those who have not adequately studied this subject." *Biometrika*, 10: 1914, 181-187.

(12) POYER, G. *Problèmes Généreaux de l'Hérédité Psychologique.* Paris, 1921.

(13) RICHARDSON, L. F. "Measurement of mental 'nature' and the study of adopted children." *Eug. Rev.*, 4: 1912-13, 391-394.

(14) RUCH, FLOYD. *On the Defensibility of Certain Abridgments of the Stanford Revision of the Binet-Simon Tests.* M.A. thesis, University of Iowa, 1925.

(15) TERMAN, L. M. and others. *Genetic Studies of Genius*, Volume I. Stanford University, 1925.

(16) TERMAN, L. M. "The intelligence of Francis Galton in childhood." *Amer. Jour. Psych.*, 28: 1917, 209-215.

(17) THEIS, SOPHIE VAN S. *How Foster Children Turn Out.* State Charities Aid Ass'n. Publication No. 165, 1924.

(18) *Whittier Social Case History Manual.* Calif. Bureau of Juvenile Research, Bull. No. 10, 1921.

(19) WILLOUGHBY, R. R. *Family Similarities in Mental Test Abilities.* Ph.D. dissertation, Stanford University, 1926.

(20) WRIGHT, SEWALL. "Correlation and causation." *Jour. Agric. Research*, 20: 1921, 557-585.

(21) WRIGHT, SEWALL. "The theory of path coefficients." *Genetics*, 8: 1923, 238-255.

(22) YERKES, R. M. (editor). *Psychological Examining in the United States Army*, 1921. (*Mem. Nat. Acad. Sci.*, 15).

PART VIII

INTELLIGENCE AND SOCIAL CLASS

The problems connected with "deprived" groups (coloured people, working class children, etc.) are legion, and nowhere else has emotion so clouded the picture as in the discussion of the relation between IQ and class, or race. No detailed discussion of the racial problem will be given here in view of the complexity of the issues which do not allow of presentation within the confines of a single paper; the reader is referred to recent publications which give a factual account of the experimental evidence (Eysenck, 1971; Jensen, 1972; Shuey, 1966). The problem is much more amenable to empirical proof in connection with social class, and we have the excellent discussion by Sir Cyril Burt to state the main facts, and introduce us to the type of statistical calculation involved. Before turning to a consideration of some of the facts, it may be useful to deal with a view held by many people relating to the implications of genetic determination of IQ, a view which is wrong in point of fact, but has nevertheless coloured the popular imagination. The popular misconception is shown in Fig. 1, which is taken from a paper by the well-known geneticist Ching Chun Li (1971); the upper part shows the popular picture, the lower part the actual picture as modern genetics sees it.

Each part of the Fig. shows a parental and a filial generation, the former on top, the latter below. Both have the same distribution of a given trait, IQ in our case, and we are asked to imagine that the distribution of this trait is perfectly coincident with social class; in other words, the 4 brightest individuals in the parental generation are in the highest of five social classes, the 4 dullest in the lowest, and the others intermediate according to the Fig. The false picture of genetic descent is shown in the top part of the Fig., with lines of direct descent leading to an identical perfect association between IQ and social class, i.e. with the children of the lowest class group having the lowest IQs, the children of the highest class group having the highest IQs, and the children of the other class groups intermediate in IQ. Such a picture is quite impossible to reconcile with any

existing genetic model; it could only obtain if heritability of IQ were in fact zero, and the environments of the five classes differed very sharply. What actually happens when heritability is pronounced, as it is in the case of IQ, is shown in the lower part of the Fig. Of the 4 children with the lowest IQ, only 1 comes from the lowest class parents; 2 come from the class above that, and 1 comes from the "middle" class. Similarly, of the 4 children with the highest IQ, only 1 comes from the highest class parents. Children in the new "middle" class come from parents in all the 5 classes. We have already seen that more than two-thirds of Terman's gifted children, with IQs over 140, did not come from the highest socio-economic group; yet the great majority of these children ended up in that group. We have also seen that the children of this gifted group had IQs 20 points below their gifted parents, in spite of the fact that they grew up in a much better environment, comparatively speaking—at least in so far as socio-economic status can be said to be correlated with the concept of a favourable environment. Altogether fewer than 60% of adults are found to be of the same social status as their parents (in the U.S.A.; British figures are given in Burt's article). Thus the genetic model, far from generating uniformity and conformity, produces a great whirling action in which children are just about as likely to go up or down as to remain close to their parental IQ and social class. To realize this consequence of genetic theory, and to eschew the false and misleading "uniformity" model depicted in the top part of Fig. 1, is the beginning of wisdom in dealing with the question of the relation between social class and IQ.

There are many different ways in which this fact can be expressed. The clearest is perhaps by way of regression to the mean, a phenomenon we have already encountered in relation to Terman's gifted children. Using Burt's data for English parents and children, we may graph the situation as in Fig. 2; this shows clearly the degree to which children's IQs regress upward for those born of below-average IQ parents, and downward

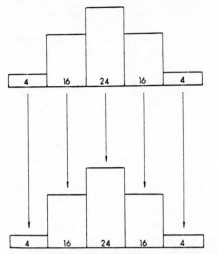

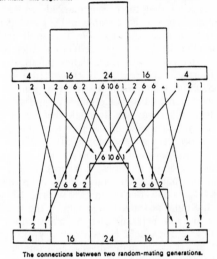

Wrong conception of heredity in a human population. Only very rigid social forces can make "like beget like."

The connections between two random-mating generations.

Fig. 1

From C. C. Li (1971). Intelligence: Genetic and Environmental Influences, *by kind permission of the author and Grune & Stratton Inc.*

for those born of above-average parents. The general formula covering the case has already been given and discussed. The close agreement of fact with prediction is most reassuring.

In our type of society, the inevitable consequence of regression of IQ, given the importance we place on educational achievement, and the high correlation between IQ and educational achievement, is a marked degree of social mobility. This is high even in the United Kingdom, although not as high as in the United States; some data from Burt (1959) may illustrate the point. Grouping fathers' and sons' social status into three broad categories, he finds the following results (Table 1):

TABLE 1

Father's Status	Son's Adult Status			
	I	II	III	Total
I	51·7	34·5	13·8	100·0
II	23·3	46·9	29·8	100·0
III	13·7	36·9	49·4	100·0

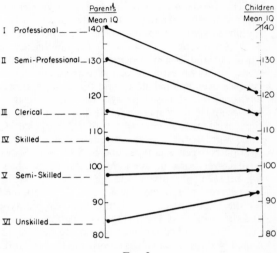

Fig. 2

In other words, less than 50% of sons have the same socio-economic status as their fathers; as many as 14% end up in the lowest class, although their parents were in the highest class, and a similar 14% end up in the highest class, although their parents were in the lowest. Is it the more intelligent who go up, and the less intelligent who go down? The paper by Waller, here reprinted, leaves little doubt that this is in fact so; social mobility upwards is strongly related to high IQ, and social mobility downwards with low IQ.* This is so even within a given family; thus holding environment (at least between-family environment, which of course is the crucial factor in arguments concerning ameliorative policies) constant makes little difference to this trend. Here then is very strong evidence to support the point made earlier that our social system is very strongly based on intelligence, and that criticisms of IQ measurements as "irrelevant" or "meaningless" are very far from the truth.

Burt has quoted several critics of the view that there are strong hereditary factors responsible for at least part of the difference in IQ between social classes, and the belief that these differences are entirely due to environmental causes is certainly strong, particularly among sociological and educational writers and theorists. Yet

* As Kerrin (1971) has shown, there is a price to pay for even upward mobility, in terms of anxiety and other emotional stress; this price should not be neglected in discussions of the subject.

it must be clear that if individual differences in intelligence are due largely to genetic factors, as we have shown them to be, then it is quite impossible for the average differences in intelligence between social classes not to include a strong genetic component. Jensen (1972) presents the statistical argument in this form:

"The correlation between phenotypes (the measurable characteristic) and genotypes (the genetic basis of the phenotype) is the square root of the heritability, or h. An average estimate of h for intelligence in European and North American Caucasian populations is ·90. An estimate of the average correlation between occupational status and IQ is ·50. A purely environmentalist position says that the correlation between IQ and occupation (or SES) is due entirely to the environmental component of IQ variance. In other words, this hypothesis requires that the correlation between genotypes and SES be zero. So we have correlations between three sets of variables: (*a*) between phenotype and genotype, $r_{pg} = $ ·90; (*b*) between phenotype and status, $r_{ps} = $ ·50; and (*c*) the hypothesized correlation between genotype and status, $r_{gs} = 0$. The first two correlations (r_{pg} and r_{ps}) are determined empirically and are here represented by the average values reported in the literature. The third correlation (r_{gs}) is hypothesized to be zero by those who believe genetic factors may play a part in *individual* differences but not in SES *group* differences. The question then becomes: is this set of correlations possible? The first two correlations we know are possible because they are empirically obtained values. The only correlation seriously in question is the hypothesized $r_{gs} = 0$. Now we know that mathematically the true correlations among a set of three variables, 1, 2, 3, must meet the following requirement:

$$r_{12}^2 + r_{13}^2 + r_{23}^2 - 2r_{12}r_{13}r_{23} < 1$$

The fact is that when the values of $r_{pg} = $ ·90, $r_{ps} = $ ·50 and $r_{gs} = 0$ are inserted into the above formula, it yields a value greater than 1·00. This means that r_{gs} must in fact be greater than zero."

(The well-known "consistency relation" used above by Jensen is discussed in some detail by Walker and Lev, 1953).

If differences in income, and in socio-economic status generally, cannot account for the observable differences in mental ability, is it reasonable to argue the other way and make intelligence responsible (at least in part) for observable differences in income? This argument is pursued by Burt in the last of the reprints in this section; only the second half of the paper is here reprinted as much of what is said in the first half would be redundant in view of our reprinting of other papers of his. Burt considers with particular care Pareto's formula, according to which income is distributed in a manner departing very far from the normal curve; many economists have considered this an argument against any relation obtaining between two things so differently distributed. Burt's suggestion to this impasse, namely that a person's output, which largely determines his income, is related to the contributory abilities by some special and possibly complex function, seems reasonable, and he adduces some evidence. It might be equally reasonable to introduce personality variables of a non-cognitive kind here; anyone who has seen the degree to which anxiety, neurosis, mental illness, or even simple fear of taking responsibility can reduce a person's "market value" in spite of high IQ will agree that some form of multiplicative relationship between IQ and favourable personality features may very well account for the immensely skewed distribution of incomes. However, this is not the place to argue the case; Burt's paper is of interest because it suggests a solution in principle to the problem posed, leaving the empirical details to be settled by suitable experiment. It is interesting to note in this connection that there is a marked tendency for business managers to have stable and somewhat introverted personalities (Eysenck, 1967), as well as being highly intelligent; it is these three factors which may be multiplicatively involved in the Pareto paradox.

The fourth of the reprints in this section asks the question, implicit in much of what has gone before: "Does intelligence cause achievement?" and answers it in a rather novel way, i.e. through the use of cross-legged analysis. In view of the fact that this type of analysis is not very widely known, and possesses considerable possibilities in relation to the analysis of causal chains of correlations, it seemed worth while including this paper, even though the conclusions may not be as clear-cut as one might have wished. Nevertheless, as the authors state, many data of the kind here analysed are routinely collected by many educational authorities, and it would be easy to carry out replications of this study in many diverse environments; the value of the results would seem likely to be high.

The last reprint in this section considers a very important social problem, which has been causing concern ever since Cattell and Burt brought it to the attention of psychologists. There seems to be a negative correlation of about − ·25 between IQ and number of children in the family; thus the duller members of society seem to breed at a greater rate than the brighter ones. If differences in IQ are largely determined by genetic causes, then one would expect the average IQ of the population to drop over time—not perhaps at a very fast rate (1 point per decade was one estimate), but nevertheless in a manner which might spell disaster to a highly industrialized civilization such as ours. Much evidence has been collected in the intervening years, and as Falek shows, the evidence is rather more reassuring than seemed likely at one time; our national intelligence is in no immediate danger. For the once, at least, a look into the future does not increase one's pessimism.

REFERENCES

BURT, C. Class differences in general intelligence: III. *Brit.J. Statist. Psychol.*, 1959, *12*, 15–33.

BURT, C. Intelligence and social mobility. *Brit. J. Statist. Psychol.*, 1961, *14*, 3–24.

EYSENCK, H. J. Personality patterns in various groups of businessmen. *Occup. Psychol.*, 1967, *41*, 249–250.

EYSENCK, H. J. *Race, intelligence and education.* (American title: The IQ Argument). London: Temple Smith, 1971. New York: Library Press, 1971.

JENSEN, A. R. *Genetics, educability, and subpopulation differences.* London: Methuen, 1972.

KERRIN, K. Social and psychological consequences of inter-generational occupational mobility. *Amer. J. Sociol.*, 1971, *77*, 1–18.

LI, C. C. A tale of two thermos bottles: properties of a genetic model for human intelligence. In: *Intelligence: genetic and environmental influences.* New York: Grune & Stratton, 1971, pp. 162–181.

SHUEY, AUDREY M. *The testing of Negro intelligence.* (2nd. Ed.). New York: Social Science Press, 1966.

WALKER, HELEN M. & LEV, J. *Statistical inference.* New York: Holt, 1953.

From C. Burt (1961). Brit. J. Statist. Psychol., *14*, 3–24, *by kind permission of the author and Scottish Academic Press*

INTELLIGENCE AND SOCIAL MOBILITY

By Cyril Burt

University College, London

The main thesis of the following paper is that, in a highly organized society, the discrepancies between the general intelligence of the children and the occupational class into which they are born is bound to produce a large and fairly constant amount of ' basic mobility ', quite apart from any deliberate changes in the political or educational structure of the society.

Since the correlation between the intelligence of fathers and sons is only about 0·50, it is evident that, when classified according to their occupational status, (i) the mean intelligence of the children belonging to each class will exhibit a marked regression towards the general mean, and (ii) the intelligence of the individual children within each class will vary over a far wider range than that of their fathers. These deductions are fully confirmed by tables compiled to show the actual distribution of intelligence among adults and children belonging to the various occupational categories. It follows that, if the frequency distribution within the several classes is to remain constant (and still more if there is to be an increasing degree of vocational adjustment among later generations), a considerable amount of social mobility must inevitably take place, involving between 20 and 30 per cent of the population. Approximate estimates are attempted of both the actual and the ideal amounts. Data obtained from the after-histories of schoolchildren, followed up in later life, are analysed to ascertain the main psychological causes tending to produce a rise or drop in occupational status.

I. The Class Distribution of Intelligence

Aim. In the course of a recent discussion on the mental differences between social classes [19, 20, 21] I argued that the apparent differences between the class-means for general intelligence were to be explained partly by the effects of social mobility in transferring abler individuals from lower classes to higher and duller individuals from higher classes to lower, and partly by the manner in which inherited or innate differences are transmitted from one generation to another. Several sociological writers, however, have questioned both these suggestions, or at any rate the way in which I assumed the two processes had actually operated. In this paper, therefore, I propose to offer more detailed evidence to support the interpretations I put forward, and at the same time to answer, so far as I can, the various objections raised against the arguments which I advanced on these various points ([19], pp. 22f, section on ' Social Mobility ').

The data which I shall analyse are drawn from two overlapping inquiries, or rather two series of inquiries: (i) cross-sectional surveys of pupils in London schools, initiated primarily for the purposes of educational or vocational guidance

Intelligence and Social Mobility

and selection; (ii) longitudinal studies of backward, gifted, and normal pupils, followed up into adult life chiefly to check the accuracy of the assessments and recommendations made while the children were still at school [4, 26]. The surveys and the subsequent inquiries were carried out at intervals over a period of nearly fifty years, namely, from 1913 onwards; and much of the data is due to the willing cooperation of numerous collaborators, particularly teachers and social workers in the service of the London County Council and colleagues or senior research-students working for the National Institute of Industrial Psychology, to all of whom I am deeply indebted.

Points of Agreement. It may help to clarify the issues involved if I begin by summarizing the major points on which both my critics and myself would, I fancy, be in general agreement.

1. During the period covered by our inquiries the population, from which our samples are drawn, and to which we intend our conclusions to apply, greatly increased in numbers, though at a diminishing rate. Both the increase itself and the diminution in the rate of increase were a continuation of processes that had been going on during the preceding half-century. Thus in 1860 the total population of England and Wales was nearly 20 million; in 1910 it was almost twice as large—36 million; and in 1960 it was 45 million [10, 11, 24].

2. During the last half-century the proportional number of children in the population steadily declined and that of the elderly steadily increased. In 1910 31 per cent of the population were boys and girls of school age (i.e. under 15) and 7 per cent men or women over 60; in 1960 only 22 per cent were of school age and 14 per cent over 60.

3. Among the lower working classes (unskilled manual labourers) both the birthrate and the deathrate were appreciably higher than among the semi-skilled, skilled, or professional classes. The number of live births per married woman averaged about 3·8 among unskilled labourers and only 1·8 in the professional classes. The differences in the mortality rates were much smaller, averaging 13·1 per 1000 among the unskilled labourers and only 10·8 per 1000 in the professional classes. For birth and death alike the absolute rates and the class differences have both appreciably diminished during the period in question. The excess of birthrate over the deathrate has been by far the most important cause of the increase in the population [11, 24].

4. During the period for which information is available there has been no great change in the average level of general intelligence. The results of the second Scottish survey indicated an actual improvement in the average score with the tests employed [7]; but I myself believe, as Sir Godfrey Thomson suggested in his preface to the report, that this was an artificial and somewhat misleading result, due partly to increased familiarity with the tests and methods of testing [8]. On the whole, a survey of the relevant evidence would appear to suggest an actual but comparatively slight decline during the period in question, approximating to a drop of 1 or 2 I.Q. points per generation [5].

Cyril Burt

5. The amount of individual variation about the average level of intelligence has apparently remained fairly constant; certainly it has not declined [6, 16]. When we compare the printed tables giving the standard deviations for complete age-groups, we usually find that in the earlier surveys it is about 12 or 13 I.Q. points and in the later as much as 16 or even more. But the apparent increase is in all probability to be explained by the fact that the later test-scales are greatly improved, and as a result decidedly more discriminative. Where the same tests have been used the figures show no appreciable change.

6. There are appreciable differences in the average level of intelligence in the different socio-economic classes, and in spite of the remarkable improvements in material and cultural conditions, the differences have altered hardly at all during the period in question [1, 3, 16].

On all these points further research and more exact information is undoubtedly required. But I believe that, as a rough provisional statement, what I have said would be accepted by most social psychologists.

Points of Disagreement. The issues on which disagreement has been most strongly expressed are those relating to the genetic hypothesis. Dr. Floud and Dr. Halsey, for example, deny that the apparent differences between the class-means for general intelligence are in any degree due to innate differences; and both contend instead for " a hypothesis of near-randomness in the social distribution of innate intelligence ". This implies that the means for all the classes would be approximately the same. Many of their colleagues have also argued that even " the apparent differences in intelligence between individuals, whether adults or children, result not from genetic causes but solely or mainly from environmental conditions ". Dr. Halsey, however, is prepared to admit that individuals may vary in innate ability; but the model he has put forward to explain how such differences are in his view transmitted and redistributed diverges widely from mine [21]. In particular he criticizes both the amount of social mobility which I had assumed and the length of time over which I assumed it had operated; his view, like that of many other social writers[1], apparently supposes that social mobility is a comparatively late phenomenon, the result more especially of recent social and educational reforms.

II. ALTERNATIVE METHODS OF ANALYSIS

Correlational Analysis and Variance Analysis. Many of the foregoing criticisms arise, I fancy, very largely from the fact that the method which I adopted in the investigations cited differed considerably from those adopted for psychological researches on heredity in the past. Most psychologists have discussed the problems of genetics in terms of the correlational procedures popularized by Karl Pearson; the investigations of my coworkers and myself were based mainly on an analysis of variance using the techniques applied by Ronald

---

[1] Most of them ignore genetic influences altogether: see the interesting papers in *Population Studies*, IX, pp. 72-81, 82-95, XI, pp. 123-136, 262-8.

Intelligence and Social Mobility

Fisher. Unfortunately such methods still seem unfamiliar to the majority of psychologists and sociologists working in this country.

The analysis of variance has numerous merits with which statistical investigators are already well acquainted; but in the field of genetics it has one special advantage over the older correlational techniques. In nearly all the earlier statistical studies heredity itself was commonly conceived as ' the tendency of like to beget like '; hence the correlation coefficient, as a measure of likeness, seemed the obvious tool. On the Mendelian theory, however, genetic influences are responsible, not only for resemblances between members of the same family, but also for differences, i.e. for individual variations. Genetic variability within families receives little or no attention from those psychological critics who still accept the Pearsonian view, and think mainly in terms of correlations; yet, as we shall see in a moment, variability within families forms one of the chief causes of mobility. Moreover, it was to a large extent the exclusive reliance on correlational analysis which was responsible for the abnormally low estimates which Pearson and his followers reached for the influence of environment. Variance techniques make it far easier to give due weight to environmental influences, and to the further complications which result from the fact that environment and heredity so often work in the same direction.

In the present paper I shall, so far as possible, avoid unfamiliar methods and formulae. Nevertheless, because I believe that researches undertaken in the near future should be deliberately planned to permit the application of these newer and more efficient techniques, I will first attempt a brief explanation of the type of procedure that would seem most appropriate, and at the same time indicate how it is related to the more familiar correlational procedures. This may to some extent help to elucidate several of the points in my recent paper which the critics have either questioned or misunderstood.

The Factorial Analysis of Variance. Let us start, rather on the lines of Fisher (*op. cit. inf.*, pp. 210f.), with the simplest type of situation—that in which only two independent components of variance are involved. To make the problem concrete let us consider the case of n identical twins, reared in different' environments, and tested or assessed for some form of educational or occupational efficiency, which we may plausibly suppose to be the result of both genetic (g) and environmental factors (e). If x_i denotes the assessment for the ith individual, r a correlation coefficient, and s^2 an estimated variance, we may write

$$x_i = g_i + e_i \qquad (i = 1, 2 \ldots n) \qquad \text{(i)}$$

Squaring and summing we obtain

$$\Sigma x^2_i = \Sigma g^2_i + 2\Sigma g_i e_i + \Sigma e_1{}^2,$$

and therefore $s^2{}_x = s^2{}_g + 2r_{ge}s_g s_e + s^2{}_e,$

or $s^2{}_x = s^2{}_g + s^2{}_e,$ \qquad (ii)

if it can be assumed that the foster-homes have been chosen in a way quite unrelated to the intellectual level of each child's own family.

Cyril Burt

If we adopt a correlational procedure, the appropriate coefficient will be the *intra-class* correlation. Accordingly, following Fisher (with a slight change of notation) let us put

$$r_{tt} = \frac{G}{G+E},\qquad\qquad\text{(iii)}$$

where G and E denote the genetic and environmental variances respectively. Now, as Fisher shows, we can obtain an unbiased estimate of r_{tt} from the two equations

$$n(1-r)s^2{}_x = \sum(x_i - \bar{x}_j)^2 = ns^2{}_w, \qquad (i = 1, 2 \ldots 2n)\qquad\text{(iv)}$$

$$(n-1)\,(1+r)s^2{}_x = 2\sum(\bar{x}_j - \bar{x})^2 = (n-1)s^2{}_b, \qquad (j = 1, 2 \ldots n)\qquad\text{(v)}$$

where x_i (as before) denotes the assessment of the ith individual, $\bar{x}_j$ the mean of the family to which that individual belongs, $s^2{}_x$ the estimated total variance, $s^2{}_w$ the variance 'within families', and $s^2{}_b$ the variance 'between families', n the number of families, and $2n$ therefore the number of twins, and r the correlation between the twins' intelligence[1].

To estimate the relative size of the contributions of G and E, however, we need two further equations. Fisher shows in the course of his discussion that

$$\overset{mn}{\sum}(x - \bar{x}_j)^2 = n(m-1)E,\qquad\qquad\text{(vi)}$$

$$\text{and } \overset{n}{\sum}(\bar{x}_j - \bar{x})^2/(n-1) = G + E/m,\qquad\qquad\text{(vii)}$$

where m is the number in each family (with twins $m = 2$). Substituting from (iv) and (v), and then solving for $G = s^2{}_g$ and $E = s^2{}_e$, we obtain

$$G = \tfrac{1}{2}(s^2{}_b - s^2{}_w),\qquad\qquad\text{(viii)}$$

$$E = s^2{}_b.\qquad\qquad\text{(ix)}$$

These then are the equations we require; and I have ventured to call the whole procedure the 'factorial analysis of variance'.[2] On substituting in equation (iii) from equations (viii) and (ix) we have for the coefficient of correlation

$$r_{ti} = \frac{s^2{}_b - s^2{}_w}{s^2{}_b + s^2{}_w},\qquad\qquad\text{(x)}$$

which sums up the relation between the results of the two alternative procedures —correlation and analysis of variance—in the simplest conceivable case.

In the foregoing problem—that of identical twins brought up in separate homes—both the variance within the family due to genetic influences and the effects of environment so far as it operates in the same direction as the genetic influences could be safely ignored. If we wish to estimate the former, we can

[1] Fisher, *Statistical Methods for Research Workers* (5th ed., 1934, chapter VII, 'Intra-Class Correlation and Analysis of Variance'. The formula for r is given on p. 212, and the equations for the sum of squares 'within families' and 'between families' will be those given in Table 39 not Table 38: cf. also [4], pp. 675f. and [14], pp. 106f.

[2] This type of analysis has wide applications in psychometrics, and may also be extended to the study of interactions: see, for example, this *Journal*, VIII, p. 116.

Intelligence and Social Mobility

take ordinary siblings brought up from birth in the *same* environment, e.g. orphanages and other residential institutions (cf. [3], pp. 90–91); and if we want to determine the effects of any correlation between environment and heredity, we can either reintroduce the correlational term r_{ge} or calculate the additional variance directly by the method described in the earlier paper [14].

Multiple Cross-Classifications. To deal with more complex situations the foregoing techniques can readily be extended to problems involving a multi-dimensional classification. In such cases, it may be noted, both the algebraic solutions and the arithmetical calculations become much simpler if the successive classifications are dichotomous. Thus, in dealing with genetical problems, it would certainly be desirable to take into account temperamental and motivational tendencies (m) as well as cognitive abilities (a). Since a general factor underlies each, we may for most purposes, treat each as supplying the basis for a further two-fold classification. In studying the influence of social class we must cross-classify both the genetic factors and the environmental according to the variations in family (f) and in social class (c): this would mean that our simple dichotomous equation (equation (i) above) must now be rewritten

$$x = g_c + g_f + e_c + e_f, \tag{xi}$$

and, if we wish to include motivational factors as well as cognitive, we must be prepared to work with eight variables, g_{ac}, g_{mc}, g_{af}, etc. In either case the derivation of the formulae will proceed much as before. But, by deciding in advance which variables we will include and which we will exclude (e.g. by arranging to keep certain conditions constant) and by avoiding so far as possible interactions or intercorrelations between the variables retained, many of the complications may be eliminated or at least reduced to insignificance.

Incidentally, we may note that with an analysis of variance it is not necessary (as it would be with a correlational procedure) to assume that the social classes themselves must be expressed by measurable quantities (e.g. by income) or ranked in linear order (e.g. in terms of prestige), as in fact has been the custom in many sociological inquiries. The method thus avoids the difficulty experienced by investigators of mobility who have endeavoured to assess or rank rural occupations on the same scale as urban and industrial[1]. The calculations would become simpler still if we were content, with several recent investigators (Lipset and Bendix [23], for example), to reduce the occupational classification in either case to a twofold division, namely, manual and non-manual.

---

[1] Glass [13], for example, in his study of social mobility in Britain, attempts to classify urban and rural populations together, and in this he is followed by L. Livi and K. Svalastoga in Italy and Denmark respectively—agricultural countries where a unidimensional classification of this kind ceases to be plausible [9]. Most other investigators classify the urban and the rural populations separately [15, 17, 18]. Even in the case of urban occupations much of the data available is expressed in terms of occupational categories which it would be very difficult to rank; in such cases, therefore, the analysis of variance, or (if Pearsonian techniques are preferred) the calculation of contingency coefficients, is far more appropriate than the calculation of correlations.

Cyril Burt

In principle, therefore, the questions with which we are concerned are essentially problems in multivariate analysis. Multivariate analysis can take several forms; and, according to the specific nature of the question we wish to answer, we may use either factor analysis, regression analysis, or discriminant analysis. But, once again, in any future research it is desirable that the investigator should keep explicitly in mind from the outset the kind of statistical techniques that are suitable for his problem and his data, and having made his choice, plan his inquiry accordingly.

In the following discussion, which is intended merely as a pilot inquiry, I shall, to begin with, confine myself primarily to assessments for general intelligence and leave motivational factors to a later section. I shall compare assessments for adults and children drawn always from the same families; but I shall adopt a moderately elaborate occupational classification. The data are too crude and limited for a detailed examination by a full analysis of variance. Moreover, in this paper it is my purpose to keep, so far as possible, to the simplest and most intelligible methods of comparison, relying largely on the percentage methods favoured by sociologists themselves. But the differences revealed, I fancy, will be sufficiently striking to lend strong support to the conclusions drawn.

III. Frequency Distributions for Adults and Children

Sources of Data. In studying the distribution of intelligence among the different occupational classes it is in my view desirable to examine, not only (as is usually done) the class-means, but the entire frequency distributions. Accordingly in Tables I and II I give frequencies both for adults and for children. For the children the bulk of the data was obtained from the surveys carried out from time to time in a London borough selected as typical of the whole county. The methods by which the assessments for intelligence were made have been described in earlier papers and in L.C.C. Reports [3, 5, 16]. For the boys who belong to the highest occupational classes, drawn for example from families who would not ordinarily send their children to Council schools, much of the data was collected in the course of work on vocational guidance at the National Institute of Industrial Psychology. The data for the adults was obtained from the parents of the children themselves. Usually our more immediate purpose was to secure practical estimates of both the average level and the range of intelligence required in the commoner types of occupation. In addition, however, when working with backward children we often wanted to see how far the backwardness was a family characteristic. And at all levels an incidental aim was to secure material for studying the problem of mental inheritance. For obvious reasons the assessments of adult intelligence were less thorough and less reliable.

The Occupational Classification. The occupational classification is much the same as that used in previous reports. It has been described by Carr-Saunders and Caradog Jones in their book on *Social Structure in England and*

Intelligence and Social Mobility

Wales ([2], Table XXXI, p. 56). Unlike the classification used in the more recent studies of social mobility it is based, not on prestige or income, but rather on the degree of ability required for the work. Class I includes those engaged in the highest type of professional and administrative work (university teachers, those of similar standing in law, medicine, education, or the church, and the top people in commerce, industry, or the civil service); class II consists of those engaged in lower professional or technical work (including most teachers, men of business, and executive clerks in the higher grades); class III of those working in intermediate types of clerical, commercial, or technical work; class IV includes those ordinarily classified as skilled workers, but it also contains an appreciable number who are engaged in commercial or industrial work of an equivalent level; class V consists of semi-skilled workers and those holding the poorest type of commercial position; class VI of unskilled labourers, casual labourers, and those employed on coarse manual work. It will be noted that the numbers in the higher groups or classes are far smaller than those in the lower. These subdivisions were in fact chosen because at the outset of our work we had in mind the proportionate numbers of children (*a*) who were transferred to Central Schools (about 12 per cent), (*b*) who were awarded junior county scholarships and transferred to what were then called secondary (i.e. grammar) schools (about 3 per cent), and (*c*) who were of exceptionally high intelligence and for the most part in attendance, not at a council school, but at one of the older public schools or at a preparatory school of similar type (about 0·3 per cent); and we wanted the occupational classification to tally so far as possible with the educational classification.

In constructing the tables the frequencies inserted in the various rows and columns were proportional frequencies and in no way represent the number actually examined: from class I the number actually examined was nearer a hundred and twenty than three. To obtain the figures to be inserted (numbers per mille) we weighted the actual numbers so that the proportions in each class should be equal to the estimated proportions for the total population. Finally, for purposes of the present analysis we have rescaled our assessments of intelligence so that the mean of the whole group is 100 and the standard deviation 15. This is done because the results of so many intelligence tests nowadays are expressed in terms of conventional I.Q.'s conforming to these requirements.

IV. Amount of Mobility

The Distribution of Adults. From the figures set out in the last column of Table I it will be seen that there are appreciable differences between the average levels of intelligence in the various classes. The average for the highest class of all—those holding the highest professional or administrative appointments—is practically 40 I.Q. points above the general level. The differences between the means for the last three classes are much smaller, largely because the numbers are far greater.

Cyril Burt

TABLE I. DISTRIBUTION OF INTELLIGENCE ACCORDING TO OCCUPATIONAL CLASS: ADULTS

	50–60	60–70	70–80	80–90	90–100	100–110	110–120	120–130	130–140	140+	Total	Mean I.Q.
I. Higher Professional									2	1	3	139·7
II. Lower Professional							2	13	15	1	31	130·6
III. Clerical				1	8	16	56	38	3		122	115·9
IV. Skilled			2	11	51	101	78	14	1		258	108·2
V. Semiskilled		5	15	31	135	120	17	2			325	97·8
VI. Unskilled	1	18	52	117	53	11	9				261	84·9
Total	1	23	69	160	247	248	162	67	21	2	1000	100·0

TABLE II. DISTRIBUTION OF INTELLIGENCE ACCORDING TO OCCUPATIONAL CLASS: CHILDREN

	50–60	60–70	70–80	80–90	90–100	100–110	110–120	120–130	130–140	140+	Total	Mean I.Q.
I. Higher Professional						1		1	1		3	120·8
II. Lower Professional				1	2	6	12	8	2		31	114·7
III. Clerical			3	8	21	31	35	18	6		122	107·8
IV. Skilled		1	12	33	53	70	59	22	7	1	258	104·6
V. Semiskilled	1	6	23	55	99	85	38	13	5		325	98·9
VI. Unskilled	1	15	32	62	75	54	16	6			261	92·6
Total	2	22	70	159	250	247	160	68	21	1	1000	100·0

Intelligence and Social Mobility

But still more striking is the wide range of individual differences within each class. With a normal distribution the range for an unselected group of 1000 cases would be (as in fact appears from the table) nearly 100 I.Q. points—i.e., from about 50 to 150; for an unselected group of 100 cases it would be about 75 to 80 I.Q. points. We should naturally expect, however, that the members of the occupational classes will form selected groups, and that their range and standard deviation will therefore be appreciably diminished. In point of fact the standard deviation within the various classes averages 9·6 (i.e. rather less than two-thirds the standard deviation of the entire group, 15). Hence the range for 100 cases would still be nearly 50 I.Q. points (as a glance at classes III to VI will confirm). Indeed, in the lowest class of all—that of unskilled workers—some of the brightest members actually display greater intelligence than the dullest members in class II, the ' lower professional '. The correlation between intelligence and occupational class therefore is by no means perfect. If we attempt to estimate it on the assumption that both distributions are in fact normal, it works out at just over 0·74. However, since the correlation must be far from linear, its precise numerical value as thus calculated can have little meaning.

The fact that the correlation is far from perfect must not be taken to imply that the duller members of the higher classes and the brighter members of the lower classes are all of necessity instances of vocational misfit. No doubt, they sometimes are. But frequently specific abilities or disabilities, and still more often qualities or infirmities of character and temperament, will fully account for the apparent discrepancies.

The Ideal Redistribution. In order to determine what is the maximum amount of interchange that ideal conditions could possibly permit, let us suppose that vocational adaptation depends solely on intelligence. Then in terms of the I.Q. scale the borderlines between the several occupational classes would be 141, 127, 115, 103, and 90 respectively, and there should be no overlapping between the successive categories. If we now reclassify the actual data for adults according to these new borderlines, we obtain the distribution set out in Table III. The number who are placed in occupations corresponding with their intelligence is shown in semi-bold. Before calculating the percentages let us pool the first three classes together to form a single group which is mainly non-manual; and let us combine the next two to form a group of skilled workers (predominantly but not entirely manual), and leave the lowest class as it is. With this threefold rearrangement (Table V) we find that only 55 per cent of the population could be regarded as correctly placed if intelligence were the sole criterion: nearly 23 per cent are in a class too high, and, with a perfect scheme of vocational selection, ought to be moved down: 22 per cent are in a class too low, and would have to be moved up.

The Distribution for Children. When we turn to the data for children (Table II), we observe that the differences between the class-means are much smaller. The average intelligence of the children in the higher groups has

Cyril Burt

TABLE III. DISTRIBUTION OF INTELLIGENCE ACCORDING TO OCCUPATIONAL CLASS: ADULTS

Rescaled

	VI 50–91	V 91–103	IV 103–115	III 115–127	II 127–141	I 141+	Total
I					2	1	3
II			1	15	14	1	31
III	1	15	38	56	12		122
IV	16	86	114	38	4		258
V	53	178	84	10			325
VI	191	46	21	3			261
Total	261	325	258	122	32	2	1000

TABLE IV. DISTRIBUTION OF INTELLIGENCE ACCORDING TO OCCUPATIONAL CLASS: CHILDREN

Rescaled

	VI 50–91	V 91–103	IV 103–115	III 115–127	II 127–141	I 141+	Total
I			1	1	1		3
II	1	4	11	9	6		31
III	11	28	51	20	12		122
IV	46	66	75	62	8	1	258
V	91	122	84	23	5		325
VI	112	105	36	7	1		261
Total	261	325	258	122	33	1	1000

TABLE V. ADULTS: PERCENTAGE IN EACH GROUP WHOSE INTELLIGENCE IS BELOW, ABOVE, OR EQUIVALENT TO THAT OF THEIR OCCUPATIONAL CLASS

	Below	Equivalent	Above	Number
Class I–III	46·2	45·5	8·3	156
Class IV–V	26·6	50·1	23·3	583
Class VI	—	73·2	26·8	261
Total population	22·7	55·4	21·9	1000

TABLE VI. CHILDREN: PERCENTAGE IN EACH GROUP WHOSE INTELLIGENCE IS BELOW, ABOVE, OR EQUIVALENT TO THAT OF THEIR OCCUPATIONAL CLASS

	Below	Equivalent	Above	Number
Class I–III	75·5	16·8	7·7	156
Class IV–V	34·8	34·3	30·9	583
Class VI	—	42·9	57·1	261
Total population	32·1	33·5	34·4	1000

fallen almost half-way towards the mean of the whole population; similarly that of the children in the lower groups has risen by a similar proportion. There is, in short, an overall regression averaging 0·52 (cf. [1], [3]). The figure is very close to the value we should expect on the assumption that the correlation between fathers and sons was due chiefly to multifactorial inheritance with assortative mating and incomplete dominance. If anything, the coefficient is slightly higher than we might expect on these grounds alone [cf. 14]. Hence environmental influences may perhaps have contributed to increase it; but, if so, the contribution must be extremely small.

The phenomenon just noted has sometimes been termed 'biological regression'; and several sociological and psychological writers have claimed that this tendency is responsible for 'the steady progress which' (so they hold) 'most populations are continually undergoing from a state of individual diversity to one of increasing individual equality', so that in the more highly civilized communities the distribution of intelligence is approaching 'near-randomness' as regards both classes and individuals. This interpretation appears to have been adopted as a corollary to the theory of 'blended inheritance' to which the majority of psychologists and sociologists still adhere[1]. A few writers, however, who recognize that the data obtained from successive generations reveal no evidence whatever for this alleged tendency towards equality, have also postulated a biological 'egression *from* the mean', which, they argue, "balances regression *towards* the mean" [22]. For this there is no need. With multifactorial inheritance this 'conservation of variance' is what we should expect.

When we look at the distribution of children's intelligence *within* the several occupational classes and compare it with that of their fathers' (Table I), we see at once that, so far from progressing towards equality, the amount of individual difference has actually increased. The standard deviation has gone up from 9·6 to 14·0, not far short of the standard deviation for the whole population (15·0). Or, to put it in another way, the range for 100 individuals selected according to occupational class has increased from 50 I.Q. for adults to nearly 75 I.Q. for their children.

One incidental consequence of this increase in variability is the appearance of bright children among the offspring of dull parents in the lower occupational classes and of dull children among the offspring of highly intelligent parents in the upper occupational classes. Consider, for example, the lowest occupational class of all. Among the adults only 20 persons out of 261 have an intelligence above the general average; among the children as many as 76, nearly four times as many—a discrepancy of 56. Dr. Floud, and others who hold as she does that differences in intelligence are due wholly to environmental advantages or disadvantages, can hardly maintain that the high level reached by these 76 boys

---

[1] This corollary from the theory of blended inheritance is mathematically deduced, and empirically disproved, in an earlier issue of this *Journal* (X, p. 56). The empirical disproof of the corollary is perhaps one of the simplest and most convincing arguments against the doctrine of blending. Clarke's 'egression' is apparently a substitute for Darwin's 'spontaneous variation'.

Cyril Burt

—all children of unskilled workers—results from the superior advantages which their home environments confer. But equally, those who adopt the traditional theory of blended inheritance, would find it quite impossible to explain the higher intelligence of these children in terms of their heredity. On the Mendelian hypothesis, however, such apparent anomalies are exactly what we should anticipate if the amount of a child's intelligence is determined mainly, or at any rate largely, by his genetic constitution, and if that in turn is the result of a chance recombination of parental genes ([14], p. 97).

Similar arguments hold good for the marked discrepancies discernible in the upper part of the distribution. In the first three occupational classes, for example, we see that among the adults only 9 out of 156 had an intelligence below the general mean, among the children as many as 39. Here again the increased numbers would be almost inexplicable on the environmental theory, but a natural consequence of the Mendelian theory of polygenic inheritance.

Consequences of the Intergenerational Changes. We have seen that two changes result from the comparatively moderate correlation that obtains between the intelligence of parents and their children: (i) the mean intelligence of the children belonging to each occupational class deviates far less than the mean of the parents from the average for the population as a whole, and (ii) the intelligence of the individual children within any one class varies over a far wider range than that of their parents. Moreover, unless their effects are in some way counteracted, both these changes will be cumulative. After about five generations the differences between the class-means would virtually vanish, and the proportional range within each class would spread out almost as widely as the proportional range of the population as a whole[1].

Now all the evidence shows (p. 5 above) that in point of fact, during the period with which we have been concerned, the occupational distribution of intelligence has remained fairly constant from one generation to the next, and it appears likely to do so in the immediate future. If therefore, when they are grown up, the children of Table IV are to exhibit the same distribution as the adults of Table I, it follows that a considerable number will have to move into a fresh occupational class. Some will go up the social ladder by one or more rungs; others will go down. One of our chief problems therefore is to assess the extent of this migration. For this purpose it will be helpful to begin by rearranging the figures for the children according to the method we have already adopted for the adults (Table III above).

Maximum Mobility. Table IV shows the distribution of the children with the scale for intelligence subdivided afresh so that the lines of division shall correspond with those we should expect between the different occupational classes if occupational efficiency depended solely upon intelligence. As before, let us group together classes I, II and III to form a non-manual group, and

---

[1] This is a simple mathematical corollary. Allowing for assortative mating and partial dominance, the correlation between occupation and intelligence after n generations would sink to approximately $0.74 \times \frac{1}{2} \times (2/3)^{n-1}$: (See [14], p. 116, eq. 23).

classes IV and V together to form a group of skilled workers, leaving class VI as it stands to form a group of unskilled workers. Then, assuming intelligence to be the sole criterion, it appears (as a little mental calculation will quickly show) that in the highest group 75 per cent of the children have an intelligence below the minimum that would be needed if they were to become efficient members of the occupational group into which they were born; on the other hand, in the lowest group 57 per cent have an intelligence well above the meagre amount required for an unskilled worker (see Table VI). In the entire sample over a third of the children have an intelligence which would apparently fit them for a higher occupational class than that of their fathers, and rather less than a third have an intelligence which would be more appropriate for a lower class.

These figures give a rough indication of the amount of movement upward or downward from one class to another which the children would have to undergo when grown up in order that the type of work they secured corresponded with their degree of intelligence—always assuming that intelligence was the sole criterion. In point of fact we know that nothing like this amount of movement actually takes place; and the figures, of course, merely indicate the *maximum* degree of mobility that is theoretically conceivable.

Actual Mobility. Let us now return to the question of fact. The ideal and most direct procedure would be to plan a longitudinal study of a large and representative sample, following up the children from school to middle life. A complete inquiry of this kind has so far never been attempted. Both in America and in this country follow-up studies have been undertaken for certain selected groups—the gifted or the backward; but for our present problem these provide at most only supplementary or confirmatory evidence. We are obliged therefore to fall back on the alternative procedure commonly adopted in similar situations; and, instead of comparing the same group at two widely diverging intervals of time, we shall compare two different groups of widely divergent ages.

Our present data supply us with two such samples. These are comparable, since the adults are the parents of the children. However, there is a difference of 28·4 years between the average age of the children and the average age of the adults; and, as we have seen, during that amount of time there would have been a variety of changes in the population. Our method of reducing the figures observed to numbers per 1000 should sufficiently allow for the change in the absolute size of the population. The differential birthrate may have entailed some slight modification in the mental quality of the population; but, in the space of three decades only, the extent of the change would, as we have seen, be almost negligible. The effects of the deathrate are largely ruled out by the fact that we have taken children who have survived to school age. Although between 1911 and 1951 the proportion of men and women over 65 very nearly doubled, this was offset by a decline in the number of boys and girls under 15: and the proportional number of males of employable age has remained much the same. The type of work available has changed appreciably: the number of those engaged in manufacturing and in professional and administrative work of various kinds

Cyril Burt

has increased; the number engaged in agriculture, in the extractive industries (mining, quarry, etc.), in domestic work, and in the distributive trades has diminished; moreover, the amount of prestige attaching to different types of occupation has altered. Nevertheless, these further changes are hardly relevant to our present problem, as we have formulated it, although in a more intensive study the bearing of all the varying conditions I have mentioned should undoubtedly be systematically examined.

Assuming then that the data in our two samples are reasonably comparable, our primary task is to determine what kind of compensating change would be necessary to bring the frequency distributions for the children (Table II) into conformity with the frequency distribution for the adults (Table I). Let us look first at the lowest occupational class of all—the unskilled workers (class VI). Among the children, it will be remembered, as many as 57 per cent have an intelligence above what is required for work of this type as against 27 per cent of the adults (Tables V and VI). Hence $(57 - 27) = 30$ per cent of the children will presumably move up to a higher occupational class as they grow up. Similarly $(75 - 46) = 29$ per cent of the upper group—that comprising classes I, II and III—will move down. In the intermediate group—classes IV and V —the changes both upward and downward will be smaller. Thus, as a comparison of the last lines of the two tables suggests, the over-all mobility will be at least $(55 - 33) = 22$ per cent. This figure I regard as indicating the minimum amount of mobility—the amount that is required to maintain what (if I may borrow a phrase from the astronomers) might be called a ' steady state '[1]. It constitutes what may be termed ' basic mobility '.

---

[1] The foregoing data and the analysis I have here attempted will, I hope, dispose of one of the strongest objections urged by Dr. Halsey [21] against the arguments brought forward by Miss Conway and myself in our endeavour to account for the wide differences in average intelligence shown by the different socio-economic classes. Dr. Halsey's criticism was that the round figures assumed for social mobility in setting up our genetic model were far too high. But our object then was of course very different from our present purpose. We merely wanted to show that, with a comparatively small amount of interchange between the several classes, a society which started from primitive conditions in which the average intelligence in the different classes was practically the same would, in the course of subsequent generations, be differentiated in such a way that the differences between the mean levels of intelligence corresponded pretty closely with those at the present day. For this purpose we deliberately assumed in our hypothetical model an amount of mobility well below that which we believed had actually occurred in order to forestall incidental criticisms on this point. In view of the figures given by sociologists themselves Dr. Halsey's criticism seemed rather surprising. But we now hope that the foregoing analysis will show that our postulated figure was well below the most probable minimum.

It has been objected that any figure for social mobility, like that given above, is bound to vary with the lines of division adopted in classifying occupations. However, as long as the basis of the classification remains unaltered, changes in the lines of division will not seriously affect the estimated figure unless the lines of division become so few and the resulting classes so large that the amount of movement is obscured. Indeed, if we imagine the various occupations to be graded according to difficulty in such a way that the distribution of the employees is approximately normal, then in theory, provided we know (i) the correlation between the intelligence of the employees and grade of the occupation, and (ii) the correlation between the intelligence of the employees' children and that of the employees themselves, the amount of mobility required to keep the population constant could be determined from the properties of the bivariate frequency distribution.

Intelligence and Social Mobility

However, as we have already seen, there was, at the time when the occupations of the fathers were recorded, considerable room for improvement in the degree of adjustment between the capabilities of the individuals and the type of employment they followed. Moreover, during the last forty years or so, as several researches in the field of vocational guidance have shown, the degree of adjustment has appreciably increased, and apparently is still increasing. Hence the actual amount of mobility is probably much greater than that which just suffices to maintain the *status quo ante*. If we may trust the most thorough of the recent inquiries [13], the overall amount of mobility would appear to be in the neighbourhood of 29 per cent—well above our minimum for a steady state, but still far below what the ideals of vocational suitability would require. Much the same figure was obtained from our analysis of after-histories (p. 19)—viz. 31 per cent.

As the reader will realize, the foregoing deductions deal only with a very limited aspect in a very limited interpretation of the rather ambiguous phrase ' social mobility '. Ordinarily the discussion of mobility treats a rise in social status as implying something more than a mere rise to a type of occupation which requires a higher I.Q. than the occupation followed by one's father[1]; and the value attached to different types of occupation as a goal for the ambitious youngster varies widely from group to group, from individual to individual, and from one period to another. Nor is intelligence the only factor which determines whether or not the ambitious youngster will succeed in achieving the vocational career at which he aims.

I propose therefore in conclusion to glance at two or three other factors which might be expected to influence the kind of occupational status which persons of varying intelligence are likely to attain, and consider what is their relative importance and how far they could affect the inferences already drawn.

V. Causal Factors

Data. Although opinions have been freely expressed about the conditions which facilitate social advancement and still more often about those which are thought to obstruct it, surprisingly little factual evidence has been obtained. The teaching of Samuel Smiles and his Victorian doctrine of ' Self-Help ' has long since faded from memory, though his biographical illustrations are by no means valueless. However, during the past fifty years the popular tendency has been to place an increasing emphasis on the external or social factors and less on the personal or psychological. But here it is principally the latter which I should like quite briefly to examine.

---

[1] As I have pointed out elsewhere, in their definitions of social class and social status different writers have relied on a wide variety of criteria ([12], pp. 37f. and refs.). The problems to which discussions of this type give rise are most readily handled by means of factor analysis. It turns out that all the criteria are positively, and indeed closely, correlated: so that a general factor must underlie them all. Hence the ideal way of allocating persons to an appropriate social class would be to use a system of weights based on a multiple regression equation. The use of such a technique of course implies that the necessary data have been collected for all the individuals concerned.

Cyril Burt

As part of the longitudinal studies of gifted and of backward children attending London County Council schools my colleagues and I have followed up into later life a large number of cases, not only of these somewhat exceptional types, but also of normal or average children who were treated as control groups. We now possess fairly detailed data for just over 200 ordinary children who have already reached an age when it is possible to say either that they have already moved out of their original class, in one direction or the other, or else that it is now practically certain that they will never do so. We have similar numbers for pupils who formerly attended central schools or won junior county scholarships as well as for pupils who were educationally subnormal. By using fractional weights for the figures obtained from these various subgroups we can compile a composite group of males which shall be reasonably representative of the total population. It includes many of the older children in the group discussed in section II—those whom we have been able to trace and follow up in their after-school life; but it includes others omitted from that group owing to lack of adequate data about their parents' abilities. For each of the sub-groups we have the following relevant information, obtained (except for vi) mainly when the children were at school: (i) the occupational class of the fathers at the time the children were born; (ii) assessments and descriptions of the home background, and particularly of the attitude of the family towards the child's social advancement; (iii) the child's own attitude, and particularly his industry, ambition, and educational and vocational aims; (iv) his level of intelligence, based on tests duly checked with the teachers and corrected where necessary; (v) his educational record (more especially his admission to a grammar school or its equivalent); (vi) his occupation when last visited.

In view of the complexity of the problem and the limitations of the data let us begin by an analysis in terms of crude percentages. For this purpose we may divide the whole composite group into three portions—(*a*) those who have remained in their original occupational class, (*b*) those who have moved up, and (*c*) those who have moved down. Similarly, it will simplify matters to reduce the assessments for intelligence to a threefold classification—(*a*) an intelligence equal to that required in the individual's original occupational class (the class of his father), (*b*) an intelligence above it, and (*c*) an intelligence below it. The other assessments can be reduced to a twofold classification, viz. (*a*) above the median and (*b*) below the median[1].

Results. The main results are shown in Table VII. The following conclusions may be drawn.

1. Of the children with an intelligence *below* the minimum required for the occupational class into which they were born none rose above it, and about a third (or rather more) dropped to a lower class. On the other hand, of those

---

[1] For much of the data in this section, and most of the calculations, I am deeply indebted to my former colleagues, Miss J. L. Hastings, Miss E. Davenport, and Mr. R. M. Weldon.

Intelligence and Social Mobility

who had an intelligence *above* the maximum required for their original occupational class nearly 60 per cent failed to rise.

2. Very few of those who were assessed as lacking in adequate motivation rose above their original class. Indeed, poor motivation was more likely than poor intelligence to contribute to a fall. On the other hand, good motivation was less certain to secure a rise.

3. A good home background, though helpful particularly during the earlier educational stages, was less effective in securing a rise than either high intelligence or strong motivation. Nor was a bad home background so fatal as seems to be commonly assumed. Nearly a quarter (24 per cent) of those who suffered from unfavourable home circumstances in childhood nevertheless succeeded in rising out of their original class.

TABLE VII. PSYCHOLOGICAL FACTORS INFLUENCING OCCUPATIONAL MOBILITY

Mobility	Intelligence			Motivation		Home Background		Educational Achievement	
	P	A	G	P	G	P	G	P	G
Up	0	12	41	2	36	24	29	18	34
Stationary	64	67	49	47	51	40	44	34	52
Down	36	21	10	51	13	36	27	48	14
	100	100	100	100	100	100	100	100	100

Mobility	Intelligence and Motivation Combined		Intelligence, Motivation, and Home Background Combined		Intelligence, Motivation, Home Background, and Educational Achievement Combined	
	P	G	P	G	P	G
Up	0	66	0	70	0	72
Stationary	32	29	23	23	18	21
Down	68	5	77	7	82	7
	100	100	100	100	100	100

Note.—P = Poor, A = Average, G = Good. The tables for 'combined' qualities include only those cases in which *all* the qualities specified were 'Poor' or 'Good'.

4. The achievement of grammar school status or (during the pre-war period) the award of a junior county scholarship, by no means sufficed to guarantee a rise in occupational class, though it often proved an important step in the child's gradual ascent. However, an appreciable number succeeded in working their way up to a higher occupational level in spite of a total lack of any formal education beyond what the elementary school could provide.

5. Two-thirds of those who have both high intelligence and strong motivation are likely to achieve an occupational rise. In fact nearly all who achieve a rise have this double characteristic. The addition of a good home background

Cyril Burt

is a further advantage; in the case of the child of the lower classes what chiefly count are the social aspirations, the ambitious aims, and the constant urging that often characterize the more earnest working-class parents; with children from higher levels it is rather the intellectual and cultural character of the home that helps. The addition of a grammar school education does not greatly increase predictability[1]: this is because most children who have good intelligence, good motivation, and good home backgrounds are pretty sure to win their way to a grammar school. Those who, despite high intelligence and good motivation, dropped to a lower occupational class were for the most part victims of ill health, either mental or physical. As the tables indicate, there was actually an increase in this type of failure among those who in addition enjoyed a good home and a good education; the increase, as the case-histories would show, is accounted for by the larger number who break down from nervous ill health.

There are many other possible factors of a somewhat miscellaneous kind which have not been included in the foregoing summary—e.g. the variations in the openings available at different times or in different regions, the effects of a wife and family, or of friends, acquaintances, or patrons able to help and wielding personal influence. From time to time we encountered evidence of such factors; but as determinants of individual mobility they seemed to be of much less importance than those we have discussed.

An Analysis by Factors and Variances. The relations between the five main variables can be roughly expressed by means of correlation coefficients. For this purpose we have assessed mobility in terms of the degree of movement as well as the direction, allotting ± 1 point for a movement to the class above or below, ± 2 points for a movement over two classes, and so on. The correlations obtained are shown in Table VIII. The correlations between social mobility and the various causal conditions are product-moment coefficients; the correlations of the causal conditions with each other are averaged tetrachorics.

The raw correlations between social mobility and the four main causal conditions differ but little in magnitude; but the partial correlations (last row of Table VIII) differ appreciably. The correlation with intelligence is by far the highest of the three (0·38); the correlation with motivation is somewhat smaller (0·29); and the correlations with home background (0·17) and educational achievement (0·05) almost negligible. These figures thus fully confirm the conclusions already reached. The partial regression equation for predicting mobility is

$$S = 0.346I + 0.272M + 0.158H + 0.149E,$$

where S denotes social mobility, I intelligence, M motivation, H home background, and E educational achievement. The multiple correlation is 0·628.

---

[1] Education, and particularly the type of education (e.g. entrance at a public school followed by Oxford or Cambridge), are unquestionably influential in determining a rise at the highest levels of all; but in a survey of the total population such cases appear by comparison few in number and exceptional in type.

Intelligence and Social Mobility

This rather modest value is no doubt due to the fact that, as we have seen, various minor factors may be operative in individual cases[1].

Table IX gives the results of the factor analysis. The matrix of correlations between the four causal conditions was first subjected to a group factor analysis, the lines of division between the groups being determined by a preliminary bipolar analysis. The correlations between social mobility, etc., and the resulting factors were then computed by the usual formula. In determining the meaning of the factors we have relied partly on the case-histories of a few

TABLE VIII. CORRELATIONS BETWEEN SOCIAL MOBILITY AND RELATED CONDITIONS

	1	2	3	4	5
1. Social Mobility	—	0·481	0·402	0·396	0·378
2. Intelligence	0·481	—	0·133	0·236	0·413
3. Motivation	0·402	0·133	—	0·376	0·162
4. Home Conditions	0·396	0·236	0·376	—	0·363
5. Educational Record	0·378	0·413	0·162	0·363	—
Social Mobility (partial correlation)	—	0·379	0·286	0·174	0·047

Note.—The partial correlations give the correlation between social mobility and the condition specified when the effects of the other three conditions are held constant.

TABLE IX. CORRELATIONS OF SOCIAL MOBILITY AND RELATED CONDITIONS WITH GROUP FACTORS

Factor	I	II	III	IV
1. Social Mobility	0·443	0·417	0·294	0·166
2. Intelligence	0·782	0·000	0·405	0·000
3. Motivation	0·000	0·731	0·329	0·000
4. Home Conditions	0·302	0·514	0·000	0·287
5. Educational Record	0·528	0·216	0·000	0·323

typical individuals who have obtained exceptionally high or exceptionally low factor measurements for each of the factors. The first factor appears to be essentially an intellectual factor; and the second a factor of incentive. The last two are based on a bipolar factor which apparently distinguishes variations that are mainly genetic from variations that are mainly environmental But the precise interpretation of factor III remains somewhat obscure[2].

[1] The method is similar to that adopted in an earlier memorandum and subjected to considerable criticism: for a reply see [6], pp. 278f.

[2] Factors I and II must each of them be partly determined by genetic characteristics. Factor III seems to imply some overlap or linkage between the genetic characteristics that make for intelligence and stability of character respectively—perhaps due merely to the fact that intelligence is an ingredient of stability, or perhaps due to some selective conditions influencing the genetic basis of both.

Cyril Burt

Between them the four factors contribute about 48 per cent of the total variance for mobility: of this, factor I contributes nearly 20 per cent, factor II 17 per cent, factor III 9 per cent, and factor IV barely 3 per cent.

Owing to the imperfect nature of the data and the methods of calculating the correlations it seems very doubtful whether much value can be attached to the figures thus obtained. We give them chiefly in the hope that their short-comings may encourage fresh investigators to plan a more systematic set of longitudinal studies, with the method of analysis kept carefully in view from the very outset, and so in the end reach a more reliable basis of comparison[1].

VI. Summary and Conclusions

1. As a convenient criterion for vocational adjustment it is assumed that, if the available occupations are grouped in order of the difficulty of the work they entail, and if the men engaged on them are grouped in order of intelligence, then there should be a perfect correspondence between the two series. Judged by this criterion it appears that well over 20 per cent of the male adults in this country have a higher intelligence than is requisite for the work they are doing and that about the same number have an intelligence which is inadequate. Many of the discrepancies, however, are accounted for by individual differences in qualities of personality or character or in special abilities or aptitudes relevant to the work concerned.

2. Owing to the imperfect correlation between the intelligence of parents and the intelligence of their children the discrepancies between the children's intelligence and the occupational category of the parents are still greater. This follows from the multifactorial theory of inheritance, and is amply confirmed by the data here examined. The figures indicate that an overall mobility of about 22 per cent is needed to keep the distribution of intelligence approximately constant from one generation to another within each occupational category. If the distribution of character-qualities could also be taken into account, a still higher figure would no doubt be obtained. There is, moreover, considerable evidence to suggest that the degree of general vocational adaptation is improving; and, partly for this reason, it is estimated that the total amount of inter-generational mobility must be nearer 30 per cent.

3. Of the various causal factors affecting the individual's rise or fall in occupational status differences in intelligence and motivation appear to be the most influential. Differences in home background and in education seem to exercise a secondary or supplementary influence, but without the basis of the first two they are of little effect.

[1] I am much indebted to Miss Howard for assistance with the calculations involved in this section.

Intelligence and Social Mobility

REFERENCES

[1] BURT, C., SMITH, M., *et al.* (1926). *A Study in Vocational Guidance.* London: H.M. Stationery Office.

[2] CARR-SAUNDERS, A. M. and JONES, D. C. (1937). *Social Structure in England and Wales.* Oxford: Clarendon Press.

[3] BURT, C. (1942). Ability and income. *Brit. J. Educ. Psychol.,* XIII, 83–98.

[4] BURT, C. (1943). *The Backward Child.* London: University of London Press.

[5] BURT, C. (1946). *Intelligence and Fertility.* London: Hamish Hamilton.

[6] BURT, C. (1947). *Mental and Scholastic Tests.* 2nd ed. London: Staples Press.

[7] Scottish Council for Research in Education (1949). *The Trend of Scottish Intelligence.* London: University of London Press.

[8] BURT, C. (1950). The trend of Scottish intelligence. *Brit. J. Educ. Psychol.,* XX, 55–61.

[9] LIVI, L. (1950). Sur la mesure de la mobilité sociale. *Population,* V, 65–76.

[10] Registrar-General (1951). *Census of England and Wales: 1951.* London: H.M. Stationery Office.

[11] Registrar-General (1951). *Decennial Supplement: England and Wales.* London: H.M. Stationery Office.

[12] BURT, C. (1953). *Contributions of Psychology to Social Problems.* London: Oxford University Press.

[13] GLASS, D. V. (1954). *Social Mobility in Britain.* London: Routledge and Kegan Paul.

[14] BURT, C. and HOWARD, M. (1956). The multifactorial theory of inheritance and its application to intelligence. *Brit. J. Statist. Psychol.,* IX, 95–131.

[15] TULDER, J. J. M. VAN, (1956). Occupational mobility in the Netherlands. *Trans. World Congr. Sociol.,* III, 209–218.

[16] FLOUD, J. E. and HALSEY, A. H. (1956). *Social Class and Educational Opportunity.* London: Heinemann.

[17] Japanese Sociological Research Committee (1957). *Social Stratification and Social Mobility.* Tokyo: Japanese Sociological Association.

[18] JANOWITZ, M. (1958). Social stratification and mobility in Western Germany. *Amer. J. Sociol.,* LXIV, 6–24.

[19] BURT, C. (1959). Class differences in general intelligence. *Brit. J. Statist. Psychol.,* XII, 15–34.

[20] CONWAY, J. (1959). Class differences in general intelligence. *Brit. J. Statist. Psychol.,* XII, 5–14.

[21] HALSEY, A. H. (1959). Class differences in general intelligence. *Brit. J. Statist. Psychol.,* XII, 1–4.

[22] CLARKE, A. D. B., CLARKE, A. M., and BROWN, R. I. (1960). Regression to the mean. *Brit. J. Psychol.,* LI, 105–118.

[23] LIPSET, S. M. and BENDIX, R. (1960). *Social Mobility in Industrial Society.* London: Heinemann.

[24] Registrar-General (1960). *Statistical Review for 1959.* London: H.M. Stationery Office.

[25] FLOUD, J. and HALSEY, A. H. (1961). Homes and schools: social determinants of educability. *Educ. Research,* III, 83–86.

[26] BURT, C. (1961). The gifted child. *The Yearbook of Education.* London: Evans. (In the press).

From J. H. Waller (1971). Social Biology, *18*, 252–259, *by kind permission of the author and University of Chicago Press*

Achievement and Social Mobility: Relationships among IQ Score, Education, and Occupation in Two Generations

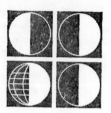

Jerome H. Waller*

Dight Institute for Human Genetics
University of Minnesota
Minneapolis, Minnesota

Cyril Burt (1961) has set forth the following hypothesis with regard to social mobility (or "social promotion"):

> . . . in a highly organized society, the discrepancies between the general intelligence of the children and the occupational class into which they are born is bound to produce a large and fairly constant amount of "basic mobility," quite apart from any deliberate changes in the political or educational structure of the society.

Several studies of the IQ test scores of adult males in various occupational classes have established that stratification of IQ by social class exists and is also accompanied by considerable variation within each class (Higgins, 1961; Bajema, 1968). When IQ scores of the children of these adults were examined in the Higgins (1961) study, the phenomenon of filial regression toward the mean was apparent within each class. Since IQ test scores measure, albeit imperfectly and in a general way, a quantitative trait with a significant genetic component (Erlenmeyer-Kimling and Jar-

vik, 1963), a large part of this observed regression may consist of "biological regression" attributable to the segregation and assortment of the genes influencing the trait. If the distribution of IQ by occupational class has not changed substantially between generations (and there is no evidence that it has), some occupational mobility of individuals must occur prior to adulthood in order for the distribution of the filial generation to approach that of the parental generation.

Burt (1961) presented rather similar data from his British sample, and it was with regard to that sample that the above-quoted hypothesis was framed. Rigorous comparison of Burt's (1961) data with that of Higgins (1961) is not possible because Burt adjusted both the mean and standard deviation of each generation in the construction of his tables, and because his actual sample size was not stated.

In a pilot study conducted by Young and Gibson (1963), 47 males "in their twenties" resident in Cambridge, England were interviewed and their fathers were traced. The results of a comparison between

* Present address: Department of Biostatistics, Graduate School of Public Health, University of Pittsburgh, Pittsburgh, Pennsylvania.

Achievement and Social Mobility

father's and son's IQ score showed the same regression phenomenon, and also the change of class status expected on the Burt hypothesis. Perhaps more importantly, when distance of movement was examined on a six-point class scale and related to the amount of difference between the IQ scores of fathers and sons, it was found that greater distance of movement was associated with greater difference in test score. The results of Gibson's recent study (1970) of 35 Cambridge scientists, their brothers, and their fathers, substantiated this association.

Duncan (1968) proposed a path diagram which represents the dependence of achieved status upon family background and intelligence. This was an extension of an earlier basic model of the process of social stratification (Blau and Duncan, 1967, p. 170). It was Duncan's contention that before one can evaluate the mechanism of "intelligence regression" described above, one should deal with a multiple-variable approach in which status itself is the dependent variable. Accordingly, he constructed a model utilizing information from various sources, all of which pertained to the United States male population of ages 25–34. The methodology employed was that developed by Sewall Wright (1921) which utilized systems of correlation coefficients interpreted causally on the basis of criteria external to the numerical analysis itself.

Achieved status was scaled according to Duncan's (1961) socioeconomic index of occupational status. When status was the dependent variable and four "predetermined" variables ("early" intelligence, number of siblings, father's education, and father's occupation) were considered in relation to that status, it was found that intelligence contributed substantially to the explained variance in the other three "entirely apart from the joint contribution shared by all four variables" (Duncan, 1968, p. 10). Of the 42% of variance in education accounted for by all four variables, 16%, or more than one-third, was due to intelligence alone; of the 28% of variance in occupational status explained by the multiple regression, about 9%, or nearly one-third, was attributed solely to intelligence; and of the 11% of variance in earnings due to multiple regression, 5%, or almost half, was accounted for by intelligence.

Duncan's (1968) summary stated the substance of the relationship quite cogently:

> If intelligence affects achievement, and if intelligence is not perfectly predictable from information on the status and circumstances of the family of origin, then intelligence will produce variation in achievement that is unrelated to the status of that family. The "meritocratic" principle has a guarantee built into it that status will not be perfectly transmitted between generations.

While it has been observed that there is a considerable stratification of IQ by social class, the presence of variability in IQ within each class coupled with the independent contribution of IQ to the variance in educational attainment, occupation, and earnings mitigates against the fixity of the individual's class position and provides a springboard for many persons to leave the class of their origin and hence to be socially mobile.

The objectives of the present study were these: to test whether the Burt hypothesis was supported by evidence from data pertaining to a sample of fathers and sons in the United States, and to illustrate the effect of intelligence (as measured by IQ test score) upon achieved status of the sons.

MATERIALS AND METHODS

The sample of this study consists of 131 fathers and their 173 sons and was taken from the much larger population studied by E. W. and S. C. Reed (1965). The present sample is representative of white males in the state of Minnesota, insofar as the only criteria for inclusion were that the sons be 24 years of age or older and that an IQ score be available for father and son. The scores had been obtained when the individuals were in school. Mean age at testing in years for the fathers was 15.90 ± 0.52 s.e. and for the sons, 13.38 ± 0.20 s.e. Group tests had been employed in the majority of cases; these included versions of the Otis and Kuhlmann tests. Occupation and education were reported by the fathers in response to a mailed questionnaire that was patterned after the OCG supplement (Occupational Changes in a Generation) to the 1962 Current Population Survey of the U.S. Bureau of the Census (see Blau and Duncan, 1968, Appendix B). In most cases educational attainment could be verified from school reports on file at the Dight Institute for Human Genetics.

Although the original records were compiled from data on families directly related to persons living in the state of Minnesota, 12 other states and one foreign country were represented in the present addresses of the 131 fathers in this sample. Among the 173 sons, 119 were residing in Minnesota: of the remaining 54, 18 were in

military service, 1 was in a foreign country, 2 were unknown, and 33 were distributed among states other than Minnesota at the time of this study.

Educational attainment and occupational level were coded using the Hollingshead (1958) system. Since this scale calls for size and/or value of farm for rating of occupational level of farmers, and since this information was unavailable, no persons listing this occupation could be included.

RESULTS

The distribution of IQ test scores is shown in Table 1 for the 131 fathers and their 173 sons. Comparison of the first two columns of means, in which all subjects are classified according to the social class (SES) of the father, demonstrates the observed regression toward the population mean for the scores of the sons. Comparison of the first and third columns of this table demonstrates the relative stability of the distribution of IQ test score by social class (SES) over the two generations.

The correlation matrix (Table 2) gives the zero-order Pearsonian correlation coefficients among IQ test score, education, number of siblings, and occupational level for 131 fathers and 170 sons (note that in this table the combined index, SES,

TABLE 1

RELATIONSHIP BETWEEN IQ TEST SCORE AND SOCIAL CLASS IN TWO GENERATIONS*

SOCIAL CLASS OF FATHER	FATHERS		SONS BY SOCIAL CLASS OF FATHERS		SONS	
	No.	$\overline{X}$ ± s.e.	No.	$\overline{X}$ ± s.e.	No.	$\overline{X}$ ± s.e.
I	1	(140)	1	(127)	7	114.43 ± 4.46
II	19	113.53 ± 2.62	26	109.04 ± 2.34	29	112.14 ± 2.34
III	43	105.56 ± 1.65	54	104.81 ± 1.72	67	105.99 ± 1.71
IV	53	93.57 ± 1.89	66	101.20 ± 1.88	58	96.87 ± 1.83
V	15	81.00 ± 4.44	26	90.88 ± 3.35	12	88.00 ± 3.84
Total sample	131	99.30 ± 1.44	173	103.06 ± 1.16	173	103.06 ± 1.16

* Social class (SES) divided according to the Hollingshead (1958) rating, a composite of occupational level and educational attainment.

Achievement and Social Mobility

TABLE 2

Correlation Matrix for 170 Father-son Pairs*

Variable	2	3	4	5	6	7	8	$\bar{x} \pm$ s.d.	s.e.
1. Occupational level of son†	0.724	0.497	—0.202	0.369	0.482	0.430	—0.169	4.241 ± 1.541	0.118
2. Educational level of son†	...	0.519	—0.222	0.456	0.528	0.467	—0.183	3.453 ± 1.217	0.093
3. IQ score of son	...	...	—0.224	0.340	0.324	0.360	—0.277	102.900 ± 14.439	1.107
4. Number of siblings of son	...	...	...	—0.111	—0.088	—0.104	0.231	2.653 ± 1.947	0.149
5. Educational level of father†	...	...	...	...	0.582	0.709	—0.374	4.494 ± 1.237	0.095
6. Occupational level of father†	...	...	...	...	...	0.569	—0.006	4.276 ± 1.535	0.118
7. IQ score of father	...	...	...	...	...	...	—0.244	98.424 ± 17.307	1.327
8. Number of siblings of father	...	...	...	...	...	...	...	3.837 ± 2.440	0.246

* $N = 170$ except for number of siblings of father, where $N = 98$.
† Occupational level and educational level ranked after Hollingshead (1958). Rank of 1 is high; 7 is low.

is not used). In addition, the correlation between the IQ test score of 84 fathers and their occupational level of origin was $r = + 0.026$. In each case the occupational level of origin was that of the male parent at age 16 of the subject. Three institutionalized retarded sons were omitted from this analysis; hence the total number of sons is reduced.

Since an individual born into the highest social class (Class I) can only remain there or move down, and an individual born into the lowest class (Class V) can only remain there or move up, the sample was restricted to the 146 father-son pairs in which the father was of Class II, III, or IV. The mean IQ scores for this sample were 100.57 ± 13.62 (s.e. $= 1.27$) for the 115 fathers, and 103.84 ± 14.38 (s.e. $= 1.19$) for their 146 sons.

The data of this study show a consistent association between father-son difference in IQ score and father-son difference in social achievement, whether the latter difference is measured in terms of ISP score or social class. The Hollingshead Index of

Social Position (ISP score) was calculated for all fathers and sons. This index provides a rating from 11 (high) to 77 (low) which can be treated as a continuous variable. The correlation between father-son difference in IQ score and father-son difference in ISP score for the total sample is $r = + 0.291 \pm 0.080 \, S_r$. For the restricted sample that includes only the fathers in Classes II, III, and IV with their sons, $r = + 0.368 \pm 0.066 \, S_r$. The exclusion of sons born into the extreme classes thus slightly increases the value of the correlation coefficient and at the same time provides a more rigorous test of the Burt hypothesis.

Table 3 shows the relationship between father-son difference in IQ score and change in social class of the sons for the sample of 170 pairs. Table 4 is confined to the sample of 146 pairs, and shows the same relationship. These latter data are represented graphically in Figure 1, in which the cases of father-son difference greater than 37.5 points are omitted. The negative and positive extremes held three

TABLE 3

RELATIONSHIP OF FATHER-SON IN IQ SCORE TO FATHER-SON DIFFERENCE IN
SOCIAL CLASS, FOR THE TOTAL SAMPLE*

RANGE OF DIFFERENCE IN IQ SCORE (SON MINUS FATHER)	SON LOWER IN SOCIAL CLASS		SAME		SON HIGHER IN SOCIAL CLASS		TOTAL
	No.	% ± s.e.	No.	% ± s.e.	No.	% ± s.e.	
+22.6 to +52.5	3	11.11 ± 18.14	4	14.81 ± 17.76	20	74.07 ± 9.80	27
+ 7.6 to +22.5	5	11.11 ± 14.05	28	62.22 ± 9.16	12	26.67 ± 12.77	45
− 7.5 to + 7.5	7	12.28 ± 12.41	24	42.11 ± 10.08	26	45.61 ± 9.77	57
− 7.6 to −22.5	11	36.67 ± 14.53	13	43.33 ± 13.74	6	20.00 ± 16.33	30
−22.6 to −52.5	7	77.78 ± 15.71	1	11.11 ± 31.43	1	11.11 ± 31.43	9
−52.6 to −67.5	2	(100%)	0	... ...	0	... ...	2
Total sample	35	20.59 ± 6.83	70	41.18 ± 5.88	65	38.24 ± 6.03	170

* The error term is the standard error of a proportion, $\sigma = \sqrt{\dfrac{pq}{N}}$.

TABLE 4

RELATIONSHIP OF FATHER-SON DIFFERENCE IN IQ SCORE TO FATHER-SON DIFFERENCE IN
SOCIAL CLASS, FOR FATHERS OF CLASSES II, III, AND IV ONLY*

RANGE OF DIFFERENCE IN IQ SCORE (SON MINUS FATHER)	SON LOWER IN SOCIAL CLASS		SAME		SON HIGHER IN SOCIAL CLASS		TOTAL
	No.	% ± s.e.	No.	% ± s.e.	No.	% ± s.e.	
+22.6 to +52.5	3	16.67 ± 21.52	3	16.67 ± 21.52	12	66.67 ± 13.61	18
+ 7.6 to +22.5	5	11.63 ± 14.34	26	60.47 ± 9.59	12	27.91 ± 12.95	43
− 7.5 to + 7.5	8	16.00 ± 12.96	23	46.00 ± 10.39	19	38.00 ± 11.14	50
− 7.6 to −22.5	10	40.00 ± 15.49	12	48.00 ± 14.42	3	12.00 ± 18.76	25
−22.6 to −52.5	7	87.50 ± 12.50	1	12.50 ± 33.07	0	... ...	8
−52.6 to −67.5	2	(100%)	0	... ...	0	... ...	2
Total sample	35	23.97 ± 7.22	65	44.52 ± 6.16	46	31.51 ± 6.85	146

* The error term is the standard error of a proportion, $\sigma = \sqrt{\dfrac{pq}{N}}$.

and two cases respectively; hence the percentages would be misleading. The three sons with the greatest negative differences moved down. At the other end, one of the two sons with the greatest positive differences moved down; the other, up.

When the occupational level of the son is taken as the dependent variable and the remaining variables in Table 2 are taken to be the independent variables, 56.25% of the variance in occupational level is accounted for by linear prediction from the 7 "predetermined" variables (the multiple R for the system is 0.75).

It is also useful to consider both education and occupational level of the sons as separate dependent variables, in order to assess the relative roles of the son's IQ score and number of siblings, and the education and occupation of the father as

Achievement and Social Mobility

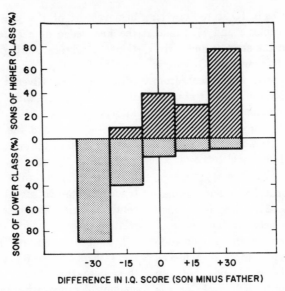

FIG. 1.—Percentage of sons moving up or down from their father's social class by differences in IQ score.

independent variables in each case. Table 5 gives the results of these analyses.

DISCUSSION

The data of the present study support the hypothesis that father-son differences in social position are attributable in some degree to father-son differences in ability as measured by IQ test score. Since IQ tests were originally designed with the objective of predicting success in school (and to a lesser degree, in society), it is not surprising that the two measures of ability (IQ score and occupational achievement) are associated. As Burt (1961) pointed out and as the data of this study show (Table 1), there is a difference in the distribution of IQ scores by a subject's social class of origin vs. the subject's own class. The "basic mobility" required by the hypothesis to restore the original occupational distribution of IQ scores is asso-

TABLE 5

STANDARDIZED REGRESSION COEFFICIENTS OF EDUCATION AND
OCCUPATIONAL LEVEL ON PREDETERMINED VARIABLES*

| | ACHIEVED STATUS | |
PREDETERMINED VARIABLE	Educational Attainment (2)	1967 Occupational Level (1)
IQ test score (3)	0.343	0.353
Number of siblings (4)	—0.101	—0.088
Father's education (5)	0.137	0.044
Father's occupation (6)	0.329	0.334
(Coefficient of determination)	(0.44)	(0.37)

* Based on correlations in Table 3.

ciated with differences in IQ score between fathers and sons (Tables 3 and 4). Figure 1 demonstrates that the amount and direction of father-son difference in IQ score is directly associated with movement from the social class of origin. This is also reflected in the correlation between father-son difference in IQ score and father-son difference in social position ($r = + 0.368$ for the sample of 146 sons).

Upon examining the correlations among IQ score, educational level, and occupational level (Table 2), there is a small apparent difference between the two generations in the roles played by education and IQ score as contributors to achieved status. Whereas the correlation between IQ score and occupational level for the fathers is $+ 0.569$, the value for the sons is lower, at $+ 0.497$. This difference is not statistically significant at the 0.05 level, but one may infer that the IQ score of the fathers is somewhat more closely associated with their achievement than is that of their sons, when achievement is measured by occupational level. A large part of this difference is attributable to the difference in age of the subjects when their occupation was rated. The mean age of the fathers at the time of the study was 52 years, but that of the sons was only 27 years. Hence the fathers had opportunity for (intra-generational) mobility. If the sons are followed up some 25 years from now, the correlation should even more closely resemble that of the fathers.

The relationship between education and occupation for the two generations also differs, but in the opposite direction. The correlation between educational level and occupational level is $+ 0.582$ for the fathers and $+ 0.724$ for the sons (Table 2). Again, difference between generations is not significant at the 0.05 level. In this case, the inference that education is more closely associated with the occupational achievement of the sons is supported by the knowledge of a change in the educational structure during this generation, specifically the advent of compulsory education laws. Given the higher correlation of IQ score with education for the fathers ($r = + 0.719$) than for the sons ($r = + 0.568$) and the higher mean educational level of the sons (3.45 vs. 4.49), it may be inferred that in the earlier generation the subjects with higher IQ scores tended to stay in school longer than their contemporaries. The first-order partial correlation between education and occupation ("holding IQ constant") is $+ 0.308$ for the fathers and $+ 0.628$ for the sons. In these data, then, there is evidence that the amount of formal education is more closely associated with the occupational level of the sons than with that of the fathers.

The correlation between IQ score and occupational level of origin for the two generations is not significantly different: for the sons, $r = + 0.324$ and for the fathers $r = + 0.206$. The probability of obtaining these two values when sampling from the same population is $P = 0.58$. This rather low correlation is consistent with the observed variability in mean IQ score within social classes and the regression toward the population mean of the sons born into each class (Table 1).

There are at least two points of interest in interpreting the results in Table 5. First, the two largest contributions to the explained variance in both education and occupational level are the IQ test score of the son and the occupational level of the father. Of the 44% of the variance in education accounted for by all four variables, 11.8%, or over one-fourth, is due to intelligence alone; and of the 37% of variance in occupational level explained by the multiple regression, 12.5%, or about one-third, is attributable solely to intelligence. The father's occupational level contributes 10.8%, or over one-fourth, of the total variance in education accounted for in the multiple regression. It contributes 12.5%, or about one-third, of the explained variance in occupational level of the son.

Second, the large independent contribution of IQ test score supports the notion that intelligence will produce variation in achievement that is unrelated to the status of the family of origin. Hence, status, as measured here by occupational level, is not perfectly transmitted between generations.

Thus the data of the present study illustrate quite well the process of achievement as outlined in the model of Duncan (1968).

SUMMARY

The present study of 173 males and their 131 fathers, representative of the nonfarm white population of Minnesota, supports the hypothesis that social mobility is correlated with the discrepancies between the general intelligence of sons (as measured by IQ test scores) and the social class into which they were born. A multiple regression analysis performed on these data illustrates the independent contribution of intelligence to the variance in two achieved statuses, educational attainment and occupational level. The substantial correlation between father-son difference in IQ score and father-son difference in social position ($r = + 0.368$), and the relationship between the magnitude (and direction) of IQ score difference and the distance (and direction) of social mobility both support the view that differences in ability provide a "springboard" that enables individuals to be socially mobile and that to some degree prevents social classes in an open society from congealing into castes.

ACKNOWLEDGMENTS

I am grateful to Dr. V. Elving Anderson, Dr. Carl J. Bajema, and Dr. Irving I. Gottesman for their helpful suggestions during the course of this investigation, and to Dr. S. C. Reed for his review of the manuscript. Dr. Reed graciously allowed access to the basic material for this study. The help of Mr. Arthur LeGasse of the University of Pittsburgh, in setting up the multiple regression analysis, is gratefully acknowledged.

This investigation was supported by the Behavior Genetics Training Program of the National Institutes of Health (Grant MH 10679), and by the Charles M. Goethe Memorial Fund in Genetics.

REFERENCES

BAJEMA, C. 1968. Relation of fertility to occupational status, IQ, educational attainment, and size of family of origin: A follow-up study of a male Kalamazoo public school population. Eugen. Quart. 15:198–203.

BLAU, P. M., and O. D. DUNCAN. 1967. The American occupational structure. Wiley and Sons, New York.

BURT, C. 1961. Intelligence and social mobility. Brit. J. Stat. Psychol. 14:1–24.

DUNCAN, O. D. 1961. A socioeconomic index for all occupations. In Albert J. Reiss, Jr. (ed.), Occupations and social status. Free Press of Glencoe, Glencoe, New York.

———. 1968. Ability and achievement. Eugen. Quart. 15:1–11.

ERLENMEYER-KIMLING, L., and L. F. JARVIK. 1963. Genetics and intelligence: A review. Science 142:1477–1478.

FALCONER, D. S. 1960. Introduction to quantitative genetics. Ronald Press, New York.

GIBSON, JOHN B. 1970. Biological aspects of a high socio-economic group. I. IQ, education, and social mobility. J. Biosoc. Sci. 2:1–16.

HIGGINS, J. V. 1961. An analysis of intelligence of 1,016 families. Ph.D. Thesis, University of Minnesota, Minneapolis.

HOLLINGSHEAD, A. B., and F. C. REDLICH. 1958. Social class and mental illness. Wiley and Sons, New York.

REED, E. W., and S. C. REED. 1965. Mental retardation: A family study. Saunders, Philadelphia.

YOUNG, M., and J. GIBSON. 1963. In search of an explanation of social mobility. Brit. J. Stat. Psychol. 16:27–36.

WRIGHT, SEWALL. 1921. Correlation and causation. J. Agric. Res. 20:557–585.

From A. Falek (1971). Social Biology, *18*, 550–559, *by kind permission of the author and University of Chicago Press*

Differential Fertility and Intelligence: Current Status of the Problem

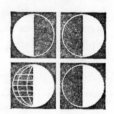

Arthur Falek

Division of Human Genetics, Georgia Mental Health Institute, and Department of Psychiatry, Emory University, Atlanta, Georgia

In 1940 Raymond B. Cattell reported that parents with higher IQ scores were inclined to have smaller families than those with lower measured intelligence. He indicated that the differential birth rate with regard to intelligence would, in time, result in a lower IQ in the general population. This finding supported earlier observations by Lentz (1927) and Maller (1933), among others, of an inverse relationship between family size and test performance. According to Cattell, the rate of decline in the United States and Great Britain was between 1.0 and 1.5 points per decade. Confirmation of Cattell's findings was presented by Burt in 1946 with a warning that the rate of decline in the English population was between 1.3 and 2.5 points per generation. While this estimate was even greater than that indicated by Cattell, Burt found actual evidence for a decline of only 0.9 points per generation in a twenty-year period ending in 1939.

In contrast to these observations, Smith (1942), on the basis of comparative IQ scores on children tested in Honolulu in 1924 and in 1938, advised that in his study there was a gain of 20 points in those evaluated 14 years later. To test his prediction, Cattell in 1950 compared the IQ scores of ten-year-old children recorded in Birmingham, England in 1936 with those obtained for ten-year-old children tested in that city in 1949. Instead of the expected decrease in IQ, he found that the more recent population showed an average gain of 1.28 IQ points. Further support for this conclusion was presented in the study of Scottish children (Scottish Council for Research in Education, 1949) in which the IQ results on some 87,000 eleven-year-old children tested in Edinburgh in 1932 were compared with the scores of approximately 71,000 Edinburgh children of the same age in 1947. Once again the average performance improved with a mean gain of 2.3 points. A survey of intelligence test performance of American high-school students in a twenty-year period by Finch (1946) also indicated improvement—despite the marked increase in the proportion of students enrolled in high school during the period of the study.

Evidence of an increase in IQ in the more recent generation was reported by Tuddenham (1948) for an adult population. To conduct this study, a random sample of 768 men drafted into the army in World War II was also administered the Army Alpha Examination of World War I. While correlation between the two tests (Army Alpha of World War I and

Differential Fertility and Intelligence

Army General Classification Test of World War II) was $r = 0.90$, the median raw score of the World War I exam was reported as 62 and that of the World War II exam was measured at 104. A raw score of 62, however, was only at the 22 percentile of World War II men and a raw score of 104 was at the 83 percentile of World War I men.

While Tuddenham emphasized that this marked increase was the result of better educational facilities, improved quality of instruction, and the development of mass media communications, his findings also inferred that the norm of reaction, the genetic response to environmental conditions, for measured intelligence was significantly improved with intellectual stimulation. While this study supported Cattell's suggestion of the need for constant revision of the IQ test to prevent obsolescence of test content and to maintain test norms, the marked improvement in test performance of the more recent generation casts doubt on Cattell's initial observation of a rapid drop in the national intelligence. The contradictory findings about changes in the IQ from one generation to the next (Cattell paradox) indicated the need for a newly constructed research design.

Penrose (1963) in his classic text, *The Biology of Mental Defect*, noted that in 1625 Bacon in his essay "Of Parents and Children," stated, "the noblest works and foundations have proceeded from childless men." Short in 1750 observed, "The most laborious part of mankind are also the most fruitful in proportion to their numbers; and the most voluptuous, idle, effeminate and luxurious are barrenest; hard labor makes the poor fruitful," and in 1869 Galton noted that a surprisingly large number of the ablest men left no descendants. Penrose was of the opinion that if this decrease in the proportion of intelligent persons had been occurring for

even one century it would have been readily detected. He indicated that the negative relationship between IQ and family size as well as the positive correlations in intelligence between mates and relatives were compatible with a genetic equilibrium in which the average intelligence level remains constant. This conclusion was based on Gorer's observation (1947) that differential fertility and intelligence was a natural process consistent with a stable genetic equilibrium and Galton's (1869) positive comparison of giants and dwarfs with men of large and small intellect with regard to their reproductive deficiencies. The admitted oversimplified statistical model to support this hypothesis was that of a single additive gene pair in a population which had complete assortative mating, reproductive advantage of the heterozygote population over the homozygote superior one, and a nonreproductive severely retarded population.

To replace genes for intelligence lost because of the relatively low fertility of the superior group, Penrose indicated the necessity of a high birth rate in the inferior group. In this manner genetic principles would also work against intellectual decline from generation to generation. He described as more realistic hypotheses those employing an indefinite number of gene loci with additive effects which were in stable equilibrium. Dobzhansky (1962) suggested that one mechanism to maintain intelligence would be a balanced polymorphism, with the mediocrities the heterotic heterozygotes and the superior and inferior people the two kinds of homozygotes. This would support Penrose (1963).

The mode of inheritance proposed by Penrose, however, did not resolve the paradox presented by the Cattell studies. The resolution of the Cattell paradox was first reported by Higgins, Reed and Reed (1962) and is one of many significant findings in the well-known volume, *Men-*

tal Retardation: A Family Study, co-authored by Elizabeth and Sheldon Reed. Elizabeth Reed's excellent paper in this symposium presents in summary fashion some of the salient points from her book including that on the resolution of the Cattell paradox.

The resolution of that paradox was possible because the investigators had insight about the basis for the paradox and collected the data necessary to resolve it. In summary, the negative correlation between family size and intelligence disappeared when the single and nonreproductive siblings of the parents were included in the analyses. The investigators found that the higher reproductive rate of lower IQ parents was offset by the large number of their siblings who never reproduced as compared with siblings of higher IQ parents. The essence of the study reported by Higgins, Reed, and Reed (1962) was that intelligence in the population was not decreasing at a significant rate and, in all likelihood, would remain static from one generation to another.

Shortly after that publication, Bajema (1963) on the basis of life-history data on a school population from Kalamazoo County, Michigan, also reported a positive relationship between intelligence and fer-tility (Table 1). This positive relationship, more pronounced in the latter than in the former study, was attributed by the author to differentials in reproductive rates in contrast to differentials in marriage rates with intelligence found by Higgins, Reed, and Reed (1962). While Bajema also found an extremely small rate of increase in intelligence from one generation to another, he suggested that there was a dynamic relationship between intelligence and fertility. It was his opinion that during the twentieth century this association would become an increasingly more positive one.

How, in fact, can it be determined whether human intelligence is changing from generation to generation? If there are changes, what are the factors that play important roles and will it be possible to influence them for the benefit of mankind? From a behavioral geneticist's point of view, necessary information in this regard includes: (1) evidence that genetic factors are significant; (2) approximations of heritability; (3) information relative to assortative mating patterns; and (4) estimates of the number of gene loci involved as well as (5) measurement data on the genetic consequences of selection pressure.

A summary of the evidence on genetic

TABLE 1

BIRTHRATE ACCORDING TO MEASURED INTELLIGENCE OF PARENT GENERATION*

STUDIES	MEASURED INTELLIGENCE						
	0–55	56–70	71–85	86–100	101–115	116–130	>130
Higgins, Reed, and Reed (1962)							
No. offspring	29	74	203	583	778	269	25
Birthrate	1.38	2.46	2.39	2.16	2.26	2.45	2.96
Bajema (1963)†							
No. offspring	...	3	75	427	344	107	23
Birthrate	...	0.00	2.05	2.30	2.08	2.51	3.00

* Fertility of parental sibs included.
† Adapted from Bajema.

Differential Fertility and Intelligence

factors in intelligence was reported by Erlenmeyer-Kimling and Jarvik in 1963. Their review of 52 studies involving some thirty thousand correlations emphasized the significant role of the genotype in mental functioning. To be certain, heritability of the IQ is still under investigation. In a recent paper McCall (in press) examined the relative heritability of the general level of IQ and contrasted it to the pattern of IQ change over age in sib-sib and parent-child pairs compared to unrelated matched controls. Within the boundaries established by the genome for an individual's intelligence level as measured by IQ test scores, McCall observed fluctuating patterns of change over age. The low parent-child correlation for the IQ obtained in that study was unusual and was possibly due in part to the method used for smoothing intelligence scores as well as to the variety of measures incorporated into the IQ assessments for the parent-child evaluations.

Operational intelligence has been described by Carter (1966) as due to the interaction of genetic endowment and environment. Although the genetic endowment cannot be measured independent of the environment, the proportion of the total variance in intelligence scores due to genetic factors has been reported. Heritability has been determined by Roberts (1961) to be between one-half to three-quarters of the variance in IQ scores, and Huntley (1966) found that 70%, and possibly more, of operational intelligence was due to genetic factors.

Estimates with regard to the coefficient of assortative mating in intelligence range from 0.40 to over 0.70. Huntley (1966) suggested that in Western society the positive correlation between the phenotypes of the spouses was at least as high as between parent and child (0.50 to 0.56) or sibs (0.47 to 0.55). The number

of gene loci which compose the genetic variance for intelligence was estimated by Spuhler (1962) as from 6 to 22 loci, assuming polygenic inheritance without dominance. This approximation could be increased by 50% if complete dominance occurs, and even further if unequal gene effects are assumed.

Based on estimated number of gene loci, coefficient of assortative mating, heritability, and the degree of dominance of each locus, it is possible to predict the genetic effects of human assortative mating for the trait under investigation. This method of evaluation was recently employed by Adams (1969) to investigate the genetic consequences of cultural adaptation to a number of traits including intelligence. According to Adams, the effect of positive assortative mating is remarkably limited from one generation to another if heritability is estimated at 0.45 and the phenotypic correlation for the trait in question, intelligence, is approximately 0.50, no matter whether the number of loci is in the range of 5 or 10 in number (Fig. 1). In such a situation, equilibrium is rapidly achieved with the maintenance of a high degree of heterozygotes. If the estimate of heritability, however, is markedly increased over 0.50 and the number of gene loci is relatively small, equilibrium is not achieved and the per cent of heterozygotes decreases as the coefficient of assortative matings increases. However, as first reported by Wright (1921) and reemphasized by Crow and Felsenstein (1968), unless the number of gene loci is small or the degree of assortative mating very intense, the increase in homozygosity is slight, while the increase in variance is large.

In our own culture, intellectual ability as measured by scholastic achievement has become an important component in mate selection. Since intelligence is a

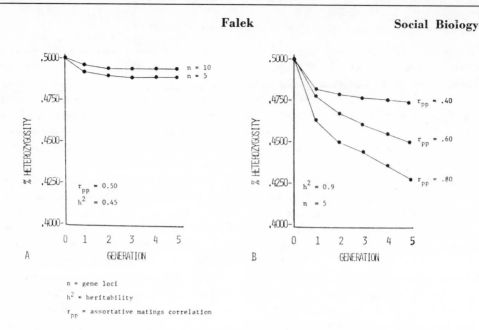

n = gene loci

h^2 = heritability

r_{pp} = assortative matings correlation

FIG. 1.—Effects of heritability and assortative mating on heterozygosity (from Adams, 1969).

cornerstone for intellectual achievement, if heritability of this trait is estimated at approximately 70% (Huntley, 1966), either a high level of assortative mating as measured by scholastic achievement or a small number of gene loci for the trait in question would result in a polarization of intelligence in the population with a marked loss of heterozygotes. If, with these conditions, marital partners with lower intelligence were to reproduce less frequently than those with higher intelligence, there would be a significant rise in the intellectual level of the population from one generation to another. However, evidence from Reed and Reed (1965), Bajema (1963), Kiser (1968), Garrison, Anderson, and Reed (1968), indicated no overwhelming preponderance of assortative matings with regard to intelligence or educational level. Furthermore, as has been stated previously, the number of gene loci which combine to express the trait intelligence is estimated from 6 to 33 or more. These findings signify that the polarization of intelligence within a few gen-

erations to those with either high or low IQ is not to be expected.

A different approach to an evaluation of the change in intelligence under conditions of natural selection was obtained by Falconer (1966). His approach introduced an estimate of the heritability of fitness as well as that of intelligence into the analysis. The genetic correlation between intelligence and reproductive fitness was estimated with data obtained by Higgins, Reed, and Reed (1962) and Bajema (1963). Falconer found a positive selection differential with regard to differential fertility and intelligence of 0.5 IQ points in the former study and 0.3 IQ points in the latter investigation. These results however, indicated an increase in the IQ of only one to two-tenths of a unit per generation. If correct, the conclusion to be drawn would confirm the suggestion by Higgins, Reed, and Reed (1962) that the IQ remains static from one generation to another.

It is possible, of course, that in actuality changes in the IQ from one generation

Differential Fertility and Intelligence

to another are somewhere between that ascertained by Falconer (1966) and that which could be projected by an assumption of intense assortative mating or a relatively small number of gene loci. With more recent data, it would be possible to determine whether there has been any change in differential selection. Fortunately, new information is now available from a follow-up of a sample of the population reported by Reed and Reed (1965). The families investigated were drawn from the original Minnesota program where (1) an IQ score was available for both parents, and (2) the mother was born before January 1, 1928. These results, therefore, signify changes in the population a decade after those reported by Higgins, Reed, and Reed (1962). The information reported by Waller (1971) confirms the expected positive marital assortment for IQ score and education achievement in a population which had reached maturity just prior to the middle of the century.

Waller (personal communication) was kind enough to send the author his data on the average number of children of each individual in the parental generation subdivided according to IQ for comparison with that reported by Higgins, Reed, and Reed (1962) and Bajema (1963). When the data from the three studies are placed in graph form alongside each other (Fig. 2), much similarity is observed in the results of the three, and there is no evidence of a bimodal distribution. The shallow U-shaped portions of the curves in both of the earlier studies can be replaced by a common line. This would emphasize the similarity of the linear increase in average number of children with increase in the parental IQ in the populations studied in Minnesota and Michigan. Waller's findings indicate that one decade later the direction of natural selection with regard to ability as measured by the IQ test score continued to demonstrate a slight reproductive advantage to those with the higher scores. The small dip in the number of children per person at IQ 116–130 varies in direction from that obtained by the other two investigators, but no significance

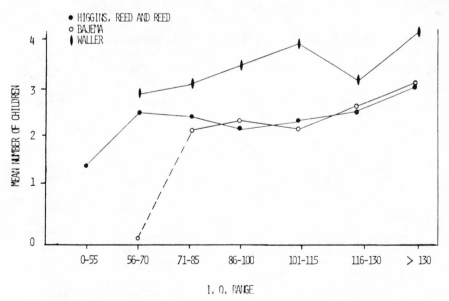

Fig. 2.—Differential fertility and intelligence.

is attributed to it, since at the next parent IQ range, the frequency of offspring is once again in positive direction. A further sampling artifact observed in this graphic comparison is the apparent consistent increase in reproduction across all parental IQ groups in the Waller study. When the size of each individual's own completed family was compared with that of his or her own family, that study, in fact, showed a decline of about 0.5% in mean completed family size in one generation among persons with one or more children.

Charting the average number of offspring per person in relation to IQ, including the nonreproductive individuals in the parental generation, however, does not account for all of the important biologic variables which affect population growth. As pointed out by Bajema (1963), to estimate the direction and intensity of natural selection in human populations with regard to a trait such as intelligence, mortality rates up to the end of the childbearing period, as well as generation length, also require investigation. A means

of simultaneously evaluating differentials in fertility, mortality, and generation length in each parental subsample divided according to IQ score was first employed by Bajema (1963) and then by Waller (1971). In addition to this statistic (the intrinsic rate of natural increase), both investigators presented separate data on generation length (parental age at birth of mid-child) and relative fitness (ratio of the growth rate of each of the phenotypic groups in comparison to the optimum phenotypic group). While data from the Bajema study indicated a slight positive relationship between IQ level and generation length (those with higher IQ's had a longer span between generations), Waller found neither a positive relationship nor a discernible negative one in his population. As shown in Table 2, in both investigations the parental group with the highest IQ scores was the optimum one with the largest rate of increase and highest levels of fitness. In these studies the direction of change was a positive one, as natural selection seemed to confer repro-

TABLE 2

INTRINSIC RATE OF NATURAL INCREASE, AVERAGE GENERATION LENGTH, AND FITNESS ACCORDING TO PARENTAL IQ

Parental IQ Range	Intrinsic Rate of Natural Increase	Average Generation Length (Yrs.)	Fitness (Av. No. Offspring/ Person)
Bajema (1963)			
–120	+0.0089	29.42	1.0000
105–119	+0.0039	28.86	0.8614
95–104	+0.0003	28.41	0.7771
80–94	+0.0075	28.01	0.9484
69–79	–0.0100	28.76	0.5774
Total sample	+0.0039	28.49	...
Waller (1971)			
131–150	+0.0299	26.59	1.0000
116–130	+0.0198	27.74	0.8218
101–115	+0.0213	27.91	0.8597
86–100	+0.0205	28.26	0.8520
71–85	+0.0211	28.12	0.8067
56–70	+0.0188	27.58	0.8073
Total sample	+0.0212	27.97	0.8504

ductive advantage on parents with the highest IQ scores.

Do the consistent findings of the three studies complete the story? Is it now possible to leave this area of social biology with confidence that in the long run the more intelligent will inherit the earth? Before we become too complacent, it would be best to determine the limitations of the three investigations as well as what other information needs to be ascertained.

Imposed on the reported reproductive advantages is Galton's law of filial regression toward the mean. Family studies indicate that children of parents with the highest or lowest IQ's will have measurement scores approximately 10 points below or above their parents. The rationale for these observations is that the unique combinations of circumstances, biologic and environmental, which produced such parents would not be expected to reoccur in their offspring. It would be of importance to obtain the IQ scores for children as well as parents in future studies designed in similar fashion to those of Higgins, Reed, and Reed (1962), Bajema (1963), and Waller (1971). The inclusion of the additional information would permit an investigation as to whether and to what extent reproductive advantages to parents with the highest intellect is meaningful with regard to an advance in the IQ from one generation to the next.

Certainly, the findings on children reported by the Cattell (1940) and Scottish studies (Scottish Council for Research in Education, 1949) as well as those of soldiers tested by Tuddenham (1948) support an increase in the IQ from a former generation to the more recent one. It would be of value to investigate soldiers now drafted into the United States Armed Forces in similar fashion to that reported by Tuddenham to determine whether measured intelligence has increased over the past quarter of a century.

It should be noted that the three most recent studies on differential fertility and intelligence were conducted on white middle-America populations. Bajema (1963) further reports that all of the persons in his study were of the Protestant faith. Waller's (1971) data are based on a follow-up of a subsample of the Minnesota population investigated by Higgins, Reed, and Reed (1965). It is, of course, the only comparative study available at present to indicate the direction of differential fertility and intelligence during the middle of the twentieth century. Comparative data on recent changes in differential selection should also be obtained from an investigation of the offspring of persons born and tested in Kalamazoo County, Michigan, a decade after those evaluated by Bajema (1962). While a study of a school population would eliminate reproductive data on noneducable retardates, the results of the proposed investigation would permit a second comparison of two populations born in the same area ten years apart.

As part of his investigation of a subsample of the Minnesota population, Waller (1971) examined several environmental factors. He reports that his correlation matrices for the relationships among IQ score, education, socioeconomic status, and family size are not much different from that obtained by other investigators. This should be but a first step in the inclusion for study of specified environmental variables which may influence natural selection and survival in human populations. As Dobzhansky (1962) has clearly stated, "Darwinian fitness is measurable only in terms of reproductive proficiency." While in lower organisms this can be readily measured by comparative counts of the offspring according to designed parental subdivisions, in human populations cultural influences and intellectual awareness play significant roles in the control of reproduction. In addition to the environmental factors reported by Waller (1971), cultural elements which may also be of importance with regard to reproduction include religion, availability of contraceptive devices, social philosophy, prior determination by the couple about family size, general physical and mental health of offspring and parents, discomfort of the mother during pregnancy and delivery, as well as the verbal influences of those in the local milieu. At present, all that is available is a superficial summary of these many variables which, in all likelihood, have unequal amounts of input into the makeup of differential fertility as it compares with intelligence. To disregard these variables may result either in fortuitous relationships or those which should not be projected from a specific to a more generalized population.

What then of the three most recent studies in this area? Of importance is the consistent observation of a positive relationship between IQ and family size. Whatever the trend, static or dynamic, the data of Higgins, Reed, and Reed (1965), Bajema (1963), and Waller (1971) may be the foundation stones in the development of a program to bring about improvement in human intelligence. Since reproductive individuals in the dull and retarded groups oftentimes have large families with a substantial proportion of the children probably unplanned and often unwanted, Carter (1966) suggested that family-planning programs in these popu-

lations would be likely to increase the positive fertility differential. Falconer (1966) estimated that if family planning were to spread into the lower intelligence group, the differential in natural selection would increase.

An attempt should be made to test these statistically derived determinations. A two-pronged attack will be necessary to obtain meaningful results. The environmental aspect requires an upgrading of educators and facilities in those school systems below educationally acceptable standards as well as the development of infant and early child care centers for those born into intellectually deprived households. Such programs should permit each child the opportunity to attain his highest level of achievement.

The genetic approach should be through the development of family-planning programs that will be attractive to and accepted by reproductive individuals of low intelligence. A program of incentive awards for maintaining small families should be incorporated into the educational curriculum for retardates. In her paper in this volume Reed reported that 83% of retardates are born to parents both of whom have an IQ of 70 or over. To permit the program every chance for success it would be important to provide counseling and information with regard to family planning to parents of severely affected children. In such manner, directed family-planning programs as well as effective educational opportunities may bring this important aspect of human evolution under human control.

REFERENCES

ADAMS, M. S. 1969. Genetic consequences of cultural adaptation. Med. Clinics No. Amer. **53**: 977.

ALSTROM, C. H. 1961. A study of inheritance of human intelligence. Acta Psychol. Neurol. Scand. **36**:175.

BACON, F. 1625. Essayes or Counsels Civill and Morall. VII. Of parents and children.

BAJEMA, C. J. 1963. Estimation of the direction and intensity of natural selection in relation to human intelligence by means of the intrinsic rate of natural increase. Eugen. Quart. **10**:175.

Differential Fertility and Intelligence

BURT, C. 1946. Intelligence and fertility. Hamilton, London.

CARTER, C. O. 1966. Differential fertility and intelligence. *In* J. E. Meade and A. S. Parkes (eds.), Genetic and environmental factors in human ability. Oliver and Boyd, Edinburgh.

CATTELL, R. B. 1940. Effects of human fertility trends upon the distribution of intelligence and culture. Yearb. Nat. Soc. Study Educ. **39** (Part I):221.

————. 1950. The fate of national intelligence: Tests of a thirteen-year prediction. Eugen. Rev. **42**:136.

CROW, J. F., and J. FELSENSTEIN. 1968. The effect of assortative mating on the genetic composition of a population. Eugen. Quart. **15**:84.

DOBZHANSKY, T. 1962. Mankind evolving. Yale Univ. Press, New Haven.

ERLENMEYER-KIMLING, L., and L. F. JARVIK. 1963. Genetics and intelligence: A review. Science **142**:1477.

FALCONER, D. S. 1966. Genetic consequences of selection pressure. *In* J. E. Meade and A. S. Parkes (eds.), Genetic and environmental factors in human ability. Oliver and Boyd, Edinburgh.

FINCH, F. H. 1946. Enrollment increases and changes in mental level. Appl. Psychol. Monogr. 10.

GALTON, F. 1869. Hereditary genius. London, MacMillan.

GARRISON, R. J., V. E. ANDERSON, and S. C. REED. 1968. Assortative marriage. Eugen. Quart. **15**:113.

GORER, P. A. 1947. Genetic factors and population. *In* G.E.W. Walstenhalme (ed.), Child health and development. J. and A. Churchill, London.

HIGGINS, J. V., E. W. REED, and S. C. REED. 1962. Intelligence and family size: A paradox resolved. Eugen. Quart. **9**:84.

HUNTLEY, R. M. C. 1966. Heritability of intelligence. *In* S. E. Meade and A. S. Parkes (eds.), Genetic and environmental factors in human ability. Oliver and Boyd, Edinburgh.

KISER, C. V. 1968. Assortative mating by educational attainment in relation to fertility. Eugen. Quart. **15**:99.

LENTZ, T. F., JR. 1927. Relation of I.Q. to size of family. J. Ed. Psychol. **18**:486.

MALLER, J. B. 1933. Vital indices and their relationship to psychological and social factors. Hum. Biol. **5**:94.

McCALL, R. B. Intelligence quotient pattern over age: Comparisons among siblings and parent-child pairs. Science (in Press).

PENROSE, L. S. 1963. The biology of mental defect. Grune and Stratton, New York.

REED, E. W., and S. C. REED. 1965. Mental retardation: A family study. W. B. Saunders, Philadelphia.

ROBERTS, J. W. F. 1961. Multifactorial inheritance in relation to human traits. Brit. Med. Bull. **17**:241.

SCOTTISH COUNCIL FOR RESEARCH IN EDUCATION. 1949. The trend of Scottish intelligence. Univ. London Press, London.

SHORT, T. 1750. New Observations, natural, moral, civil, political and medical. On City, Town and Country Bills of Mortality. London.

SMITH, S. 1942. Language and non-verbal test performance of racial groups in Honolulu before and after a fourteen year interval. J. Genet. Psychol. **36**:51.

SPUHLER, J. N. 1962. Empirical studies on quantitative human genetics. *In* Proceedings of the seminar on the use of vital and health statistics for genetic and radiation studies. United Nations, New York.

TUDDENHAM, R. D. 1948. Soldier intelligence in World Wars. I and II. Amer. Psychol. **3**:54.

WALLER, J. H. 1971. Differential reproduction: Its relation to I.Q. test score, education and occupation. Soc. Biol. **18**:122.

WRIGHT, S. 1921. Systems of mating III. Assortative mating based on somatic resemblance. Genetics **6**:144.

From W. D. Crano, D. A. Kenny and D. T. Campbell, J. Educ. Psychol., *63*, 258–275. *Copyright* (1972), *by kind permission of the authors and the American Psychological Association*

DOES INTELLIGENCE CAUSE ACHIEVEMENT?:

A CROSS-LAGGED PANEL ANALYSIS[1]

WILLIAM D. CRANO[2]

Michigan State University

DAVID A. KENNY AND DONALD T. CAMPBELL

Northwestern University

The literature of cognitive development has produced two opposing models of mental growth. One holds that the acquisition of concrete mental skills causes the later development of higher order organizational schema or rules. The contrasting model postulates a progression in which the initial acquisition of larger schema results in the increased capacity to acquire new concrete skills. While both probably operate to some extent, an attempt was made in this research to determine the *preponderant* developmental sequence. The scores of 5,495 students who had taken intelligence and achievement tests in both fourth and sixth grades were analyzed through the use of the cross-lagged panel correlation technique. For students of suburban schools ($N = 3,994$), the abstract-to-concrete causal sequence predominated, while among inner-city school children, the opposite held. The specific causal relationships between skills assessed on the various subscales of the tests employed, the value of the cross-lagged panel correlation technique in causal analysis, and an extensive methodological examination and qualification of this analytic model are presented.

The original impetus for the development of intelligence tests was provided by the call for a diagnostic tool with which to discriminate between normal and retarded children. Research was therefore focused upon the problems of measurement, not theory building. In one of their early statements, for example, Binet and Simon (1905) specifically avoided any speculation concerning the possible relationships between social or physiological variables and intelligence. Their task, as they envisioned it, was one of measurement, not speculation.

Even in Binet's time, however, scientists were not content to address themselves solely to the still-to-be-resolved problems of intelligence measurement. Considered of greater importance were questions about the relationship between intelligence and achievement, and whether one of these factors was in some way responsible for the generation or development of the other. To many of the early psychologists, two possibilities were immediately apparent: first, that intellectual advancement was a function of an organism's progression from the acquisition of concrete specific skills to the generation of higher order abstract rules (which we shall define as intelligence), contrasted with the view that the ability for abstract thought was a constant quality whose development was facilitated through the organism's interaction with the environment. If we might use the terms intelligence and achievement loosely, the problem could be restated in the following way: Does the acquisition of specific skills or the learning of specific information (achievement) result in an increased ability for abstraction (intelligence), or is the

[1] This research was supported by National Science Foundation Grant GS–1309X. We wish to express our gratitude to Joel Aronoff, Hiram Fitzgerald, and Nancy Hammond for their assistance at various phases of this investigation.
[2] Requests for reprints should be sent to William D. Crano, Department of Psychology, Olds Hall, Michigan State University, East Lansing, Michigan 48823.

progression more accurately described as one in which intelligence causes achievement, that is, does the greater ability to form abstractions result in a greater amount of concrete information being absorbed and retained?

It would be a mistake to view these possibilities as being mutually exclusive. Quite possibly, the causal sequence might operate in both directions, with the acquisition of concrete specific skills causing the development of higher order abstract rules which in turn give rise to yet additional concrete acquisitions. While this reciprocal dependence might well operate, one sequence may predominate. The primary focus of this report is the investigation of the preponderant causal sequence.

The question of preponderance is not at all novel. As Thorndike (1903) observed,

A human being is ... the sum of an original nature acted on by antenatal influences and the later environment. The first problem of educational science concerns the *relative shares* of these agencies in determining human thought and conduct [p. 40].

Although scientists have confronted the question of preponderance or "relative shares" since Thorndike's time, they have lacked the necessary analytic tools to resolve it. Despite this fact, the social and political importance of this question has forced many scientists into premature speculation concerning its probable solution. Thus Galton (1892), responding within the historic and social confines of 19th century England, would state long before the development of even marginally reliable intelligence tests,

I have no patience with the hypothesis occasionally expressed, and often implied, especially in tales written to teach children to be good, that babies are born pretty much alike, and that the sole agencies in creating differences between boy and boy, and man and man, are steady application and moral effort. It is in the most unqualified manner that I object to pretensions of natural equality.... I acknowledge freely the great power of educational and social influences in developing active powers of the mind, just as I acknowledge the effect of use in developing the muscles of a blacksmith's arm, and no further [p. 12].

Galton saw clearly the importance of environmental influences in the development of potential; inherited mental "powers," however, were seen to be the preponderant causal component in the intelligence-achievement sequence. This view, influenced undoubtedly by Galton's cousin, Charles Darwin, has been forcefully defended in today's psychology by Cyril Burt (1944, 1949), among others.

As partial proof of the importance of genetic inheritance in the determination of intelligence differences, scientists of this persuasion point to the impressive volume of studies demonstrating that animals of greater problem-solving acuity, greater speed, greater longevity, etc., can be obtained through a carefully controlled breeding process.

Even more pertinent are the results of numerous studies of twins reared separately. If the concrete-to-abstract causal sequence predominated, then the intelligence or achievement test scores of twins assigned at random to different learning environments would not be expected to correlate beyond chance levels. Erlenmeyer-Kimling and Jarvik's (1963) review of the last 50 years of twin studies, however, demonstrates that this expectation is clearly in opposition to the obtained results. The relationship between the intelligence test scores of twins reared apart has been consistently greater than that of test scores of siblings reared apart, and clearly stronger than that obtained between scores of nonrelated persons.[3]

Other scientists, of course, find it more worthwhile to emphasize the importance of environmental influences over genetic factors. Piaget (1950, 1952), for example, recognized the fundamental importance of inborn processes ("elementary sensorimotor mechanisms," or "reflexes"), but relegated to them a relatively minor role in the determination of intelligence and achievement in the normal child. These reflexes (sucking, grasping, orientation to light, arm waving to strong stimulation, etc.), ubiquitous in all but the most severely physically retarded child,

[3] The interpretation of these findings must be tempered in light of the fact that the twins studied in the investigations reviewed by Erlenmeyer-Kimling and Jarvik (1963) were not typically assigned *at random* to different learning environments, and thus, similar environmental influences might be at least partially responsible for similarities of test scores.

could hardly be made to explain the wide range of individual differences in evidence even among "normal" persons. Piaget conceptualized intelligence, or the ability to deal in abstractions, as a dynamic developmental phenomenon, rather than a fixed genetically inherited quality. Further gains in intelligence could be effected by the acquisition of specific skills, information, and rules which, with other concrete skills, information, and rules, combined in the formation of higher order, abstract, generalized principles (i.e., intelligence). Piaget conceptualized a causal sequence in which the acquisition of specific skills (achievement) combined with other specific skills in generating more abstract cognitive rules (intelligence).[4]

Between the extremes of the genetic and environmentalist positions all shades of opinion are represented. The continuing controversy within this area serves to indicate that the fundamental question of preponderance of influence in the determination of intelligence and achievement differences has yet to be resolved satisfactorily. A consideration of current educational practices, however, would seem to belie this proposition. Each year throughout the United States, for example, hundreds of thousands of dollars are spent on the standardized tests used in elementary schools. In these testing programs, there is a heavy investment not only in intelligence tests, but also in achievement tests, which purportedly mark the progress of the student and the accomplishments of the educational process. The use of intelligence tests is based on the assumption that such instruments tap a dimension distinct from the one measured in the achievement test—that intelligence is a prerequisite for achievement. Intelligence tests are expected to measure better than past achievement a student's potentialities for future achievement. If statements of a causal nature were to be made, intelligence

would be seen as one of the causes (although possibly only one of many) of subsequent achievement. Clearly the reverse is not usually held among educational test specialists. Rarely would one find advocated the thesis that present achievement is one of the causes of later intelligence scores. But if the usual assumptions are wrong—if so-called intelligence tests are just another (more generalized) form of achievement test—then important revisions in research policy would necessarily follow. Surely it is conceivable, given the continuing controversy surrounding the preponderance of causation issue, that the usual assumptions could indeed be wrong, but how is one to investigate the validity of these assumptions?

As discussed above, the probable cause of controversy regarding the preponderance of causation was not the ill will or small-mindedness of our scientific predecessors, but rather a lack of proper methodological tools with which to confront this issue. The principal drawback is that the question of preponderance is basically a correlational one. Assuming that achievement and intelligence could be independently measured, the ideal study would examine the relationship between these two factors and the changes in their relationship over time. The word *relationship* here should be emphasized, as it clearly points up the correlational nature of this "ideal" investigation. Certainly, other, more powerful statistical techniques have been employed in research of this type, but often with less than adequate justification (e.g., Hunt, 1961, has discussed the misuse of analysis of variance techniques in this field). For many years however, it has been the rule that, "correlation does not imply causation." This old saw, bothersome though it has been, was nevertheless valid.

With the recent development of the cross-lagged panel correlational technique, however, inferring causal relationships on the basis of correlational results has become possible. (For a description of this technique, more extensive and technical than that to be presented in this report, see Campbell, 1963; Campbell & Stanley, 1963; Pelz & Andrews, 1964; Rozelle & Campbell, 1969.) This method is based upon one of science's

---

[4] Other positions consistent with the concrete-to-abstract causal sequence were developed by Ferguson (1954, 1956) and Hunt (1961), among others. Support for even the most radical environmentalist hypothesis could be drawn from the work of Scott (1964), who demonstrated the dramatic effects of early sensory deprivation upon the later development of a wide range of organisms.

DOES INTELLIGENCE CAUSE ACHIEVEMENT

most useful rules of causal inference, that of time precedence: In every science, when a given event consistently precedes the occurrence of another, and the reverse does not hold, one of only two possibilities is entertained: (*a*) Event 1 is presumed to be a cause (possibly only one of many) of Event 2; or (*b*) both Event 1 and Event 2 are the effects of some more general cause(s).

It is the aim of all experimental design to negate the possibility of the second alternative. By controlling the application of the independent variable, the experimenter is assured that its occurrence was not dependent upon some more general prior event, and, thus, any differences occurring between experimental and control subjects can be attributed to the presence or absence of the independent variable. In this way, the second alternative (i.e., that Events 1 and 2 are both effects of some more general cause) is rendered implausible (see Crano & Brewer, in press).

But how does the concept of time precedence impinge in correlational investigations? Clearly, correlational techniques can be employed to study the strength of a relationship between variables, but no reliable causal estimate can be made from a single coefficient of correlation taken independently. Suppose, however, that one had available correlational information relating two variables at *more than one point in time*. For the sake of later exposition, let us assume that the two variables of interest were individuals' scores on achievement and intelligence tests, administered (approximately) simultaneously, at least twice (say, 2 years apart, in Grades 4 and 6), and that every possible relationship between these scores had been calculated. The resulting matrix of correlations could be presented in the manner employed in Figure 1.

On the basis of much prior experimentation, we would expect the unlagged, synchronous correlations (i.e., $r_{I_4 A_4}$, $r_{I_6 A_6}$) and the lagged autocorrelations (i.e., the test-retest correlations $r_{I_4 I_6}$, $r_{A_4 A_6}$) to be quite large, if the tests employed were reliable. From the perspective of causal inference, however, the correlations crossed and lagged over time (i.e., $r_{I_4 A_6}$, $r_{A_4 I_6}$) provide information of critical importance.

Let us consider the three possibilities arising from a comparison of $r_{I_4 A_6}$ with $r_{A_4 I_6}$. If high intelligence test scores in Grade 4 are consistently followed by high achievement test scores in Grade 6, but the converse is not true (i.e., that high A_4 scores are not consistently followed by high I_6 scores), then we would expect $r_{I_4 A_6}$ to be greater than $r_{A_4 I_6}$. If, on the other hand, achievement was the precursor of intelligence, then the pattern of correlational differences would be reversed (i.e., $r_{A_4 I_6} > r_{I_4 A_6}$). As was stated above, the presence or change in a variable (e.g., an intelligence test score) *consistently followed* by a change in status (either a gain or loss) of another variable (e.g., an achievement test score) satisfies the time-precedence notion of causality. Thus, if $r_{I_4 A_6} > r_{A_4 I_6}$ (and if all other factors were constant) we could assume that the causal vectors were in the direction of intelligence causing later achievement. This would of course not rule out some type of reciprocal causation operating as a feedback loop, with, for example, gains in intelligence causing later gains in achievement scores which in turn trigger later gains in intelligence, etc., but would rather demonstrate that the preponderance of causation was in the direction of intelligence causing later achievement. Such a finding would be an exciting confirmation of long-held but untested beliefs of the causal efficacy of intelligence in partially determining achievement.

It is possible, of course, that no causal relationship exists between intelligence and achievement, or that both of these qualities are the *effect* of some more general causal influence. In either case, no differences between the cross-lagged values would be expected (i.e., $r_{I_4 A_6} = r_{A_4 I_6}$). Such a result would provide little justification for the

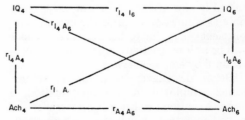

Fig. 1. Output presentation mode—schematic representation.

separate status of intelligence tests, in that it would not support the assumption that intelligence is a predictor of later achievement in a way in which achievement itself is not.

A final outcome, that the cross-lagged difference was opposite that usually predicted, that is, achievement better predicts later intelligence, and thus the classical notions of causality would be more correct if reversed, is also a possibility. This result (i.e., $r_{A_4I_6} > r_{I_4A_6}$) would also be exciting, and one perhaps anticipated by psychological learning theory and recent formulations of intelligence as presented by Bruner (1966), among others.

As discussed above, intelligence may be epitomized as an adaptive flexibility in responding to novel problems presented by the environment (and sampled in intelligence tests), while achievement is more directly related to the mastery of adaptive skills in dealing with familiar tasks (such as school subjects). Many studies have shown that habits and skills learned in specific settings generalize to more novel stimuli and settings. When any novel task is presented, the repertory of available skills, hunches, and insights is greater if the pool of specific past achievements is large and diverse. If we conceive of such learning processes as continuing throughout the school years, then it follows that this year's specific learning achievements will generalize into next year's increased ability to solve novel problems, that is, into next year's "intelligence." Intelligence would thus be viewed as a very general distillate of past achievements.

Regardless of one's theoretical stance, the cross-lagged panel correlation technique provides a realistic choice among the three alternative causal possibilities noted above. Actions taken on the basis of the results obtained in this investigation will vary, probably as a function of prior theoretical commitments, but unlike before, these actions will be at least partially grounded in or constrained by empirical evidence.

Before describing the tests and subject sample employed in this investigation, a word of caution regarding the generalization of this analytic technique to other questions of a causal nature is in order, since the appar-

ent simplicity of this method can be deceiving. As Rozelle and Campbell (1969) noted, the cross-lagged panel correlation does not always enable an unambiguous decision between two competing causal hypotheses, because, in fact, four competing hypotheses exist in situations of this type. Suppose, returning to the previous example, that $r_{I_4A_6} > r_{A_4I_6}$. Would this result necessarily imply that the preponderance of causal effects was in the direction of intelligence causing future achievement? It would not, unless some needed qualifications were first postulated.

Of the four simple cross-causal relations that are possible between intelligence and achievement, we have assumed that two are so implausible that they can be disregarded. Specifically, we reject the two possible negative relationships: high achievement causes later intelligence losses (low achievement causes later intelligence), and high intelligence causes a subsequent decline in achievement (low intelligence causes high subsequent achievement).

In the present investigation, the possibilities involving a negative relationship between intelligence and achievement are extremely implausible, and for the moment will be deleted from the list of probable competing hypothesis. There is much empirical evidence supportive of this action. The results of numerous investigations, for example, have demonstrated that rarely, if ever, will achievement and intelligence scores be negatively correlated. Thus, we will oppose two of the four potential hypotheses, without any undue concern regarding the plausibility of the remaining two (The viability of this assumption will be examined in a later section of this paper).

In many other investigative situations amenable to cross-lagged panel analysis, the degree of existing knowledge regarding the general relationship between the two variables of interest is so restricted that none of the four competing hypotheses can arbitrarily be discarded. In Rozelle and Campbell's (1969) study of the causal relationship of grades and class attendance, for example, three of the four possible competing hypotheses were viewed as plausible, and two were "confirmed" in the judgment of the investigators. In situations of this type (and the present study is not one of them) the cross-lagged panel technique must be employed with extreme caution (see Kenny, 1970; Rickard, in press; Sandell, 1971).

Assuming that the general relationship between intelligence and achievement is both positive and substantial, we may then proceed to a discussion of the tests and samples employed in the present investigation.

METHOD

Sample

The data on which the analyses were based were provided by the Board of Education of the Milwaukee Public Schools. In Grades 4, 6, and 8, both intelligence and achievement tests are administered to all public school children. Within any given test year, the two tests are administered with a minimum of time lag between them. In the present investigation, relations between intelligence and achievement test scores of children attending fourth grade in the academic year 1963–64, and sixth grade 2 years later, were investigated. A total of 5,495 complete sets of data were collected. That is, 5,495 children who had (in 1963–64) completed both intelligence and achievement tests in their fourth year of elementary school and also, 2 years later, completed (parallel forms of) these tests in the sixth grade, comprised the subject sample.

Tests

Level three of the Lorge-Thorndike intelligence test (1957 version) was administered to the sample. All children in Grade 4 received the same form of the intelligence test. In the sixth grade, an alternate form of the Level 3 test was employed. In the construction of this instrument, the authors attempted to generate tests aimed at the assessment of behavioral characteristics "which they would describe as intelligent [Lorge & Thorndike, 1957, p. 12]." The tasks purportedly dealt with the ability to employ abstractions and general concepts, entailed the interpretation, use, and recognition of the relationships among symbols, required flexibility and the ability to employ novel patterns of concepts, and, finally, focused upon power rather than speed (see Lorge & Thorndike, 1957, pp. 12-13).

This instrument consists of both verbal and nonverbal batteries. Within the verbal battery were tasks that involved completion, verbal classification, arithmetic reasoning, and vocabulary. This test consisted of 90 items for which 34 minutes were alloted. The nonverbal battery (79 items, 27 minutes' administration time) was entirely pictorial or numeric, and consisted of tests involving pictoral classification and analogy, as well as numeric relationships.

The Iowa Tests of Basic Skills constituted the achievement test battery administered to the sample. Alternate forms of this test were employed in the fourth and sixth grade test administrations. These tests "provide for the measurement...of certain *skills* involved in reading, work-study, language, and arithmetic [Manual, Iowa Tests of Basic Skills, 1956]." This device consists of the following subscales:

Vocabulary. The 38 items (46 for the sixth grade test) of this subtest consist of a stimulus word in context which the respondent is to match with one of four definitions provided. A total of 17 minutes is alloted for this test.

Reading Comprehension. In this test, respondents are provided a selection to read, varying in length from a few sentences to an entire page. The function of this test is to determine the ability of the student to apprehend the meaning of the communication, to draw appropriate inferences, to grasp the significance of the information provided, etc. The fourth grade test consists of 68 items, the sixth grade, 76. Administration time for both is 55 minutes.

Language. This test consists of four separate subscales, concerned with spelling, punctuation, capitalization, and usage. The format of all items employed in these scales is similar. Respondents are presented with a series of stimuli, one of which might be in error. The task of the subject is to identify this error. In the Spelling subscale (38–46 items, 12 minutes' administration time), for example, four words are presented, and one of these may be misspelled.[5] In both the Capitalization and Punctuation subscales, one or two sentences extending over three lines of equal length are presented. The respondent is to identify the line on which a capitalization or punctuation error occurs. Both the capitalization and the punctuation test consist of 39 (42) items; the former is administered in 15 minutes, while the latter is allocated 20. Language Usage items consist of 3 sentences, one of which could contain a usage error. Tested on this subscale was the use of the pronouns, verbs, adjectives, and adverbs. In addition, the avoidance of double negatives and redundancies, commonly misused homonyms and miscellaneous word forms was investigated. In both grades sampled, this test consists of 32 items, with a 20-minute time allowance.

Work-Study Skills. This test is composed of three subscales. The skills assessed in these tests "are those which have been traditionally classified as 'work-study' skills and which are of crucial importance to self-education in out-of-school and postschool activities [Manual, 1956, p. 64]." The first of these instruments is concerned with Map Reading. Within this test, a number of different types of maps are presented to the student, and questions concerning distances, directions, locations and map legends are provided. The test consists of

---

[5] The first value refers to the number of items in the fourth-grade test; the second, to the number of items in the sixth-grade test.

W. D. CRANO, D. A. KENNY, AND D. T. CAMPBELL

27 (40) multiple-choice questions, with a time limit of 30 minutes. The second component of the work-study skills test is concerned with Graph and Table Reading. In this section of the test, at least five different types of illustrative figures are employed (e.g., pictographs, line graphs, circle graphs, various tabular materials, etc.). Respondents must interpret the illustrations and sometimes perform arithmetic operations in generating the appropriate response. This test is composed of 24 (28) items, and is administered in 20 minutes. The final component of the work-study test investigates the student's Knowledge and Use of Reference Materials. Test items deal with the proper use of "the parts of a book, the globe, current magazines, the dictionary, the encyclopedia, and an atlas [Manual, 1956, p. 67]." A total of 52 (59) items are employed in this test, with 30-minutes' administration time allotted.

Arithmetic. The final section of the Iowa Tests was concerned with the assessment of arithmetic skills. This test is composed of two subscales. The first deals with the student's grasp of Arithmetic Concepts. The logic of arithmetic computation is examined in this subtest. Mastery of concepts involving the number system, whole numbers, decimals, fractions, ratios and percentages, standard measures, and geometric figures is examined in this test of 36 (45) items, for which 30 minutes is allotted. In the Arithmetic Problem Solving subscale of the Arithmetic Skills test, actual computational expertise is assessed. All the items in this test are of the word-problem variety. None involve mere calculation, but demand that the student read the item and respond to the relevant aspects under investigation. This test is composed of 27 (31) items, and can be administered in 30 minutes.

In total, the Iowa Test of Basic Skills consists of 425 (487) items administered in 4 hours and 39 minutes of working time. The Lorge-Thorndike intelligence test is composed of a total of 164 items, and can be administered in 61 minutes.

TAB

MEANS, STANDARD DEVIATIONS, AND MATRIX OF INTERCORRELA

	1	2	3	4	5	6	7	8	9	10	11	12	13	14
1. Vocabulary (4)a	1.0													
2. Read Comp (4)	743	1.0												
3. Spelling (4)	593	584	1.0											
4. Capitalization (4)	602	628	635	1.0										
5. Punctuation (4)	500	549	544	651	1.0									
6. Usage (4)	697	678	573	611	557	1.0								
7. Map Reading (4)	560	577	437	497	434	513	1.0							
8. Graphs (4)	613	642	483	565	511	575	616	1.0						
9. References (4)	591	630	548	597	518	567	563	605	1.0					
10. Ar. Concept (4)	614	624	514	576	525	579	588	651	590	1.0				
11. Ar. Problem (4)	534	572	499	556	502	528	487	585	577	654	1.0			
12. Composite Ach (4)	822	858	689	740	659	769	696	763	754	787	736	1.0		
13. Verbal IQ (4)	767	735	663	646	548	698	593	650	640	664	585	807	1.0	
14. Nonverbal IQ (4)	527	552	452	528	471	504	510	562	499	572	492	626	673	1.0
15. Composite IQ (4)	703	702	606	641	556	654	603	663	621	676	589	782	901	920
16. Vocabulary (6)	752	706	503	538	469	675	546	591	542	572	486	740	718	521
17. Read Comp (6)	713	723	504	553	487	450	561	624	559	602	527	745	716	556
18. Spelling (6)	596	577	733	575	511	581	428	472	537	497	476	653	672	428
19. Capitalization (6)	590	592	569	645	574	603	474	537	537	553	501	677	639	524
20. Punctuation (6)	561	563	550	576	562	590	448	501	509	534	496	644	620	499
21. Usage (6)	656	631	535	555	495	707	458	535	513	525	485	683	675	502
22. Map Reading (6)	523	529	373	461	411	453	511	528	461	527	447	586	559	501
23. Graphs (6)	497	505	367	450	381	449	460	530	445	501	432	563	529	469
24. References (6)	649	664	549	636	558	622	544	629	609	626	584	744	712	599
25. Ar. Concept (6)	570	561	454	522	469	519	508	575	498	604	535	650	623	550
26. Ar. Problem (6)	507	523	434	513	457	473	439	529	488	550	534	600	568	478
27. Composite Ach (6)	737	733	585	636	570	700	587	658	616	653	586	799	766	603
28. Verbal IQ (6)	708	680	582	593	509	666	560	611	572	626	550	749	816	634
29. Nonverbal IQ (6)	525	534	438	520	458	504	498	548	481	562	493	611	649	726
30. Composite IQ (6)	659	649	546	595	516	627	566	618	563	634	558	727	784	730
M	4.17	3.96	4.33	4.18	4.11	3.95	4.05	3.81	4.26	4.04	4.08	4.06	99.2	98.1
σ	.900	.979	1.10	.896	.973	1.15	.897	.884	.874	.860	.696	.774	14.5	15.7

a Decimal points for all correlations less than 1.0 have been omitted. The parenthesized figure following the title of each test refers

DOES INTELLIGENCE CAUSE ACHIEVEMENT

RESULTS

The matrix of correlations among the various subscales employed in this investigation with means and standard deviations for each subscale, over both measurement sessions, is presented in Table 1. Normed grade equivalents, based upon the number of correct items answered per scale, are the basic unit of data of the Iowa achievement tests. In the Lorge-Thorndike test, raw item scores were adjusted by the respondent's age in forming the IQ scores used in this analysis. In addition to these values, composite scores for both the intelligence and the achievement tests consisting of a simple average of their respective subscale scores were derived, and are also presented in Table 1.

With this information, an estimate of the viability of one of the assumptions necessitated by the use of the cross-lagged panel technique can be made. As was noted earlier, this approach, in and of itself, does not enable the investigator to choose between one of two hypotheses, but rather between pairs of logical possibilities. In the present investigation, however, one hypothesis of each of these competing pairs (i.e., the negative relationships) was discarded as extremely implausible. Information consistent with this assumption is presented in Table 1. The direction of correlations between fourth and sixth grade tests, for example, is uni-

LE 1
TIONS FOR ALL SUBTEST AND COMPOSITE SCORES, TOTAL SAMPLE

15	16	17	18	19	20	21	22	23	24	25	26	27	28	29	30
1.0															
674	1.0														
693	819	1.0													
597	591	588	1.0												
634	614	637	660	1.0											
610	580	604	625	722	1.0										
640	695	681	622	655	671	1.0									
579	578	626	434	514	477	485	1.0								
546	543	585	418	492	462	472	580	1.0							
717	679	735	650	706	683	673	635	620	1.0						
641	610	644	521	596	582	575	610	585	709	1.0					
571	537	589	498	564	529	527	555	551	674	673	1.0				
747	858	865	699	757	731	773	707	682	833	775	723	1.0			
796	738	750	648	647	631	695	572	546	732	642	577	790	1.0		
755	551	589	464	557	562	542	529	501	648	599	517	650	731	1.0	
828	691	716	597	644	638	663	588	559	738	663	584	770	932	923	1.0
98.9	5.91	6.08	6.21	6.57	6.26	6.00	5.98	6.12	6.36	5.97	5.95	6.06	99.6	99.8	99.7
13.8	1.38	1.18	1.29	1.62	1.82	1.87	1.26	1.16	1.14	.809	.926	1.09	15.4	14.5	14.0

to the administration year of the particular test. More complete titles and descriptions for each subscale are provided in the text.

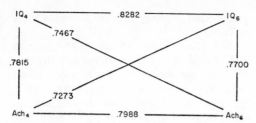

FIG. 2. Cross-lagged panel results of the inter-relations of intelligence and achievement test composite scores.

formly positive. In fact, not a single negative relationship appeared in the entire matrix of correlations.

Additional confirmatory information can be obtained by considering the composite score relationship of the synchronous un-lagged IQ and achievement tests. The correlation between these contiguously administered tests is positive and significant at both measurement periods

$$(r_{I_4A_4} = .7815, r_{I_6A_6} = .7700; p < .001,$$

$$df = 5493 \text{ for both correlations}).[6]$$

Both of these findings serve to render implausible the rival hypothesis that a negative relationship exists between intelligence and achievement as measured on the tests employed in this investigation. We are thus in a position to investigate the remaining possibilities, namely, that the causal relationship is predominately in the direction of intelligence affecting later achievement, or, of achievement influencing later intelligence.

A number of analytic options is available in this study, but none is completely desirable. One of the most obvious of these consists of a comparison of the crossed and lagged composite score correlations $(r_{I_4A_6}, r_{A_4I_6})$. Again, we must emphasize the probable reciprocal causal dependence between these two dimensions. It seems highly probable that both of the possible causal relationships operate to some extent, in a type of feedback system. The test between the cross-lagged coefficients simply

enables some estimate concerning the preponderant cause-effect relationship to be made. The pattern of relationships necessary for this comparison is presented in Figure 2. The cross-lagged correlations are both positive and substantial, and suggest a feedback system in which both operations affect one another to a great extent. A comparison of the cross-lagged correlations indicates, however, that the predominant causal sequence is that of intelligence causing later achievement. A test of this inequality revealed that the obtained difference between $r_{I_4A_6}$ and $r_{A_4I_6}$ was statistically significant ($t = 2.941$, $df = 5492$, $p < .01$, two-tailed).[7] For the total group of respondents, then, the preponderant causal sequence is apparently in the direction of intelligence directly predicting later achievement to an extent significantly exceeding that to which achievement causes later intelligence.

The same causal sequence may not, of course, operate in all groups. Of extreme importance today, for example, is the question of whether the pattern of causal relationships obtained from data on students in inner-city schools would be similar to that obtained from a suburban sample. To consider this question, schools were divided into core and suburban samples. A core school was one that was eligible for comprehensive programs of aid under Title 1 of the Elementary and Secondary Education Act, for the 1967–68 school year. Upon recalculating the matrix of correlations for both core and suburban samples, it was found that among suburban students, the intelligence-causes-achievement sequence based on a consideration of composite scores clearly predominated ($r_{I_4A_6} = .7329$, $r_{A_4I_6} = .7049$, $t = 3.479$, $df = 3991$, $p < .001$, two-tailed). Within the core sample, the direction of differences between the cross-lagged correlations was opposite to that of the suburban group ($r_{I_4A_6} = .6086$, $r_{A_4I_6} = .6180$, $t = -.521$, $df = 1498$, $p > .05$). Although this finding was not

[6] The relationship between the intelligence and achievement tests employed in the present investigation appears to be consistent over time. A test of significance between these two correlations disclosed that the null hypothesis that $r_{I_4A_4} = r_{I_6A_6}$ could not be rejected ($z = 1.52$, $p > .05$).

[7] This test was based upon a correction of the usual t test between correlations, suggested by Pearson and Filon (1898), which takes into account the indirect correlation between the arrays under comparison, which are modified by the four other relevant values (see also Peters and VanVoorhis, 1940, p. 185).

statistically significant, the directional differences between the core and suburban samples might be used to stimulate a good deal of theoretical speculation regarding the nature of the predominant causal sequence in relatively advantaged and relatively deprived groups.

Before undertaking an action of this type, however, one should be aware of the limitations which the use of composite scores imposes. The Iowa tests composite, for example, consists of the average score of 11 widely varying subscales. It seems unlikely that such a heterogeneous combination could prove meaningful. Two students sharing the same composite score, for example, might well have completely different patterns of correct and incorrect responses. Similarly, in the Lorge-Thorndike intelligence test composite, verbal and nonverbal skills are combined to give the overall average. The meaningfulness of such an average is certainly open to question. Thus, any speculation based upon the composite score data presented above must be tempered by extreme caution.

One solution to the composite-score problem is an investigation of the relationships among individual subscales of the tests employed. In both the Iowa tests and the Lorge-Thorndike, the internal reliability coefficients of individual subscales are quite large. We might assume, therefore, that all items within any given subscale focus upon the same ability. In addition to providing a solution to the problems generated by the use of composite scores, such an approach enables a more precise investigation of the various relationships that exist among the various skills or abilities tapped by the components of the two tests which were employed.

To investigate the relationships among the individual subtests for the entire subject sample, a total of 78 t tests between all possible pairs of cross-lagged correlation coefficients is necessitated. In calculating 78 nonindependent t tests, however, the choice of an appropriate alpha level is a definite problem. Several solutions are available (e.g., one might correct for multiple nonindependent comparisons through a modified Newman-Keuls approach) but the most conservative appears to be that suggested by

Campbell, Miller, Lubetsky, and O'Connell (1964). To generate an appropriate comparison using this approach one must determine a value that would occur only once in 100×78 times, given a true difference of zero. To determine this quantity, one would derive the z value corresponding to a probability of $1/(100 \times 13 \times 12/2)$, or $p = .00012820$. For such a probability, a corresponding z value of 3.6559 is required. Similarly, the necessary value for $p = .05$ would be based upon a calculation of $1/(20 \times 13 \times 12/2)$, or $p = .00064102$, $z = 3.2202$. With these corrected values, we can begin to investigate the pattern of causal relationships within the total sample of subjects, and within the two subgroups, the core and suburban samples.

Before examining the differences between all possible pairs of cross-lagged correlation coefficients, however, a final comment on this technique is in order. One of the major assumptions of the cross-lagged panel technique is that of "stationarity" (Rozelle & Campbell, 1969), that is, that the common factor structure of the tests employed at both points in time remains constant. A necessary consequence of such an assumption is that the synchronous correlations are equal at both points in time (e.g., $r_{I_4A_4} = r_{I_6A_6}$). An examination of Table 1, however, reveals that the synchronous correlations change more than would be expected by sampling error alone, and we must therefore conclude that the common factor structure changes over time.

Two different sources of change can be made to account for the synchronous correlation differences, changes in kind, and changes in amount. With changes in kind, the loading of a test on one common factor changes while the test's loading on another common factor remains the same or changes in the opposite direction. A good example of changes of kind is provided in infant intelligence tests. These tests tend to measure motor skills more than mental ability, while for older children, the opposite holds. Suppose that intelligence (I) and some motor skill (M) were measured at ages 1 and 5 for the same subject sample. If $r_{I_1M_5}$ was greater than $r_{I_5M_1}$, we could not conclude that intelligence causes motor skill, but rather that the two measures of motor skills

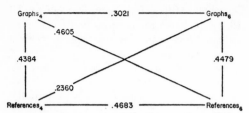

FIG. 3. Uncorrected cross-lagged correlations between Graphs and Tables and References subscales for core school respondents.

correlate more highly than a measure of motor skill with mental ability.

With changes in amount, all the loadings of a test change by a multiplicative constant. In a sense, the common factor structure of the tests does not change, but there are changes in the amount of communality and, therefore, uniqueness. Consider, for example, the pattern of intercorrelations presented in Figure 3.[8] On the basis of the cross-lagged correlations alone, it seems obvious that the ability to read graphs and tables predicts the ability to use references. These same results could have occurred, however, if (a) the reliability of the References test decreased from Grade 4 to 6, while that of the other test increased, or, (b) the specific variance of the References test increased over time, and decreased for the test of graph and table interpretation.

To test the viability of these alternatives, we could inspect the synchronous correlations of each of these two variables with all the other variables employed in this investigation at both measurement periods. Such an analysis bolsters the plausibility of the alternatives noted above, since, in every case *except* that under consideration, the synchronous correlations involving the References test declined from grade four to six, while those of the Graphs and Tables test increased. Given this systematic shift in synchronous correlations, we felt it plausible to assume that the bulk of the changes in factor structure were changes of amount, not kind.

Clearly, some means of correcting for differential reliability or specificity deviations that might occur between measurement periods is necessary if the full value of the cross-lagged panel technique is to be

[8] These data were taken from the core sample.

realized. The simplest solution available consists of a correction for attenuation of the cross-lagged values. Although this solution has the advantage of simplicity, it corrects only for reliability changes and cannot be used to control for any changes in the specificity of tests that might occur over time.

A more satisfying solution would involve a factor analytic approach. Within the fourth- and the sixth-grade measurement sessions, a separate factor analysis of the matrix of test correlations could be computed. If the assumption of "changes of amount only" is valid, then the cross-lagged correlations would be equal if corrected by the ratio of appropriate communalities, as presented in the following formulae:

$$r'_{x_4 y_6} = r_{x_4 y_6} \cdot \sqrt[4]{\frac{h^2_{x_4} \cdot h^2_{y_6}}{h^2_{x_6} \cdot h^2_{y_4}}},$$

and,

$$r'_{y_4 x_6} = r_{y_4 x_6} \cdot \sqrt[4]{\frac{h^2_{y_4} \cdot h^2_{x_6}}{h^2_{y_6} \cdot h^2_{x_4}}}.$$

Conceptually, this solution seems ideal; the wide dispersion of communality estimates generated by various factor analytic techniques, however, renders this approach inoperable in practice.

A more intuitive solution to the problem of the estimation of communality ratios was thus employed in the present investigation. For each variable pair, the synchronous correlation at Grade 4 ($r_{x_4 r_4}$) was divided by the synchronous correlation of these same variables at Grade 6. The resulting matrix of ratios should be single factored if the "change of amount" assumption is valid (see Kenny, 1970, for a more formal mathematical development of these arguments). Spearman's (1927) "two factor" technique was employed in the solution of this matrix

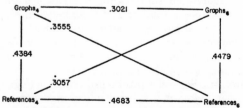

FIG. 4. Corrected cross-lagged correlations between Graphs and Tables and References subscales for core school respondents.

DOES INTELLIGENCE CAUSE ACHIEVEMENT

TABLE 2
Corrected Cross-lags and t Values: Total Group, Core, and Suburban Schools, Respectively

Comparison X	Y	$r_{X_4Y_6}$	$r_{Y_4X_6}$	t	$r_{X_4Y_6}$	$r_{Y_4X_6}$	t	$r_{X_4Y_6}$	$r_{Y_4X_6}$	t
Vocabulary with	Read Comp	.7065	.7118	−.723	.5721	.5845	−.627	.6899	.6942	−.479
Vocabulary with	Spelling	.5965	.5023	9.320	.4944	.4308	2.721	.5940	.4832	9.189
Vocabulary with	Capitalizing	.5914	.5369	5.263	.4768	.4530	.992	.5551	.4980	4.408
Vocabulary with	Punctuation	.5344	.4930	3.594	.4342	.4441	−.389	.5035	.4442	4.149
Vocabulary with	Usage	.6562	.6740	−2.099	.5193	.5791	−2.787	.6397	.6458	−.582
Vocabulary with	Map Reading	.5202	.5483	−2.456	.3519	.4099	−2.060	.4898	.5179	−2.005
Vocabulary with	Graphs	.5342	.5497	−1.385	.3496	.3996	−1.749	.5170	.5236	−.488
Vocabulary with	References	.6026	.5839	1.851	.4479	.4573	−.373	.5836	.5593	1.975
Vocabulary with	Ar. Concept	.5702	.5719	−.168	.4113	.4374	−.996	.5417	.5366	.389
Vocabulary with	Ar. Problem	.5054	.4880	1.467	.3548	.3897	−1.256	.4767	.4486	1.931
Vocabulary with	Verbal IQ	.7164	.7090	1.027	.6133	.5884	1.317	.6942	.6897	.496
Vocabulary with	Nonverbal IQ	.5134	.5317	−1.760	.4220	.4090	.530	.4557	.4844	−2.182
Read Comp with	Spelling	.5825	.4988	8.063	.4941	.4240	2.983	.5770	.4794	7.855
Read Comp with	Capitalizing	.5982	.5472	4.956	.5031	.4871	.694	.5609	.5067	4.189
Read Comp with	Punctuation	.5408	.5071	2.945	.4691	.4556	.546	.5061	.4625	3.062
Read Comp with	Usage	.6377	.6431	−.603	.5203	.5473	−1.233	.6164	.6135	.265
Read Comp with	Map Reading	.5313	.5589	−2.453	.3545	.4251	−2.539	.5076	.5310	−1.704
Read Comp with	Graphs	.5480	.5748	−2.452	.3678	.4201	−1.872	.5338	.5571	−1.784
Read Comp with	References	.6220	.5965	2.621	.4769	.4857	−.367	.6066	.5719	2.930
Read Comp with	Ar. Concept	.5656	.5965	−2.998	.4275	.4757	−1.896	.5332	.5658	−2.542
Read Comp with	Ar. Problem	.5259	.5244	.126	.3906	.4230	−1.204	.4985	.4920	.467
Read Comp with	Verbal IQ	.6942	.7006	−.846	.6028	.5871	.819	.6679	.6805	−1.312
Read Comp with	Nonverbal IQ	.5272	.5624	−3.414	.4241	.4654	−1.722	.4776	.5180	−3.083
Spelling with	Capitalizing	.5697	.5740	−.424	.4923	.4860	.281	.5567	.5719	−1.241
Spelling with	Punctuation	.5227	.5376	−1.325	.4784	.4332	1.845	.5032	.5360	−2.420
Spelling with	Usage	.5351	.5812	−4.503	.4979	.5083	−.469	.5100	.5723	−5.054
Spelling with	Map Reading	.3712	.4299	−4.445	.2351	.3113	−2.520	.3599	.4164	−3.600
Spelling with	Graphs	.3946	.4390	−3.434	.2398	.3085	−2.265	.3922	.4352	−2.836
Spelling with	References	.5364	.5789	−3.970	.4365	.4793	−1.733	.5347	.5751	−3.192
Spelling with	Ar. Concept	.4532	.4979	−3.786	.3288	.3971	−2.513	.4440	.4861	−2.979
Spelling with	Ar. Problem	.4314	.4786	−3.787	.3263	.3843	−2.092	.4201	.4660	−3.088
Spelling with	Verbal IQ	.5885	.6643	−8.646	.5756	.5902	−.780	.5614	.6627	−9.480
Spelling with	Nonverbal IQ	.4282	.4372	−.790	.4127	.3931	.823	.3814	.3963	−1.056
Capitalizing with	Punctuation	.5475	.6045	−5.539	.4951	.5388	−1.978	.5182	.5733	−4.307
Capitalizing with	Usage	.5546	.6032	−4.739	.4748	.5230	−2.112	.5242	.5658	−3.241
Capitalizing with	Map Reading	.4584	.4769	−1.457	.3118	.3309	−.644	.4318	.4444	−.818
Capitalizing with	Graphs	.4833	.5003	−1.381	.3314	.3626	−1.064	.4661	.4704	−.290
Capitalizing with	References	.5887	.5794	.899	.4784	.4523	1.059	.5733	.5561	1.369
Capitalizing with	Ar. Concept	.5211	.5548	−2.994	.4117	.4523	−1.564	.4898	.5158	−1.862
Capitalizing with	Ar. Problem	.5101	.5035	.548	.4008	.4090	−.305	.4870	.4682	1.280
Capitalizing with	Verbal IQ	.5995	.6324	−3.523	.5537	.5294	1.166	.5599	.6005	−3.411
Capitalizing with	Nonverbal IQ	.5076	.5368	−2.648	.4676	.4494	.767	.4539	.4900	−2.569
Punctuation with	Usage	.5204	.5611	−3.642	.4606	.4987	−1.593	.4835	.5293	−3.306
Punctuation with	Map Reading	.4296	.4279	.126	.3143	.3099	.143	.3951	.3970	−.112
Punctuation with	Graphs	.4309	.4432	−.929	.2900	.3075	−.576	.4066	.4214	−.930
Punctuation with	References	.544¹	.5221	1.911	.4426	.4111	1.206	.5223	.5022	1.433
Punctuation with	Ar. Concept	.4929	.5088	−1.316	.4288	.3953	1.255	.4501	.4819	−2.134
Punctuation with	Ar. Problem	.4781	.4742	.310	.3713	.3896	−.653	.4526	.4446	.519
Punctuation with	Verbal IQ	.5408	.5834	−4.005	.5029	.5011	.076	.4956	.5546	−4.419
Punctuation with	Nonverbal IQ	.4706	.4850	−1.188	.4185	.4073	.437	.4212	.4428	−1.427
Usage with	Map Reading	.4507	.4604	−.768	.2880	.3343	−1.556	.4139	.4250	−.719
Usage with	Graphs	.4827	.4975	−1.213	.3056	.3598	−1.836	.4611	.4725	−.779
Usage with	References	.5768	.5532	2.219	.4539	.4373	.657	.5519	.5297	1.706
Usage with	Ar. Concept	.5183	.5256	−.643	.4189	.3985	.770	.4735	.4923	−1.344
Usage with	Ar. Problem	.4704	.4877	−1.415	.3653	.3889	−.856	.4313	.4549	−1.572
Usage with	Verbal IQ	.6738	.6679	.714	.5976	.5721	1.321	.6453	.6433	.197

TABLE 2—Continued

Comparison		$r_{X_4Y_6}$	$r_{Y_4X_6}$	t	$r_{X_4Y_6}$	$r_{Y_4X_6}$	t	$r_{X_4Y_6}$	$r_{Y_4X_6}$	t
X	Y									
Usage with Nonverbal IQ		.4929	.5130	−1.839	.4283	.4195	.362	.4342	.4651	−2.240
Map Reading with Graphs		.4964	.4883	.666	.2677	.2993	−1.045	.4977	.4756	1.537
Map Reading with References		.5067	.4947	1.004	.3176	.3220	−.150	.4946	.4822	.861
Map Reading with Ar. Concept		.5102	.5253	−1.278	.3091	.3490	−1.360	.4983	.5026	−.305
Map Reading with Ar. Problem		.4396	.4464	−.521	.2729	.2868	−.453	.4182	.4260	−.492
Map Reading with Verbal IQ		.5696	.5501	1.786	.4246	.3467	2.808	.5449	.5331	.888
Map Reading with Nonverbal IQ		.4900	.5096	−1.634	.3586	.3147	1.500	.4531	.4863	−2.248
Graphs with References		.5430	.4154	2.403	.3555	.3057	1.704	.5378	.5153	1.667
Graphs with Ar. Concept		.5345	.5394	−.437	.3244	.3341	−.330	.5306	.5351	−.336
Graphs with Ar. Problem		.4899	.4665	1.873	.3185	.2534	2.134	.4781	.4664	.794
Graphs with Verbal IQ		.5746	.5622	1.153	.4135	.3434	2.496	.5599	.5600	−.006
Graphs with Nonverbal IQ		.4985	.5152	−1.414	.3331	.3079	.850	.4766	.5086	−2.254
References with Ar. Concept		.5367	.5809	−4.092	.3897	.4314	−1.578	.5179	.5618	−3.357
References with Ar. Problem		.5241	.5435	−1.706	.3555	.3991	−1.574	.5168	.5316	−1.093
References with Verbal IQ		.6234	.6531	−3.246	.5265	.5194	.318	.6006	.6373	−3.274
References with Nonverbal IQ		.5076	.5678	−5.437	.4284	.4465	−.717	.4660	.5355	−5.051
Ar. Concept with Ar. Problem		.5482	.5368	1.043	.4032	.3945	.335	.5290	.5185	.790
Ar. Concept with Verbal IQ		.6343	.6151	2.036	.5282	.4609	2.846	.6003	.5906	.824
Ar. Concept with Nonverbal IQ		.5504	.5617	−1.055	.4211	.4197	.055	.5117	.5266	−1.105
Ar. Problem with Verbal IQ		.5590	.5590	0.000	.4727	.4150	2.273	.5248	.5359	−.831
Ar. Problem with Nonverbal IQ		.4844	.4861	−.139	.4146	.3304	3.060	.4370	.4580	−1.404
Verbal IQ with Nonverbal IQ		.6274	.6658	−4.508	.5810	.6149	−1.848	.5697	.6152	−4.042

(see Harman, 1960), and the resulting communality estimates were employed in correcting the cross-lagged correlations for reliability and specificity changes, through the use of the correction formulae presented above.[9] Employing these communality estimates in the correction formulae generally lessens the differences between the cross-lagged values. In the illustration comparing reference versus graph and table interpretation, for example, the correction process has reduced the difference in cross-lagged correlation values from .22 to .05 (see Figure 4).

The same general approach was employed in investigating all possible subscale relations obtained over the total sample, and

[9] The procedure employed here is not a true factor analysis, because many of the ratios entered in the matrix will exceed unity. Nevertheless, it was felt that the procedures outlined by Spearman could legitimately be employed in this analysis, because we assumed that for each variable the unique factor loadings can freely change over time, while all the orthogonal common factor loadings change by some constant. That is,

$$A_t = KA_{t+k},$$

where A_t are the common factor loadings at time t, A_{t+k} are the common-factor loadings at time $t + k$, and K is a diagonal matrix of communality ratios (see Kenny, 1970).

also within the core and suburban subsamples.[10] A series of t tests was computed on the difference between all pairs of corrected cross-lagged values, and these results are summarized in Table 2.

A more graphic representation of the results obtained for the suburban sample is presented in Table 3. Again, it must be stressed that the t test differences noted in these tables are based upon the corrected cross-lagged correlation coefficients, and the significance levels employed have been corrected for multiple comparisons. Thus it seems likely that these results, if erroneous, will be conservatively biased.

DISCUSSION

In the statistical comparison of composite IQ and achievement test scores presented earlier, the predominant causal sequence over all subjects was in the direction of intelligence causing later achievement. Dividing the total sample into core and suburban subunits, however, revealed that this se-

[10] Within the bounds of sampling error, the matrix of ratios of synchronous correlations appeared to be single factored, thus supporting our assumption of "changes in amount only" in the factor structure.

DOES INTELLIGENCE CAUSE ACHIEVEMENT

TABLE 3

PATTERNS OF CAUSAL INTERRELATIONS: SUBURBAN SAMPLE

Cause variable	Effect variables												
	1	2	3	4	5	6	7	8	9	10	11	12	13
1. Vocabulary			**	**	**								
2. Reading comprehension			**	**									
3. Spelling													
4. Capitalization													
5. Punctuation				**									
6. Usage			**	*	*								
7. Map reading			*										
8. Graph and table													
9. References													
10. Arithmatic concept									*				
11. Arithmatic problems													
12. Verbal IQ			**	*	**				*				
13. Nonverbal IQ									**			**	

* $p < .05$ (i.e., $p < .00064102$, $t > 3.2202$, as discussed in text).
** $p < .01$ (i.e., $p < .00012820$, $t > 3.6559$).

quence held only within the suburban sample; if any relationship existed in the core sample, it was opposite to that of the suburban group.

Given the dangers involved in the use of composite scores, it is perhaps wise to focus upon the more specific subscale relationships before commenting upon this result. With 13 subtest scores employed in this investigation, 78 comparisons are possible. Having adjusted alpha to account for these multiple comparisons, 22 significant differences were found in an analysis involving all subjects (Table 2). (Without the alpha adjustment, 33 of 78 t values would have reached the $p < .05$ level.) Within the suburban sample, 17 comparisons were significant; among the core students, however, not even one of the 78 t values was significant.

The results of the analysis of the total group thus provide a somewhat misleading impression, since the significant causal relations obtained depend almost completely upon differences that exist within the suburban sample.[11] A further indication of the lack of comparability of the core and suburban groups can be gained through a consideration of the differences in causal directionality that exist among the various subscale

[11] This is understandable, since the suburban group constitutes 73% of the total sample.

comparisons in these two groups. In almost 40% of the 78 subscale comparisons, the signs of the obtained t values differ between core and suburban samples. The difference between the core and suburban groups in mere numbers of significant causal relationships is quite striking, as is the directional difference in the composite-score comparison; neither of these findings, however, is as compelling as the fact that causal directionality of the relationships between various concrete and abstract activities differs between these groups almost 40% of the time. On the basis of these results, it is clear that a *combination* of the data from the core and suburban subjects can be extremely misleading. These findings should thus be approached with extreme caution. For this reason, the following discussion will be focused upon results obtained for the two subgroups separately.

There are probably a number of potential approaches in explaining the causal discrepancies in the findings above, and one of the most promising is an investigation of the results obtained from the suburban sample. A plausible explanation of these findings can lead to a more complete understanding of the lack of significant causal effects within the core group.

The Iowa Tests of Basic Skills is composed of 11 subtests, the first 6 of which clearly depend upon linguistic abilities (see Table 3). While the general focus of these subtests is similar, the skills which they assess vary in degree of abstractness. On the basis of both the descriptive manual provided for the Iowa tests (1956), and an investigation of the specific items that constitute the various linguistically oriented subscales, it would seem that the tests of Vocabulary, Reading Comprehension, and Language Usage appear to represent scales that assess abilities more abstract than those tapped in the Spelling, Capitalization, and Punctuation subtests. If this evaluation is correct, then the results in Table 3 indicate that the acquisition of the more general, abstract cognitive abilities causes later gains in more specific linguistic skills. In addition to supporting this abstract-to-concrete explanation of linguistic development, data in Table 3 also demonstrate the causal ineffectiveness of the concrete skills in generating abstract abilities. Both Vocabulary and Language Usage, for example, appear to function as causal determinants of Spelling, Capitalization, and Punctuation skills; Reading Comprehension is somewhat less effective, and apparently affects only Spelling and Capitalization.

Results consistent with these findings are to be found in a consideration of the effects of the test of Verbal IQ. This subscale of the Lorge-Thorndike intelligence test is a clear attempt to assess skills considerably more abstract than those measured in the Spelling, Capitalization, and Punctuation subscales of the Iowa tests. As demonstrated in Tables 2 and 3, the more abstract abilities tapped in the Verbal IQ test serve as causal determinants of these concrete skills, just as did those assessed in the tests of Vocabulary and Reading Comprehension.

A review of the remaining scales of the Iowa Tests provides relatively little information concerning possible causal relationships among the various skills assessed through this device. Both the Work-Study and the Arithmetic subtests assess relatively abstract skills. The subscales of these tests, however, are only minimally effective as predictors of other skills.

Much the same might be said of the nonverbal portion of the Lorge-Thorndike intelli-gence test, perhaps the most abstract of all the scales employed in this investigation; such an assessment of the causal efficacy of this scale, however could be extremely misleading. The results indicate that nonverbal intelligence does not directly influence the acquisition of the concrete skills. But as data in Tables 2 and 3 show, nonverbal intelligence apparently causally influences verbal IQ, an ability which, in turn, is a predictor of many of the more concrete linguistic skills (spelling, capitalization, punctuation, reference usage).

The findings indicate that an abstract-to-concrete causal sequence of cognitive acquisition predominates among suburban school children. The positive and often statistically significant cross-lagged correlation values (Table 2) also indicate that the concrete skills act as causal determinants of abstract skills; their causal effectiveness, however, is not as great as that of the more abstract abilities. Taken together, these results suggest that the more complex abstract abilities depend upon the acquisition of a *number* of diverse, concrete skills, but these concrete acquisitions, taken independently, do not operate causally to form more abstract, complex abilities. Apparently, the integration of a number of such skills is a necessary precondition to the generation of higher order abstract rules or schema. Such schema, in turn, operate as causal determinants in the acquisition of later concrete skills.

A review of Tables 2 and 3 lends support to this observation. None of the more specific concrete skills assessed in the various subtests employed in this investigation (Spelling, Capitalization, Punctuation, Reference Usage, Arithmetic Problem Solving) functions as a major causal determinant in either the core or suburban sample. The more abstract abilities (Vocabulary, Reading Comprehension, Language Usage, Verbal and Nonverbal IQ), however, are clearly effective in determining later, more specific achievement.

This pattern of findings might be explained in terms of a simple statistical artifact, in that there would appear to be a greater possibility for test-specific irrelevancies to cancel in tests involving more complex cognitive operations. The tests that

DOES INTELLIGENCE CAUSE ACHIEVEMENT

focus upon the assessment of a single skill or acquisition seem to be more vulnerable to the accumulation of such error (i.e., test-specific bias), which would vary from administration to administration. The attendant test-retest reliabilities of such tests would be adversely affected, and this, in turn, would lessen the chances of obtaining significant *t* differences in the tests employed in the assessment of preponderant causal relationships. The rather impressive reliabilities of the tests, as reported in the technical manuals (Lorge & Thorndike, 1957; Iowa Manual, 1956), and the reliability–specificity correction process described earlier, however, severely limit the plausibility of this alternative.

A more probable explanation of the results obtained is that the preponderant causal sequence is indeed most accurately described as a progression from the abstract to the concrete. The ability to form abstractions (i.e., to employ general complex rules or schema) results in the absorption and retention of more concrete information and skills. The opposite sequence holds, but in an attenuated fashion. A specific concrete acquisition, perhaps a necessary component in the formation of a more general rule, is causally ineffective unless it can be integrated with other concrete acquisitions in generating a more abstract cognitive schema. Taken independently, *specific* concrete skills and information are not effective determinants of abstract rules. Apparently, the acquisition of a combination of diverse (concrete) skills is a necessary, but not sufficient, condition for the formation of abstractions.

This observation might provide a key to the explanation of the complete lack of significant causal relations in the core sample. The assimilation of specific concrete skills may proceed within the core schools at a pace so retarded that the integration necessary for the generation of abstract schema simply cannot take place. If this is so, then the orderly feedback sequence of skill acquisition and integration would be disrupted.

Some evidence supportive of such an interpretation is available. Statistical tests comparing the average scores of *each* of the achievement subscales for the core and suburban subsamples were performed on the data used in this investigation. At the fourth-grade level, differences in normed grade equivalents between core and suburban achievement test scores for each subscale were highly significant, with suburban children outscoring core school students. These differences not only were maintained at the sixth-grade level, but in 10 of 11 subscales, were greater than those noted in the fourth grade. In 7 of these 10 instances, the *t* ratio had also increased from fourth- to sixth-grade test administrations. The suburban school children greatly outperformed the core students in the fourth grade, and lengthened their lead when tested 2 years later.

Discontinuities in this type of scholastic achievement have been noted many times in the past (Harlem Youth Opportunities Unlimited, Inc., 1964; Hentoff, 1966; Kohl, 1968; Kozol, 1967); the contribution of this apparently redundant finding of the present investigation lies in its potential utility in generating an understanding of the dynamics involved in the short-circuiting of the intelligence–achievement sequence of cognitive acquisition in evidence among educationally deprived groups. To be sure, the mere assimilation of concrete academic skills is retarded within the core schools. This is unfortunate, since the core-school children—the products of this educational system—have, in absolute terms, less of the information which is necessary for survival in today's society. The ramifications of this deprivation, however, are even more devastating, since the data of this investigation indicate that a retardation in the mere accumulation of specific skills and information results in an attenuation of the rate at which higher order cognitive organization principles are formed.

In any study that investigates issues as complex as those discussed here, alternative explanations are almost always available. Thus, the reader should be aware of some of the more persuasive limitations on the generalization of the findings presented above. The ideal study of this type would have employed very young children as the primary respondents to obtain a more definitive picture of the intelligence–achievement relationship, unaffected by the interaction of concrete and abstract cognitive functions occurring over time. Unfortunately, the reliable assessment devices necessary for such an investigation simply do not exist (see Bayley, 1955). Results of tests of children younger than those in the present investigation, and appropriate for use in a cross-lagged panel investigation, may well be available, but whether these data would have been any less susceptible to potential temporal-interactional confounding than those employed is debatable.

Another, perhaps more telling, objection that could be raised in response to the findings of this investigation concerns the choice of achievement test employed. The Iowa Tests of Basic Skills is not an example of the typical achievement test. In his review of the Iowa tests, for instance, Herrick (1959) commented:

This test battery cannot be considered as an achievement battery in the usual sense of measuring knowledge in the common content areas of the elementary school curriculum.... The focus of these tests is on the evaluation of the generalized intellectual skills ... not on content per se [p. 16].

Both Morgan (1959) and Remmers (1959) made similar evaluations and each emphasized the strong resemblance between the content of the Iowa tests and that found in most group tests of intelligence. A critic of the present investigation could employ this marked similarity to question the obtained results, since both of the assessment devices focused upon the same general skills and abilities; thus, any causal differences obtained (between conceptually identical scales) could be considered artifactual.

Such an argument, however, would force the critic to posit a number of extremely tenuous assumptions. For example, the degree of generality of the achievement test must closely approximate that of the intelligence test if this alternative is to be entertained. In certain subtests, this proposition might prove acceptable. Many of the achievement subscales, however, quite obviously do not approximate the degree of generality of the intelligence test. Further, these relatively concrete tests of specific acquisitions are the very ones that most often prove to be determined by the more general cognitive skills. In view of these findings, the use of a more concrete achieve-

ment assessment device would likely have enhanced the differences obtained. The abstract-to-concrete causal sequence suggested by the data of the present investigation, that is, would probably be demonstrated even more clearly in a study involving the use of an instrument focused upon the knowledge of very concrete specific skills and information.

Such a supposition need not be left to speculation. Most educators would agree that the testing policy of the schools sampled in this investigation is not an unusual one. Educational systems throughout the country commonly employ both intelligence and achievement batteries in the systematic assessment of their students' accomplishments. The cross-lagged panel correlational technique enables the educator to test the wisdom of this strategy, to decide between competing test batteries, and thus gradually to improve the quality of his assessment operations independent of test constructors' often inflated claims.

The use of this method in a systematic program of investigation would not necessarily demand a great deal of the educator, since, in many school situations, the necessary data are already available. If, for example, only a minimal temporal separation exists between the administration of two or more standard assessment devices (IQ tests, achievement tests, etc.), and such tests are administered two, three, four, or more times throughout the students' academic careers, then the basic raw data needs for the proper use of the cross-lagged panel analysis are satisfied.[12]

If educators throughout the country were to embark on an investigative program of this type, a more certain assessment of the sequence of cognitive development could result. Arising through the combined efforts of numerous investigators, employing many different tests and diverse subject populations, these combined results would prove quite resistant to counterargument. Clearly, the reliable confirmation of either of the two competing causal hypotheses discussed

---

[12] Ideally, information detailing item difficulties over the entire scale, or subscale reliabilities (split half, Kuder-Richardson, etc.) for each wave of testing would also be obtained.

above would have massive implications for educational policies and practices.

It is our hope that this paper, and the analytic technique that has been proposed, will stimulate a program of this nature. The problem to which this report has been addressed is a real and important one and the data for its solution are already available—all that remains is their proper employment.

REFERENCES

BAYLEY, N. On the growth of intelligence. *American Psychologist,* 1955, **10,** 805–811.

BINET, A., & SIMON, T. Méthodes nouvelles pour le diagnostic du niveau intellectuel des anormaux. *L'Année Psychologique,* 1905, **11,** 191–244.

BRUNER, J. S. *Toward a theory of instruction.* New York: W. W. Norton, 1966.

BURT, C. Mental abilities and mental factors. *British Journal of Educational Psychology,* 1944, **14,** 85–94.

BURT, C. The structure of the mind: A review of the results of factor analysis. *British Journal of Educational Psychology,* 1949, **19,** 100–111 and 176–199.

CAMPBELL, D. T. From description to experimentation: Interpreting trends as quasi-experiments. In C. W. Harris (Ed.), *Problems in measuring change.* Madison: University of Wisconsin Press, 1963.

CAMPBELL, D. T., MILLER, N., LUBETSKY, J., & O'CONNELL, E. J. Varieties of projection in trait attribution. In G. A. Kimble (Ed.), *Psychological monographs general and applied.* Washington, D.C.: American Psychological Association, Inc., 1964.

CAMPBELL, D. T., & STANLEY, J. C. Experimental and quasi-experimental designs for research on teaching. In N. L. Gage (Ed.), *Handbook of research on teaching.* Chicago: Rand McNally, 1963.

CRANO, W. D., & BREWER, M. B. *Principles of research in social psychology.* New York: McGraw-Hill, in press.

ERLENMEYER-KIMLING, L., & JARVIK, L. F. Genetics and intelligence: A review. *Science,* 1963, **142,** 1477–1479.

FERGUSON, G. A. On learning and human ability. *Canadian Journal of Psychology,* 1954, **8,** 95–112.

FERGUSON, G. A. On transfer and the abilities of man. *Canadian Journal of Psychology,* 1956, **10,** 121–131.

GALTON, F. *Hereditary genius.* London: Macmillan, 1892.

Harlem Youth Opportunities Unlimited, Inc. *Youth in the ghetto: A study of the consequences of powerlessness and a blueprint for change.* New York: Haryou, 1964.

HARMAN, H. H. *Modern factor analysis.* Chicago: University of Chicago Press, 1960.

HENTOFF, N. *Our children are dying.* New York: Viking Press, 1966.

HERRICK, V. E. Tests and reviews: Achievement batteries. In O. K. Buros (Ed.), *The fifth mental measurement yearbook.* Highland Park, N. J.: Gryphon Press, 1959.

HUNT, J. McV. *Intelligence and experience.* New York: Ronald Press, 1961.

KENNY, D. A. Cross-lagged and common factors in panel data. Paper presented to the conference on structural equations, University of Wisconsin, 1970.

KOHL, A. *36 children.* New York: Signet, 1968.

KOZOL, J. *Death at an early age.* New York: Houghton Mifflin, 1967.

LORGE, I., & THORNDIKE, R. L. The Lorge-Thorndike intelligence tests: Examiner's Manual. Boston: Houghton Mifflin, 1957.

Manual for administrators, supervisors, and counselors, Iowa Tests of Basic Skills. Boston: Houghton Mifflin, 1956.

MORGAN, G. A. V. Tests and reviews: Achievement batteries. In O. K. Buros (Ed.), *The fifth mental measurement yearbook.* Highland Park, N. J.: Gryphon Press, 1959.

PEARSON, K., & FILON, L. N. G. Mathematical contributions to the theory of evolution. *Transactions of the Royal Society* (London), Series A, 1898, **191,** pp. 259, 262.

PELZ, D. C., & ANDREWS, F. M. Detecting causal priorities in panel study data. *American Sociological Review,* 1964, **29,** 836–848.

PETERS, C. C., & VAN VOORHIS, W. R. *Statistical procedures and their mathematical bases.* New York: McGraw-Hill, 1940.

PIAGET, J. *The psychology of intelligence.* London: Routledge and Kegan Paul, 1950.

PIAGET, J. *The origins of intelligence in children.* New York: International Universities Press, 1952.

REMMERS, H. H. Tests and reviews: Achievement batteries. In O. K. Buros (Ed.), *The fifth mental measurement yearbook.* Highland Park, N. J.: Gryphon Press, 1959.

RICKARD, S. The assumption of causal analyses for incomplete causal sets of two multilevel variables. *Multivariate Behavior Research,* in press.

ROZELLE, R. M., & CAMPBELL, D. T. More plausible rival hypotheses in the cross-lagged panel correlation technique. *Psychological Bulletin,* 1969, **71,** 74–80.

SANDELL, R. G. Note on choosing between competing interpretations of cross-lagged panel correlations. *Psychological Bulletin,* 1971, **75,** 367–368.

SCOTT, J. P. The effects of early experience on social behavior and organization. In W. Etkin, (Ed.), *Social behavior and organization among vertebrates.* Chicago: University of Chicago Press, 1964.

SPEARMAN, C. The abilities of man. London: Macmillan and Co. Ltd., 1927.

THORNDIKE, E. L. *Educational psychology.* New York: Lemcke and Buechner, 1903.

THORNDIKE, E. L. *The original nature of man.* New York: Columbia University Press, 1913.

(Received January 25, 1971)

From C. Burt (1943). Brit. J. Educ. Psychol. 13, 83-98. *By kind permission of the author and Scottish Academic Press*

Ability and Income

THE RELATION BETWEEN THE DISTRIBUTION OF ABILITY AND THE DISTRIBUTION OF INCOME.

So far I have argued that differences in income, and in economic and social advantages generally, cannot form the sole or even the main cause of the observable differences in mental ability. Is it, then, reasonable to conjecture that these differences in innate mental ability may after all form the main cause, though not perhaps the only cause, of the wide differences in income or earnings? If that were so, the first and most obvious consequence would be that the distribution of individual ability would resemble the distribution of private incomes.

Accordingly, in our surveys of mental ability, one of the first questions to decide (if I may quote the terms of my earlier *Report*) was this[1]: "Is intelligence distributed like income, where those who have little are the commonest type and those who have much are few and far between? Or is it distributed like height and other physical characteristics, where the average type is the commonest, and the dwarfs and the weaklings are almost as rare as the giants and the strong?" As we have seen, the results obtained seemed definitely to favour the latter hypothesis; and with this general conclusion most psychologists, I imagine, would now agree. If, however, we accept the theory of a normal (or nearly normal) distribution, how are we to account for an amazing disparity between the ascertainable curve for incomes and the assumed curve for general ability?

From the figures published by the Board of Inland Revenue and other authorities we may calculate that the average income in this country is about £180; the figures for surtax show that more than sixty persons have incomes of above £100,000, and the largest incomes

---

[1] *Distribution of Educational Abilities* (1917), pp. 34 *f.* and Fig. 6; *Mental and Scholastic Tests* (1921), p. 162 and Fig. 24. My conclusion in these and other cases was that the distributions were "only *approximately* normal": on applying the recognised statistical test for 'goodness of fit,' the departure from normality proved to be significant in every instance (P always less than ·01). Dearborn (*Intelligence Tests*, 1928) reproduces for comparison curves from various investigations in America: "In all," he says, "the distribution is symmetrical and continuous" (and, one might add, approximately normal); "practically the same range and distribution of individual differences in intelligence which were found by Burt in the schools of London are found in the schools of Boston" (p. 85; cf. pp. 150 *et seq.*). In a paper on 'The Mental Differences between Individuals' (*Brit. Ass. Ann. Rep.*, 1923, p. 229), Fig. 1, I later gave results for 8,599 adults. Here the conclusion was the same—approximate normality only. (I may add that data from intelligence tests now being applied in the Army seem in complete conformity with these earlier inferences.) More recently, however, Thorndike has applied the same test of significance to pooled distributions for the sixth, ninth, and twelfth grades in American schools and for freshmen at American colleges: he obtains, in every case, P= ·9999 or more (*Measurement of Intelligence*, 1927, pp. 521-56; cf. pp. 271-87). Here, however, it seems important to recall the criticisms passed by Fisher and others on such high values for P: "extremely close agreement throws as much suspicion on the hypothesis or the technique as extreme disagreement" (cf. *Statistical Methods*, p. 83).

Ability and Income

of all run to over half a million.[1] In the graph for the distribution of intelligence (*The Distribution of Abilities*, Fig. 6), the printer has allowed about two inches for the frequencies below the average ; to plot a frequency-curve for incomes on such a scale would require a graph running to over 500 feet in length. To put it another way, if human stature, instead of obeying the normal curve, followed that of incomes, then our richest millionaires would be giants three miles tall, with heads like Mount Blanc capped in perpetual snow.

Prof. Pigou has endeavoured to reconcile the two different distributions in the following way. He agrees that " on the face of things we should expect that, if people's capacities are distributed according to the Gaussian curve of error, their incomes will also be distributed in the same way." But, as he points out, a normal distribution of capacity might easily hold good within the more or less homogeneous groups that have been examined, without holding good of the composite population as a whole. " Brain-workers may constitute one homogeneous group, hand-workers another, but jointly they do not ; thus the normal law would rule in each separately, but not in both together."[2] The wider psychological surveys, however, put this suggestion out of court. Intelligence tests have now been applied to large and comprehensive samples, including school children of every social grade, adults of almost every occupation, and (within the last year or two) thousands of recruits for the Army. The results make it perfectly clear that, although the distribution of ability does not perfectly conform with the normal curve, nevertheless the amount of skewness is much too slight to bear out the explanation Prof. Pigou has suggested. The deviations from normality exhibited by different distributions can be readily compared by computing the appropriate functions of the higher moments (beta-functions) ; for the normal curve $\beta_1 = 0$, $\beta_2 = 3$; for most distributions of intelligence quotients, β_1 lies between $0 \cdot 0$ and $0 \cdot 2$, and β_2 between 2 and 4 ; for curves of income in Great Britain at various dates, $\beta_1 = 1 \cdot 2$ (approximately), $\beta_2 = 50,000$ or more.

Of the few other economists who have touched upon the psychological problem, the majority seem disposed to abandon the notion of a normal distribution altogether. In particular, Pareto, and still more Pareto's followers in the United States, have declared that the elongated curves of income-distribution can be no economic accident, but represent an iron law resulting from an " inexorable biological fact."

Carl Snyder, for instance, has recently come to the following conclusion : " Where differences of attainment are concerned, the frequencies do *not* follow the pattern of the normal curve : the number of persons superior to the mode tends to be much smaller than the number inferior. The explanation is obvious. High achievement is always due to a combination of *several* fundamental faculties : hence, the number of persons with exceptional artistic ability (for example) is far less than the number with average talents " ; and, to support this view, he cites Seashore's figures for the distribution of musical ability.[3]

Similarly, Prof. Harold Davies maintains that " the Pareto law is only one example of a much more general law of inequality, which we might refer to as the *law of the distribution of special abilities*. . . . One of the strongest arguments *against* the Binet I.Q. as a measure for the higher levels, is the fact that abilities as measured by it are made to conform to the normal curve." With the Binet scale " the addition of a unit at a high level is considerably *more* difficult than the addition of a unit at a low level." On the other hand, " in playing billiards the addition of one billiard to a run of x is no more difficult than the addition of one billiard to a run of x' " ; similarly, in working for an income, " it is not improbable that to add one dollar to actual income is approximately the same at each level," e.g., whether your income is \$100,000 or only \$1,000. Hence, he believes, the symmetrical curve of I.Q.'s does a flagrant injustice to the actual spread of high abilities towards the upper end of the scale.[4]

[1] These figures are based on the latest accessible returns. For earlier years, and for a discussion of the sources of information, see Colin Clark, *National Income and Outlay* (1937), p. 109 *et seq.*, and refs.

[2] *Economics of Welfare*, 1924, pp. 608-9. Pigou and Hugh Dalton (*The Inequality of Incomes*, 1920, p. 128) both insist that " the facts of bequest and inheritance of property " must tend to skew the curve of income still further. The same objection was urged against Pareto's claim (that the ' law ' of income-distribution is the direct result of a ' biological fact ') by Benini (*Principii di Statistica Metodologia*, 1906, pp. 310 *et seq.*). However, it now seems generally agreed that, although the inheritance of property must unquestionably magnify the pre-existing asymmetry in the income-curve, it cannot account for that asymmetry entirely, or even to any large extent.

[3] *Capitalism the Creator* (1940), chaps. xiv. and xv.

[4] *The Analysis of Economic Time Series* (1941), p. 427.

CYRIL BURT

It seems, therefore, incumbent on the psychologist to examine more closely this general law of inequality,' which these writers propose to substitute for the normal law. Pareto[1] has expressed his 'universal law' for the distribution of earnings by a simple mathematical equation, $N = \dfrac{C}{x^a}$, where N is the number of persons whose income exceeds x units, and C a constant; the index or exponent, a, measures the inequality of the incomes: according to Pareto, its value cannot vary greatly from 1·5; according to the actual data it appears never to fall below 1 and seldom to be greater than 1·67.[2] Assuming the variables to be continuous, and differentiating Pareto's equation, we can express his formula in terms more familiar to the statistical psychologist. We obtain $y = \dfrac{aC}{x^{a+1}}$, where y denotes the proportionate number of persons having an income of $f(x \pm \frac{1}{2}dx)$. Such an equation describes, not a symmetrical, but a J-shaped curve, belonging to Pearson's Type XI.[3] In old schemes of marking a J-shaped distribution seems often to have been tacitly assumed: the vast majority of pupils merely 'passed'—i.e., satisfied the minimum requirements; a smaller proportion were awarded a third class; fewer still a second; and fewest of all a first; while one or two individuals, standing out from the rest, achieved a 'mark of distinction.' In the moral sphere, too, as F. H. Allport has noted, what he terms the 'J-curve of conforming behaviour' is apt to "appear in place of the chance-biological (normal) curve."[4] Many of these distributions can be plausibly fitted by means of the foregoing formula.

But I am tempted to simplify Pareto's formula still further, and to suggest that, in the case of income at any rate, the initial value of a is approximately unity and that it is augmented to 1·5, or rather more, by various artificial circumstances, peculiar to the country or the time (e.g., the manner in which property is inherited and taxed). If this were done, the fundamental law would reduce to a simple law of the inverse square, viz., $y = \dfrac{C}{x^2}$; and therefore $N = \dfrac{C'}{x}$, or $Nx =$ Constant.

To the psychologist, familiar with the text-book curves for the distributions of mental abilities, all these equations may wear an unaccustomed aspect. Yet analogous laws are by no means difficult to find in the physical world. Thus, with a gas expanding adiabatically, $P = \dfrac{C}{V^a}$; and the rate of decrease of pressure (P) per unit increase of volume (V) is consequently $\dfrac{aC}{V^{a+1}}$, where a is never less than 1, and never exceeds 1·67. If we put $a=1$ (as in isothermal expansion) we have $PV =$ Constant, the equation known to every schoolboy as the formula

[1] *Cours d'economie politique* (1897), II, pp. 299-345. Both Bowley and Stamp have shown that (with certain reservations) the law is applicable to British incomes. Lord Stamp fitted Pareto's formula to the early returns of the British super-tax; and, on the strength of the discrepancies, informed the Inland Revenue authorities that they must have missed over 1,000 payers in certain classes. He adds: "They promptly went and found them!" (*Wealth and Taxable Capacity*, p. 83.)

[2] Most observers, however, seem now agreed that, instead of remaining relatively constant, it has (during the past half century at any rate) shown a discernible tendency to decline: cf. A. L. Bowley, *ap. Select Committee on Income Tax*, 1906; *Evidence*, p. 81.

[3] For the fitting of such a type, see Elderton, *Frequency Curves*, p. 110. Elderton, curiously enough, remarks that he has "not come across a distribution really represented by Type XI."

[4] *J. Soc. Psych.*, V (1934), pp. 141 *et seq.* What about those who do not conform, or who fail in the examination, or have incomes below the mode? These have to be treated as rare exceptions beyond the pale of the J-law: in the same way the initial rise of pressure in experiment on Boyle's law, and the extreme cases in experiments on Weber's law, used to be treated as exceptions to the theoretical curve, not as part of it. It would seem better, however, to meet the difficulty by regarding the Pareto equation as a first approximation to a Type V or VI formula: an instructive modification of this kind has indeed been proposed by one of his Italian followers (Amoroso, 'Ricerche intorno alla curva dei redditi,' *Ann. di Matem.* II, 1925, pp. 123-60). The psychologist would probably think first of rescaling the base line by taking a logarithmic function of income, and then using the ordinary formula for the normal distribution; and, in point of fact, except for the highest incomes of all, this device has been claimed to give a very plausible fit (Gibrat, *Les inégalités économiques*, 1931): but the fit is a poor one for British incomes.

Ability and Income

for Boyle's law.[1] The non-mathematical reader will perhaps more easily grasp the implication of the simplified expression I have proposed if he recalls the numerous examples of the law of the inverse square occurring in other fields : e.g., its appearance in measuring the attractive force of gravitation, magnetism, electric charges, heat, light, and sound, radiation, and the like, and, indeed, any effect radially and uniformly distributed from some central point. In sound, for instance, the intensity or loudness of a noise diminishes in inverse proportion to the square of the distance of the receiver from the source.

The analogies from physical dynamics are, I venture to think, not so far fetched as they may seem. In estimating the mental output of a human being or a human community, it is natural to begin by imagining a simplified working model, just as in thermodynamics we start from the notion of an ideal machine. And the calculations appropriate to such a model will naturally be expressed in terms of familiar dynamic concepts, whether or not they obey the familiar laws. Unfortunately, in discussions on what may conveniently be termed psycho-dynamics, owing to a confusion between the metaphorical and the strict meanings of the terms, ' capacity for work ' has been identified with mental ' energy ' ; and mental ' energy ' in turn has been identified with ' general intelligence ' as measured by the usual tests. At the same time, amount of work is measured by actual output ; and since, in physics, energy as capacity for work is itself measured by amount of work done on actual trial, psychologists have apparently assumed that the distribution of output (and therefore the distribution of payment for output) should follow the same law as the distribution of mental capacity, whether or not that is expressed by the Gaussian or ' normal ' curve. This I hold to be a fallacy.

If I take a large number of my students, I find that, with intelligence-tests or academic examinations, the marks measuring their ' ability ' conform pretty closely with the normal curve.[2] Yet, when I collect records of their output as psychologists in later life, I find that the frequency-curve is not even approximately normal, but J-shaped ; and this holds good in many other fields of human output for which detailed data are available. May I give one simple illustration of a type that every reader can verify for himself ?

Let us take the latest publication of sufficient size on educational psychology—Prof. Valentine's *Psychology of Early Childhood*—and let us study the output records of the chief workers in this sphere as shown in the index of authors. It contains just over 200 names. How great have been the contributions of these writers as assessed by the number of references to the works of each one ?

An exponential law (like that of cooling or diminution of pressure with increase of altitude) yields a very poor fit. Let us therefore turn to the figures deducible from the simplified formula suggested above, viz., $y = \dfrac{1}{x^2} \cdot \dfrac{1}{\sum \frac{1}{x^2}}$ or in percentages, $y = \dfrac{100}{1 \cdot 645 \, x^2} = \dfrac{60 \cdot 8}{x^2}$, where

x is the number of references, and y the number of psychologists whose output has been sufficiently large or important to be referred to x times. The actual and the calculated frequencies are shown in Table III. Now the fit is surprisingly close.

Should frequency of reference be thought to indicate qualitative value rather than quantitative amount, it is quite as easy to procure a direct measure of individual output from the indexes of various psychological journals. In general, the exponent of x, namely $(a+1)$, hovers between 1·5 and 2·6, exactly as the simplified version of Pareto's formula requires.[3]

It appears evident, then, that individual output as thus assessed does not follow the normal curve, although individual ability conceivably may. But I venture to suggest that the apparent inconsistency between the two distributions vanishes directly we recognise that the functional relation between output (as effect) and capacities (as causes)

---

[1] Other parallels are the law relating rate of working and resistance in an electrical conductor circuit, and the laws of friction in mechanical processes. At the Ministry of Munitions, during the last war, I found that the ' output ' of the heavier howitzers (number of rounds fired during its life) and the ' output ' of accidents among munition workers both gave frequency-distributions conforming approximately to the formula just cited.

[2] Miss Harwood has recently analysed the marks of many groups of candidates sitting for two or three typical university academic examinations over a period of years ; and finds that, even when no instructions are given the examiners about the allotment of such marks, they nevertheless show an approximately normal distribution, i.e., the prior attempt to admit only suitable candidates on entrance has not skewed the distribution so much as might be supposed.

[3] I may add that Miss Stevenson has recently analysed a number of output-curves in this way ; and further confirmed this result.

CYRIL BURT

may be of many different kinds, and indeed is more likely to be indirect and complex than immediate or simple. Thus, we may willingly grant, with Snyder, that " achievement of a high sort " is the ultimate resultant of a " *combination* of fundamental faculties " (or abilities). But then we must go on to observe that everything really depends on *how* they are combined.

TABLE III.—FREQUENCY CURVE FOR OUTPUT IN EDUCATIONAL PSYCHOLOGY.

No. of References (x)	1	2	3	4	5	6	7	8

No. of Psychologists (y) :
  (i) Actual ....
  (ii) Calculated ....
	121
	122·1
		32
		30·0
			12
			13·6
				9
				7·6
					6
					4·9
						2
						3·4
							4
							2·5
								2
								1·9

No. of References (x)	9	10	11	12	13	14	15	16

No. of Psychologists (y) :
  (i) Actual .....,..............
  (ii) Calculated ....
	3
	1·5
		2
		1·2
			1
			1·0
				2
				0·9
					1
					0·7
						1
						0·6
							0
							0·5
								0
								0·5

No. of References (x)	17	18	19	20–23	..	24	..	27

No. of Psychologists (y) :
  (i) Actual ....
  (ii) Calculated ....
	0
	0·4
		1
		0·4
			1
			0·3
				0
				0·3
					..
					..
						1
						0·2
							..
							..
								1
								0·2

Ordinarily, having assumed that the measurements for the independent ' factors ' are distributed among the different individuals in accordance with the normal curve, we make the further assumption that these ' factor-measurements ' combine by simple addition. Now I suggest that, where we are dealing, not with a complex mental *ability*, but with a complex mental *output*, it would be quite as reasonable (at least in many instances, though possibly not in all) to *multiply* as to add. It is a simple matter to show how this will lead from a normal curve for the components to a J-shaped curve for the products. Take factor-measurements for two factors only, and imagine that each is distributed into five classes (allotted marks of 0, 1, 2, 3, 4 respectively) and that distribution obeys the binomial law (i.e., the frequencies are proportional to 1, 4, 6, 4, 1). Combine the marks for these two factors by multiplying them instead of summing them ; and then redistribute the final marks into five classes as before. We arrive at the frequencies shown in Table IV (*b*).

TABLE IV.—FREQUENCY DISTRIBUTION OBTAINED BY MULTIPLYING THE COMPONENT FACTOR-MEASUREMENTS.

Measurement.	Frequencies (*in Percentages*).	
	(*a*) *For Each Factor.*	(*b*) *For Two Factors Combined.*
0—1 .... 1—2 .... 2—3 .... 3—4 .... 4—5	6·25 25·0 37·5 25·0 6·25	49·6 36·0 10·9 3·1 0·4
TOTAL.........	100·0	100·0

What particular function should be chosen in any given case is a point to be determined by the concrete and empirical nature of the processes concerned, not by some abstract *à priori* principle, laid down once and for all. Thus, bodily height, width, and depth are each of them (in

Ability and Income

the case of most animals) normally distributed, or nearly so : but, since these ' factors ' must be highly correlated (otherwise the individuals could not preserve approximately the same shape) it follows that volume, and therefore weight which depends upon volume, and pressure which depends on weight, will be estimated better by multiplying rather than by adding. This, indeed, is likely to be the case with any varying characteristic which (like measurements involving time, to take one obvious instance) has an absolute zero of its own.[1] If, for example, one of the ' factors ' is speed, industry, or retentiveness, the deviations must tend to augment those due to mere intelligent insight, by a process more akin to multiplication than to addition. Or consider the effect of blindness on the number of runs scored by one cricketer, or of doubling the speed of leg-movement of those of another : the change in score would not be correctly estimated by just *adding* the changing measurements. In short, when it comes to computing actual output, we seem to be faced with something like the converse of Weber's law : so long as we are measuring sensory *capacity* in the laboratory, we proceed from the physical stimulus to the consequent mental change, and, in so doing, we encounter the well-known phenomenon of *diminishing* returns ; but when we are measuring *output* in industry, in commerce, or in any intellectual field, we virtually proceed from mental capacity to a consequent physical change ; and there we meet with the opposite phenomenon of *increasing* returns.

The practical corollary seems plain. The tacit habit of treating the symmetrical curve of mental ability as entailing a corresponding symmetry in the curve of mental output has hitherto led us to underrate, and to underrate very grossly, the extraordinarily high output of which the super-normal child should eventually be capable. It follows that the ultimate return to the community that would be gained by investing public funds in the tasks of discovering and educating those super-normal individuals is far above what we have hitherto been inclined to expect. Every psychologist, therefore, should readily endorse the pronouncements of the few economists who have expressed an opinion on this point : " No extravagance," says Marshall, " is more prejudicial to the growth of national wealth than the wasteful negligence which allows genius that happens to be born of lowly parentage to expend itself in lowly work ; and there is no change that would conduce so much to a rapid increase in that wealth as an improvement in our schools and scholarships such as would enable the clever son of a poor man to rise gradually till he has the best education the age can give."[2]

IV.—SUMMARY.

Since teachers and administrators will be interested solely in the practical inferences, while psychologists will ask rather for the evidence on which those inferences are based, it will perhaps be convenient to summarise the technical arguments first, and then set down the practical outcome in as simple and non-technical language as possible.

The problem with which we have been concerned is the relations between intelligence, on the one hand, and economic conditions, on the other. All who have discussed this issue, no matter which side they take, assume that ' intelligence ' is one of the most important factors both in educational progress and in social and industrial efficiency ; but no final agreement can be reached, unless both parties to the controversy accept the same definition of ' intelligence.' By ' intelligence ' is here understood an innate factor entering in various degrees into every mental process that involves cognition—not (as some writers would suggest) any complex set of performances as measured by a recognised scale of intelligence tests.

A.—*Technical conclusions.*

(1) When this distinction is made, it appears that differences in ' intelligence,' defined as an *innate* factor, can only be assessed *approximately* by the raw measurement

[1] This would seem to be Pareto's own explanation. In his later work he writes : " au-dessus de la moyenne il n'y a pas de limite de hauteur ; il y a une limite au-dessous " ; and he claims that this is so both for income and for ability, as measured, for example, at ordinary scholastic examinations (*Manuel*, 1927, p. 385).

[2] *Principles of Economics*, p. 213. Cf. Pigou, *loc. cit.*, p. 707 : " Stupidly organised investments in children's capacities, like other stupidly organised investments, will yield little return : well-organised investments, especially investments adjusted to the natural abilities of the children affected, hold out large promise."

Cyril Burt

of ' intelligence,' automatically obtained by applying one of the recognised scales. Hence for the study of theoretical questions like the present, as well as for the practical diagnosis of individual cases, it is necessary to adjust the calculated I.Q. (or whatever mark or score is used) in the light of other relevant information, including supplementary tests of a practical type. Obviously, for research purposes, such adjustments must not be too arbitrary or subjective ; nor must they beg the question at issue in the research.

(2) Measured by these adjusted I.Q.'s intelligence appears to be distributed—approximately, though not exactly—in conformity with the symmetrical ' curve of error.' On the other hand, the distribution of personal income does not present, even approximately, any such symmetrical curve, but rather a highly skewed J-shaped curve, which can be fitted by a law of the inverse square (or some low power of that order) such as could be deduced from what economists know as ' Pareto's equation.'

(3) The discrepancy can best be reconciled, not by substituting a new law of ability for the normal law, but by regarding earned income as depending mainly on output, and output as related to the contributory abilities by some special and possibly complex function. This suggestion is confirmed by observing that, in many intellectual fields at any rate, the distribution of the output itself approaches the J-shaped curve (shown by income) rather than the symmetrical curve (shown by measurements of intelligence).

(4) The particular function relating the output of different individuals to their respective abilities requires to be determined empirically for each important type of work whether scholastic or industrial. There are, however, indications that such functions will be similar to those already encountered in dealing with the work or output of physical machines.

B.—*Practical conclusions.*

(1) The foregoing results support the view that the wide inequality in personal income is largely, though not entirely, an indirect effect of the wide inequality in innate intelligence.

(2) They do not support the view (still held'by many educational and social reformers) that the apparent inequality in intelligence of children and adults is in the main an indirect consequence of inequality in economic conditions.

(3) Nevertheless, mental output and achievement, as distinguished from sheer innate capacity, are undoubtedly influenced by differences in social and economic conditions. In particular, the financial disadvantages under which the poorer families labour annually prevent three or four thousand children of superior intelligence from securing the higher education that their intelligence deserves.

(4) The most striking instances of this are to be found at the final stage of education. With the available data a simple calculation shows that about 40 per cent of those whose innate abilities are of university standard are failing to reach the university ; and presumably an equal number from the fee-paying classes receive a university education to which their innate abilities alone would scarcely entitle them.

PART IX

THE BIOLOGICAL
BASIS OF INTELLIGENCE

From the very beginning of the intelligence testing movement, efforts have been made to relate IQ as tested to some brain features which might be thought of as causally involved in the production of intelligent behaviours. Brain size itself is of course the first variable that suggests itself, and indeed there does appear a slight but definite relationship. Tyler (1956, p. 622) has summarized the evidence as follows: "Eleven studies have been made of the relationship between intelligence . . . and cranial capacity. In all instances, the correlations have been positive, although small, ranging from ·08 to ·34." Of course, head size is a very rough guide to brain size (because of different skull thickness, differing proportions of white and grey matter, differing body size, differing arrangement of convolutions, etc.), and even brain size does not take into account the number of cells per cubic inch and other microscopic and macroscopic details of the cortex. One might say that no really serious effort has in fact been made to relate IQ and brain anatomy, so that the positive but slight correlations found so far are encouraging but not sufficient to give us more than the most indirect of hints as to the real extent of any relations there might be. Perhaps it is the need for interdisciplinary and longitudinal research that has put off researchers; whatever the cause, very little is known about this aspect of the body-mind relation.

Another physiological variable which was thought to be related to intelligence was speed of neural transmission, and early investigators attempted to measure it through the latency of certain reflexes, such as the patellar tendon reflex—without much success. Roth (1964) has shown that it is the increase in latency with increase in complexity of signal (log. of number of alternative responses) which correlates with intelligence, dull subjects showing a more marked increase than bright ones. This interesting approach has been shown by Jensen (unpublished) to give replicable results, but very little has been done to exploit its theoretical significance.

The great breakthrough came during the second World War, when a junior sergeant tester in the British Army, engaged on statistical analysis of test data, found himself with nothing to do; following the Army principle that one must at least appear to be busy in case someone noticed one's idleness and gave one something even more unpleasant to do, he started correlating any sets of data he could lay his hands on. He was rather surprised when he discovered a significant correlation among these meaningless data, and when he went to see just what it was that he had correlated, he found that it was IQ, on the one hand, and number of teeth missing, on the other. This correlation of $-·63$ was quickly verified by correlating the same variables on other samples, and still constitutes the highest correlation between intelligence and a physical feature of the human organism that has ever been discovered. Unfortunately the causal chain is unlikely to go from the possession of teeth to the possession of intelligence; social class (at that time at least, i.e. before the national health service had come into being) determined very largely the dental care lavished on a person's teeth, and as we have seen social class is also highly correlated with intelligence. There may also be a possibility that more intelligent people, irrespective of class, take greater care of their teeth. Eysenck (1947) has reported data to show that intelligent people tend to be larger in body size than dull ones; they also tend to be leptomorphic in body build. These relationships are not strong, and they too have never been followed up.

Of more interest to many investigators has been the electroencephalogram, and in particular the alpha wave. This is often regarded as some kind of homeostatic energy system, possibly some rhythmic excitement level in the dendritic layers of the cortex. As Cattell (1971) has pointed out, "like a flywheel it betokens energy 'resting', ready to be used. . . . When a person perceives, concentrates, or thinks, the simple oscillation is wiped out as by some kind of discharge. Furthermore, it has been noted that its very existence depends on the existence of a sufficiently large volume of associational cortex, i.e. cortex not directly concerned to cope with sensorimotor immediate experience as such." Cattell develops interesting hypotheses regarding alpha waves as indirect measures of the "cortical associational neuron mass" which he conceives to be basic to fluid intelligence, and which calls to mind Thomson's theory of number of "bonds" as determining IQ score, revisited and revised recently by Maxwell (1972). But the sad truth is that in adults there is no simple relation between alpha rhythm and ability measures (Lindsley, 1961). With children, as Cattell notes, there are correlations ranging from ·3 to ·6, but these are with M.A. rather than with IQ, i.e. they seem to be related to maturation. This whole field is ripe for more intensive study.

One aspect of EEG work has been rather more promising, and has been more fully developed in recent years, namely the so-called evoked potentials, i.e. the waves of negative and positive electricity evoked by a sudden stimulus. These waves are quite characteristic for a given person, both in shape and latency, and it has been suggested that they are connected with referring input to analyzing mechanisms, and with establishment of memory engrams; possibly they might be measures of the "speed of processing" bits of information as these enter the cortex. Cattell points out that "it seems reasonable to suppose that they are concerned not only with memorizing but also with the *evaluation* of the stimulus—its referral to the sorting in the sensory area, and also with the eduction of relations. For they appear when relations are demanded with other sensory areas, as when one presents a standard perceptual intelligence problem. Now a smaller total cortical apparatus, like a smaller computer, might be expected to take longer to process a fixed number of relations up to the required level for solution, as presented by a standard test problem." Ertl's (1966) original observations did in fact show a correlation of about $-·7$ between intelligence and a latency measure (taken from stimulus presentation to third wave crest). In spite of the high reliability of evoked potential latencies such a high relationship is intrinsically unlikely, and hence the original observation met with incredulity. However, later work by Ertl and Schafer (1969) and others showed that correlations of rather more modest magnitude (i.e. in the neighbourhood of ·3) could be reproduced with some reliability. The most careful and large-scale study in this field, carried out by Shucard and Horn, is reprinted here as the first paper in this section; it will be found to throw much light on the whole subject. Certainly the results leave little doubt that we can now identify at least one of the physiological features correlated with intelligence, and the high reliability of this measure, together with the difficulty Ertl has reported in changing the latency by any environmental manipulation, suggests that studies of heritability could with advantage be undertaken in this area (cf. Osborne, 1970).

Work in our own laboratories has given strong support to the results reported by Ertl and Schafer, and by Horn, with some interesting additional findings. Using 93 adults, randomly sampled, Hendrickson (1972) administered the AH4 test of intelligence, which gives a verbal, a spatial and a total score; she also determined latencies and amplitudes of evoked potentials in response to sounds of 3 different intensities. (Intensity did not markedly affect the issue, and consequently her results quoted below are for all intensities combined). Table 1 lists the correlations; a value of ·20 is required for significance at the 5% level, and of ·27 at the 1% level. It will be seen that both latency (negatively) and amplitude (positively) are correlated with intelligence; more so with verbal than with spatial intelligence, and possibly most of all with total intelligence score. The average size of the correlations range from ·3 to ·5 for latency (P and N stand for positive and negative portions of the wave, and the numbers stand for the first, second and third waves respectively). The average size of the correlations range from ·3 to ·45 for amplitude, when we are considering verbal ability, and from ·1 to ·25 when we are considering spatial ability. It should be borne in mind that latency and amplitude are essentially uncorrelated; we can therefore sum their inverse hyperbolic tangent values in order to predict intelligence. Quite roughly, such a combined score of latency and amplitude would correlate with verbal intelligence between ·5 and ·6; this is not a kind of value which one would reject as unimportant. In order to gain some idea of the "true" correlation between evoked potential and verbal intelligence, we would have to correct these coefficients for attenuation; this would give a value in excess of ·6, and possibly approaching ·7.

We can take this statistical consideration a step further; both amplitude and latency were found to be correlated significantly with personality variables (extraversion, neuroticism, etc.) which themselves do not correlate with intelligence (Eysenck, 1971). That means that these personality measures can be used as suppressor variables, thus raising the observed correlations above ·70. But the g saturation of the intelligence test used is not likely to be above ·8 at the most, so that a perfect measure of g could not correlate with the test above this value; certainly ·7 or thereabouts comes pretty close to this optimal value, suggesting that the evoked potential is not very far removed from being a perfect physiological measure of g. Such a conclusion is of course premature, in the absence of repeat studies demonstrating similar relationships, of similar size; earlier work as noted above, has usually given somewhat lower values. But this is likely to be due to the prevalent use of visual stimuli; our use of auditory stimuli seems to rule out certain artefacts which cloud the picture. However that may be, complex chains of statistical correction of observed data are always suspect and it would be wiser not to make premature claims for the evoked potential as a measure of IQ. The main reason for introducing these calculations here is simply that raw, uncorrected coefficients seriously underestimate the true relationships; a decision as to whether our corrections have tended to exaggerate them must be left to future work. In any case, there can be no doubt that at long last a serious step has been taken in the direction of identifying the physiological basis of intelligence.*

TABLE 1

Latency:	Verbal	Spatial	Total
P_1	−·41	−·39	−·44
N_1	−·44	−·38	−·45
P_2	−·48	−·44	−·50
N_2	−·34	−·35	−·38
P_3	−·41	−·29	−·38
N_3	−·29	−·25	−·30
Amplitude:			
A_3	·31	·10	·22
A_4	·95	·25	·37
A_5	·31	·19	·27

Correlations between Verbal, Spatial and Total scores on the AH4 test intelligence, and evoked potential latency and amplitude.

Numerical subscripts refer to successive waves; P and N, to positive and negative deviations respectively.

An entirely different approach to the general problem of the biological basis of intelligence is offered in our second reprint. Here a group of investigators has been concerned for many years with the brain chemistry accompanying and underlying intelligent behaviour and with the hereditary and environmental influences which determine and change this brain chemistry. The paper quoted goes into considerable historical detail concerning the growth and general philosophy of this project, and there is no need for any detailed discussion of it here. One can only express one's admiration for the tenacity with which the workers in this team have followed up the important clues they have unearthed; it seems sad that others have not followed their lead. The general philosophy underlying their work seems eminently suited to the problems posed by intelligence measurement as a whole, and its genetic and environmental basis in particular. The argument will be found to be somewhat complex, but it would be idle to expect the solution to such a profound problem to be easy.

* It is important to add that in some unpublished sesearch from our laboratory, J. Rust found very high heritabilities for amplitude and latency of evoked potentials, going up to 90% for amplitude, and somewhat lower (up to above 80%) for latency. This is added evidence for the heritability of intelligence.

The last paper is somewhat related to the preceding one; if biochemical activity in the cortex determines and accompanies intelligent activity, then one would expect chemical agents, administered to the organism (rat or human) to be able to alter the biochemical balance for better or worse. There is no difficulty about the "worse"; but that is not our aim. Can we increase intellectual activity, improve problem-solving ability, and thus "up" IQ by the administration of drugs? For many years the possible use of glutamic acid for this purpose has been debated and investigated; the paper here reprinted seems to offer a resolution of the apparently contradictory experimental findings. The authors find that the drug improves performance of dull rats (and probably humans), but does not affect the performance of average or bright rats (and probably humans). This may not be a world-shaking conclusion, but it does seem to demonstrate once and for all that intelligence can be improved by drug administration, and if this is possible in principle, there seems no reason why other drugs should not be discovered which might raise the IQ level even of above-average organisms. Even if this should prove impossible, it is surely a cause for rejoicing that a remedy may be in existence for general dullness. This whole subject of the biological basis of intelligence is likely to come much more to the fore in the next few years; now that we have a reasonably firm basis on which to proceed, it is likely that our knowledge in this field will advance by leaps and bounds.

REFERENCES

CATTELL, R. B. *Abilities, their structure, growth, and action.* Boston: Houghton Mifflin, 1971.

ERTL, J. P. Evoked potentials and intelligence. *Rev. de l'Universite d'Ottowa*, 1966, *36*, 599–607.

ERTL, J. P. & SCHAFER, E. W. P. Brain response correlates of psychometric intelligence. *Nature*, 1969, *223*, 421–422.

EYSENCK, H. J. *Dimensions of personality.* London: Routledge & Kegan Paul, 1947.

EYSENCK, H. J. Relation between intelligence and personality. *Percept. & motor Skills*, 1971, *32*, 637–638.

HENDRICKSON, ELAINE. Experimental investigation of individual differences in cortical evoked response. London: Unpublished Ph.D. thesis, 1972.

LINDSLEY, D. B. The reticular motivating system and perceptual integration. In: D. E. Sheer (Ed.) *Electrical stimulation of the brain.* Austin: Univ. of Texas Press, 1961.

MAXWELL, A. E. Factor analysis: Thomson's sampling theory recalled. *Brit. J. math. statist. Psychol.*, 1972, *25*, 1–21.

OSBORNE, R. T. Heritability estimates for the visual evoked response. *Life Sciences*, 1970, *9*, II, 481–490.

ROTH, E. Die Geschwindigkeit der Verarbeitung von Information und ihr Zusammenhang mit Intelligenz. *Ztschr. f. angew. & experim. Psychol.*, 1964, *11*, 616–622.

TYLER, L. E. *The psychology of human differences.* New York: Appleton-Century-Crofts, 1956.

From D. W. Shucard and J. L. Horn, J. Comp. Physiol. Psychol., 78, 59–68. *Copyright* (1972), *by kind permission of the authors and the American Psychological Association*

EVOKED CORTICAL POTENTIALS AND MEASUREMENT OF HUMAN ABILITIES[1]

DAVID WM. SHUCARD[2] AND JOHN L. HORN

University of Denver

A consistent pattern of reliable correlations of the order of from −.15 to −.32 was found between measures of intelligence and measures of visual average evoked potential latency recorded from the frontoparietal scalp. Measures of fluid and crystallized intelligence correlated to about the same magnitude with evoked potential latency measures. There were significant correlations between measures representing simple cognitive processes (e.g., motor–perceptual speed) and evoked potential latency. The average size of ability–latency correlations as well as the number of significant correlations increased as conditions of evoked potential testing which tend to impose alertness on subjects were relaxed.

Since Berger's (1929) discovery of the electroencephalographic (EEG) technique for monitoring neural activity of the central nervous system (CNS), investigators have attempted to show that variations in this activity reflect processes which are related to intellectual function. Reviews of the evidence in this area by Ellingson (1956, 1966), Vogel and Broverman (1964, 1966), Vogel, Broverman, and Klaiber (1968), and Shucard (1969) indicate a lack of agreement concerning the relationship between brain-wave phenomena and intellectual abilities in the normal range, although brain damage and retardation often coexist and are indicated both by EEG measurement and psychological test scores.

Recently, the visual average evoked potential (AEP) has shown promise of reflecting differences in intellectual function. Relationships have been found between the latency of visual AEP peaks (LAEP) recorded from the scalp and scores obtained on the Wechsler-Bellevue, Primary Mental Abilities (PMA), and Wechsler Intelligence Scale for Children (WISC) tests (see Barry & Ertl, 1965; Chalke & Ertl, 1965; Ertl, 1968; Ertl & Schafer, 1969). Correlations between abilities and LAEP measures ranged

from −.10 to −.88. The largest correlations were found for the latency of AEP components occurring between 100 and 500 msec. (LAEP 3 and LAEP 4). Corroborating results were reported by Plum (1968) and Weinberg (1969). Rhodes, Dustman, and Beck (1969) also found a trend in the same direction for late AEP components.

Although these studies demonstrated a relationship between AEP measures and human abilities (*a*) the relationship has not been replicated over a broad range of the population; (*b*) the studies were based on omnibus measures of intelligence rather than on measures of different kinds of intelligence, thus rendering it impossible to isolate the variables which may be responsible for a finding of correlation between AEP measures and intelligence; and (*c*) the findings have not been integrated in a coherent theory.

The purpose of this investigation was to study the relationships which AEP measures (particularly LAEP) may have with operationally independent forms of intelligence, as indicated in the theory of fluid and crystallized intelligence (See Horn, 1968, 1970a, 1970b). The aim was to allow for a more detailed analysis of the AEP–intelligence relationship. Further, because previous investigations suggested that AEP measures might be related to speed of responding and changes in attention or arousal (see Donchin & Lindsley, 1966; Jane, Smirnov, & Jasper, 1962; Lansing, Schwartz, & Lindsley, 1959; Monnier, 1952;

---

[1] The research reported in this article is based on a dissertation submitted to the Faculty of the University of Denver, Department of Psychology, in partial fulfillment of the requirements for the PhD.

[2] Requests for reprints should be sent to David Wm. Shucard, Department of Behavioral Science, National Jewish Hospital, 3800 E. Colfax Avenue, Denver, Colorado 80206.

DAVID WM. SHUCARD AND JOHN L. HORN

TABLE 1
LIST OF TESTS SELECTED TO MEASURE Gf, Gc, Gs, AND Gv WITH INDICATIONS OF PRIMARY AND SECOND-ORDER FACTORS

Testing order	Test	Number of items	Testing time	Primary factor	Second-order factor	Similar to Wechsler scale	Similar to PMA tests
1	Follow the line—Vz	80	4	Vz	Gv		S
2	Canceling numbers—P	50	4	P	Gs	COD	
3	Mixed operations—N	20	3	N	Gc		N
4	Necessary operations—R	15	5	R	Gc-Gf	ARIT	R
5	Letter series (speed)—Isp	40	7	I	Gf		R
6	Letter series (level)—Ilv	18	10	I	Gf		R
7	Matrices (speed)—CFRsp	20	5	CFR	Gf	BLKD	R
8	Matrices (level)—CFRlv	18	8	CFR	Gf-Gc	BLKD	R
9	Common analogies (speed)—CMRsp	20	6	CMR	Gf-Gc	R	
10	Common analogies (level)—CMRlv	15	6	CMR	Gf-Gc	R	
11	Abstruse analogies (level)—ACMRlv	15	6	CMR	Gc	INF	V
12	Nonsense syllogisms—Rs	15	4	Rs	Gc	R	V
13	Vocabulary—V	24	6	V	Gc	VOC	V
14	Controlled associations—Fa	4	4	Fa	Gc		
15	Letter span forward—Msf	12	5	Ms	Gf	DIG	M
16	Number span backward—Msb	12	5	Ms	Gf	DIG	M

Note.—Most of the abbreviations for primary abilities are either those suggested by French, Ekstrom and Price (1963) or Guilford (1967) or are minor variations on these.

Morrell & Morrell, 1966; Rhodes et al., 1969; Vaughan, Costa, Gilden, & Schimmel, 1965), the role of these variables in the relationship between LAEP and intelligence was also investigated.

METHOD

Description of the Sample

The sample consisted of 108 paid subjects obtained from businesses, personal contacts, welfare agencies, and universities in the Denver area. Their ages ranged 16-68 yr. old. There were 60 males and 48 females. In acquiring this sample an attempt was made to achieve variation in occupation, age, sex, and socioeconomic class, in order to ensure that there would be satisfactory variance in the abilities and AEP measurements.

Group Testing

A battery of 16 ability measures was administered to groups of between 20-30 subjects.

The tests used to measure intellectual abilities are listed in Table 1. Also included in the table is a summary of primary and second-order factors obtained in previous investigations which utilized these tests. The tests were selected to provide for reliable and broadly valid measurement of fluid intelligence (Gf) and crystallized intelligence (Gc) and simpler processes, such as apprehension span (Ms), visual perceptual speediness (P), and visualization (Vz). In addition, entirely new tests were constructed in accordance with the principles described by Furneaux (1952, 1961) to provide for

separate speed and level measurements of fluid intelligence in induction (I), conceptual configural relations (CFR), and conceptual semantic relations (CMR). Furneaux had provided for separate speed and level scores only in a letter series test (I). Here, operationally independent speed and level measurements were obtained through the use of matrices and verbal analogies tests, as well as through the use of letter series.[3]

Individual Testing

Apparatus. The apparatus for the EEG and AEP recordings was a Model 78 Grass 16-channel polygraph, 12 channels of which were utilized in this study. Thirteen Grass gold-plated electrodes were attached to various areas on the subject's head and were connected to the amplifiers or polygraph channels by way of a jack box located in the room with the subject.

A Larkins evoked response programmer (ERP) triggered a Grass Model PS-1 photostimulator set

[3] The basic idea of Furneaux's technique is to provide, on the one hand, a measure in which the complexity or difficulty with which one successfully copes is assessed (in the level, or power measure) and, on the other hand, the average rate of successfully solving problems of moderate difficulty (as the speed measure). The level measure is obtained by cycling items according to difficulty and grading the subject according to difficulty level worked successfully, regardless of the number of problems solved. In obtaining the speed measure, a record of the speed at which the subject worked is kept and from this is derived an estimate of the rate of production of correct answers.

EVOKED POTENTIALS AND INTELLIGENCE

at an intensity of 1 producing a 10 μsec. flash of light. The lamp itself was encased in a wooden box and packed with insulating material to prevent the subject from hearing the click produced by the activation of the lamp.

Two of the EEG channels were connected to a Nuclear Data Enhancetron 1024 and monitored on a Tektronix 564 storage oscilloscope. The ERP also activated the Enhancetron to sweep.

The AEP measures were plotted on a Mosley Model 2-D-2M X-Y plotter, and a Grass Model SWC-1 square-wave calibrator and Hewlett Packard attenuator were used in calibration of the plotter.

A marker device leading from the ERP to one of the polygraph recording channels was used to indicate onset of Enhancetron sweep. A microswitch connected to a series of timers located on the ERP was utilized in measuring the subject's reaction time (SRT).

All of the apparatus was housed in a copper-shielded and grounded room approximately 12 × 15 ft. The equipment was separated from the subject by a sliding cooper-screened door which in turn was covered with a dark curtain to prevent the subject from seeing the equipment lights, the experimenter, and the apparatus.

An air-conditioning fan served as a masking device which prevented the subject from hearing extraneous sounds.

Procedure. Prior to the start of a test session a 5-μv. square-wave calibration signal was put through the entire system, averaged over a 1 sec. sweep time for 100 trials, and printed out on the X-Y plotter.

The electrodes were attached to the subject's scalp using electrode cream. These were located in the following positions (according to the 10-20 international system): F_4, C_4, P_4, O_2, F_3, C_3, P_3, O_1. Three additional electrodes were used to monitor the subject's eye movements and a ground electrode was located on the forehead. An A_1 electrode (left ear lobe or mastoid area directly behind ear) was used as a reference for checking electrode impedence.

Following attachment of the electrodes, the subject was placed on a bed in a supine position with head resting on a pillow and tilted slightly forward. The photostimulator lamp was located directly overhead approximately 11 in. from the subject's eyes.

The AEP amplifiers had a band pass of 3-200 Hz. with specific 60 Hz. filtering. Electrode impedence was measured periodically throughout the course of the experimental session and maintained below 5,000 ohms. After the initial measure of electrode impedence all lights were turned off. The only remaining sources of light were from equipment in the experimental room. A flashlight covered with a red filter was used whenever illumination was needed.

The subject was instructed to keep his eyes focused on a circular luminous disc approximately 1 in. in diameter attached 3-3.5 in. in front of the center of the stimulator lamp. This procedure was utilized so that the subject would not have to focus directly at the lamp but rather have his eyes in a comfortable position with the lids partially closed.

Testing conditions. Twenty-four adaptation trials were presented at the beginning of an experimental session. These consisted of two sets of 12 flashes (one set with the subject's eyes closed, the other with eyes open) which occurred randomly with an interstimulus interval (ISI) of 1-4 sec. This random ISI was maintained for all experimental conditions. These 24 trials were used to acquaint the subject with the experimental situation, to allow the subject's eyes to dark-adapt further, and to acquire an index of the subject's EEG with eyes closed.

The EEG was recorded between the following pairs of electrodes: F_4-C_4, C_4-P_4, P_4-O_4, F_4-P_4, F_3-P_3, F_3-C_3, C_3-P_3, and P_3-O_1. Eye movements were measured between FP_1-PG_2, and from PG_2-FP_2.

The AEP was recorded between F_4-P_4 and F_3-P_3. The F_4-P_4 placement is equivalent to that used by Ertl (1968; Ertl & Schafer, 1969). The AEP measures for both cerebral hemispheres were recorded simultaneously by means of the dual input option provided by the Enhancetron.

Three experimental conditions followed the adaptation trials. In each condition the amplifier settings and electrode placements were the same as previously described. The AEPs were obtained for 100 light flashes for each of the three conditions.

In the first condition, called the "high extrinsic activation" (HEA) condition, the subject was required to press a button in response to the light stimulus which occurred 250 msec. *after* the Enhancetron began the sweeps upon which the AEP record was based. The equipment was wired to eliminate recordings that might result from false anticipations, i.e., button presses occurring before onset of the stimulus. The SRT was recorded for these 100 trials.

The second condition was the "medium extrinsic activation" (MEA) condition. The subject was required to keep count of the light flashes. In all other respects, this condition was like HEA. It occurred 5-10 min. after the HEA condition.

The third condition was the "intrinsic activation" (IA) condition. The subject was required to lie quietly and attend to the light stimulus. This condition followed the MEA condition by 5-10 min.

The EEG and eye-movement recordings provided an index of alertness based upon traditional techniques. The records obtained in each condition were rated by a highly experienced EEG expert[4] who used a 6-point scale to represent different arousal states. A score of 1 indicated EEG signs

[4] Grateful thanks are extended to David Metcalf for performing this function as well as providing laboratory facilities and much helpful advice throughout the course of the study.

DAVID WM. SHUCARD AND JOHN L. HORN

associated with drowsiness, a score of 6 indicated signs of extreme alertness, and scores between these extremes indicated intermediate levels of alertness.

In addition to EEG and eye-movement measures of alertness, an attempt was made to obtain subjective measures of alertness during the evoked potential session through the use of a brief questionnaire administered to the subject following each experimental condition.

AEP Scoring and Preliminary Data Analysis

The latencies and amplitudes of the first five AEP peaks and troughs were determined for all conditions of the study by measurements in millimeters which were converted to milliseconds (for latencies) and microvolts (for amplitudes). A complete description of the procedures for determining the AEP components is provided in a separate article (Shucard, Horn, & Metcalf, 1971); hence, these will be described only briefly here. A 250 msec. Enhancetron sweep preceding onset of the stimulus was used to establish a maximum base rate of activity (base-line band) in this period and two-thirds of this base-line band was then used as the unit of change in potential needed to indicate an AEP component. The application of this procedure is illustrated in Figure 1.

Once AEP components were identified, latency and amplitude (AEPA) measures were obtained and from these the various representative LAEP and AEPA variables were selected for use in the final analysis (see below).

Several analyses were carried out prior to the main analysis in order to establish reliabilities, esti-

mate the independence (or lack of same) of subsets of variables, combine variables (to reduce the number of variables), and choose the most salient and theoretically meaningful measures for further analysis. In these analyses only the internal structure of variables was considered. That is, the selection of a variable for use in the final analysis was based on its reliability and on how well it represented those variables in the domain (behavioral or physiological) from which it came. For example, the interrelationships among the various LAEP measures were considered on their own without calculating the correlation between those measures and the ability measures.

As a rough check on the assumption that the selected tests would measure separate factors identifiable as Gf and Gc, a factoring of the 16 measures derived from the ability tests was carried out. The number of factors was estimated as two according to the procedure suggested by the Horn (1965) modification of the Guttman-Kaiser-Dickman rationale for estimating the number of factors. The first two principal components were determined and rotated, first in accordance with the Varimax (Kaiser, 1958) criterion, then by the Promax procedure (Hendrickson & White, 1964) with power set arbitrarily at 5, and finally by visual plot, taking account of the positive manifold considerations suggested by Thurstone (1947).

The results were quite similar for all three rotations. The variance for the two factors was about the same (4.60 and 4.52 for Gf and Gc, respectively) and the correlation between the two dimensions was about .50 (as determined from the visually rotated solution). In general, the results provided good support for the expectations con-

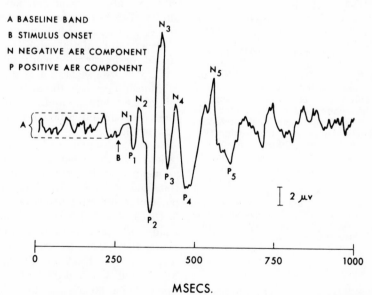

Fig. 1. Illustration of AEP scoring for an actual subject used in this study.

TABLE 2

ABILITY MEASURES COMBINED TO FORM BROAD ABILITY VARIABLES

Ability variable	Test measures combined to yield ability variable
Omnibus general ability (G)	All ability measures listed below
Fluid intelligence (Gf)	Number correct on number span backward test (Msb)
	Speed, level, and accuracy[a] on letter series speed test (Isp, Ilv, Iac, respectively)
	Speed and level on matrices test (CFRsp, CFRlv)
	Speed and level on common analogies (CMRsp, CMRlv)
Fluid intelligence speed (Gfsp)	Isp, CFRsp, CMRsp
Fluid intelligence level (Gflv)	Ilv, CFRlv, CMRlv
Crystallized intelligence (Gc)	Number correct on wide range vocabulary test (V)
	Performance on nonsense syllogisms test (Rs)
	Level of performance on abstruse analogies test (ACMRlv)
	Number correct on mathematical mixed operations test (N)
	Performance on mathematical word problems test (R)
	Number correct on verbal association test (Fa)
Perceptual speediness (Gs)	Number correct on crossing out numbers test (P)
Visualization (Gv)	Number correct on line following test (Vz)
Association fluency (Fa)	Fa
Memory span (Ms)	Msb

[a] A measure obtained by rescoring the letter series speed test for number correct.

cerning which tests would measure Gf and Gc (see Table 1).

The factoring served mainly to attest to the hardiness of the Gf-Gc factorial distinction and to provide support for the plan to combine test scores to yield broad measures of Gf and Gc. Table 2 illustrates the test scores used in the factor analysis and the manner in which they were combined to yield the broader ability measures used in the final analyses. The ability variables were operationally defined as the sum of the unweighted standard scores of number span backward (Msb), induction-speed (Isp), level (Ilv), and accuracy or number of correct answers on the induction speed test (Iac), conceptual figural relations (CFRsp and CFRlv), and conceptual semantic relations (CMRsp and CMRlv). Crystallized intelligence was measured by the unweighted sum of standardized subscores representing the abilities known as verbal comprehension (V), formal reasoning (Rs), esoteric conceptual relations (ACMRlv), numbers (N), general reasoning (R), and association fluency (Fa). Clearly, both Gf and Gc represent reasonably good measures of intelligence as this concept is usually conceived and operationalized. Separate measures of perceptual speediness (P or Gs), visualization (Vz or Gv), associational fluency (Fa), and memory span (Ms) were also included in the final analyses as well as separate measures for scores obtained under Furneaux-type speed conditions (Gfsp) and Furneaux-type level conditions (Gflv).

RESULTS

The selected measures were intercorrelated by the product-moment procedure.

There are several things worth noting about the results. First, the correlations were in the "expected" direction. That is, all but 2 of 300 correlations between ability measurements and AEP latency for both negative and positive peaks obtained across all three experimental conditions were negative: Long AEP latency was associated with low ability, short latency with high ability. The correlations ranged between .05 and −.32, with most hovering around −.15. With a sample of 100 subjects, correlations of .195 or larger are significant at the .05 level. Thus the suggestion is that there is a relationship between the cortical evoked potential and human abilities, but that the linear correlation which represents this is not very large.

Second, the number of noteworthy correlations with later component LAEP measurements was different for the three conditions under which AEPs were obtained. In particular, directing attention to the LAEP 3, LAEP 4, and LAEP 5 measures derived from both positive and negative components, there were 9 correlations of .19 or larger in the HEA condition, 11 in the MEA condition, and 32 in the IA condition (there being 60 possible under each condition). More specifically, if only correlations

DAVID WM. SHUCARD AND JOHN L. HORN

TABLE 3

INTERCORRELATIONS AMONG ABILITY AND POSITIVE LAEP MEASURES

LAEP measure	Ability measure								
	G	Gf	Gc	Gv	Gs	Fa	Gfsp	Gflv	Ms
HEA condition									
P₁	18	13	*23*	*19*	05	*25*	06	15	12
P₂	15	12	*21*	08	08	18	07	04	18
P₃	13	11	15	07	08	12	03	09	09
P₄	*22*	*19*	*21*	*19*	*21*	10	16	16	12
P₅	17	16	15	14	17	01	15	12	14
MEA condition									
P₁	11	08	*20*	03	00	*28*	00	00	*26*
P₂	14	09	*22*	03	06	*25*	05	04	13
P₃	13	09	18	08	04	07	04	06	11
P₄	*24*	*20*	*25*	*23*	*20*	10	13	*19*	14
P₅	13	09	14	11	12	00	07	09	07
IA condition									
P₁	*21*	*20*	*19*	18	17	12	11	*19*	11
P₂	*20*	17	*25*	07	06	*21*	13	09	*19*
P₃	*19*	*19*	18	13	11	10	13	11	*26*
P₄	*26*	*24*	*22*	*22*	*24*	13	*20*	18	*24*
P₅	*26*	*25*	*23*	*19*	*19*	10	*22*	*20*	*20*

Note.—All correlations are in the negative direction and have decimal points removed. Significant correlations are in italic.

with G, Gf, and Gc are considered, 3 of 18 correlations were .19 or larger for the HEA condition, 4 of 18 were of this size for the MEA condition, and 14 of 18 were this large for the IA condition (the other correlations in this case were very near to .19). Considering only the positive LAEP 3, LAEP 4, and LAEP 5 measures, three of nine correlations were significant with G, Gf, and Gc for the HEA condition. In the IA condition, on the other hand, eight of the nine correlations were significant. These relationships are illustrated in Table 3.

Because there were no major differences between the results obtained with negative and positive AEP peak latency measures, only the results for the positive peaks are presented in Table 3. Significant correlations have been italicized in order to focus attention on the pattern of noteworthy correlations. It is this pattern which appears to be significant in the present study, not any particular "significant" correlation. It appears that when AEP measures are recorded under conditions which would seem to produce low alertness, low arousal, or low attention to stimuli, the correlations between latency of the evoked potential and intellectual abilities are increased relative to correlations obtained under conditions of externally enforced arousal, alertness, or attention.

There were no patterns of significant correlations between amplitude AEP measures and abilities, although amplitude measures correlated around .3 to .4 with independent latency measures. Amplitude did not correlate at a noteworthy level with reaction time or with the EEG ratings of arousal; that amplitude measures very likely have something to do with arousal–attention, however, is indicated by the finding that mean amplitude, over the entire sample, decreased significantly between the HEA and IA conditions ($t = 2.66$, $df = 214$, $p < .01$ for left hemispheric measures; $t = 2.22$, $df = 214$, $p < .05$ for right hemispheric measures).

The EEG ratings of arousal had significant negative correlations with the LAEP measures obtained for the N_1 component in each of the three conditions in which the AEP was recorded (a high arousal score being associated with a short AEP latency), but these ratings did not correlate to a noteworthy degree with the ability measures or any other LAEP measures.

The magnitude of correlations between late LAEP measures and Gf was, in general, no larger than the magnitude of the correlations between LAEP and Gc. The sum of all the Gf correlations with LAEP measures was 1.73 for the IA condition, while the corresponding sum for Gc was 1.72.

There were no noteworthy differences between the LAEP correlations obtained for the separate speed and level component measures of Gf. The correlations in these cases tended to be somewhat lower than the correlations obtained for the overall Gf measure, this probably reflecting the somewhat lower reliabilities of the component measures.

The correlations between LAEP measures and the simple perceptual speediness (Gs), visualization (Gv), and memory span (Ms) variables also were somewhat lower than the correlations between LAEP and Gf and Gc. Once again this could reflect lower reliability for the elementary tests as compared to the broader composite measures.

These results indicate that LAEP relates not only to complex intellectual abilities such as Gf and Gc, but also to processes that are as simple as those represented by Gs, Ms, and Gv. If the correlation between LAEP and the complex measures is due primarily to the relation between LAEP and the simpler processes, then partialing the variance associated with a simple measure in the correlation between LAEP and the complex measure should reduce the correlation substantially, perhaps to zero.

Partial correlations between LAEP and Gf and Gc were calculated using each of the above-mentioned simple variables, individually and collectively, in the partialing. For example, in the correlation between LAEP and Gf, visualization (Gv) was partialed first by itself, reducing the correlation (absolute value) between the average latency for positive peaks and Gf in the IA condition from .26 to .17. When Gv was partialed in company with Ms, the correlation was reduced further to .08, a correlation that is not significantly different from zero. The results from the partialing analysis are summarized in Table 4.

The results indicate that the partialing of any one of the simple variables reduced the correlation between LAEP and Gf or Gc by about .10; that is, the correlations tended to be reduced from a value larger than the "significance" level to a value below this— the above-mentioned reduction from .26 to .17 being typical. Partialing of two or more variables tended to reduce the correlation by about another .05 to .10. There was some suggestion that the Gf–LAEP correlations were reduced more by this partialing than were the Gc–LAEP correlations, but the differences were small and one would not want to imply that this was any more than a trend that needs to be examined more carefully in follow-up study.

The correlations between LAEP and simple reaction time (SRT) were, in general, quite small (absolute value), and in a direction indicating that long latency of the evoked potential was associated with fast reaction time. Partialing reaction time did

TABLE 4
PARTIAL CORRELATIONS BETWEEN ABILITY MEASURES AND AVERAGE LATENCY FOR POSITIVE PEAKS IN THE IA CONDITION

Variable partialed	Abilities							
	G	Gf	Gc	Gv	Gs	Gfsp	Gflv	Ms
O	28	26	25	21	21	21	20	25
Gv	18	17	17		10	12	07	20
Gv + Ms	11	08	12		07	08	04	
O	28	26	25	21	21	21	20	25
Ms	18	16	17	14	24	13	16	
O	28	26	25	21	21	21	20	25
Gfsp	18	16	16	12	09		09	19
O	28	26	25	21	21	21	20	25
SRT	31	30	28	23	24		22	26
O	28	26	25	21	21	21	20	25
Gs	18	17	18	11		10	10	20
Gs + SRT	22	20	21	14		13	12	21
Gs + SRT + Ms	15	12	15	12		09	08	
Gs + SRT + Ms + Gv	11	07	12			07	03	
O	28	26	25	21	21	21	20	25
Age	21	19	22	14	12	13	13	21

Note.—Decimal points are omitted, all correlations are negative.

not affect the correlations between LAEP and abilities to any noteworthy extent.

Since age varied in this sample of subjects, the relationship between LAEP and abilities was considered with age partialed. It can be seen that the effect of partialing age out of this relationship was to reduce the correlations, although the overall relationship between LAEP and Gf and Gc was maintained. The removal of age appeared to have its major influence on the less complex abilities such as visualization, perceptual speed, intellectual speed, and intellectual level.

DISCUSSION

The results of this study indicate that the relationship between latency of the evoked potential and intellectual abilities is a replicable phenomenon and that LAEP may mirror long-term central nervous system differences. The general trends of the correlations in all conditions, and particularly in the IA condition, support the findings of other investigators.

The fact that the correlation between abilities and LAEP measures did not approach a magnitude comparable to that found in previous studies until the low-arousal (IA) condition was imposed, indicates that the relationship is due, in part, to evoked potential individual differences which appear most reliably when conditions producing arousal are uniformly low. Under conditions which impose arousal, the LAEP for duller subjects becomes more comparable to that for brighter subjects and the correlation between LAEP and ability drops. A number of interpretations of this finding are possible.

The interpretation stemming from the original hypothesis is that bright subjects—subjects who score relatively high on tests that are widely accepted as indicating intelligence—tend to maintain their alertness even during the rather boring IA condition, whereas the duller subjects tend to be less able or perhaps less willing to maintain alertness during the IA condition. This implies then, that short evoked potential latency represents, in part, intellectual alertness that can be either self-induced or induced by external conditions. According to this interpretation, brighter subjects are better able to remain alert throughout conditions of low arousal, whereas dull subjects do not or cannot thus motivate themselves. However, they can be forced to a level of alertness comparable to that of bright subjects by requiring them to perform a task that demands attention to the stimulus producing the evoked potential. This interpretation suggests that the longer the testing session over which AEPs are obtained (i.e., the more stimulus presentations) the higher will be the correlation between LAEP and measures of intelligence. This implication is consistent with previous results in which larger numbers of stimulus presentations were used and larger correlations were obtained.

There is, however some evidence which questions the above interpretation. This evidence suggests that the brighter subjects have a tendency to be *less* alert during the IA condition than the duller group. First, the positive correlation between evoked potential latency and amplitude measures indicates that lower evoked potential amplitude is associated with shorter latency. Second, correlations between ability measures and the subject's report of how awake he was during the IA condition were all in the negative direction and ranged from −.31, −.32 and −.20 for G, Gf and Gc, respectively. These relationships indicate that higher ability subjects, more frequently than the duller subjects, reported they were not very alert during the IA condition. Of course the self-report measure of alertness may indicate only that brighter subjects are better able to admit low alertness or are more aware of their change in alertness in going from previous conditions to the IA condition. Nevertheless, the negative correlations between self-reported awakeness and ability measures along with the positive correlation between evoked potential amplitude and latency, suggest that brighter subjects may have been less alert than duller subjects in the IA condition. The interpretation is consistent with the notion that brighter people show greater plasticity or flexibility. According to this notion when higher ability subjects are instructed to relax (as in the IA condition) after completing the more demanding previous tasks (HEA and MEA), they do a better job of relaxing than do the subjects of lesser ability.

This notion of increased flexibility among brighter individuals is not incompatible with the hypothesis that bright subjects are more capable than dull subjects of intrinsically activating themselves. The data suggest that not only are bright subjects more capable of activating themselves but they also have greater ability to decrease their level of activation relative to the duller subject. In other words, brighter subjects are more capable of regulating their state of alertness so that this is appropriate for a particular task. This interpretation in terms of plasticity is consistent with the results obtained by Dinand and Defayolle (1969).

It is important to note that none of these interpretations completely explains the latency–abilities relationship. However, it does appear that changes in the subject's state associated with the experimental conditions influence the magnitude of the relationship between LAEP and abilities and this in part accounts for the results of previous studies. At a practical level, the results suggest that to use LAEP as a predictor of intelligence the arousal state of the subject should be reduced and the conditions of AEP measurement should be carefully defined.

The findings also indicate that LAEP correlates about as much with narrower abilities, such as Gs, Gv, and Ms as with G, Gf, and Gc, although the former are more age dependent. This suggests that what is common to LAEP, to simple abilities and to the complex abilities is some process that can be understood and made operational in terms of relatively simple tests. Support for this implication is provided by partial correlation results indicating that when linear components of the simple abilities are partialed, the correlations between LAEP measures and complex abilities are substantially reduced.

REFERENCES

BARRY, W. M., & ERTL, J. P. Brain waves and human intelligence. In F. B. Davis (Ed.), *Modern educational developments: Another look.* New York: Educational Records Bureau, 1965.

BERGER, H. Uber das elektrekephalogramm des menschen. *Archiv für Psychiatrie und Nevenkrankheiten*, 1929, **87**, 527–570.

CHALKE, F. C. R., & ERTL, J. P. Evoked potentials and intelligence. *Life Sciences*, 1965, **4**, 1319–1322.

DINAND, J. P., & DEFAYOLLE, M. Utilisation des potentiels évoqués moyennés pour l'estimation de la charge mentale. *Agressologie*, 1969, **10**, 525–533.

DONCHIN, E., & LINDSLEY, D. B. Average evoked potentials and reaction times to visual stimuli. *EEG Clinical Neurophysiology*, 1966, **20**, 217–223.

ELLINGSON, R. J. Brain waves and problems of psychology. *Psychological Bulletin*, 1956, **53**, 1–34.

ELLINGSON, R. J. Relationship between EEG and test intelligence: A commentary. *Psychological Bulletin*, 1966, **65**, 91–98.

ERTL, J. P. Evoked potentials, neural efficiency and I.Q. Paper presented at the International Symposium for Biocybernetics, Washington, D.C., 1968.

ERTL, J. P., & SCHAFER, E. W. P. Brain response correlates of psychometric intelligence. *Nature*, 1969, **223**, 421–422.

FRENCH, J. W., EKSTROM, R. B., & PRICE, L. A. *Manual for Kit of Reference Tests for Cognitive Factors.* Princeton, N. J.: Educational Testing Service, 1963.

FURNEAUX, W. D. Some speed, error and difficulty relationships within a problem solving situation. *Nature*, 1952, **170**, 37–38.

FURNEAUX, W. D. Intellectual abilities in problem solving behavior. In H. T. Eysenck (Ed.), *Handbook of abnormal psychology.* New York: Basic Books, 1961.

GUILFORD, J. P. *The nature of human intelligence.* New York: McGraw-Hill, 1967.

HENDRICKSON, A. E., & WHITE, P. O. Promax: A quick method of rotation to oblique simple structure. *British Journal of Mathematical Statistical Psychology*, 1964, **17**, 65–70.

HORN, J. L. A rationale and test for the number of factors in factor analyses. *Psychometrika*, 1965, **30**, 179–185.

HORN, J. L. The organization of abilities and the development of intelligence. *Psychological Review*, 1968, **75**, 242–259.

HORN, J. L. Organization of data on life-span development of human abilities. In P. B. Baltes & L. R. Goulet (Eds.), *Life span developmental psychology.* New York: Academic Press, 1970 (a).

HORN, J. L. Personality and ability theory. In R. B. Cattell (Ed.), *Handbook of modern personality theory.* New York: Aldine, 1970 (b).

JANE, J. A., SMIRNOV, G. D., & JASPER, H. H. Effects of distraction upon simultaneous auditory and visual evoked potentials. *EEG Clinical Neurophysiology*, 1962, **14**, 344–358.

KAISER, H. F. The Varimax criterion for analytic rotation in factor analyses. *Psychometrika*, 1958, **23**, 187–200.

LANSING, R. W., SCHWARTZ, E., & LINDSLEY, D. B. Reaction time and EEG activation under alerted and nonalerted conditions. *Journal of Experimental Psychology*, 1959, **58**, 1–7.

MONNIER, M. Retinal and motor responses to photic stimulation in man: Retinocortical time and optomotor integration time. *Journal of Neurophysiology*, 1952, **15**, 469–486.

MORRELL, L. K., & MORRELL, F. Evoked potentials and reaction times: A study of intra-individual variability. *EEG Clinical Neurophysiology*, 1966, **20**, 567–575.

PLUM, A. Visual evoked responses: Their relationship to intelligence. Unpublished doctoral dissertation, University of Florida, 1968.

RHODES, L. E., DUSTMAN, R. E., & BECK, E. C. The visual evoked response: A comparison of bright and dull children. *EEG Clinical Neurophysiology*, 1969, **27**, 364–372.

SHUCARD, D. W. Relationships among measures of the cortical evoked potential and abilities comprising human intelligence. Unpublished doctoral dissertation, University of Denver, 1969.

SHUCARD, D. W., HORN, J. L., & METCALF, D. An objective procedure for the hand scoring of scalp average evoked potentials. *Behavioral Research Methods and Instrumentation*, 1971, **3**, 5–7.

THURSTONE, L. L. *Multiple factor analyses.* Chicago: University of Chicago Press, 1947.

DAVID WM. SHUCARD AND JOHN L. HORN

Vaughan, H. G., Jr., Costa, L. D., Gilden, L., & Schimmel, H. Identification of sensory and motor components of cerebral activity in simple reaction-time tasks. *Proceedings of the 73rd Annual Convention of the American Psychological Association*, 1965, **1**, 179–180.

Vogel, W., & Broverman, D. M. Relationship between EEG and test intelligence: A critical review. *Psychology Bulletin*, 1964, **62**, 132–144.

Vogel, W., & Broverman, D. M. A reply to "Relationship between EEG and test intelligence: A commentary." *Psychology Bulletin*, 1966, **65**, 99–109.

Vogel, W., Broverman, D. M., & Klaiber, E. L. EEG and mental abilities. *EEG Clinical Neurophysiology*, 1968, **23**, 166–175.

Weinberg, H. Correlation of frequency spectra of averaged visual evoked potentials and verbal intelligence. *Nature*, 1969, **224**, 813–815.

(Received December 16, 1970)

From M. R. Rosenzweig (1964). Kansas Studies in Education, *14*, 3–34, *by kind permission of the author and University of Kansas*

Effects of Heredity and Environment on Brain Chemistry, Brain Anatomy, and Learning Ability in the Rat[1]

Mark R. Rosenzweig
Professor of Psychology, University of California, Berkeley

Why does a researcher in animal behavior and physiology presume to address a group interested in mental retardation? In my own case, at least, it is certainly not because I bring solutions to the problems in this field. Rather it is because I believe that only a broad attack on understanding of the physiology of learning will eventually provide knowledge applicable to many questions about learning, including those of mental retardation. Believing this, I would like to tell you about some research underway on the physiology of learning, while cautioning you against expecting early applications to mental retardation. Although this research was not undertaken with retardation in mind, I am happy to be able to describe it here, and I look forward to your comments and reactions.

Before coming to the research, let us consider briefly how retardation is related to learning, and secondly, why animal subjects must be employed in many approaches to the study of brain mechanisms in learning. Since these questions are relevant to several of the presentations in this symposium, I feel called upon, as the first speaker, to bring them up at the outset. Retardation is often defined in terms of a range of scores on an intelligence test. Some workers use the I.Q. range of 50-75; for others, it is anything below 75. The intelligence test items reflect chiefly the knowledge already acquired by the individual; to some extent they may also indicate the ability to solve novel problems. The retarded child shows an increase from year to year in the number of test items he can answer successfully, but the increase is slower than that of the normal child. Furthermore, the retarded child arrives at a ceiling of mental age, about three per cent of American children apparently being destined not to reach a mental age of 12. Retardation is thus characterized by slowness in rate of learning and limitation in complexity of what can be learned. Understanding of retardation could undoubtedly be deepened and extended by finding what physiological processes in the brain underlie learning and how these processes can be facilitated or inhibited.

Research on the physiology of learning is being pursued in many laboratories, both psychological and physiological, and chiefly with animal subjects. The use of animal subjects complements and extends the scope of research with human subjects. It permits experimentation on hereditary factors in learning ability—experiments which the long human life span would make extremely time-consuming, even if they could otherwise be arranged. It permits the use of physiological and surgical interventions which can be better

---

[1] This research was supported in part by grants from U.S. Public Health Service, Surgeon General's Office, and National Science Foundation. It also received aid from the U.S. Atomic Energy Commission.

Kansas Studies in Education

controlled and evaluated than the hereditary and clinical accidents that occur in man. It permits complete control over the environment and training of the subjects, thus facilitating research on the effects of early experience on both cerebral development and later learning ability. For these reasons, the greatest amount and generally the most technically refined research on the physiology of learning is being done with animals.

The wealth of material from animal experimentation is reflected in J. McV. Hunt's recent book, *Intelligence and Experience* (1961).* Hunt cites both animal and human studies in attempting to decide whether it is correct to regard a person's intelligence as fixed and its development as predetermined. (This is a question to which we will return in the latter part of this paper.) Hunt gives a prominent place in his discussion to Hebb's (1949) theories and to animal experiments of the McGill psychological laboratory.

At the same time, it must be recognized that many workers in the field of retardation have been inclined to doubt the relevance of animal studies, when they have mentioned them at all. Thus in reporting various approaches to determining effects of early education of the mentally retarded, Kirk (1958) gave least space to animal studies. He described briefly two experiments from the McGill laboratory "as items of interest with no reference to their application to human development. . . . Designs of experiments with animals can be made much more rigid than those with humans, but it is not known whether inferences from the results are applicable to humans in a natural environment" (pp. 6-7). The caution in extrapolation from one form to another is undoubtedly justified. But I am not convinced (and the organizers of this conference apparently are also not convinced) that the widespread neglect of animal studies is therefore also justified. The rest of this paper will therefore present experimental material that may be of interest and may stimulate the thinking of workers in retardation, even if it cannot be applied directly.

The research will show how both heredity and environment affect brain measures and learning ability. Most of it employs two special strains of rats from our Berkeley colonies. The results come from a collaborative program begun in 1953 and directed by three investigators—Dr. Edward L. Bennett, a biochemist, Dr. David Krech, an experimental psychologist, and myself, a physiological psychologist.[2] Let us consider first hereditary determinants of learning ability and of cerebral measures; environmental determinants will be taken up in a later section of this paper.

---

* A complete citation of all references mentioned may be found in the Bibliography at the end of the article.

[2] Thanks are due to Hiromi Morimoto, Marie Hebert, Barbara Olton, and Ann Orme for help with the chemical analyses and to Carol Saslow for help with the statistical analyses.

Effects of Heredity and Environment

HEREDITARY DETERMINANTS OF LEARNING ABILITY
AND OF CEREBRAL MEASURES

Many of you have heard of the maze-bright and maze-dull strains of rats developed at Berkeley by Robert C. Tryon (1940, 1942, 1963). The present descendants of these strains differ significantly in a large number of behavioral and physiological characteristics. Whether such strains can be considered to differ generally in intelligence is a rather complex question which merits our attention. Because information about these strains is scattered in many references, it will be useful to gather some of this material here, and new unpublished findings will also be added. The currently existing strains are the S_1 and S_3, descendants respectively of the Tryon maze-bright and maze-dull strains. Information about their hereditary background will be given before describing their present status.

TRYON'S GENETIC SELECTION EXPERIMENT

Tryon began his classical study in 1929, taking off from a preliminary investigation of Tolman (1924) and using a 17-unit automatic maze developed by Tolman, Tryon, and Jeffries (1929). Tryon tested a large number of male and female rats of heterogeneous stocks. Males and females with low error scores were then bred together, and so were males and females with high error scores. Among the offspring of the low-error group, those who themselves made few errors were kept for breeding. Similarly, in the other group, those who made many errors were mated. The selective breeding was continued over many generations. By the seventh generation, there was very little overlap between the "bright" and "dull" lines, and further selection through many more generations did not increase the separation. (Tryon's 1940 paper—which appeared in a symposium somewhat like the present one —carried the account through the 18th selected generation, and his 1942 paper, through the 22nd selected generation.) The experiment demonstrated that selection for maze-solving ability could be accomplished in only a few generations, and later experiments have confirmed this (Heron, 1935, 1941; Thompson, 1954). Early in the experiment Tryon introduced color-coding to prevent accidental intermixing of the strains; that is, among the maze-brights, he kept one line with gray coats, and among the maze-dulls, a line with black coats. There were also white lines of both maze-brights and maze-dulls.

With animals of the 22nd generation, Tryon sought to test the possibility that motivational differences between the strains might account for the difference between their error scores in the maze. He therefore ran the following groups: (1) 71 maze-bright rats with "normal" hunger motivation (i.e., receiving the standard goal ration used throughout the selection experiment), (2) 43 maze-brights that had been satiated with extra rations, (3) 71 maze-dulls with "normal" hunger, and (4) 57 maze-dulls whose motivation was heightened because they were on reduced rations and consequently

Kansas Studies in Education

showed a weight loss. The results, which have never before been published, are shown in Figure 1. It is apparent that degree of hunger motivation scarcely affected the error score of either strain (although it did have some effect on running speed). While the satiated maze-brights made slightly higher error scores than those who were normally motivated, they made considerably fewer errors than the dull groups with either normal or heightened hunger. The two dull groups did not differ at all in scores, despite the considerable difference in motivation to run the maze; motivation was evidently not what the dull strain needed to improve their performance.

FIGURE 1

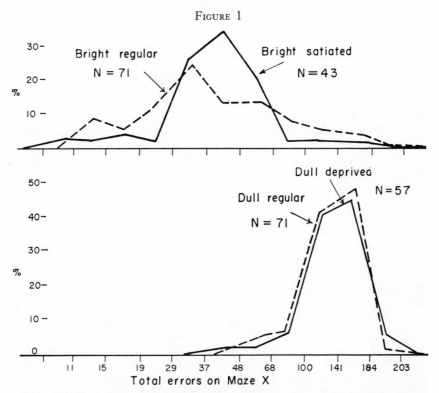

Error scores of Tryon maze-bright and maze-dull rats run under varying motivational conditions. In the maze-bright strain (upper part of figure), rats satiated with extra food did not make many more errors than rats run under the normal deprivation condition. In the maze-dull strain (lower part of figure), rats run under increased deprivation did not differ in error scores from rats run under the normal deprivation condition. Regardless of motivational state, the maze-brights made many fewer errors than the maze-dulls. These results, obtained by Tryon with animals of the 22nd selected generation, have not been published previously.

Other investigators made further observations with the Tryon lines during and shortly after the termination of selection. Krechevsky (1933) studied the "hypotheses" of animals of the seventh selected generation, using an

Effects of Heredity and Environment

unsolvable problem in an apparatus that offered both visual and spatial cues. He reported that the "brights" tended to vary their hypotheses more than the "dulls" and that the "brights" responded more in terms of the spatial cues while the "dulls" responded more to the visual cues.

Hamilton (1935) looked for anatomical differences between the two lines, examining members of the eleventh and twelfth selected generations. Of the several measures of body size and weight taken, Hamilton reported, ". . . brain weight is the only variable in which the bright animals are significantly and consistently greater than unselected animals, and in which dull animals are consistently and significantly smaller than normal animals" (p. 69). (As we will see, the situation is quite different with respect to the S_1 and S_3 lines.)

In 1940, animals of the nineteenth selected generation were placed in the departmental colony as two separate breeding groups, with no further selection pressure. Only the gray maze-brights and the black maze-dulls were taken, so that there would be no chance of accidental intermixing of the lines. Tryon carried on his selection program for several more generations, but did not obtain increased separation of the lines.

Searle (1941, 1949) attempted to determine whether Tryon's maze-bright animals were generally superior to the maze-dulls in learning ability or whether the superiority was confined to the test employed in the selection program. He used animals from the colony stocks, three generations after the Tryon lines had been established in the colony. Ten maze-bright, ten maze-dull, and ten animals of a crossed line were given a variety of tests of learning, activity, and emotional behavior, and patterns of behavior were determined by correlational techniques. This was Searle's conclusion:

"No evidence was found that a difference exists between the Brights and Dulls in the learning capacity *per se*. A detailed study of the behavior profiles indicated that the Brights are characteristically food-driven, economical of distance, low in motivation to escape from water, and timid in response to open space. Dulls are relatively disinterested in food, average or better in water [escape] motivation, and timid of mechanical apparatus features. It is concluded that brightness and dullness in the original Tryon Maze may be accounted for in large part by such motivational and emotional patterns. Although indications exist that the two strains may also be differentiated with reference to certain basic "cognitive" tendencies, the procedures followed in this experiment were not sufficiently analytical to indicate their nature" (1949, p. 323).

It should be noted that Tryon's experiment in which food motivation was varied (cited on p. 5 above) was done at almost the same time as Searle's experiment and employed much larger groups of animals. Tryon's conclusion, it will be recalled, was that error scores were practically independent of food motivation in both strains.

THE S_1 AND S_3 LINES

In 1950 the descendants of the Tryon maze-bright animals were renamed

Kansas Studies in Education

the S_1 line and the descendants of the maze-dulls, the S_3 line. It was clear that in the absence of maintained selection pressure and with the consequent possibility of genetic drift, the resemblance of the existing lines to their ancestors was indeterminate. Because of this, we have not claimed to work with the Tryon lines but only with their descendants.

BEHAVIORAL DIFFERENCES BETWEEN THE S_1 AND S_3 LINES

Since we wanted to test possible relations between brain chemistry and learning ability, we decided to see whether the S_1 line was superior to the S_3 line in learning. We first found that with the unsolvable problems in the Hypothesis Apparatus the S_1 animals responded more in terms of the spatial cues and the S_3 more to the visual cues (Rosenzweig, Krech, & Bennett, 1958), just as Krechevsky had reported for the maze-bright and maze-dull strains in 1933. Furthermore, since all animals tended to respond visually at first in this apparatus, we interpreted the subsequent testing of spatial hypotheses by the S_1s as more adaptive than maintenance of the (unprofitable) visual hypothesis by the S_3s (Rosenzweig *et al.* 1958, p. 351). The original Tryon maze was no longer available, so we tested the two lines under hunger motivation in several alley mazes—the Lashley III maze, the Hebb-Williams maze, and the Dashiell checkerboard maze. The results are shown in Table 1.

On each test the S_1s scored significantly fewer mean errors than the S_3s. Lashley had shown that brain-injured rats made more errors than normals on his III maze, and we found S_3s to make more errors on it than the S_1s. McGaugh and his collaborators have also found the S_1 to excell the S_3 line on the Lashley III maze when trials are massed; with single daily trials, the difference disappears (McGaugh, Westbrook, & Burt, 1961; McGaugh, Westbrook, & Thomson, 1962). On the Dashiell maze, Krechevsky (1937) had found that brain-lesioned rats made more errors and stayed more at the periphery than did normals. In our recent work we found the S_3 line to differ from the S_1 line in the same directions that brain-injured rats differ from normal controls. (See the Dashiell maze results in Table 1.) On the Hebb-Williams maze the S_1s were again superior to the S_3s. It thus appears that the S_3 line learns significantly more slowly than the S_1 line over a variety of alley mazes, suggesting a general difference in problem-solving ability.

The facilitating effects of stimulant drugs on learning may also differentiate the S_1 and S_3 strains, although the findings here are rather complex and show a good deal of situational specificity. McGaugh, Westbrook, and Burt (1961) tested S_1 and S_3 rats in the Lashley III maze, administering either a synthetic strychnine-like compound or a control injection before the daily set of trials. The results, given in the upper part of Table 2, showed that (a) the control S_1s made less than half as many errors as the S_3s, and (b) the drug apparently had no effect on S_1s but improved the learning of S_3s strikingly. McGaugh *et al.* interpreted the results in terms of the perseveration-consolidation hypothesis. They suggested that the S_3s are inferior learners because there is insufficient post-trial reverberation of neural activity and therefore incomplete consolidation. The drug, "by facilitating CNS activity,

Effects of Heredity and Environment

TABLE 1

Mean Errors of S_1 and S_3 Strains on Behavioral Tests and Significance of
Differences

Test	S_1 Strain	S_3 Strain	P
Hebb-Williams			
Errors	66	78	<.01
(N)	(37)	(39)	
Dashiell			
Errors	24	33	<.01
Periph. Units	3.2	3.9	<.01
(N)	(28)	(27)	
Lashley III			
Errors	19	42	<.01
(N)	(14)	(14)	

TABLE 2

Mean Error Scores on Lashley III Maze, with Strain, Drug, and
Spacing of Trials as Variables

	Controls		Drug Injected		Strain	Drug	S×D
	S_1	S_3	S_1	S_3			
Massed trials;	12.9	33.2	15.7	17.3	<.05	<.01	<.05
pre-test injections.	(7)	(13)	(11)	(12)	(including a third strain)		
(McGaugh et al., 1961)							
Single daily trials;	19.4	17.8	5.3	14.9	N.S.	<.005	<.01
post-test injections.	(5)	(12)	(6)	(11)			
(McGaugh et al., 1962)							

increases the amount of intertrial reverberation in the S_3. . . . The effect
of this is to equalize the amount of consolidation occurring on each trial and
thus to eliminate strain differences in learning" (McGaugh et al., 1961, p. 504).
In a further experiment (McGaugh, Westbrook, & Thomson, 1962), the rats
were run for a single trial a day and injections were administered after the
trial. Here (see the lower part of Table 2) the control S_1s were not superior
to the S_3s, but the experimental (drugged) S_1s made far fewer errors than
the S_3s. In discussing these results the authors suggested that in the prior
experiment the S_1 rats might not have showed improvement because their
performance was already near the ceiling for massed trials. The later experiment, they suggested, might indicate strain differences in the effect of the
drug on the total amount of consolidation. In both experiments, we may
note, when one strain was superior—whether this occurred under the control
or experimental condition—it was the S_1 strain that was superior to the S_3.

Kansas Studies in Education

Electroconvulsive shocks given within 30 minutes after each single daily trial impair learning of the Lashley III maze, and the deleterious effect is more pronounced on S_3 than on S_1 rats (Thomson, McGaugh, Smith, Hudspeth, & Westbrook, 1961). This is true even though unshocked control animals of the two strains do not differ in spaced learning. The authors of this experiment suggested that the strain differences in electroconvulsive effect were due to differences in post-trial consolidation, and that the differences in consolidation rate might be mediated by the strain differences in cerebral acetylcholine concentration and acetylcholinesterase activity that will be described on pp. 13-15. (Another possible reason for the difference is that S_3 animals, although having the higher seizure threshold, have more severe seizures than the S_1s—see below, p. 17.)

The S_1 line has also been found to be less active than the S_3 line in rotating wheels (unpublished results of Gordon Pryor). This is similar to one of the findings made by Searle when he compared the Tryon maze-bright and maze-dull strains.

Behavioral differences of quite another sort between the S_1 and S_3 strains were reported by Whalen (1961). He quantified various aspects of the mating behavior of nine males of each of the two strains and found the S_1 to be superior to the S_3 in "mean copulatory efficiency" ($P<.01$). This may, in fact, not be unrelated to the sorts of adaptive behavior we have been considering, since Anderson (1938) found that measures of sexual activity in the male rat correlated significantly with measures of maze-learning ability.

Not all of the available evidence, it should be noted, points to the superiority of the S_1 over the S_3 line. Petrinovitch (1963), using a six-unit visual discrimination apparatus, found the S_1s to be slightly but not significantly better than the S_3s. Strychnine significantly improved learning of both strains, but, while the improvement was somewhat greater for the S_1s, the difference between strains was again not significant.

Rowland and Woods (1961) constructed a replica of the Tryon 17-unit maze at Hollins College, Virginia, and they tested ten S_1 and twelve S_3 animals. They found the S_3s to make significantly *fewer* errors than the S_1s ($P<.025$). While this striking reversal must be taken into account, we believe that a replication under better conditions is in order before much weight is to be put upon the result. For one thing, the number of animals run was small, and, more importantly, there is some reason to believe that they were not functioning at their best. We had shipped animals from Berkeley to Virginia to be used as breeders. For some reason, they did not reproduce well. Therefore eight of the S_1 and eight of the S_3 animals shipped from Berkeley were tested at about 210 days of age. Four S_1 and four S_3 bred at Hollins College were tested at about 90 days of age; two of the S_1s refused to run. It would seem worthwhile to test a larger sample of animals about whom questions of health or emotional status could not be raised.

We have also recently found the S_3 animals to make fewer errors than the S_1s, under rather special test conditions. In order to test problem-solving

Effects of Heredity and Environment

without using hunger motivation, we have constructed an automatic programmed apparatus in which we can present similar sequences of choices to those used in the Krech Hypothesis Apparatus. The rat runs the automated maze to avoid or escape shock. We call the new device ATLAS (Automated Test of Learning And Solving), but so far it has not taken much of a weight off our shoulders. In the manual Hypothesis Apparatus, we have shown (Krech, Rosenzweig, & Bennett, 1962) that animals raised in a complex environment do significantly better than animals raised in a restricted environment. Also, over a series of reversal problems alternating between light and dark cues, the first few were increasingly more difficult and then the animals found the problems increasingly easier. The S_1 and S_3 lines are now being compared (by Lewis Klein) on the reversal discrimination problem, and preliminary results show the S_1s to do somewhat better than the S_3s. In ATLAS, contrary to results with the manual apparatus, the rats tend to make more and more errors on successive problems throughout the problem series; they often seem to ignore the problems we set and to concentrate on escaping the shock swiftly rather than on avoiding it. Furthermore, animals raised in the complex environment actually made significantly more errors in ATLAS than did littermates raised in the restricted environment. The S_1 animals made significantly more errors than the S_3 in the automated maze. (These unpublished results with ATLAS were obtained by Hal Markowitz, James Sorrells, and Frank Harris.) We are now analyzing the data further to determine whether ATLAS can be considered a test of problem-solving ability or whether animals actually receive less shock by ignoring the formal problems that are presented.

The results with different testing devices indicate that caution must be used in generalizing from one situation to another. In spite of the consistent results shown in Table 1, we cannot assert that the S_1 strain will be superior to the S_3 in all problem-solving situations.

Cerebral Differences between the S_1 and S_3 Lines

As they do on specific behavioral measures, the S_1 and S_3 strains differ significantly on a number of cerebral measures—anatomical, chemical, and physiological. Several of the cerebral differences indicate that the S_1 animals, as compared with the S_3, have greater cerebral excitability and a greater capacity to sustain neural activity, but again, as in the behavioral case, the interpretation of the differences is not always simple or clear.

Acetylcholinesterase activity. Our first measures were of activity of the enzyme acetylcholinesterase (AChE) which plays an important role in transmission at many synapses in the central nervous system. When a nerve impulse reaches the end of a neuron, it causes liberation of a chemical mediator or transmitter substance; this chemical messenger diffuses across the synaptic gap in a fraction of a millisecond and initiates excitation of the post-synaptic membrane. At many synapses, the transmitter substance is acetylcholine (ACh). At other synapses, other chemical mediators are used. Even where

Kansas Studies in Education

ACh is not the transmitter, it may play a role in the liberation of the actual transmitter (Koelle, 1962). When ACh is released, it must be destroyed quickly in order that the one-to-one input-output relation across the synapse be preserved. AChE breaks down ACh with great speed. We soon found the S_1 brains to exceed the S_3 brains in AChE activity per unit of tissue weight (Rosenzweig *et al.*, 1958), as can be seen in Table 3. (The number of cases on which each value is based is shown in parentheses below the value.) We then decided to breed selectively for high and low cerebral AChE activity, and a few generations of selection sufficed to breed high and low AChE lines from two foundation stocks (Roderick, 1960). Within the new pairs of strains, behavioral differences were not large, but the strains with *lower* AChE activity tended to do somewhat better on maze tests. In order to characterize the transmitter systems better, we then measured ACh concentration as well.

TABLE 3

Mean Cerebral Values of S_1 and S_3 Strains and Significances of Differences

	S_1 Mean	S_3 Mean	P signif. at or beyond level shown
ACh concentration (in total brain minus cerebellum)[1]	27.3 (16)	24.1 (19)	.001
AChE activity per unit of wt. (total brain minus cerebellum)[1]	168.3 (11)	153.5 (10)	.01
ChE activity per unit of wt. (total brain)[2]	4.12 (12)	3.64 (12)	.001
Serotonin concentration (total brain minus cerebellum)[2]	594 (10)	478 (10)	.01
Total brain wt.[2]	1678 (12)	1912 (12)	.001
Electroshock seizure threshold[3]	23.4 (18)	24.3 (18)	.05
Picrotoxin[4] Seizure threshold, mdn.	1.35	1.80	.02
Lethal dose, mdn.	3.95 (12)	3.05 (15)	.002

[1] Rosenzweig, *et al.*, 1960. [3] Woolley, *et al.*, 1961.
[2] Unpublished data from our laboratory. [4] Burt, 1962.

Acetylcholine concentration. The S_1 line has a significantly greater concentration of ACh than the S_3 line, as Table 3 shows. Moreover, the relative difference in ACh is greater than the relative difference in AChE activity, so that the ratio ACh/AChE is higher in the S_1 than in the S_3 line. In the

Effects of Heredity and Environment

pairs of lines bred for high and low AChE activity, on the contrary, there was little or no difference in ACh concentration. In those lines, then, the ACh/AChE ratio is higher for the low AChE line of each pair. The ratio has the dimension of time required for ACh to be hydrolyzed by AChE, under our conditions of analysis. Within all three pairs of strains (S_1-S_3, and the two Roderick pairs) a higher ratio is associated with better problem solving (Rosenzweig, Krech, & Bennett, 1960). This may mean that somewhat slower hydrolysis and longer action of ACh at the synapse is beneficial, and further tests of this hypothesis are in progress.

Cholinesterase activity. As well as the specific enzyme, AChE, there is a non-specific enzyme that also hydrolyzes ACh. The non-specific enzyme is called cholinesterase (ChE). In the nervous system, ChE is found especially in glial cells while AChE is found principally in neurons. Overall, AChE activity in the brain is much greater than ChE activity. We have recently found the S_1 strain to have significantly more ChE activity than the S_3 strain, just as the S_1s have the greater AChE activity. This may be of functional importance, since the possibility of an active role of the glial cells in learning has recently been suggested by several investigators.

Serotonin. A substance which may be a synaptic mediator and on which much research is being done currently is serotonin. One hypothesis is that it inhibits emotional behavior; another is that it modulates the rate of breakdown of ACh. Gordon Pryor, in our laboratory, has recently found the S_1 strain to have significantly more serotonin per gram of brain than the S_3 strain. Results of one of his unpublished experiments are given in Table 3.

Brain weight. The brains taken for chemical analysis were first weighed, and the S_1 brains were found to be significantly *lighter* than the S_3 brains. Values from a typical experiment are presented in Table 3. (The ChE activity values in the table are based on the same animals.) We have previously shown how brain weights of the two strains develop from about 30 to 150 days of age, the S_3 weights being about one-tenth greater all along the way (Bennett, Rosenzweig, Krech, Karlsson, Dye, & Ohlander, 1958). It will be recalled that Hamilton had found that that the brains of the Tryon maze-bright animals (from which the S_1 are descended) weighed *more* than those of the maze-dulls (from which the S_3 are descended). These contrasting sets of results, perhaps better than any other, emphasize the necessity of considering the present S_1 and S_3 lines to be different from the Tryon lines. The results also indicate that absolute brain weight is not a correlate of learning ability. This conclusion is supported by the finding that the Minnesota maze-bright and maze-dull strains did not differ in brain weight (Silverman, Shapiro, & Heron, 1940). (*Changes* in brain weight may be another matter, as we shall see in a later section.)

The difference of brain weight between the S_1 and S_3 lines does not reflect a difference in body weight, since the two strains are quite similar in body weights. (The Tryon maze-bright line was heavier in both body weight and brain weight than the maze-dull line.)

Kansas Studies in Education

Electroshock convulsive thresholds. Thresholds of seizures with electroshock have been used to study the maturation of brain excitability and the effects of chemical agents on brain excitability. We decided to see whether strain differences existed in these thresholds. The results showed clearly that the S_1 line has significantly lower thresholds than the S_3 and that the two lines have different patterns of convulsive activity (Woolley, Timiras, Rosenzweig, Krech, & Bennett, 1961). The thresholds are given in Table 3. The two pairs of high and low AChE strains were also tested (Woolley *et al.,* 1963) and in each case the strain with greater AChE activity had a significantly lower convulsive threshold than the low-AChE strain from the same foundation stock. In five of the six strains, females had significantly lower thresholds than the males.

Picrotoxin seizure thresholds. Burt (1962) determined both the minimal dose of picrotoxin required to produce seizures and the lethal dose. Significantly less of the drug was needed to produce seizures in S_1s than in S_3s, and in females than in males. These findings are consistent with those on electroshock thresholds which we have just seen. The lethal doses, which were reported only for the males, were significantly *higher* for the S_1 than for the S_3 animals. It is not clear why the S_1s, although their convulsive thresholds are lower, can nevertheless tolerate larger doses than the S_3s without a lethal effect. Perhaps related to the greater mortality of the S_3 animals is the fact that with electroshock as well as with picrotoxin, when stimulation was well above threshold but below the lethal dose, the S_3s had more severe seizures than the S_1s.

Lactic dehydrogenase activity, and percent protein. With strain differences appearing in so many measures, it is worth reporting that there are some aspects in which the S_1 and S_3 brains cannot be distinguished. One of these is in the activity of the enzyme lactic dehydrogenase, which is important in one of the metabolic pathways for utilization of glucose. Using 59 male S_1s and 47 male S_3s, we found significant differences in AChE activity but essentially no difference in lactic dehydrogenase activity (Bennett *et al.,* 1958). Similarly, the percentage of protein in the brain does not differentiate the two strains (Bennett, Rosenzweig, Krech, Ohlander, & Morimoto, 1961).

ARE THERE ANY INTRINSIC RELATIONSHIPS BETWEEN THE BEHAVIORAL AND CEREBRAL DIFFERENCES?

The results we have considered show clearly that there are significant hereditary differences between the S_1 and S_3 lines in both behavior and brain measures. While the existence of the differences is not in doubt, their interpretation is more hazardous. The S_1 animals do solve most problems that we have presented more readily than do the S_3s, but a greater variety of problems and of motivational conditions should be explored before we will be able to generalize about the "intelligence" of the two lines. And perhaps, as Tryon and Searle have claimed, it will not prove possible to generalize, behavior in each situation depending upon a number of specific characteristics. The brains of the S_1 animals are more readily excited, electrically and chemically, than are those of the S_3s, and the S_1 brains are more richly provided with the synaptic transmitter, acetylcholine, and its enzyme of degradation, acetylcholinesterase, than are the S_3s. It is premature to conclude that where behavioral superiority of the S_1s is found, it is due to the greater excitability and chemical endowment of their brains. The long continued inbreeding of the lines may have fixated many characteristics that have nothing to do with maze-solving ability. The possibility of causal relations between brain measures and problem-solving is, however, strengthened by further experiments that we do not have time to discuss here but can only mention. These experiments have shown significant correlations between individual differences in brain chemistry and problem-solving scores *within* single strains (Rosenzweig *et al.*, 1958, pp. 351-3; Krech *et al.*, 1962). Work along this line is continuing in our laboratories.

Environmental Determinants of Cerebral Measures and of Learning Ability

After having studied\ for several years how strain and individual differences in brain chemistry might determine differences in behavior, we decided a few years ago to extend our search and see whether there might be an inverse relation—effects of experience on brain chemistry. Tryon (1940) had projected a study of effects of environmental variations on his two strains: "What sorts of environmental variables of a psychological and biologically pathological character will make hereditarily bright animals dull, and hereditarily dull animals bright?" (p. 118). Although Tryon did not carry out such a study, by now a great number of experiments with animals and human subjects have indicated that richness of training and experience can benefit later problem-solving and intelligence. Many of these studies are cited by Hunt (1961). Is it possible that these types of experience also produce measurable changes in the brain? If so, can it be determined whether the effects of experience on later behavior are actually mediated by the cerebral changes? These were the additional questions we decided to attack.

Effects of Environmental Complexity and Training on Cerebral Measures

Reasons for Predicting Effects of Experience on Brain Chemistry

We have already mentioned our interest in the ACh-AChE system, which is the most thoroughly studied and best known chemical transmitter system in the brain. In the case of many enzymes, synthesis of the enzyme is enhanced by presence of the substrate, and we therefore predicted that increased liberation of the substrate ACh through activation of the nervous system would lead to increased activity of the enzyme AChE. We pointed out that Burkhalter, Jones, and Featherstone (1957) had demonstrated in a chick lung preparation that addition of ACh led to increased activity of AChE. Such modification had not been shown directly in the nervous sys-

Kansas Studies in Education

tem, but in our first publications on this subject—the 1959 Pittsburgh Symposium (Rosenzweig, Krech, & Bennett, 1961) and Krech, Rosenzweig, & Bennett, (1960)—we cited some studies of other workers suggesting that change of AChE activity can be produced in neural tissue: Removal of one optic vesicle from frog larvae led to deficiency of AChE activity in the contralateral optic lobe. This deficiency in AChE activity was chiefly restricted to layers with dense synaptic networks, and an enzyme not specifically involved in neural transmission—succinoxidase—was not significantly affected by the experimental procedure (Boell, Greenfield, & Shen, 1955). Similarly, unilateral transection of the cerebellar peduncles in the rat caused a significant drop in AChE activity of the cerebellar cortex, the drop being greater on the side ipsilateral to the cut than on the contralteral side (Sperti & Sperti, 1959). While both of these studies reduced the neural activity of the brain regions assayed, Pepler and Pearse (1957) attempted to increase neural activity in hypothalamic nuclei of rats by putting animals of one experimental group on a high salt diet and by using lactating rats in another experimental group. In the nuclei related to water excretion and to lactation, the experimental animals were found to have higher AChE activity than control animals.

More recently, Briggs and Kitto (1962) have also hypothesized that enzyme "induction" in the brain may be basic to learning. Referring to our work among others, they have suggested that the reported involvement of RNA in learning may be only what is required to effect altered synthesis of AChE. Smith (1962) has proposed much the same hypothesis.

Our prediction, then, was that enriching the experience of animals would lead to greater central neural activity; that this, in turn, would lead at some central synapses to greater liberation of ACh, and that increased concentration of the substrate would lead to greater activity of AChE.

BEHAVIORAL METHODS

Our basic experimental design called for giving littermate rats differential experience and then sacrificing them for analysis of brain AChE activity. Because we could not predict how much experimental treatment might be necessary to produce observable cerebral effects, we included differences of both home cage environment and formal training, and we maintained these differences over a prolonged period.

The experimental conditions have been described in detail (Krech *et al.*, 1960; Rosenzweig, Krech, Bennett, & Diamond, 1962), so they will be stated only briefly here: One male animal chosen at random from a litter was put at weaning (about 25 days of age) in the Environmental Complexity and Training (ECT) group. Such a group consisted of ten to twelve animals. They lived in a large home cage provided with "toys." Every day they explored an open field apparatus. After about 30 days with this schedule, daily formal training was added. The animals were trained successively in the Lashley III maze, the Dashiell checkerboard maze, and the Krech hypothesis apparatus. Training was for small sugar pellet rewards; food and water were available *ad lib* in the home cage. Each ECT animal had a littermate in the Isolated Condition (IC). The IC rats lived in individual cages where they could not see or touch another animal. The isolation cages were opened a few times a week for addition of food, and the isolated animals were removed for weighing about once a week. It should be remarked that our isolation condition was not as strict as that in Melzack's experiments (to be described later in this symposium) and the behavioral effects on our rats were not at all as severe as those on his dogs. In some experiments, a third animal from each litter led a normal colony life—the Social Condition (SC). In the standard experiments, the differential behavioral conditions were maintained for about 80 days—from 25 to 105 days of age. Variants of the standard conditions will also be described later.

DISSECTION OF BRAIN AND CHEMICAL ANALYSIS

At the conclusion of the behavioral phase of an experiment, the animals were taken to the chemical laboratory and sacrificed for analysis of the brains. The animals were identified only by code numbers which did not reveal what behavioral treatment they had received. The dissection procedures have been described in detail (Rosenzweig *et al.*, 1962). Standard samples of the visual and somesthetic areas of the cerebral cortex were marked off with the aid of a small plastic T-square, as shown in Figure 2. The samples were circumscribed with a scalpel, and peeled from the underlying white matter. Rat cortex can be peeled off rather cleanly from the white matter, as we have shown (see Fig. 1 in Krech, Rosenzweig, & Bennett, 1963). The third sample consisted of the remaining dorsal cortex. The fourth section, labeled "ventral cortex," also includes such associated tissue as the hippocampus, the amygdala, and the corpus callosum. The last sample consisted of all the rest of the brain and included medulla, cerebellum, and olfactory bulbs as well as the core of the cerebrum; this sample is called Subcortex II. As each sample was removed, it was weighed accurate to 0.1 mg and was then frozen on dry ice and stored at —20°C. in a deep freeze until chemical analysis.

The main chemical measure to be reported includes all enzymatic activity that hydrolyzes ACh. This includes both the specific enzyme, AChE, and the less specific enzyme, cholinesterase (ChE). We have shown (Rosenzweig *et al.*, 1958; Bennett, Krech, & Rosenzweig, 1963) that over 95 per cent of the activity in the rat brain is due to AChE, so we will call the overall activity AChE. Our standard procedures of analysis, using an automatic titrator, have been described previously (Rosenzweig *et al.*, 1958). The nomenclature of these enzymes has been confused, and in the past many workers, including ourselves, have referred to both of them as "cholinesterase." Now that a standard terminology has been recommended by the Commission on Enzymes of the International Union of Biochemistry (1961), we are following recommended usage.

Kansas Studies in Education

FIGURE 2

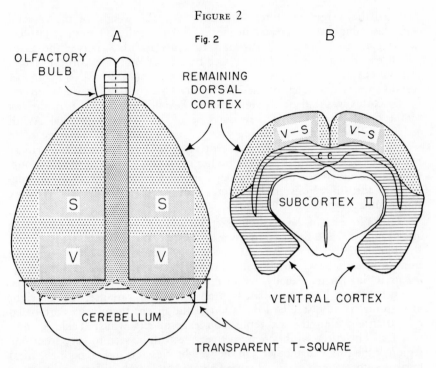

A   Fig. 2   B

OLFACTORY BULB

REMAINING DORSAL CORTEX

V–S   V–S

C C

SUBCORTEX II

S   S

V   V

VENTRAL CORTEX

CEREBELLUM

TRANSPARENT T-SQUARE

Diagrams of the rat brain showing the parts into which it is divided for analysis in our experiments. Fixed samples of visual cortex (V) and of somesthetic cortex (S) are delimited with the aid of a calibrated plastic T-square. (Reprinted from Rosenzweig *et al., J. Comp. Physiol. Psych.*, 1962, 55, 429-37, with permission of the American Psychological Association.)

RESULTS WITH STANDARD ECT AND IC CONDITIONS

Clear effects on brain chemistry were shown in the first experiments comparing brains of littermates kept under enriched or restricted conditions for 80 days after weaning (Krech *et al.*, 1960). These experiments were conducted with rats of six different strains, all of which showed similar effects. In the earlier experiments, only four brain samples were taken. Since then we have used especially the Berkeley S_1 strain, and during the last few years we have accumulated data on 67 littermate S_1 pairs from whom the five brain regions were analyzed.

Effects on AChE activity and tissue weight, S_1 strain. In our earlier experiments, we were puzzled to find that the ECT animals, as compared with their IC littermates, had significantly higher AChE activity in the subcortex but significantly lower AChE activity in the cortex (Krech *et al.*, 1960). The measure of enzymatic activity used in that report was AChE activity *per unit of wet weight of tissue,* a frequently employed measure. Realizing that this measure is as much a function of weight as of enzymatic activity, we later

Effects of Heredity and Environment

analyzed the weight measures and found that the weight of the cerebral cortex was significantly greater in the ECT than in the IC animals (Rosenzweig *et al.*, 1962). For the 67 pairs of S_1 rats, *total* AChE activity of the cortex has increased with enriched experience by 2.2 per cent, but cortical weight increased by 4.8 per cent, so activity per unit of weight decreased by 2.4 per cent in the cortex. (Each of these differences between ECT and IC means for the cortex was statistically significant at beyond the .05 level.) In the rest of the brain (Subcortex II), the increase of 2.1 per cent in total AChE activity with enriched experience was not accompanied by an increase in weight (there was, in fact, 0.9 per cent loss), so subcortical AChE activity per unit of weight was 3.1 per cent higher in the ECT than in the IC group. (While the difference between groups in subcortical weight was not significant, the differences in both total and relative AChE activity were significant at beyond the .001 level.)

Results for each of the five brain sections and for certain combined regions are given in Table 4. For each measure and region, the means of the ECT and IC animals are given. Next is the quotient of these means. Then comes the number of cases in which the value for the ECT animal exceeded the value for its IC littermate. Finally, we give the significance of the difference between ECT and IC groups, based on an analysis of variance. To the right of each mean is the standard deviation of the mean; these values are based on variance within the six replication experiments which Table 4 summarizes. The effects of differential experience can be seen to vary from one region of the cortex to another. On the weight measure and on both chemical measures, the sample of visual cortex shows the largest differences between experimental groups, and the sample of somesthetic cortex shows the smallest closely. In all six experiments, for example, the relative difference between the ECT and IC means was greater for the sample of visual cortex than for the sample of somesthetic cortex—and this for all three measures. On the weight measure, the visual cortical sample was heavier for the ECT than for the IC animal in 53 of the 67 littermate pairs (79 per cent), while for the somesthetic sample, ECT exceeded IC in 43 of the 67 pairs (64 per cent). The greatest consistency was found for total cortex where the ECT animal exceeded its IC littermate in weight in 55 of the 67 cases (82 per cent). The distribution of differences in weight of total cortex between ECT and IC littermates is given in Figure 3. It is clear that these differences in cortical weight are not distributed around zero in a random fashion but rather, in most cases the ECT weight is greater than the IC weight. In contrast, the distribution of differences·in subcortical weight, shown in the lower part of the figure, does not depart significantly from a random distribution.

Where an intermediate SC group was used, the cerebral results generally fell between those of the ECT and IC groups. This indicates that in relation to colony conditions, an enriched environment and training lead to *increases* in cortical· weight and in AChE activity throughout the brain, while impoverished conditions lead to *decreases* on these measures.

TABLE 4

Statistics on Brain Weights and Acetylcholinesterase Activity of 67 Littermate Pairs of S_1 Rats Raised in Environmental Complexity and Training (ECT) or in the Isolated Condition (IC)

| | CORTEX | | | | | | | | | | REST OF BRAIN (Subcortex II) | | TOTAL BRAIN | | Total Cortex (Subcortex II) (×1000) | |
| | Visual Sample | | Somesthetic Sample | | Remaining Dorsal | | Ventral | | Total | | | | | | | |
	M	S.D.	M	S.D.	M	S.D.	M	S.D.	M	S.D.	M	S.D.	M	S.D.	M	S.D.
WEIGHT (mg)																
ECT	62.4	4.1	47.3	3.3	284	18	307	25	701	32	943	42	1644	66	744	32
IC	58.0	4.8	45.8	2.7	271	16	295	27	670	32	952	39	1621	65	704	26
ECT/IC	1.076		1.033		1.049		1.041		1.048		.991		1.014		1.057	
ECT>IC[a]	53/67		43/67		49/67		46/67		55/67		31/67		46/67		55/67	
P	<.001		<.05		<.001		<.01		<.001		N.S.		<.01		<.001	
TOTAL AChE ACTIVITY[b]																
ECT	37.7	3.5	34.8	2.6	212	16	340	34	623	44	1795	109	2416	126	348	26
IC	35.9	4.0	34.1	2.5	206	17	334	26	610	35	1759	96	2367	114	348	22
ECT/IC	1.050		1.021		1.028		1.018		1.022		1.021		1.020		1.001	
ECT>IC[a]	47/66		39/67		41/66		40/66		45/64		43/66		43/63		33/63	
P	<.001		N.S.		<.05		N.S.		<.05		<.001		<.001		N.S.	
AChE ACTIVITY PER UNIT OF WEIGHT[c]																
ECT	60.2	3.8	73.4	3.1	74.6	3.7	111.3	7.1	88.9	4.3	190.5	11.5	147.0	7.1	468	26
IC	61.8	4.2	74.2	3.4	76.0	4.3	114.1	8.6	91.1	4.4	184.8	11.2	145.9	7.1	494	30
ECT/IC	.974		.989		.982		.975		.976		1.031		1.008		.946	
ECT>IC[a]	20.5/66		29.5/67		23.5/66		26.5/66		23/64		49/66		33/63		15/63	
P	<.001		N.S.		<.01		<.05		<.01		<.001		N.S.		<.001	

[a] Number of littermate pairs in which the ECT value is greater than the IC value.

[b] Given in terms of moles acetylcholine $\times 10^8$ hydrolyzed per minute, under our standardized assay conditions.

[c] Given in terms of moles acetylcholine $\times 10^{10}$ hydrolyzed per minute per mg tissue, under our standardized assay conditions.

Effects of Heredity and Environment

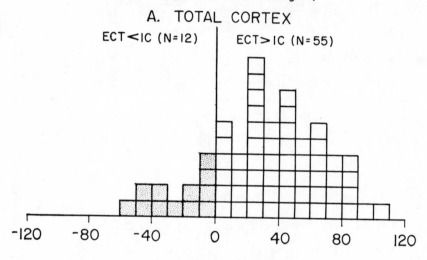

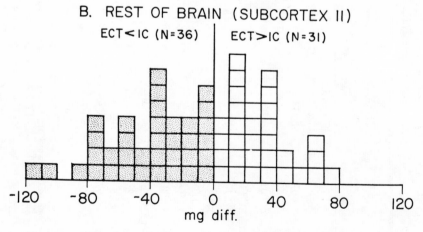

Differences in weight of brain tissue in 67 pairs of littermates of the S_1 strain (ECT weight minus IC weight). Each square represents the weight of tissue from an ECT animal minus the weight of tissue from its IC littermate. For total cortical tissue, the ECT animal has the greater weight in 82 per cent of the pairs, while in the rest of the brain the groups do not differ.

Kansas Studies in Education

ECT-IC differences in the S_3 strain. In our original report on effects of differential experience (Krech *et al.*, 1960), we found smaller effects among 20 littermate pairs of S_3 animals than among 9 pairs of S_1s. Since then, in the experiments in which the five sections of the brain were taken, two experiments have been run with S_3 animals. In each case, the cerebral effects among the S_3s were smaller than those found among S_1s run at the same time. The combined values for the two S_3 experiments are presented in Table 5; this table is set up in the same way as was Table 4 for the S_1 animals.

TABLE 5

Effects of ECT and IC on 21 Littermate Pairs of S_3 Rats Run from from 25 to 105 Days of Age

	TISSUE WEIGHT (mg)		
	Total Cortex	Rest of Brain (Subcortex II)	Total Brain
ECT	774	1074	1848
IC	758	1082	1840
Pairs, ECT>IC	14/21	7/21	12/21
ECT/IC	1.021	.992	1.004
P	<.05	N.S.	N.S.
	TOTAL AChE ACTIVITY		
ECT	598	1801	2399
IC	594	1772	2366
Pairs, ECT>IC	10/21	13/21	12/21
ECT/IC	1.006	1.016	1.014
P	N.S.	N.S.	N.S.

In order to facilitate comparisons of the magnitudes of the ECT-IC differences between the two strains, Table 6 has been prepared. This table shows the percentage by which the ECT mean exceeded the IC mean for each of the measures. It will be seen that for each of the measures in the table, the effect was smaller for the S_3 than for the S_1 line. The interaction of strain and condition is not statistically significant, however, and further experiments are therefore in progress to determine whether the ECT-IC effects are consistently smaller in the S_3 than in the S_1 strain. The completion of these experiments has demonstrated that the brains of the S_1 animals are significantly more modifiable than those of the S_3s (Rosenzweig, Krech, & Bennett, 1964).

MEASUREMENTS OF CORTICAL DEPTH

The surprising finding of an increase in weight of the cortex as a consequence of enriched experience demanded further investigation. Since this

Effects of Heredity and Environment

TABLE 6

*Effects of ECT and IC on Brain Weight and Total AChE Activity
of S_1 and S_3 Rats*

(Percentage Differences between Means, ECT minus IC)

		CORTEX			REST OF BRAIN (Subcortex II)	TOTAL BRAIN
WEIGHT	Visual Sample	Somesthetic Sample	Remaining Dorsal	Ventral		
S_1 (67 pairs)	7.6***	3.3*	4.9***	4.1**	−0.9	1.4**
S_3 (21 pairs)	5.1	0.0	1.8	2.2	−0.8	0.4
TOTAL AChE ACTIVITY						
S_1 (67 pairs)	5.0***	2.1	2.8*	1.8	2.1***	2.0***
S_3 (21 pairs)	4.2	−1.9	0.9	0.3	1.6	1.4

*P<.05, **P<.01, ***P<.001

effect was found even with our standard samples of visual and somesthetic cortex where the surface areas of the samples were held constant, we interpreted the change as one probably occurring in the thickness or depth of the cortex. To test this, we prepared further ECT and IC groups of S_1 animals and delivered them to our neuroanatomical collaborator, Dr. Marian C. Diamond. Dr. Diamond has found the depth of cortex of ECT rats to exceed that of their IC littermates by 6.2 per cent in the visual region and by 3.8 per cent in the somesthetic region (Diamond, Krech, & Rosenzweig, in press). In both cortical regions, the increases in depth were statistically significant at beyond the .01 level. These relative differences in depth correspond well with the relative differences we have found in tissue weight for the same regions (see Table 4). This correspondence of results supports the use of tissue weight as a measure of cortical development in experiments where the tissue must be consumed for chemical analysis. Further histological investigations are also in progress in our laboratories to determine what changes occur in brain cells and in cerebral vasculature as a consequence of differential experience. There are changes in the size of cortical blood vessels that indicate an increased blood supply in the ECT animals.

Changes in ChE with differential experience. In recent experiments we have measured separately the ChE and AChE activities in the brains of ECT and IC animals of both strains (Bennett *et al.*, 1963). To determine ChE and AChE activity we have used a modification of the spectrophotometric method described by Ellman, Courtney, Andres, and Featherstone (1961). AChE activity is measured using acetylthiocholine as the substrate. To measure ChE activity, AChE is first inhibited by a highly specific agent, and butyrylthiocholine is used as the substrate. The results of these analyses have confirmed that our previously announced findings can all be attributed to AChE activity. ChE activity is not only very minor compared with AChE activity, but the *change* in enzymatic activity with experience is also almost completely due to AChE.

Although the contribution of ChE activity to our overall results is thus negligible, ChE activity nevertheless shows its own pattern of change with differential experience. Table 7 gives the relative differences between ECT and IC means for both AChE and ChE activities per unit of weight of tissue. AChE activity per unit weight is lower for the ECT group than for the IC group in the cortex and higher in the subcortex, as we have noted previously. For ChE activity per unit of weight, on the other hand, the ECT animals have significantly higher values than their littermates in the cortex; the subcortex shows no significant differences between groups, although the S_3 animals show a decrease of 3.3 per cent.

The possible significance of the results with ChE lies in the fact, mentioned above, that while AChE is known to occur chiefly in neurons, ChE predominates in glial cells. The occurrence of a significant change in ChE activity with experience may therefore indicate that the glia as well as the neurons participate in cerebral changes with experience. Some additional support for this possibility comes from our histological investigations which suggest an increase in the ratio of glia to neurons in the cortex following enriched experience.

RESULTS WITH VARIANT AND CONTROL EXPERIMENTS

Rather than allow ourselves on the basis of these experiments to accept the rather startling conclusion that differential experience can alter brain chemistry and brain anatomy, we have sought to devise and test alternative interpretations for these findings.

Control experiments for differential handling and activity. It was apparent from the outset that the ECT animals received more handling and engaged in more locomotor activity than their IC littermates. The ECTs are handled every day, while the ICs are handled on the average of only once a week for weighing (and less often in the later stages of the experiment). Handling, at least before weaning, has been shown to produce physiological and behavioral differences in rats. We therefore did a control experiment in which twelve S_1s and twelve S_3s were given several minutes of handling daily while their littermates experienced no handling at all between weaning and sacrifice. The results are being reported elsewhere in detail (Rosenzweig *et al.,* in preparation). They give no indication that differential handling affects our brain measures. A more extensive replication would be desirable, but we have no reason to believe that differential handling can account for our results.

Differential handling introduced *before weaning* may affect the brain. Tapp and Markowitz (1963), working in our laboratories, handled S_3 rats on

Effects of Heredity and Environment

TABLE 7

Effects of Differential Experience on AChE and ChE Activity/mg[1]

(Expressed as Percentage of Difference between Means, ECT minus IC)

AChE Activity (with AcCh)

EXP.	STRAIN	Total Cortex	Subcortex	Total Brain	Total Cortex Subcortex
I	S_1	−2.6	3.5**	1.0	−6.0****
II A	S_1	−0.7	2.6**	1.1	−3.1**
II B	S_3	−3.0**	3.1**	1.1	−5.9****
% cases, ECT>IC		42	79	55	17

ChE Activity (with BuSCh)

EXP.	STRAIN	Total Cortex	Subcortex	Total Brain	Total Cortex Subcortex
I	S_1	5.7**	−1.0	0.0	7.1**
II A	S_1	5.7****	0.2	1.5	5.6****
II B	S_3	4.9***	−3.3	−1.3	8.1***
% cases, ECT>IC		82	44	58	78

AChE Activity (with AcSCh)

	Total Cortex	Subcortex	Total Brain	Total Cortex Subcortex
	−2.6**	2.6	0.8	−5.4*
	−0.9	2.2**	0.7	−2.8**
	−2.6*	1.8	0.0	−4.2**
	29	56	50	21

N=12 littermate pairs in each experiment

*P<.10
**P<.05
***P<.01

[1] From Bennett, et al., 1963.

Kansas Studies in Education

days two through ten *post partum*. These animals developed differences in cerebral weight and AChE activity, as compared with rats from unhandled litters, but the pattern of changes was quite distinct from that seen in our experiments with differential experience.

The ECT animals appeared to be more active than their isolated littermates, although this is based on inadequate observation since we tried to stay away from the IC animals as much as possible. Further evidence for such a difference in activity is the fact that the ECT animals weighed about seven per cent less than the ICs at sacrifice, although all animals had food available *ad lib*. Among rats as among men, an active life is known to result in a lighter, lither form. To test whether differential activity might account for the results we observed, we ran two experiments (Rosenzweig *et al.*, in preparation). In each, animals of one set were confined in small individual living cages; each of these animals had a littermate who could go freely from his cage to a rotating wheel. Comparison of the brain measures of the inactive and active groups showed essentially no differences. Zolman and Morimoto (in preparation) ran a similar activity control experiment for shorter periods of ECT-IC experience that they found to be effective in producing brain changes; their control test also showed no cerebral effects of locomotor activity in the running wheels.[3] We conclude on the basis of all present evidence that neither differential handling nor differential locomotor activity can account for the ECT-IC effects.

Social grouping. Our experimental conditions are also distinguished by the number of animals living together, the ECT cages containing ten to twelve rats; the SC cages, three; and the IC animals being solitary. The number of animals caged together has been shown to affect certain physiological measures, and this is not a matter of the cage-space per animal. We have begun experiments to determine whether social grouping contributes to the ECT-IC effects.

Effects of differential experience among younger and older animals. All of the results we have considered so far were obtained with animals put in the differential conditions at weaning (about 25 days of age). It occurred to us that perhaps the ECT condition was only stimulating and accelerating the growth and development that are characteristic of young animals. In this case, the cerebral effects would not be expected among mature animals. To test this possibility, we put S_1 animals into the ECT, SC, and IC conditions at 105 days of age (the age at which the animals were sacrificed in our standard experiments). Rats of 105 days of age can be considered adult, since they mature sexually at about 70 days, and since brain growth, which never stops completely in the rat, has fallen to a low rate by that age. Prior

---

[3] It may be that activity in a rotating cage does not provide the best possible control condition, since such activity shows little or no correlation with activity in an open field and since the S_1 strain is not very active in wheels. Another control experiment in which the active animal had access to an open field would now seem desirable.

Effects of Heredity and Environment

to the experiment, the animals had lived under colony conditions. Two replications were run, each with twelve sets of triplets. A summary of the results is given in Table 8. It is apparent that the ECT-IC differences were at least as great among the mature as among the younger animals. We conclude that the effects of differential experience do not depend critically upon the (post-weaning) age at which the experience is given.

TABLE 8

Effects of ECT and IC on Brain Weight (mg) of Younger and Older S_1 Rats
(Percentage Differences between Means, ECT minus IC)

| Days Run and N (pairs) | Visual Sample | CORTEX | | | | REST OF BRAIN (Subcortex II) | TOTAL BRAIN |
		Somesthetic Sample	Remaining Dorsal	Ventral			
25-105 days (67 pairs)	7.6***	3.3*	4.9***	4.1**		−0.9	1.4**
105-185 days (24 pairs)	10.7***	2.3	5.4**	6.0**		2.4*	3.9***

*P<.05, **P<.01, ***P<.001

Effects of shorter periods of differential experience. The 80-day period of the standard experiments was settled on originally in the hope that it would be sufficiently long to produce measurable effects. Once these effects had been obtained, experiments were undertaken to determine how they developed over time; in these experiments, different sub-groups were exposed to the experimental conditions for different lengths of time. The results are being presented in detail elsewhere (Zolman & Morimoto, in preparation; Rosenzweig *et al.*, in preparation). Here it is enough to say that significant changes in cortical weight appear after only a few weeks in the different environments but that significant changes in total AChE activity require over 60 days.

HYPOTHESIZED GROWTH OF BRAIN CELLS INDUCED BY EXPERIENCE

Having found consistent changes in cortical weight and depth and in AChE and ChE activity following differential experience, we have been trying to evolve testable hypotheses about changes at the level of brain cells that could account for the changes that we observe in the rather gross blocks of tissue we analyze. Let us sketch briefly here an account that we are now attempting to test. It is framed in terms of increased branching of neurons and multiplication of glia as consequences of increased cerebral activity.

The great neuroanatomist Ramón y Cajal long ago (1895) suggested that cerebral exercise might increase the ramifications of neurons in the brain, thus permitting greater interrelations of mental processes. At the same time he knew that a talented person and even a genius might not have an excep-

Kansas Studies in Education

tionally large brain and might even have a brain of less than average weight. He therefore went on to suppose that, to maintain a fixed cerebral volume while neural processes expanded, there might be a diminution of cell body volume or of the neuroglial framework. We would like to take up Cajal's hypothesis of neural ramification with cerebral activity, but dropping, because of our findings, the restriction that cerebral volume remain unchanged.

As we conceive of this possibility, the outgrowths of neurons would add both bulk and total AChE activity. The volume of the soma might also increase as the extensions of the cell grew, but the growth of the processes would be more important, since the volume of somata is only a small fraction of the bulk of the brain. Ready growth of neural ramifications in the normal brain is suggested by the observations of Rose, Malis, & Baker, (1961). Where one neuron touches another, the membrane is likely to become rich in AChE, as Geiger and Stone (1962) observed in cultures of human brain cells. Previously functional synapses may also become richer in AChE as increased liberation of ACh induces greater synthesis of AChE. Growth of neural processes is probably accompanied by growth and multiplication of glia cells. The glia support the neurons mechanically, form the neural sheaths, and may also exchange metabolites with the neurons. Growth and multiplication of glia would contribute both bulk and ChE activity. Growth of neural prolongations and of associated glial cells with increased cerebral activity would thus account for increased tissue bulk, increased total AChE and ChE activity —all of the changes we have observed in the cortex with enriched experience. If greater growth occurred in the glia than in the neurons, this could account for the rise in ChE activity surpassing that of AChE activity at the cortex.

At the subcortex, enriched experience leads to an increase of AChE but not of ChE activity, and—among the younger animals, at least—it does not cause an increase in tissue volume. Clearly the cellular changes must be different in the cortex and subcortex. Perhaps the subcortical change is restricted to synaptic AChE activity.

Beyond our primary findings, what evidence exists and what is being obtained to test this neural-outgrowth hypothesis? The only further piece of evidence we now possess is that the ratio of number of glial cells to number of neurons increases with the ECT condition. This has been found in both the visual and somesthetic areas in both of our histological studies, but the differences were not statistically significant. Further histological studies are now in progress or in preparation to test aspects of this formulation: (a) Paul Coleman at the University of Maryland is measuring dendritic branching in cortical cells of some of our ECT and IC pairs. (b) Brains of new ECT and IC groups will be imbedded so that accurate measurements can be made of the size of glia and neural somata. Further counts of glia and neurons and measurements of blood vessels will also be made on these brains. These anatomical studies are slow and painstaking, but they offer hope of providing valuable information about how the brain reacts to environmental conditions.

Effects of Heredity and Environment

EFFECTS OF DIFFERENTIAL EXPERIENCE ON PROBLEM-SOLVING ABILITY

While our research on effects of experience has concentrated upon cerebral effects, we have also been interested in effects on problem-solving ability. Many experimenters have shown that rats maintained in an enriched or complex environment make fewer errors, when later tested for learning, than rats maintained in an impoverished or restricted environment. There were several reasons for repeating such experiments in our laboratory: (1) We wanted to be sure whether such behavioral effects would occur with *our* strains of rats kept in *our* versions of enriched and impoverished environments. (2) The difference in problem-solving efficiency of rats from complex and restricted environments has been ascribed by some workers to differences in exploratory tendencies (Woods, Fiske, & Ruckelshaus, 1961). According to this interpretation, rats from complex environments have largely satiated their exploratory tendencies and will settle down readily to solve a maze, while rats coming from a restricted environment will explore a new situation eagerly, and while exploring they will inevitably be piling up a sizeable error score. We hoped to be able to measure learning ability without the contaminating effects of systematically different exploratory tendencies. (3) If these two objectives could be attained, then it would be worthwhile determining in greater detail whether the differential environments affected later learning equally or even similarly in the two strains. Cooper and Zubek (1958), testing McGill bright and dull animals in the Hebb-Williams maze, have demonstrated that strains may respond quite differently to the same environmental conditions. They reported that scores of bright animals were not improved by environmental enrichment (extending from 25 to 65 days of age), but that the scores were impaired by environmental restriction; conversely, their dull animals were benefited by enrichment but were not harmed by restriction. In fact, animals of both strains from the enriched environment had almost equally good scores (suggesting a possible ceiling effect), and animals of both strains from the impoverished environments had identically poor scores. Only when coming from the usual colony condition did the strains differ, the brights then being as able as animals from the complex environment and the dulls being as slow to learn as animals from the restricted environment.

So far we have made good progress on the first two problems listed above, and we hope soon to start on the third. We have used a reversal discrimination problem in the Hypothesis Apparatus to test 15 littermate pairs of S_1s; one animal of each pair was kept from 25 to 55 days of age in our ECT condition and the other, in the IC condition (Krech *et al.*, 1962). The person doing the testing had not been involved in the environmental stage of the experiment and did not know whether a particular animal came from the ECT or the IC condition; this precluded both experimentor bias and also transfer on the part of the animal from earlier to later handler. The results, in Figure 4, show that the groups did not differ on the simple initial problem of going through all lighted alleys. When each animal reached criterion,

Kansas Studies in Education

FIGURE 4

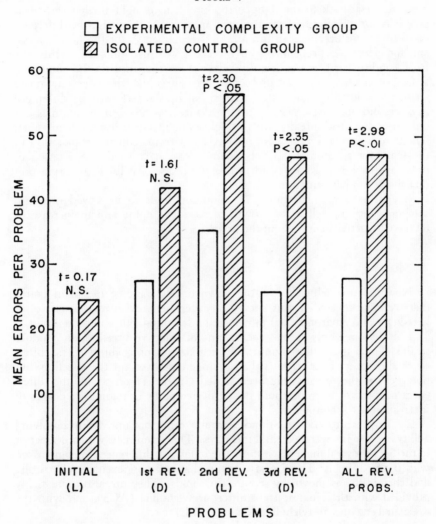

Mean errors on reversal-discrimination problems of S_1 animals that had previously spent one month in either a complex environment (open bars) or in isolation (hatched bars). While the two groups do not differ on the initial problem, the complex experience group is superior on all the reversal problems. The reversals were between light-correct problems (L) and dark-correct problems (D) in the Krech Hypothesis Apparatus. (Reprinted from Krech *et al., J. Comp. Physiol. Psychol.*, 1962, 55, 801-7, with permission of the American Psychological Association.)

it was shifted to the opposite, dark-correct problem. Here difficulty increased and a difference between groups began to appear, but it was still not significant. Reversal back to the light-correct problem brought further difficulty, especially for the restricted-environment animals. At this point the difference between groups became significant, and it remained so for the next reversal and for errors per problem on all reversal problems combined. Thus, the ECT condition led to significantly better scores than did the IC condition, at least on the more difficult problems. We believe that the interpretation in terms of exploratory tendencies is ruled out by the fact that the difference in scores did not arise when the testing device was novel to the animals but only after they had already run through its eight alleys hundreds of times. The thorough pretraining was probably effective in reducing exploration in the maze for all animals. Twelve pairs of S_3s have so far been tested in this way (by Lewis Klein), and in this strain also, the ECT condition produced superior performance.

It appears, then, that the ECT condition leads to improved problem-solving ability as well as to growth of cortical volume and to increase of total AChE activity throughout the brain.

Summary

Now let us conclude by setting down briefly some of the main points that we have covered in this survey of experiments with rats on effects of hereditary and environmental influences on learning ability and the brain.

1. It requires only a few generations of selective breeding to produce strains of rats that differ significantly in maze-learning ability. The differences also appear in other tests than the one employed for the selection, but how general they are has not been settled. In the Tryon strains the differences in speed of learning could not be overcome by changing the degree of motivation of the animals.

2. The present Berkeley S_1 and S_3 strains differ not only in maze-solving ability but also in several cerebral measures. The S_1 animals, who are superior to the S_3s in several maze tests, show the following differences in comparison with the S_3 animals: The S_1s have brains that are more excitable electrically and chemically, as shown by seizure thresholds. They are also more richly provided with the synaptic transmitter, acetylcholine (ACh), and with the associated enzyme, acetylcholinesterase (AChE).

3. The possibility was discussed that the differences in ability and the cerebral differences are intrinsically related. The finding of correlations within strains between learning scores and cerebral measures supports this possibility. More research is needed to give a definitive answer to this question.

4. For both the S_1 and S_3 strains, animals given enriched experience perform better on a problem-solving test than animals whose experience was restricted.

Kansas Studies in Education

5. Animals given enriched experience (ECT) develop brains that differ measurably in several respects from those of littermates kept in an impoverished environment (IC). The enriched-experience animals have

    a. Heavier and thicker cerebral cortices,

    b. Greater total AChE activity throughout the brain, and

    c. Greater ChE activity in the cortex but not in the subcortex.

Animals kept in an intermediate colony environment (SC) are found to have brain measures that are in most cases intermediate between those of the ECT and IC groups.

6. The differences between ECT and IC groups in cortical weight and cerebral AChE cannot be attributed to either differential handling or loco-motor activity. Furthermore, they appear as readily in mature as in younger animals. Thus the anatomy and chemistry of the brain appear to be more responsive to experience than had been supposed. (The changes in ChE activity with experience have been found too recently for control experiments to have been performed.)

7. Whether the cerebral changes with differential experience (described in 5) actually mediate the changes in problem-solving ability (described in 4) is, again, a matter requiring further research.

We wish to emphasize that the behavioral and cerebral variations that we are studying are not gross or "abnormal." They can be detected only by the use of accurate and refined tests, but they are none the less real on that account. Similarly, in the field of mental retardation, many cases cannot be detected by casual observation, and in many, no gross pathology of the brain can be found, so that subtle deviations must be sought.

We are hopeful that further research on relations between learning ability and brain measures in animals will eventually help in the understanding of physiological mechanisms of learning. Our understanding will not be complete until it encompasses individual differences in learning ability among men, ranging from the gifted to the retarded.

BIBLIOGRAPHY

Anderson, E. E. Interrelationship of Drives in the Male Albino Rat. II. Intercorrelations between 47 Measures of Drives and Learning. *Comp. Psychol. Monogr.*, 1938, *14*, 1-119.

Bennett, E. L., Rosenzweig, M. R., Krech, D., Karlsson, H., Dye, N., & Ohlander, A. Individual, Strain and Age Differences in Cholinesterase Activity of the Rat Brain. *J. Neurochem.*, 1958, *3*, 144-152.

Bennett, E. L., Rosenzweig, M. R., Krech, D., Ohlander, A., & Morimoto, H. Cholinesterase Activity and Protein Content of Rat Brain. *J. Neurochem.*, 1962, *6*, 210-218.

Bennett, E. L., Krech, D., & Rosenzweig, M. R. Effects of Environmental Complexity and Training on Acetylcholinesterase and Cholinesterase Activity in Rat Brain. *Fed. Proc.*, 1963, *22*, 334. (Abstract)

Boell, E. J., Greenfield, P., & Shen, S. C. Development of Cholinesterase in the Optic Lobes of the Frog (Rana pipiens). *J. Exp. Zool.*, 1955, *129*, 415-451.

Briggs, M. H. & Kitto, G. B. The Molecular Basis of Memory and Learning. *Psychol. Rev.*, 1962, *69*, 537-541.

Burkhalter, A., Jones, M., & Featherstone, R. M. Acetylcholine-cholinesterase Relationships in Embryonic Chick Lung Cultivated in Vitro. *Proc. Soc. Exp. Biol.*, 1957, *96*, 747-750.

Burt, G. S. Strain Differences in Picrotoxin Seizure Threshold. *Nature*, 1962, *193*, 301-302.

Cooper, R. M. & Zubek, J. P. Effects of Enriched and Restricted Early Environments on the Learning Ability of Bright and Dull Rats. *Canad. J. Psychol.*, 1958, *12*, 159-164.

Effects of Heredity and Environment

Diamond, M. C., Krech, D., & Rosenzweig, M. R. The Effects of an Enriched Environment on the Histology of the Rat Cerebral Cortex. *J. Comp. Neurol.*, in press.

Ellman, G. L., Courtney, K. D., Andres, V. N., Jr., & Featherstone, R. M. A New and Rapid Determination of Acetylcholinesterase Activity. *Biochem. Pharmacol.*, 1961, 7, 88-95.

Freedman, A. M., Willis, A., & Himwich, H. E. Correlation between Signs of Toxicity and Cholinesterase Level of Brain and Blood during Recovery from Di-isopropyl Fluorophosphate (DFP) Poisoning. *Amer. J. Physiol.*, 1949, 157, 80-87.

Geiger, R. S. & Stone, W. G. Demonstration of the Presence of Cholinesterases in Long-term Cultures and Subcultures of Adult Mammalian Brain Cells. *Fed. Proc.*, 1962, 21, 366. (Abstract)

Hamilton, J. A. The Association between Brain Size and Maze Ability in the White Rat. Unpublished Ph.D. thesis, Univ. Calif., 1935.

Hebb, D. O. *The Organization of Behavior*. New York: Wiley, 1949.

Heron, W. T. The Inheritance of Maze Learning Ability in Rats. *J. Comp. Psychol.*, 1935, 19, 77-89.

Heron, W. T. The Inheritance of Brightness and Dullness in Maze Learning Ability in the Rat. *J. Genet. Psychol.*, 1941, 59, 41-49.

Hunt, J. McV. *Intelligence and Experience*. New York: Ronald Press, 1961.

International Union of Biochemistry. *Report of the Commission on Enzymes*. New York: Pergamon Press, 1961.

Kirk, S. A. *Early Education of the Mentally Retarded*. Urbana, Ill.: Univer. of Illinois Press, 1958.

Koelle, G. B. A New General Concept of the Neurohumoral Functions of Acetylcholine and Acetylcholinesterase. *J. Pharmacy Pharmacol.*, 1962, 14, 65-90.

Krech, D., Rosenzweig, M. R., & Bennett, E. L. Effects of Environmental Complexity and Training on Brain Chemistry. *J. Comp. Physiol. Psychol.*, 1960, 53, 509-519.

Krech, D., Rosenzweig, M. R., & Bennett, E. L. Relations between Brain Chemistry and Problem-solving, among Rats Raised in Enriched and Impoverished Environments. *J. Comp. Physiol. Psychol.*, 1962, 55, 801-807.

Krech, D., Rosenzweig, M. R., & Bennett, E. L. Effects of Complex Environment and Blindness on Rat Brain. *Archives of Neurology*, 1963, 8, 403-412.

Krechevsky, I. Hereditary Nature of "Hypotheses." *J. Comp. Psychol.*, 1933, 16, 99-116.

Krechevsky, I. Brain Mechanisms and Variability: I. Variability within a Means-end-readiness. *J. Comp. Psychol.*, 1937, 23, 121-138.

McGaugh, J. L., Westbrook, W., & Burt, G. Strain Differences in the Facilitative Effects of 5-7-diphenyl-1-3-diazadamantan-6-01 (1757 I.S.) on Maze Learning. *J. Comp. Physiol. Psychol.*, 1961, 54, 502-505.

McGaugh, J. L., Westbrook, W. H., & Thomson, C. W. Facilitation of Maze Learning with Posttrial Injections of 5-7-diphenyl-1-3-diazadamantan-6-01 (1757 I.S.). *J. Comp. Physiol. Psychol.*, 1962, 55, 710-713.

Pepler, W. J. & Pearse, A. G. E. The Histochemistry of the Esterases of Rat Brain, with Special Reference to Those of the Hypothalamic Nuclei. *J. Neurochem.*, 1957, 1, 193-202.

Petrinovich, L. Facilitation of Successive Discrimination Learning by Strychnine Sulphate. *Psychopharmacologia*, 1963, 4, 103-113.

Ramón y Cajal, S. *Les Nouvelles Idées sur la Structure du Système Nerveux chez L'homme et chez les Vertébrés*. Edition française revue et augmentée par l'auteur. (Trans. by L. Azoulay) Paris: C. Reinwald, 1895.

Roderick, T. H. Selection for Cholinesterase Activity in the Cerebral Cortex of the Rat. *Genetics*, 1960, 45, 1123-1140.

Rose, J. E., Malis, L. I., & Baker, C. P. Neural Growth in the Cerebral Cortex after Lesions Produced by Monoenergetic Deuterons. In Rosenblith, W. A. (Ed.), *Sensory Communication*. Massachusetts, M.I.T. Press & New York: Wiley, 1962. Pp. 279-301.

Rosenzweig, M. R., Krech, D., & Bennett, E. L. Brain Enzymes and Adaptive Behavior. In Ciba Foundation Symposium on the *Neurological Basis of Behavior*. London; J. & A. Churchill, 1958. Pp. 337-355.

Rosenzweig, M. R., Krech, D., & Bennett, E. L. A Search for Relations between Brain Chemistry and Behavior. *Psychol. Bull.*, 1960, 57, 476-492.

Rosenzweig, M. R., Krech, D., & Bennett, E. L. Heredity, Environment, Brain Biochemistry, and Learning. *Current Trends in Psychological Theory*. Pittsburgh: Univer. Pittsburgh Press, 1961. Pp. 87-110.

Rosenzweig, M. R., Krech, D., & Bennett, E. L. Strain Differences in Cerebral Responses to Environmental Complexity and Training. *Fed. Proc.*, 1964, 23, 255 (Abstract).

Rosenzweig, M. R., Krech, D., & Bennett, E. L. Modifying Brain Chemistry by Enrichment or Impoverishment of Experience. In Newton, G. (Ed.) *Readings in Early Experience*. In press.

Kansas Studies in Education

Rosenzweig, M. R., Krech, D., Bennett, E. L., & Diamond, M. C. Effects of Environmental Complexity and Training on Brain Chemistry and Anatomy: a Replication and Extension. *J. Comp. Physiol. Psychol.*, 1962, *55*, 429-437.

Rowland, G. L. & Woods, P. J. Performance of the Tryon Bright and Dull Strains under Two Conditions in a Multiple T-maze. *Canad. J. Psychol.*, 1961, *15*, 20-28.

Searle, L. V. A Study of the Generality of Inherited Maze-brightness and Maze-dullness. *Psychol. Bull.*, 1941, *38*, 742. (Abstract)

Searle, L. V. The Organization of Hereditary Maze-brightness and Maze-dullness. *Genet. Psychol. Monogr.*, 1949, *39*, 279-325.

Silverman, W., Shapiro, F., & Heron, W. T. Brain Weight and Maze Learning in Rats. *J. Comp. Psychol.*, 1940, *30*, 279-282.

Smith, C. E. Is Memory a Matter of Enzyme Induction? *Science*, 1962, *138*, 889-890.

Sperti, L. & Sperti, S. Effects of Chronic Lesions of the Peduncles on Cerebellum Cholinesterase Activity, in the Albino Rat. *Experientia*, 1959, *XV*, 441.

Tapp, J. T. & Markowitz, H. Infant Handling: Effects on Avoidance Learning, Brain Weight, and Cholinesterase Activity. *Science*, 1963, *140*, 486-487.

Thompson, W. R. The Inheritance and Development of Intelligence. *Proc. Assoc. Res. Nerv. Ment. Dis.*, 1954, *33*, 209-231.

Thomson, C. W., McGaugh, J. L., Smith, C. E., Hudspeth, W. J., & Westbrook, W. H. Strain Differences in the Retroactive Effects of Electroconvulsive Shock on Maze Learning. *Canad. J. Psychol.*, 1961, *15*, 69-74.

Tolman, E. C. The Inheritance of Maze-Learning Ability in Rats. *J. Comp. Psychol.*, 1924, *4*, 1-18.

Tolman, E. C., Tryon, R. C., & Jeffress, L. A. A Self-recording Maze with an Automatic-delivery Table. *Univ. Calif. Publ. Psychol.*, 1929, *4*, 99-112.

Tryon, R. C. Genetic Differences in Maze Learning Ability in Rats. *Yearbk. Nat. Soc. Stud. Educ.*, 1940, *39*, Part I, 111-119.

Tryon, R. C. Individual Differences. In Moss, F. A. (Ed.), *Comparative Psychology* (revised ed.). New York: Prentice-Hall, 1942. Pp. 330-365.

Tryon, R. C. Experimental Behavior Genetics of Maze Ability and a Sufficient Polygenic Theory. *Amer. Psychologist*, 1963, *18*, 442. (Cited by title)

Whalen, R. E. Strain Differences in Sexual Behavior of the Male Rat. *Behavior*, 1961, *18*, 199-204.

Woods, P. J., Fiske, A. S., & Ruckelshaus, S. I. The Effects of Drives Conflicting with Exploration on the Problem-solving Behavior of Rats Reared in Free and Restricted Environments. *J. Comp. Physiol. Psychol.*, 1961, *54*, 167-169.

Woolley, D. E., Timiras, P. S., Rosenzweig, M. R., Krech, D., & Bennett, E. L. Sex and Strain Differences in Electroshock Convulsions of the Rat. *Nature*, 1961, *190*, 515-516.

Woolley, D. E., Timiras, P. S., Rosenzweig, M. R., Krech, D., & Bennett, E. L. Strain Differences in Seizure Responses and Brain Cholinesterase Activity in Rats. *Proc. Soc. Exp. Biol. Med.*, 1963, *112*, 781-785.

From K. R. Hughes and J. P. Zubek (1956). Canad. J. Psychol., *10*, 132–138, *by kind permission of the authors and the Canadian Psychological Association*

EFFECT OF GLUTAMIC ACID ON THE LEARNING ABILITY OF BRIGHT AND DULL RATS: I. ADMINISTRATION DURING INFANCY[1]

K. R. HUGHES AND JOHN P. ZUBEK
University of Manitoba

IN 1944 Zimmerman and Ross (27), working at Columbia University, reported that the feeding of glutamic acid to young rats resulted in a considerable improvement in maze-learning ability. Later another group of Columbia workers (2) reported beneficial effects on the performance of rats in a complex reasoning problem. Extension of this work to mentally retarded children has suggested that glutamic acid may increase the IQ as measured by standard intelligence tests (1, 4, 8, 16, 20, 25). A number of negative studies have also been reported, however (5, 6, 10, 13, 15, 24).

Since the early Columbia studies, every single attempt to verify the positive animal findings has failed (3, 7, 11, 12, 17, 21, 23). Perhaps the most crucial of these animal studies was carried out by Stellar and McElroy (21), who duplicated every possible feature of the original Zimmerman and Ross experiment (except strain) and still obtained negative results. As a result of such findings the original enthusiasm about the possibilities of glutamic acid has almost disappeared, and little or no investigation, at either the animal or the human level, is now being done.

One important variable, which has been overlooked in the animal research on the effects of glutamic acid, is that of differences in learning ability from one strain to another. Examination of the learning scores of the Zimmerman and Ross control animals shows that they made many more errors than did the control animals of Stellar and McElroy, though tested on an identical maze and under similar conditions (36.5 *vs.* 13.4 errors). It would thus appear that the former group of workers was using a much duller strain of animals than was the latter. If this is the case, then differences between strains in initial learning ability may be the cause of the conflicting data, for it is conceivable that glutamic acid may facilitate the learning ability of dull animals but have no effect on bright ones. An obvious test of this hypothesis would be to obtain strains of bright and of dull rats and determine whether glutamic acid has a differential effect on the two groups, improving the learning ability of

[1]This research was supported by a grant-in-aid from the National Research Council of Canada.

CANAD. J. PSYCHOL., 1956, **10** (3).

EFFECT OF GLUTAMIC ACID ON LEARNING

the dull animals, but having no effect on the bright ones. Since such strains were available in the colony at Manitoba, it was decided to use them in an experimental test of the hypothesis.

EXPERIMENT I

The first experiment was largely an exploratory study to determine whether glutamic acid has any effect on the maze-learning ability of a strain of dull rats.

Subjects. Thirty-one naïve, hooded rats of the McGill dull strain (F_{10}) were used. These animals had been selectively bred for dullness on the Hebb-Williams maze. They were divided into an experimental group containing 18 rats (6 males, 12 females) and a control group containing 13 rats (7 males, 6 females).[2]

Apparatus. The 12 problems of the Hebb-Williams closed-field maze were used in the manner described by Rabinovitch and Rosvold (18).

Procedure. The 31 animals of the dull strain were weaned at 25 days of age, and both the experimental and the control groups were placed on a normal colony diet (Fox chow pellets). In addition to this food, the experimental animals were given a daily supplement of 5 grams of wet mash, containing 200 mg. of monosodium glutamate, while the controls received the 5 grams of wet mash, but without any added glutamate. This feeding procedure was continued for 40 days. At 65 days of age the food supplement was discontinued, and all animals began their adaptation and preliminary sessions on the Hebb-Williams maze. The 12 problems were then presented, two problems per day, approximately 9 hours apart. Eight trials were given on each problem. The learning score of each animal was the total number of error zones entered in the 12 maze problems. Time scores were also kept. Time was recorded from the moment the animal passed through the entrance door until it took its first bite of food.

Results

The mean error and time scores for the dull experimental and control groups are given in Table I. It can be seen that the dull experimentals made fewer errors than did the controls. This difference is statistically significant ($t = 3.02$, $p < .01$). The dull experimentals also showed better time scores than the controls. This difference is also significant ($t = 3.17, p < .01$).

TABLE I

MEAN ERROR AND TIME SCORES OF DULL EXPERI-
MENTAL AND CONTROL RATS IN EXPERIMENT I

	Dull experimental	Dull control
Mean errors	107.6	144.9
Mean time (secs.)	407.2	541.1

[2]The uneven sex matching was due to accidental loss of several cages of animals. There were no significant differences between the performances of males and females in any of the groups.

HUGHES & ZUBEK

Experiment II

Since these results were the first positive ones to be obtained since the early Columbia studies it was decided to repeat the entire procedure with another group of dull animals, in order to be certain that glutamic acid really has a beneficial effect on maze-learning ability. A bright strain was also used in this experiment to see whether it would fail to show improvement.

Subjects. Twenty-four naïve, hooded rats of the McGill dull strain (F_{11}) were used. These were divided at weaning (25 days) into an experimental group containing 13 rats (7 males, 6 females) and a control group containing 11 rats (5 males, 6 females). A group of 19 hooded rats of the McGill bright strain (F_{11}) was also used. These were divided at weaning into an experimental group containing 8 animals (6 males, 2 females) and a control group of 11 animals (5 males, 6 females).

Procedure. The dull experimentals and bright experimentals received a daily supplement of 200 mg. of monosodium glutamate (in 5 grams of wet mash) for 40 days, while the dull and bright controls received a placebo supplement (plain wet mash). Following the adaptation and preliminary sessions all four groups of animals were tested on the 12 problems of the Hebb-Williams test at the rate of two problems a day, approximately 9 hours apart.

TABLE II

MEAN ERROR AND TIME SCORES OF DULL AND BRIGHT, EXPERIMENTAL
AND CONTROL RATS IN EXPERIMENT II

	Dull		Bright	
	Experimental	Control	Experimental	Control
Mean errors	127.5	164.0	116.5	117.0
Mean Time (secs.)	601.8	850.0	372.0	391.5

Results

Table II summarizes the error and time scores of the dull and bright, experimental and control groups. From the table we see that the dull experimentals again made significantly fewer errors ($t = 2.16$, $p > .01 < 0.5$) and took significantly less time ($t = 3.05$, $p < .01$) in learning the maze problems than did the dull control animals. However, glutamic acid does not seem to have had any effect on the bright strain, the error scores of the experimental and control groups being almost identical. The time scores show the bright experimentals as slightly superior, but the difference is not statistically significant ($t = 0.99$, $p > .10$).

Discussion

The results of the two experiments indicate that glutamic acid does have a beneficial effect on dull rats and can increase their learning ability considerably. On the other hand, this substance does not influence the learning ability of bright animals. It thus appears that a possible explanation for the conflicting reports in the literature on animals lies in the overlooked variable of differences between strains in initial learning ability. The workers at Columbia may, for some reason, have possessed an animal strain that was much duller than the strains in other laboratories. These duller animals would, in the light of the present results, show improvement in learning ability, while the brighter ones used by other investigators, e.g. Stellar and McElroy (21), would not. Both Stellar and McElroy and Porter and Griffin (17), in reporting their negative studies, suggested that the effects of glutamic acid might be specific to the Sherman strain kept at Columbia University. This suggestion, however, was never followed up, and the question of "strain specific effects" remained unanswered.

These findings on the differential action of glutamic acid are in line with the clinical data. In no case has glutamic acid benefited human subjects of normal or above normal intellectual ability (1, 25). The positive results have always been obtained with a mentally retarded sample. It is not surprising, therefore, that when an analgous selection of animal subjects was made the results should turn out to be the same.

What is the mechanism underlying this improvement in learning ability? One possibility is that the acid mediates its effect simply by alleviating some pre-existing dietary deficiency of glutamate. This, however, seems not to be the case. First, rats are known to be able to synthesize glutamic acid in quantities sufficient to meet their bodily requirements. Secondly, Porter and Griffin (17) have demonstrated that animals raised on diets deficient in glutamic acid show no improvement in learning ability following excess glutamate supplementation. A much more likely hypothesis is offered by Zimmerman et al. (26), who suggest that the improvement in learning ability may be due to the facilitatory effect of glutamic acid upon certain metabolic processes underlying neural activity. In support of this view they cite Nachmansohn et al. (14), who have shown that glutamic acid is important in the synthesis of acetylcholine, a chemical substance necessary for the production of various electrical changes occurring during neural transmission. Nachmansohn reports that the rate of acetylcholine formation could be increased four to five times by adding glutamic acid to dialysed extracts of rat brain. More recent work (22) has shown that the concentration of this acid in the brain is disproportionately high, as compared with the concentration of other amino acids or with its concentration in other body tissues. Furthermore, of all the amino acids, glutamic acid alone is capable of serving as the respiratory substrate of the brain in lieu of glucose. This further points to the involvement of glutamic acid in neural function. Finally, Sauri (19), using rats, found that the acid exerts its main action on the cerebral cortex, lowering the threshold of excitability. All this clearly points to the importance of glutamic acid in cerebral metabolism.

Zimmerman's suggestion still does not account for the differential effect of glutamic acid on the learning ability of the two strains of animals. However, if we assume that the cerebral metabolism of the dull rats is defective in some way, while that of the bright rats is normal, then glutamic acid might facilitate or improve the defective cerebral meta-.bolism of the dull animals, while having no particular effect on the normal metabolism of the bright ones. A relationship between cerebral metabolism and mental functioning has been demonstrated by Himwich and Fazekas (9). In a careful study of tissue preparations from the brains of mentally retarded persons, they were able to show that these tissues were incapable of utilizing normal amounts of oxygen and carbohydrates. For example, in cases of mongolian idiocy and phenylpyruvic oligophrenia, the brain removed much less than the normal amounts of oxygen and glucose from a given volume of blood passing through it. In other words, the cerebral metabolism of these mentally retarded patients was defective. In the light of this work it would be of importance to know something about the cerebral metabolic state of the two animal strains, and especially of the glutamate-fed dulls. Since the necessary biochemical techniques are already available, this should not present too much of a problem.

The experimental findings of this study raise a number of questions. How permanent is the improved learning ability? Will it continue without further supplements of glutamic acid, or must the acid diet be continued for the improvement to last? Will dosages of acid greater than 200 mg. per day still further improve learning ability? What is the role of age? Will administration of glutamic acid to adult animals also produce improvement, or must it be given during infancy? Some of these questions we hope to answer in the near future.

SUMMARY

The purpose of this experiment was to study the effect of glutamic acid on the maze-learning ability of bright and dull rats (McGill strain).

Each strain of animals was divided into an experimental and control group at the time of weaning (25 days). The dull experimentals and bright experimentals received a daily supplement of 200 mg. of monosodium glutamate (in 5 grams of wet mash) for 40 days, while the dull and bright controls received a placebo supplement. Following the usual adaptation and preliminary sessions, the animals were tested on the 12 problems of the Hebb-Williams maze at the rate of two problems a day.

The results indicate that glutamic acid can increase the learning ability of dull rats considerably. It does not, on the other hand, affect the learning ability of bright rats.

Possible mechanisms underlying the improvement are discussed.

REFERENCES

1. ALBERT, K., HOCH, P., & WAELSCH, H. Glutamic acid and mental deficiency. *J. nerv. ment. Dis.*, 1951, **114**, 471–491.
2. ALBERT, K., & WARDEN, C. J. The level of performance in the white rat. *Science,* 1944, **100**, 476.
3. BRAIDER, LUCY M. The effect of the administration of L(+) glutamic acid in learning in the albino rat. M.Sc. thesis, Univer. Pittsburgh, 1949.
4. DU PLESSIS, D. L. The effect of glutamic acid on the I.Q., the scholastic achievement and the physical condition of the mentally retarded pupil. *J. soc. Res.* (Pretoria), 1953, **4**, 137–145.
5. ELLSON, D. G., FULLER, P. R., & URMSTON, R. The influence of glutamic acid on test performance. *Science*, 1950, **112**, 248–250.
6. ERNSTING, W. De behandelung van geestelijk achtergebleven kindern met glutaminezuur. *Ned. Tijdschr. Geneesk.*, 1949, 93, 1044–1054.
7. HAMILTON, H. C., & MAHER, EILEEN B. The effects of glutamic acid on the behaviour of the white rat. *J. comp. physiol. Psychol.*, 1947, **40**, 463–468.
8. HARNEY, SISTER MAUREEN. *Some psychological and physical characteristics of retarded children before and following treatment with glutamic acid.* Washington, D.C.: Catholic Univ. of America Press, 1950.
9. HIMWICH, H. E., & FAZEKAS, J. F. Cerebral metabolism in mongolian idiocy and phenylpyruvic oligophrenia. *Arch. Neurol. Psychiat.* (Chicago), 1940, **44**, 1213–1218.
10. LOEB, H. G., & TUDDENHAM, R.D. Does glutamic acid administration influence mental function? *Pediatrics*, 1950, **6**, 72–77.
11. MARX, M. H. Effects of supranormal glutamic acid on maze learning. *J. comp. physiol. Psychol.*, 1948, **41**, 82–92.
12. MARX, M. H. Relationship between supranormal glutamic acid and maze learning. *J. comp. physiol. Psychol.*, 1949, **42**, 313–319.
13. McCULLOCH, T. L. The effect of glutamic acid feeding on cognitive abilities of institutionalized mental defectives. *Amer. J. ment. Def.*, 1950, **55**, 117–122.
14. NACHMANSOHN, D., JOHN, H. M., & WALSH, H. Effect of glutamic acid on the formation of acetylcholine. *J. biol. Chem.*, 1943, **150**, 485–486.
15. OLDFELT, VERA. Experimental glutamic acid treatment in mentally retarded children. *J. Pediat.*, 1952, **40**, 316–323.
16. PORTA, V. La valutazione dell'intelligenza col test di Rorschach. *Arch. Psicol. Neurol. Psichiat.*, 1951, **12**, 337–349.
17. PORTER, P. B., & GRIFFIN, A. C. Effects of glutamic acid on maze learning and recovery from electroconvulsive shocks in albino rats. *J. comp. physiol. Psychol.*, 1950, **43**, 1–15.
18. RABINOVITCH, M. S., & ROSVOLD, H. E. A closed-field intelligence test for rats. *Canad. J. Psychol.*, 1951, **5**, 122–128.

19. SAURI, J. J. Accion del acido glutamico en el sistema nerviosa central. *Neuroropsiquiat.* (Buenos Aires), 1950, **1**, 148–158.

20. SCHWÖBEL, G. Untersuchungen über die Beeinflussbarkeit psychischer Funktionen durch Glutaminsäure. *Nervenarzt*, 1950, **21**, 385–396.

21. STELLAR, E., & McELROY, W. D. Does glutamic acid have any effect on learning? *Science*, 1948, **108**, 281–283.

22. WAELSCH, H. Glutamic acid and cerebral function. In ANSON, M. L., EDSALL, J. T., & BAILEY, K. (eds.), *Advances in protein chemistry*, pp. 301–339. New York: Academic Press, 1951.

23. ZABARENKO, L. M., PILGRIM, F. J., & PATTON, R. A. The effect of glutamic acid supplementation on problem solving of the instrumental conditioning type. *J. comp. physiol. Psychol.*, 1951, **44**, 126–133.

24. ZABARENKO, R. N., & CHAMBERS, G. S. An evaluation of glutamic acid in mental deficiency. *Amer. J. Psychiat.*, 1952, **108**, 881–887.

25. ZIMMERMAN, F. T., BURGEMEISTER, BESSIE B., & PUTNAM, T. J. A group study of the effect of glutamic acid upon mental functioning in children and adolescents. *Psychosom. Med.*, 1947, **9**, 175–183.

26. ZIMMERMAN, F. T., BURGEMEISTER, BESSIE B., & PUTNAM, T. J. Effect of glutamic acid on the intelligence of patients with mongolism. *Arch. Neurol. Psychiat.* (Chicago), 1949, **61**, 275–287.

27. ZIMMERMAN, F. T., & ROSS, S. Effect of glutamic acid and other amino acids on maze learning in the white rat. *Arch. Neurol. Psychiat.* (Chicago), 1944, **51**, 446–451.

PART X

THE PARADIGM AND ITS CRITICS

In the preceding sections we have been concerned with the elaboration and documentation of the model of intelligence which is presented by modern psychology; in this section we must deal with some criticisms which are frequently offered of this model. It would have been very useful if we could have followed the fashion adopted in the other sections, of choosing two or three outstanding papers to represent current views; unfortunately this is not possible because detailed, and particularly quantitative, criticisms of the model or paradigm are hard to find. There is of course no dearth of criticisms of specific points, usually suggesting improvements or slight changes in certain estimates or constants; but this is not what would be appropriate here. The model as such is indeed often criticised, but only *en passant*, and most frequently by persons who have little knowledge of the facts on which the model is based. Such criticism is not very useful, and is in any case too discursive to be answered in any meaningful fashion. Yet clearly no scientific model can escape criticism; indeed, it is quite undesirable that it should. Consequently I have tried to gather together some representative criticisms which I have found in the writings of well-known psychologists; these have then been presented on the following pages, together with such comments and answers as seemed appropriate. I have at times had recourse to arguments derived from the modern philosophy of science, primarily because critics often doubt the scientific nature of measurement in this field; a discussion of such questions naturally demands that certain groundrules be agreed on and followed.

There is one general criticism which is often voiced by laymen and experimental psychologists alike. Thus Zangwill (1950) has this to say: "Intellectual testing is a technology whose theoretical foundations are distinctly insecure. . . . Tests of ability find a variety of uses at the present day and have real and important applications to education and personnel selection. But, at the present stage of development, it would be unwise to suppose that they furnish more than a broad indication of

mental status. Exactly what such tests measure is decidedly problematical. The basic procedures, moreover, can hardly be said to derive from established scientific principles." In another place, Zangwill takes up the question of just why he has decided to dismiss the theory and practice of mental testing as a mere technology. His answer, which as he admits may reflect bias, is as follows: "Science evolves in three principal stages: First, the collection of facts; second, the devising of hypotheses designed to explain these facts; and third, the submission of hypotheses thus derived to the test of experiment. Factorial analysis, he would claim, proceeds first by designing arbitrary tests of abilities; second, by assigning arbitrary scores to the results so obtained; and third, by submitting the resulting correlations to a mathematical analysis which results in the isolation of factors. These factors, whose psychological significance (if any) is unknown, are then identified with the original abilities."

Chambers (1943) castigates psychometrists even more harshly. "Too frequently mathematical psychologists build elegant and dizzy numerical edifices, forgetting in their architectural zeal the flimsy foundations upon which their fabrics stand." And again: ". . . we may say that it is at least very doubtful whether the concept of measurable quality may be applied at all to psychological qualities; it is certain that psychological qualities do not function in isolation; and it is exceedingly doubtful what is the significance of marks arbitrarily assigned to the results of a single testing on a particular occasion. It is on this very uncertain basis that the whole of the work of the factorial analysts rests." What Chambers says about "elegant and dizzy numerical edifices" has of course also been said of many other scientists; many of the comments of French physicists concerning Newton's Principia sounded very much like this (Manuel, 1968). In any case, what is involved in psychometric work of the kind discussed by Chambers is essentially the estimation of the rank of a matrix, a job hardly deserving of such hyperbole; it should not be beyond the ability of a bright sixth-form schoolboy.

Zangwill is certainly right in drawing attention to the technological aspects of intelligence testing, and the degree to which the applied side has outgrown the pure. Many studies in the field of intelligence testing are concerned with application, very few with fundamental matters; this unbalance has had undesirable effects on the development of the scientific basis of intelligence testing. Many of the applications are poor in quality, ill-considered in design, and over-ambitious in interpretation; it would not be entirely inaccurate to say that there are very few areas in psychology where so-called "research" is poorer in quality than here (clinical psychology might perhaps be the winner in these stakes, by a narrow head). But this is not really relevant to a consideration of the paradigm; this must be judged in terms of the evidence put forward in its support, using for this purpose the best-designed and best-executed studies we can find. A thousand bad studies cannot disprove or invalidate a single good one, and while the existence of the thousand bad studies casts some reflections on psychology as a profession, it cannot be used as an argument against the value of the model itself. We must therefore examine in some detail Zangwill's criticisms in the light of such studies as have been reprinted or reviewed in this volume.

Let us first look at Zangwill's "three stages" which mark the development of a scientific discipline, without quibbling too much about his somewhat idiosyncratic statement of these stages. Medawar (1967) has criticized the notion that science begins with facts; he objects to the assumption of "a logically mechanized process of thought which, starting from simple declarations of fact arising out of the evidence of the senses, can lead us with certainty to the truth of general laws." As T. H. Huxley pointed out, "those who refuse to go beyond fact seldom get as far as fact." Even the most elementary "fact" is already part of a whole system of hypotheses and theories, even though these may remain largely implicit. Measurement of length, to take only the most elementary kind of measurement which even primitive societies take for granted, is based on many assumptions; it requires a rigid instrument for carrying out the measurement, for instance, and this requirement is difficult to test in any rigorous way, and is quite difficult to state in a theoretically satisfactory manner. Measurement of length requires theoretical assumptions about the effects of temperature on the measuring instrument —otherwise the distance of Edinburgh from London would be less in the summer than in the winter! We cannot begin with a collection of "facts" because the very notion of a fact is tied up with theoretical assumptions, however elementary these may be. Is the observation of a conditioned reflex a "fact"? We observe a muscle twitch, or a sudorific discharge, or a vascular change; we *interpret* these events in terms of an experimental paradigm, and a theoretical expectation. Even the very act of seeing cannot be interpreted as a simple

factual intake of information; seeing has to be learned, and is consequently an amalgam of fact and fiction, induction and deduction, apprehension and experience. Monkeys brought up in darkness cannot see when brought into the light, even though their visual apparatus is unimpaired; the facts transmitted through sight are unrecorded through lack of an interpretative theory, built up by experience.

However that may be, let us return to the question of whether or not the creators of the intelligence model have followed the hypothetico-deductive method in their work. Spearman postulated, on the basis of previous work and previous theories, that intelligence entered as a general factor into every sort of intelligence test fulfilling certain requirements (i.e. his neogenetic laws); he deduced from this hypothesis that matrices of correlations between such tests, chosen and administered according to certain rules we have already discussed, would in effect have a rank of unity. He further showed that this rank was approximated quite closely in a number of experimental studies, bearing in mind of course the existence of sampling errors. Thurstone and Thurstone (1941), who had been highly critical of Spearman's theory, demonstrated that when they used groups of tests to define primary factors of N (numerical ability), W (word fluency), V (verbal ability), S (spatial ability), M (rote memory), and R (reasoning), these correlated together in a matrix of almost exactly rank one, as shown in Table 1 below. They even calculated the correlations of these various factors with g, and found that as one would have expected on Spearman's hypothesis R had the highest loading, and S and M the lowest. Thus Spearman's most cogent critic has provided us with the firmest support for the existence of a general factor of intellectual ability. The Thurstones state: "This finding raises the interesting question whether a unique general factor can be determined. Its interpretation here would be that the primary mental abilities are correlated by a general factor which operates through each of the primaries. Each of the primary factors can be regarded as a composite of an independent primary factor and a general factor which it shares with other primary factors." Thus Spearman's conception of "specific factors" is now labelled by Thurstone "primary factors"; these absorb the "undue similarities" between tests which Spearman suggested might cause departure from the rank one type of matrix. It is difficult to see why Zangwill would withhold approval of the general form of the argument, or its experimental verification.

It is necessary, of course, to take care regarding the correct statement of the argument. It is not right to argue, as some do, that the discovery of a low rank for matrices of intercorrelations proves that a general factor of intelligence exists. We must begin with the hypothesis postulating such a factor, plus specifics for each test; we can then deduce the rank of the matrix that should result from intercorrelating carefully chosen tests, and

TABLE 1

Primaries	N	W	V	S	M	R
N (Numerical ability)	—	·47	·38	·26	·19	·54
W (Word fluency)	·47	—	·51	·17	·39	·48
V (Verbal ability)	·38	·51	—	·17	·39	·55
S (Spatial ability)	·26	·17	·17	—	·15	·39
M (Rote memory)	·19	·39	·39	·15	—	·39
R (Reasoning)	·54	·48	·55	·39	·39	—
Correlations with g:	·60	·69	·68	·34	·47	·84

Inter-correlations between Primary Factors, and their g Saturations. (From Thurstone & Thurstone, 1941).

arrange experiments to see whether this low rank (unity) actually occurs, within sampling errors. This does not prove the existence of a general factor; as Popper (1959, 1963) has pointed out so often, the predictive success of a theory does not prove that theory to be right, it simply prolongs its life until finally falsified. Nevertheless, it does impose on critics the duty to explain the findings on the basis of a better theory; lacking such a theory (and none has been proposed so far) generalized criticisms of the kind offered by Zangwill does not really advance our understanding very much.

Let us take another point made by Zangwill, and often repeated by other writers. "Factorial analysis . . . proceeds first by designing arbitrary tests of abilities." Is this in fact true? Arbitrary means capricious, based on one's own wishes, notions, or will. But this is hardly correct. Spearman laid down very precise canons of test construction, embodying the neogenetic principles; it is possible to criticise these canons, but they can hardly be called arbitrary. Furthermore, it is noteworthy that it is precisely those tests which embody these principles to the fullest extent, i.e. such tests as Matrices, or Dominoes, which constantly achieve the highest g saturations. This is predictable in terms of Spearman's theory; here we have therefore another verification. Again, we cannot claim to have proved his theory, only to have supported it. However, such support is all a scientific theory requires, and can possibly receive from empirical research. Unless we can point to an alternative theory which makes better predictions, it would seem reasonable to accept the model as the best at present available.

Zangwill continues his sentence, quoted above, by saying: ". . . second, by assigning arbitrary scores to the results so obtained." Again, this is not true. Thurstone, Thorndike and others have spent much time and energy on working out methods of absolute scaling, determining an absolute zero point, and in general removing the taint of "arbitrariness" from the scoring of intelligence tests. Zangwill might criticize these efforts, but has not in fact done so; the mere assertion that the scores are "arbitrary" can hardly be taken as a proper

scientific criticism. They may be wrong, but they are not arbitrary!

Zangwill concludes his sentence by saying that factor analysis proceeds ". . . third, by submitting the resulting correlations to a mathematical analysis which results in the isolation of factors. These factors, whose psychological significance (if any) is unknown, are then identified with the original abilities." Here we have two criticisms. In the first instance, it is suggested that we do not know the psychological significance of our factors; indeed, we do not know whether they have any such significance or not. It is difficult to answer such a criticism, largely because it is difficult to assign any meaning to it. What is meant by "psychological significance" in this context? Who decides when we have succeeded in bestowing "psychological significance" (whatever that may mean) on anything? Does the notion of "gravitation" have any "physical significance" beyond the laws which relate physical bodies together in terms of the inverse square distance, and their reciprocal masses? Is it not sufficient for these factors to derive whatever "psychological significance" they may have from the nomological network in which they become embedded through empirical research? Why should we expect something from psychological concepts which we do not require from physical concepts?

In the second instance, these "factors are identified with the original abilities." This again is not true; such identification would be an example of reification, and as we have seen in the first section, such reification is not the aim of the psychologist. Indeed, he is the first critic of any attempts to do anything of the kind. Admittedly, some psychologists may have fallen into this trap, but I know of no well-known psychologist who would willingly reify factors in this manner. Thus the three main points made by Zangwill are all aimed at a man of straw, rather than at any actual worker in this field who has made any sizeable contribution to the model or paradigm with which we are dealing. True, this misunderstanding is widespread; it is to be hoped that the detailed discussion of some of the logical points involved in it which appeared in the first section of this book will clarify the situation.

This demand for "psychological meaning" recalls a long-continued battle in physics which has split physicists into two groups. One group demands that theories should result in concepts whose interaction can be visualized, while others have no wish to go beyond the statements of relations contained in the formulae of a given theory. A good example is the theory of heat, where we have side by side the thermodynamic and the kinetic theory. Thermodynamics deals with unimaginable concepts of a purely quantitative kind: temperature measured on a thermometer, pressure, measured as the force exerted per unit area, and volume, measured by the size of the container. Nothing is said in the laws of thermodynamics about the nature of heat. On the other side, Bernoulli, in his famous treatise on hydraulics, postulated that all "elastic fluids", such as air, consist of small particles which are in constant irregular motion, and which constantly collide with each other and with the walls of the container. This was the foundation stone of the kinetic theory of heat, which results in a picture of events which is eminently visualizable, and which gives to many people a feeling of greater "understanding", of better and more thorough "explanation" than do the laws of thermodynamics. Consider for example the "insight" which we seem to gain in looking at Cailletet's famous experiment, which originated cryogenic research, by considering his cooling device as part of a single stroke of an expansion engine! Nevertheless, many phenomena are quite untractable to kinetic interpretations even today, which yield easily to a thermodynamic solution. It seems that visualizability is a kind of bonus which may make a theory more easily acceptable, perhaps particularly to people who are visualizers, but which is a psychological interest only, not of general scientific importance. "Psychological meaning" would seem akin to this notion of visualizability; we want to have something more than the simple statistical or mathematical formulations relating facts and events together. Psychometrics eschews this need, and prefers the formalism of the thermodynamic type of solution. It is doubtful if Zangwill's criticism has any more force, therefore, than would a criticism of modern thermodynamic theory on the grounds that it was difficult to visualize just what was going on.

Of course, times change, and with them the possibility of successfully "reifying" concepts, i.e. of pointing to some physical reality underlying them. The history of the atom is of considerable interest in this connection (Nye, 1972). In the first half of the 19th century, Dumas and Berthelot dominated European science, and their refusal to recognize the actual existence of atoms was widely accepted as orthodoxy; as Dumas said, speaking of the atomic theory: "If I were master of the situation, I would efface the word atom from Science, persuaded that it goes further than experience and that, in chemistry, we should never go further than experience." (Caullery, 1948, p. 125). Wurtz and others rallied to the defence of the atom, and an international confrontation resulted at the 1860 Karlsruhe Congress; this was followed by another open confrontation at the Académie des Sciences. Even as late as 1904 Ostwald, speaking about the stoichiometrical laws of chemistry, asserted that while the atomic hypothesis had indeed been historically responsible for the deduction of the early laws, nevertheless "chemical dynamics has . . . made the atomic hypothesis unnecessary for this purpose and has put the theory of stoichiometrical laws on more secure ground than that furnished by a mere hypothesis." (Ostwald, 1904). Ostwald was joined by Mach, and even by Planck; Mach (1905) wrote that "once an hypothesis has facilitated, as best it can, our views of new facts, by the substitution of more familiar ideas, its powers are exhausted. We err when we expect more enlightenment from an hypothesis than from the facts themselves." The great exponent of the physical reality and interpretation of atoms and molecules of course was Boltzman, who could appeal successfully to many great advances which had depended entirely on atomistic theory, such as van der Waals's formula for the behaviour of fluids, the extension of Gibbs's dissociation theory, and Clausius's estimation of specific heats. Finally, of course, Perrin silenced the controversy by showing, through his studies of Brownian movement, that atoms and molecules did possess "reality" in the sense that had been denied them by the proponents of the thermodynamic view. Perhaps the work on evoked potentials summarized in the last Section will serve the same purpose with respect to intelligence; it is here that it may find "a local habitation and a name", rather than continue to be defined, as it is at present, in the same way as Maxwell's theory: "Maxwell's theory is Maxwell's system of equations." (Cohen, 1956).

The last criticisms on which Zangwill and Chambers seem to agree relates to the question of measurement, i.e. the possibility and appropriateness of measurement in the case of psychological qualities. In addition to the references to principles of scientific measurement given in the foreword, the best discussion of the problem as it concerns the psychologist, and in particular as it concerns the measurement of intelligence, is given by Burt (1941) in his book on "The Factors of the Mind." As he points out, the modern notions of measurement, like those of mathematics, are ultimately derived from Cantor's theory of classes (Mengenlehre), which in this country has been developed mainly by Russell. Following these principles, we may say that "to arrange traits, personalities, or anything else in order, it is necessary and sufficient to find a relation that is (i) connexive, (ii) asymmetrical, and (iii) transitive, and to demonstrate by empirical observation that this relation holds good of the members of the class. Thus, of x, y, and z denote possible members of the class, the requisite conditions may be formulated as follows:

(i) *Connexive Postulate*—If x and y both $< z$ or both $> z$, then either $x < y$, $y < x$, or $x = y$.
(ii) *Postulate of Asymmetry*—If $x < y$, then neither $y < x$ nor $y = x$.
(iii) *Postulate of Transitivity*—If $x < y$ and $y < z$, then $x < z$.

Here $=$ does not necessarily mean 'equals', but merely 'may always be interchanged in the argument'; and $<$ does not necessarily mean 'is less than' but merely stands for *any* relation obeying the conditions specified (e.g. such a relation as 'precedes', 'is nearer than', 'more difficult than', 'preferable to', 'commoner than', 'happier than', 'redder than', 'more beautiful than', etc.)" Burt goes on to demonstrate that these postulates can be shown to be satisfied empirically in various psychometric relations but it would take us too far afield to follow him in these specific demonstrations.

It is curious that those who take the view that measurement of intelligence is not measurement in the scientific sense at all, never take their argument beyond mere assertion; nor do they specify precisely what they mean by measurement, and in what way their definition disagrees with that of Cantor and Russell, say. No serious discussion has been offered by the critics, and consequently it is difficult to deal with their criticisms; unless we are told unequivocally and specifically what they conceive the true principles of measurement to be, and in what way intelligence measurement violates these principles, no convincing answer seems possible.

When one looks at the verbal statements sometimes made in criticism, one feels that statements about intelligence testing not being measurement are based, more than anything, on the presence of error in the establishment of a given person's IQ. This is, of course, a very naive notion; error is inherent in all scientific measurement. To imagine otherwise is to be ignorant of the very first principles of science. Painfully and slowly the size of the error is investigated, some of its causes discovered, and finally controlled. To achieve a balanced view, it is useful to read such books as Kisch (1965) on the history of scales and weights, or Knowles Middleton (1966) on the history of the thermometer; the reader will find there errors more egregious, abuses more grievous, and difficulties every bit as real, as those which he will encounter in the measurement of intelligence. One of the most interesting faults in the early thermoscopes and thermometers, for instance, was the fact that they were not sealed; until the variability of the pressure of air became known around 1650, it was not realized that in this way the instrument was measuring a mixture of temperature and barometric pressure! As Pascal wrote in his description of the celebrated barometric experiments on the Puy-de-Dôme: "From (this experiment) there follow many consequences, such as . . . the lack of certainty that is in the thermometer for indicating the degrees of heat (contrary to common sentiment). Its water sometimes rises when the heat increases, and sometimes falls when the heat diminishes, even though the thermometer remained in the same place." (1648). Having got a thermometer, however primitive, we next need a scale; it is this scale which converts a thermoscope into a thermometer. The first scales used were quite arbitrary (at least as arbitrary as critics would have us believe IQ units to be); later ones, following the work of Fahrenheit around 1726, were based on two fixed points (usually the ice point and the steam point). Such scales also made an important and unproven assumption, namely that the variable property being measured changes linearly with temperature, as for instance the position of the meniscus in a mercury thermometer.

Such a practical temperature scale (the most sophisticated expression of which is in what is now known officially as the International Practical Temperature Scale of 1948, and the subsequent (1960) text revision of that scale) "has the supreme merit, from the point of view of the user, that it can be defined in sufficient detail to be compatible with the most advanced techniques available for measuring temperature. It has the fatal flaw, from the scientific point of view, that it does not depend on any fundamental understanding of temperature, with the result that the scale is a patchwork of arbitrarily chosen thermometric parameters, fixed points and interpolation formulae." (Lovejoy, 1965, p. 793). This understanding became available only after a clear distinction had been made between the intensive quantity, temperature, and its corresponding extensive quantity, heat—a distinction which became possible only after the erroneous caloric theory had been overthrown, which regarded heat as a fluid. This overthrow was accomplished by such men as Count Rumford, Sadi Carnot, Helmholtz and others; the resulting science of thermodynamics was respectably clothed in a mathematical formalism by Clausius and William Thomson (later Lord Kelvin) by 1849. But thermodynamics tells us nothing about the atomic processes which lie at the basis of the phenomena with which it deals; for this insight we must turn to statistical mechanics as developed by Maxwell, Boltzman, Gibbs and others in the second half of the 19th century. The classical Maxwell-Boltzman statistics reveal the thermodynamic temperature T as a measure of the average random energy of the atoms and molecules (with restrictions introduced later by quantum theory in the Bose-Einstein equation). This constant improvement over the years shows how measurement is dependent on theory, and how theory is improved by having new facts due to measurement to explain. There is no point where one could say—this is not proper scientific measurement, and no point where one could say—this is. In fact, as we have seen, the kind of scale which most people would recognize as classically measuring temperature—the ordinary mercury thermometer—and which they would compare with IQ measurement to the great disadvantage of the latter, suffers from precisely the faults which intelligence measurement is supposed to suffer from, i.e. a failure to derive from a fundamental understanding of the nature of temperature. And even now, as we have noted, the formulary of thermodynamics and the reifications of statistical mechanics have by no means been completely reconciled; there is still much work to be done before we gain that profound understanding of the phenomena in question which is the aim of science—there is still lacking any great understanding, for instance, of cryogenic phenomena (Jackson, 1962; Mendelssohn, 1964; Squire, 1953; Zemansky, 1957).

Two further kinds of criticisms must be considered, at least briefly. The first of these relates to the well-demonstrated effects on learning behaviour in animals of early sensory or social deprivation; Hunt (1961, 1968) has given a good account of these experiments, and has used them in support of the view that such early deprivations may also be at the basis of learning and IQ defects in human children. Such a conclusion seems quite unwarranted; the facts are not in dispute, but it is very doubtful if they are in any way relevant to the problem of human intelligence, at least in so far as Western countries or the "Eastern Block" countries are concerned. (Too little is known about the "developing" countries in this respect to say very much about them). Deprivations, either perceptual or social, have to be pretty severe in order to have marked and lasting effects on animals; such deprivations are by no means characteristic of "deprived" children. The reader is referred to naturalistic descriptions of such "deprived" children, school drop-outs with IQs around or below 90, as are given for instance by David and McGuire (1972); sensory and social deprivation is entirely missing in these dull members of big city gangs. The contrary, if anything, would be true; these boys and girls have far more stimulation than a typical middle-class, introverted, school-attending boy or girl. Unless direct proof can be given of the notion that sensory or social deprivation is a causal factor in low IQ in any except a few very rare and unusual "Kaspar Hauser" cases, we must conclude that these animal experiments, while interesting in their own right, are quite irrelevant to the problems we are now considering.

Possibly more relevant are cross-cultural studies, e.g. those of Eskimo intelligence. Unfortunately the concept of "deprivation" is not usually well defined, but one would surely have to conclude that Eskimo children, brought up in an environment startlingly undifferentiated with respect to many stimuli we take for granted, under economic conditions which are extremely poor, and with considerable family instability and insecurity, would be unlikely to be able to compete, even on "culture fair" tests, with white children brought up under ordinary Western conditions. Yet, as several authors have shown, these Eskimos, living in the icy wastes far above the arctic circle, score at or above white Canadian norms on the Progressive Matrices (MacArthur, 1968), a finding replicated by Berry (1966) and Vernon (1965). They score much higher than Jamaican or American Negroes, although these are brought up under conditions much more closely resembling those of the white groups in question, and with a much better supply of environmental and social stimuli. Interestingly enough, Eskimos living under the most primitive conditions did better on the tests than those who lived in closer contact with whites and had become acculturated. (These studies may also serve as additional proof that the often repeated criticism that IQ tests are made by white, middle-class psychologists for white, middle-class children, and are unfair to children not belonging to this charmed circle, is mistaken. Certainly the makers of the tests employed in these studies did not have Eskimo children in mind when they constructed their test items!)

It is of course not impossible to advance ad hoc environmentalistic explanations of these startling findings (Vernon, 1965, p. 732) but these are without proof and do not have any bearing on the "deprivation" hypothesis. The point to note is that if social and sensory deprivation, or other environmental deprivation factors, are postulated to account for IQ deficits in white working-class or coloured populations, then the logic of the explanation requires absolutely that a severely deprived group, such as the Eskimos, should show evidence of IQ deficit; the fact is that they do not. (Other examples of "deprived" groups failing to fit into this environmentalistic paradigm have been given by Eysenck, 1971). Thus the "deprivation" hypothesis limps on two feet; the evidence from animal work which is brought out to support it is true but irrelevant, and the evidence from human children does not support it, but rather goes counter to it. Much further work will clearly be needed before the hypothesis can even be put into a form which will be properly testable; at the moment its proponents are far from agreed precisely what constitutes "deprivation", and how this hypothetical entity can be measured. Furthermore, it is of course not only necessary to demonstrate that deprivation (however defined and measured) affects IQ; it is required to show that the effects go beyond the "reaction range" of environmental influences defined in a previous section before the results can be regarded as in any way critical of our paradigm.

This lack of concern over the quantitative properties of the "reaction range" in assessing the adequacy of the model is widespread. Let us consider as an example the well-known case of Gladys and Helen, monozygotic twins with an IQ difference of 24 points (Newman, Freeman & Holzinger, 1937). It has been argued that if environment can make a difference of 24 points, then the observed difference in IQ of whites and blacks (15 points on the average) fades into insignificance; it has also been argued that such a very large difference is incompatible with the hypothesis of an 80%/20% distribution of the variance between heredity and environment. Even if we are willing to forget that the test used in this study was one of crystallized intelligence, rather than fluid intelligence, there is a quite clear-cut answer to this point. Gladys and Helen were one pair of twins out of a sample of 122 such pairs; given the reaction range calculated from the properties of our model (which is equal to 28 points of IQ), it would be improbable if there were not one such case with a difference of about 24 IQ points in the sample. When the observed differences between pairs of twins are plotted, they give rise to a close approximation of a Gaussian curve; this enables us to calculate the probability of finding any particular size difference in a given sample. In this case there is only 1 chance in 100 that the largest value out of 122 would have been smaller than 17 points; the finding of the largest value in this sample at a 24 point IQ difference is precisely what would be expected in terms of the model. In other words, had the Helen and Gladys case not occurred, we would have reason to doubt the adequacy of our model, as giving a prediction of monozygotic twin differences in IQ in excess of observation. That such a triumphant verification of prediction can be quoted as convincing disconfirmation of the theory in question illustrates better than anything the topsy-turvy world in which some of the critics of the model live. Nor can this case be used as relevant to the black-white difference in IQ; to do so would require us to compare a difference in means based on hundreds of thousands of cases, and hence with a vanishingly small standard error, with a difference in scores between two highly selected individuals, with a high standard error adding to their scores (quite apart from the fact that this difference is picked out *ex post facto* as the largest from a set of 122 such differences). A proper comparison would use the mean difference for all 122 cases, which is 6·60, with a S.D. of 5·20; this mean difference is reduced to 5·63 when we eliminate (as we must) the effects of errors of measurement. To pick and choose the one single largest difference for comparison, instead of the mean, is quite impossible.

Another form of "deprivation" which is often adduced as being responsible for the low IQ of groups of coloured and/or low-class subjects is malnutrition. Most favoured here is the hypothesis of a "critical period"; this states that developing organ systems are most vulnerable at the period of maximum growth. Interruption of development at a critical period is likely to be irreversible or, at the least, subsequent development is likely to be retarded; hence prenatal and early postnatal exposure to conditions of famine would in terms of this hypothesis have the most severe effects on the intelligence of the child. An excellent study is available which submits this hypothesis to searching investigation (Stein et al., 1972). Cohorts of children born at varying periods after the famine imposed by the Germans on certain regions of Holland during the war (as retribution for the participation of Dutch workers in the battle following the Arnhem landing of British paratroops) were compared with children born during the same time in other parts of Holland not exposed to famine conditions. (At their lowest point the official food rations in the famine areas fell to 450 calories, which is a quarter of the minimum standard. Death rates rose sharply, and many deaths were certified as being due to starvation).

The investigators used three dependent variables: severe mental retardation, mild mental retardation, and IQ scores; the independent variable, of course, was exposure to famine. The study population comprised 125,000 males born in the selected famine and control cities during the 3-year period 1st Jan. 1944 to 31st Dec. 1946, and who were inducted into the army at about 19 years of age. The following findings were reported: (1) "The frequency of severe mental retardation among survivors of the birth cohorts is related neither to conception nor to birth during the famine." (2) "The frequency of mild mental retardation too is related neither to conception nor to birth during the famine."

(3) With respect to the IQ test used (Raven's Matrices), "once more we failed to find an association with the period of famine." These results, as the authors indicate, "point either to a high order of protection afforded the foetus in utero, or to great resilience of the foetus in the face of nutritional insult, or to both."

These findings are sufficiently clear-cut to disprove the hypothesis of "critical growth", as far as the influence of malnutrition on intelligence is concerned. A more general disproof of the "critical period" hypothesis is given by Johnson (1963) who shows that MZ twins separated at a mean age of 2 months are less alike when later tested for IQ than MZ twins separated at a mean age of 24 months. This significant difference is in a direction contrary to that demanded by the hypothesis! Of course these results should not be taken too far; as the authors point out, "the results should not be generalized to the effects of chronic malnutrition with a different set of dietary deficiencies such as often occurs in developing countries, not to nutritional insult in postnatal life." This is true, although it must be said that if extreme degrees of malnutrition during the most vulnerable period of the child's life have absolutely no effect on his intelligence, then anyone asserting the influence of lesser degrees of malnutrition during less vulnerable periods must be prepared to produce very direct and incontrovertible evidence, ruling out all other possibilities, before much credence can be given to his beliefs. Some such evidence exists as far as developing countries are concerned, but it does not exist as far as such countries as the U.K., the U.S.S.R., the U.S.A. or the European continent are concerned. A thorough review of the evidence on malnutrition and mental deficiency is given by Kaplan (1972).

The other criticism to be considered can be put in the form that "IQ tests are simply not adequate to measure processes of thinking" (Voyat, 1970, p. 161), and that such tests as those pioneered by Piaget would be more suitable. "Piaget's approach not only allows an understanding of his intelligence functions, but describes it. Since the interest of Piaget's tests lies in describing the mechanism of thinking, they permit an individual, personalized appraisal of further potentialities independent of culture." (p. 161). Piaget views development of cognitive functions as going through certain stages—sensorimotor, preoperational, concrete operations, and formal operations; he has devised a large number of ingenious "tests" or clinical-type procedures for assessing the child's mental development as he moves through these stages, and the various sub-stages into which they can be broken down. These tests are certainly "culture fair" to about the same extent as Raven's Matrices, or the Cattell tests; Arctic Eskimos excel over white urban Canadian children to about the same extent as they do on the Matrices, and Canadian Indians do almost as well as Eskimos (MacArthur, 1968; Vernon, 1965b). Furthermore, formal schooling has no effect on the age of achieving the various component structures and skills that comprise these stages (Kohlberg, 1968; Sigel & Olmsted, 1970). However, these tests cannot be said to measure something very different from the g defined by ordinary IQ tests; Vernon (1965b) and Tuddenham (1970) have shown that correlations between IQ test items and Piaget-type test items are high. In fact, Piaget items have very high g loadings, and seem to measure little else but g; this speaks equally well for Piaget's insight into child psychology as for the Spearman-type theory of neogenesis which underlies the creation of "culture-fair", high g loading traditional test items. Along very different paths, these two approaches converge on an identical g. Far from being a criticism of ordinary intelligence testing, therefore, the work done with Piaget-type tests strongly confirms the value of the paradigm. Nor can it be said that Piaget-type tests do not show strong evidence of hereditary determination (DeLemos, 1969), or fail to show the usual white-black differences (Tuddenham, 1970); in this study oriental children also showed their usual superiority over white children (Eysenck, 1971). In all ways that have been tested, Piaget-type test items behave exactly as one would expect on the hypothesis that they were good measures of g; they certainly fit into our model perfectly. If indeed they "describe the mechanism of thinking" and are "independent of culture", then the same must be said of intelligence as tested by IQ tests.

As an alternative to Piaget-type tests, critics often suggest measures of "creativity" or "originality", of the kind popularized, e.g. by Getzels and Jackson (1962). The claim is made that there exists a pervasive dimension of individual differences, appropriately labelled "creativity", that is quite distinct from general intelligence; this "creative intelligence" is measured by "divergent", as opposed to "convergent" tests. Such claims have been severely criticized (Thorndike, 1963; Wallach & Kogan, 1965), and there is little doubt that the evidence fails to support those who believe in the existence of separate "intelligences". To take Getzel's and Jackson's own research as an example, we may look at the intercorrelations of the "creativity" tests as opposed to the "IQ" tests; on the basis of the claim one would expect high correlations within each group, zero correlations between groups. This is not found. The five creativity tests were hardly any more strongly correlated among themselves, than they were correlated with intelligence (IQ). For the boys, for instance, the correlation between the creativity battery of tests and IQ is ·26, while between the creativity tests themselves it is ·28. (These values are rather low because of restriction of range in the ability of the subjects.) "There is no evidence, in short, for arguing that the creativity instruments are any more strongly related to one another than they are related to general intelligence. The inevitable conclusion is that little warrant exists here for talking about creativity *and* intelligence as if these terms refer to concepts at the same level of abstraction. The creativity indicators measure nothing in common that is

distinct from general intelligence." (Wallach & Kogan, 1965. These authors present criticisms and reviews of other studies in the field also, on which they base their negative conclusion. They also suggest ways and means of actually measuring some aspects of creativity which in due course will no doubt become recognized aspects of general intelligence.) Just as in the case of Piaget, then, we find that the type of test suggested by critics to be better substitutes of intelligence tests are nothing but ordinary IQ tests, measuring much the same factor; there is no proper basis for criticism in this work (Nicholls, 1972.)

What, then, could one say when asked for an impartial and reasonable assessment of the present status of the measurement of intelligence? It is as easy, and as undesirable, to exaggerate what has been achieved as to underrate it. Psychologists have created a paradigm, or model, which embraces many divergent facts; this paradigm is quantitative in nature, and permits of deduction and testing. The essential features of this paradigm are that intelligence can be conceived as "innate, general, cognitive ability"; these three adjectives have been criticized and subjected to many empirical tests, which on the whole, and with certain essential qualifications, have shown them to give a good account of the facts. Measurement of this hypothetical quality, intelligence, can be undertaken with a certain degree of accuracy; such measurement is both reliable and valid. In relation to social reality measures of intelligence behave very much as one would have expected on a priori grounds, assuming intelligence to be what the model says it is; occupations requiring high intelligence are usually represented by individuals scoring higher on IQ tests than occupations requiring little intelligence, for instance, and social mobility pushes intelligent individuals upwards, dull ones downwards. Heredity plays a very important part, but so does environment; the figure assigning heredity twice as much importance as environment in our type of culture is not seriously disputed. This leaves a great deal of influence to environment; many critics have failed to realize the width of the reaction range discussed in a previous section. All observed changes in IQ can easily be accommodated within this model, given the reaction range calculated from the 80%/20% ratio of hereditary and environmental determinants of individual variance. These are very great achievements; few areas of psychology can show anything comparable. The fact that the conclusions reached go counter to what many people would have liked is irrelevant in this context; we are concerned with scientific truth, not with political meliorism.

The main criticism of "intelligence" as a unified concept would seem to lie in the points dealt with in Section V. There is a curious similarity between Spearman, whose views of intelligence have become the battle-ground over which most of the skirmishing has taken place, and John Dalton, the discoverer of the Atom (Greenaway, 1966). None of the main points that

Dalton made were true, nevertheless the Daltonian over-simplifications were well suited to the needs of chemistry during the 19th century, for they were pointing in the right direction, and they were nearly true. Atoms are not indestructible, as Dalton supposed, but the energies involved are hundreds of thousands of times those of chemical reactions. Atoms of the same element can have very different weights, as the discovery of isotopes has demonstrated, but these are so well mixed in nature as to present an almost constant average weight. They need not combine in simple whole-number ratios, as Dalton taught, but the whole-number assumption was useful for the simpler substances which were all the early chemists could hope to deal with. So, as Jones (1966) has pointed out, "all that Dalton said about atoms – apart from the bare fact of their existence, which wasn't novel – was wrong . . . yet, for all that, John Dalton, more than any other single individual, was the man who set modern chemistry on its feet. For in devising a general scientific theory, the important thing is not to be right – such a thing in any final and absolute sense is beyond the bounds of mortal ambition. The important thing is to have the right idea." (p. 496) Galton certain had the right idea, and Spearman and Burt, Terman and Thurstone put it into a form in which it could be demonstrated to be scientifically useful.

It is useful in the sense alluded to by Thomas Young in his first Bakerian lecture in 1801: "Although the invention of plausible hypotheses, independent of any connection with experimental observations, can be of very little use in the promotion of natural knowledge; yet the discovery of simple and uniform principles, by which a great number of apparently heterogeneous phenomena are reduced to coherent and universal laws, must ever be allowed to be of considerable importance towards the improvement of the human intellect."

Unfortunately, for many people – even for many psychologists – the scientific data are less important in their assessment of intelligence testing than certain extra-scientific notions which should play no part in such an evaluation. Their objections remind one strongly of the objections Goethe made against Newton's colour theory (Matthaei, 1971). Goethe could not accept the impersonal, objective, strictly scientific approach of Newton; with his poetic imagination he rebelled against what he saw as the imposition of a lifeless straitjacket upon a living thing. Matthaei gives us in detail all Goethe's objections to Newton and an account of his own colour theory; the book is of very great interest, not only as a historical account, but also because of the light it throws on many modern anti-scientific attitudes. But withall Newton was the winner; we know that he was right and Goethe wrong. Only strict, impersonal, objective scientific research, following the dictates of the scientific method, will lead us to greater knowledge and deeper insight; as the great mathematician Hilbert said: "Wir mussen wissen. Wir werden wissen." We must know – we shall know;

in the measurement of intelligence we have made a good beginning.

REFERENCES

BERRY, J. W. Temne and Eskimo perceptual skills. *Internat. J. Psychol.*, 1966, *1*, 207–222.

BURT, C. *The factors of the mind.* London: Univ. of Lond. Press, 1940.

CAULLERY, M. *La science française depuis le XVII e siecle.* Paris: Colin, 1948.

CHAMBERS, E. G. Statistics in psychology and the limitations of the test method. *Brit. J. Psychol.*, 1943, *33*, 185–192.

COHEN, R. S. Hertz's philosophy and science. In: H. Hertz. *The principles of mechanics.* New York: Dover, 1956.

DAVID, S. & McGUIRE, P. *The Paint House: words from an East End gang.* London: Penguin, 1972.

DE LEMOS, M. The development of conversation in aboriginal children. *Internat. J. Psychol.*, 1969, *4*, 255–269.

EYSENCK, H. J. *The IQ argument.* New York: Library Press, 1971. (*Race, intelligence and education.* London: Temple Smith, 1971).

GETZELS, J. W. & JACKSON, P. W. *Creativity and Intelligence.* New York: Wiley, 1962.

GREENAWAY, F. *John Dalton and the Atom.* London: Heinemann, 1966.

HUNT, J. McV. *Intelligence and experience.* New York: Ronald Press, 1961.

HUNT, J. McV. Environment, development and scholastic achievement. In: M. Dentich, I. Katz, & A. R. Jensen (Eds.) *Social class, race, and psychological development.* New York: Holt, Rinehart & Winston, 1968.

JACKSON, L. C. *Low temperature Physics.* London: Methuen, 1962.

JOHNSON, R. C. Similarity in IQ of separated indentical twins as related to length of time spent in same environment *Child Development*, 1963, *34*, 745-749.

JONES, D. E. The atomization of chemistry. *New Scientist*, 1966, *1st Sept.*, 493–496.

KAPLAN, B. J. Malnutrition and mental deficiency. *Psychol. Bull.*, 1972, *78*, 321-334.

KISCH, B. Scales and weights: a historical outline. London: Yale Univ. Press, 1965.

KOHLBERG, L. Early education: a cognitive developmental order. *Child development*, 1968, *39*, 1013–1062.

KNOWLES MIDDLETON, W. E. *A history of the thermometer.* Baltimore: John Hopkins Press, 1966.

LOVEJOY, D. R. Peculiarities and paradoxes in temperature measurement. *New Scientist*, 1964, *422*, 792–795.

MacARTHUR, R. Some differential abilities of northern Canadian native youth. *Internat. J. Psychol.*, 1968, *3*, 43–51.

MACH, E. *Erkenntuis und Irrtum.* Leipzig: J. A. Borth, 1905.

MANUEL, F. E. *A portrait of Isaac Newton.* Cambridge: Harvard Univ. Press, 1968.

MATTHAEI, R. *Goethe's colour theories.* London: Studio Vista, 1971.

MEDAWAR, P. B. *The art of the soluble.* London: Methuen, 1967.

MENDELSSOHN, K. (Ed.) *Progress in cyrogenics.* 4 vols. New York: Academic Press, 1964.

NEWMAN, H. H., FREEMAN, F. N. & HOLZINGER, K. J. *Twins: a study of heredity and environment.* Chicago: Univ. of Chicago Press, 1937.

NICHOLLS, J. A. Creativity in the person who will never produce anything original and useful. *Amer. Psychologist*, 1972, *27*, 717–727.

NYE, MARY J. *Molecular reality*. London: Macdonald, 1972.

OSTWALD, W. Elements and compounds. Faraday Lectures, 1904.

PASCAL, B. *Recit de la grande experience de l'equilibre des liquers*. Paris: Oeuvres, 1648.

POPPER, K. R. *The logic of scientific discovery*. London: Hutchinson, 1959.

POPPER, K. A. *Conjectures and reputations*. London: Routledge & Kegan Paul, 1963.

SIGEL, J. E. & OLMSTED, P. Modification of cognitive skills among lower-class black children. In: J. Vellmuth (Ed.) *Disadvantaged Child*. Vol. 3. New York: Brunner-Mazel, 1970, 300–338.

SQUIRE, C. F. *Low temperature physics*. New York: McGraw Hill, 1953.

STEIN, Z., SAENGER, G. and MARALLA, F. Nutrition and Mental Performance. *Science*, 1972, *178*, 708–713.

THORNDIKE, R. L. Some methodological issues in the study of creativity. Proceedings 1962 Invitational Conference on Testing Problems. Princeton: Educ. Testing Service, 1963.

THURSTONE, L. L. & THURSTONE, T. G. *Factorial studies of intelligence*. Chicago: Univ. of Chicago Press, 1941.

TUDDENHAM, R. D. A "Piagetian" test of cognitive development. In: B. Dockrell (Ed.) *On intelligence*. Toronto: Ontario Inst. Stud. Educ., 1970, 49–70.

VERNON, P. E. Environmental handicaps and intellectual development: II & III. *Brit. J. educ. Psychol.*, 1965a, *35*, 1–22.

VERNON, P. E. Ability factors and environmental influences. *Amer. Psychologist*, 1965b, *20*, 723–733.

VOYAT, G. IQ: God-given or man-made? In: J. Hellmuth (Ed.) *Disadvantaged child*. Vol. 3. New York: Brunner-Mazel, 1970, 158–162.

WALLACH, M. & KOGAN, N. *Modes of thinking in young children: A study of the creativity-influence distinction*. New York: Holt, Rinehart & Winston, 1965.

ZANGWILL, O. L. *An introduction to modern psychology*. London: Methuen, 1950.

ZEMANSKY, M. W. *Heat and thermodynamics*. New York: McGraw-Hill, 1957.